Assessment and Management of Orofacial Pain

Cover photograph:

Ceramic sculpture made according to Raku techniques called "La Dee Dah" by Patricia Chatlin who took up the art of Raku ceramics after sustaining a back injury and which has helped her control her back pain.

In 16th Century Japan, the Zen potter Rikyu developed a new art in ceramics, the Art of Raku. The technique was a simpler one and a more subtle one. Porous glazed ware was placed in a hot kiln, taken to orange heat, then placed with metal tongs in leaves, pine needles, or sawdust. That moment of firing is the essence of Raku: the pearl glaze, the luster, the soft crackle, the captured moment when the molten glaze and the smoking embers are one.

Today we celebrate this classical and unique pottery, where fire, earth and chance merge.

Pain Research and Clinical Management

Editorial Board

P.D. Wall *(London, UK)*[†] Chairman

M.R. Bond *(Glasgow, UK)*	Neuropsychiatry
M.J. Cousins *(St. Leonard's, NSW, Australia)*	Chronic pain
H.L. Fields *(San Francisco, CA, USA)*	Anesthesiology
M. Fitzgerald *(London, UK)*	Pediatric pain
K.M. Foley *(New York, NY, USA)*	Cancer
P.J. McGrath *(Halifax, NS, Canada)*	Pediatrics
J.M. Gybels *(Louvain, Belgium)*	Neurosurgery
R.G. Hill *(Harlow, Essex, UK)*	Electrophysiology
S.B. McMahon *(London, UK)*	Physiology
H. Merskey *(London, ON, Canada)*	Psychiatry
A.C. Williams *(London, UK)*	Chronic pain

Pain Research and Clinical Management

Volume 14

Assessment and Management of Orofacial Pain

Edited by

Joanna M. Zakrzewska
Department of Clinical and Diagnostic Oral Sciences, Oral Medicine Unit, Dental Institute, Barts and the London Queen Mary's School of Medicine and Dentistry, Turner Street, London E1 2AD, UK

Sheelah D. Harrison
Department of Oral and Maxillofacial Surgery, Eastman Dental Hospital, 256 Gray's Inn Road, London WC1X 8LD, UK

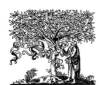

2002
ELSEVIER
AMSTERDAM • BOSTON • LONDON • NEW YORK • OXFORD • PARIS • SAN DIEGO •
SAN FRANCISCO • SINGAPORE • SYDNEY • TOKYO

ELSEVIER SCIENCE B.V.
Sara Burgerhartstraat 25
P.O. Box 211, 1000 AE Amsterdam, The Netherlands

First edition 2002

Library of Congress Cataloging in Publication Data
Assessment and Management of Orofacial Pain / edited by Joanna M. Zakrzewska and Sheelah D. Harrison. – 1st Ed.
     p. ; cm. – (Pain research and clinical management, ISSN 0921-3287; v. 14)
   Includes bibliographical references and index.
   ISBN 0-444-50984-4 (alk. paper)
   1. Orofacial pain. I. Zakrzewska, Joanna M. II. Harrison, Sheelah D. III. Series.
   [DNLM: 1: Facial Pain–diagnosis. 2. Facial Pain–therapy. WE 705 A846 2002]
 RK322 .A875 2002
 617.5'2–dc21

                                                                2002029803

British Library Cataloguing in Publication Data
Assessment and Management of Orofacial Pain. - (Pain
  research and clinical management ; v. 14)
  1.Orofacial pain 2.Orofacial pain - Treatment
  I.Zakrzewska, Joanna M.; II.Harrison, Sheelah D.
  617.5'22

  ISBN 0444509844

ISBN: 0-444-50984-4 (hardbound)
ISSN: 0921-3287 (series)

Dedication
to Professor Patrick D. Wall

who was an inspiration to us all.

Foreword

Orofacial pain represents an important clinical pain issue, affecting a large number of patients, from childhood to old age.

Orofacial pain consists of a heterogeneous sample of conditions, ranging from simple dental pain via temporomandibular disorders to classical neurological orofacial pain, such as trigeminal neuralgia and trigeminal neuropathies. These patients have traditionally been treated by different health care professionals including dentists, general practitioners, ENT physicians, psychologists, neurologists and surgeons with a different approach to history, examination, classification and treatment. It is not unusual to see the same patient being sent from one specialist to another without communication between the health care providers. The result can be frustrating and disappointing for all parties involved.

The heterogeneity of the disorders and their assessors are some of the reasons for the complexity and confusion in the area of orofacial pain. There is a great need for a comprehensive description of orofacial pain in order to understand the physiology and pathophysiology of orofacial pains and so enhance treatment. It is therefore greatly appreciated that the editors, Joanna Zakrzewska and Sheelah Harrison, together with their multidisciplinary colleagues have undertaken the difficult task of drawing together evidence from a wide range of sources in order to present a textbook of orofacial pain. They have taken a novel approach to this task in that the key facts from each chapter are summarized in easily identified tables. This ensures that both the expert and the novice find something of value in the book. There has also been a strong emphasis on ensuring that the best evidence is used and means of updating the data is provided. It is to be hoped that this book will contribute to a better understanding of the various orofacial pain conditions, their diagnosis, classification and treatment. This will, hopefully lead to improved outcomes for many orofacial pain patients.

Troels Staehelin Jensen
Professor of Experimental and Clinical Pain Research,
University of Aarhus, Denmark,
President elect of the International Association for the Study of Pain

Preface

Welcome! The overall aim of this book is to provide you with an evidence-based approach to assessment and management of dental and orofacial pain in an interactive format using a biopsychosocial model. Our objectives for the book are as shown below.

We would hope that by reading this book you will learn to:

- List and define the common and rare causes of orofacial pain using a classification system.
- Understand the factors that influence orofacial pain perception.
- Appreciate the need for and then know how to take a structured orofacial pain history which includes psychosocial factors, quality of life and compliance issues.
- Discuss the value of different investigations in the diagnosis of orofacial pain.
- Apply the principles of diagnosis and management to solving clinical problems using the biopsychosocial model.
- Evaluate critically using evidence based methodology the management of different types of orofacial pain.
- Appreciate the need for improved communications between patients and clinicians and the value of resources such as patient support groups, patient information and the internet.

This book is primarily a practical clinical book and so only includes epidemiology, aetiology and pathophysiologcal data that are relevant to the management of these conditions at the present time. It is written by practising clinicians who are experts in these areas, most of whom have written doctorates on these topics and so have an excellent working knowledge of the literature that is relevant for you as a clinician. We hope that this book will appeal to a wide range of clinicians who may be medically or dentally trained, psychologists and even patients who wish to become better informed. We hope there is something for everybody.

Sackett et al. in their book on "Evidenced Based Medicine: How to Practice and Teach EBM" put forward the view that textbooks will become obsolete in the electronic age as they are large and cannot keep up with the pace of change unless they are revised on a yearly basis. In defence of the textbook they point out that textbooks take material from a wide range of sources and integrate them so as to make it easier for the busy reader to acquire information quickly. We would hope that this book would fulfil their criteria of being a "super" textbook by providing explicit criteria for selecting its evidence, using a credible evidence search process and citing evidence in support of its recommendations. Data for the book have been collected from a wide range of medical and dental sources including pain, dentistry, oral medicine, oral and maxillofacial surgery, neurology, neurosurgery, psychiatry, psychology and anthropology. This has been possible due to the multidisciplinary team writing the book. We have provided details of web sites where you can update the information in this book and also highlighted resources such as the Cochrane Library and Clinical Evidence which are regularly updated.

The practice of continuous, lifelong and self-directed learning is made easier and more fun if you, the reader, are involved in the process rather than passively reading text. The data are presented in an easy to read manner which will enable you to access the book at any point and for short periods of time. This has been done by the use of simple text with bullet points, box sections listing key messages/summaries, interactive boxes giving you some case studies of genuine patients and lists of annotated references and further reading texts. Reading only the data in the key facts box should give you the most important facts from any chapter. The biggest stimulus to learning is the clinician faced with a patient problem and hence the use of case scenarios which may be similar to situations you have encountered. At the end of each chapter we have provided you with further resources which we hope you will use to deepen your understanding of the subject. We provide reading resources that aim at several levels, undergraduate to postgraduate, so please do not feel offended if some of the books appear to be very basic.

As this is not a book you need to read from cover to cover or in the exact order it is produced, it has inevitably led to some repetition especially in the reading material. Each chapter can be read on its own. Chapters 1–9 provide you with background information generic to all facial pain patients, some of which you may find heavy going such as Chapters 1 and 2, please do not be discouraged, read on. Chapters 10–17 are on named conditions so providing you with more specific background information as well as foreground information on assessing and managing a patient with a particular condition. We have tended to use the words chronic idiopathic facial pain and atypical facial pain synonymously and have used the generic word temporomandibular joint pain for all forms of pain around the joint. Some historical data are added in some chapters to show how the knowledge has evolved.

No such book can be written without the help of many other people. The book would never have been started but for Professor Patrick Wall's suggestion. It was a wonderful opportunity to be able to work with Pat and I enjoyed my regular visits to him to discuss progress on the book or more precisely discuss new research ideas in the field. Pat's death after only the first two chapters had been written was a great blow and so we were left to work on our own. Heather Fry and Steve Ketteridges' books on education provided us with the idea for the format we have used in this book. I am very grateful to our two trainees in oral medicine, Dr Philip Atkin and Dr Michael Escudier, for reading through many of the chapters and providing their comments and views. The structured notes and many of the measures we describe in the book were developed with their help and case studies come from patients we saw together.

This book would not be what is without the help of numerous patients, not only have we used some of their case studies but their feedback in clinics and through support groups have taught us to look on our patients as experts who can contribute significantly to a book such as this. I am grateful to our dental students who looked at resources available to patients and assessed their quality. Without the background help of my secretary, Anne Spooner, the writing would have been difficult. Not only were references ordered, retrieved and copied as necessary but manuscripts were corrected, organised and printed. I was also protected from interruptions: telephone calls and callers were carefully filtered to give uninterrupted time for writing. Dr Kate Maguire not only suggested that I look at pain in metaphors and showed me how to do it (Chapter 9) but also helped me to reflect on what I was trying to achieve when dealing with patients with facial pain. I am grateful to Dr. Sheelah Harrison for her help in planning the outline of the book.

Finally, but not least, I am grateful to my family, Jan, Konrad and Krystyna for their patience and forbearance during the year this was put together.

I hope the book will help healthcare workers to empower their facial pain patients and enable them to either become totally pain free or to come to terms with their pain just as Patricia Chatlin, the artist of the Raku ceramic on the front cover, who has suffered back pain said "pain and injury represented loss of function, self and control. . . building in clay became a metaphor for rebuilding 'Self'. Through exploration and acceptance one eventually transcends earthbound thinking and life's creative dance begins".

Joanna M. Zakrzewska

August 2002

List of Contributors

Behnam Aghabeigi

Oral Surgeon, Department of Oral and Maxillofacial Surgery, Eastman Dental Institute, 256 Gray's Inn Road, London WC1X 8LD, UK

M.S. Chong

Neurologist, The Medway Hospital NHS Trust, Gillingham, Kent, and King's College Hospital NHS Trust, London, Mapother House, London SE5 9AZ, UK

Sheelah D. Harrison

Oral Surgeon, Department of Oral and Maxillofacial Surgery, Eastman Dental Hospital, 256 Gray's Inn Road, London WC1X 8LD, UK

Toby Newton-John

Clinical Psychologist, Eastman Dental Hospital, Gray's Inn Road, London WC1X 8LD and Sub-Department of Clinical Health Psychology, University College London, Gower Street, London WC1E 6BT, UK

Joanna M. Zakrzewska

Oral Physician, Department of Clinical and Diagnostic Oral Sciences, Oral Medicine Unit, Dental Institute, Barts and the London Queen Mary's School of Medicine and Dentistry, University of London, Turner Street, London E1 2AD, UK

Contents

Assessment and Management of Orofacial Pain
Pain Research and Clinical Management, Vol. 14
Edited by J.M. Zakrzewska and S.D. Harrison
© *2002 Elsevier Science B.V. All rights reserved*

CHAPTER 1

Introduction

Joanna M. Zakrzewska[*]

Department of Clinical and Diagnostic Oral Sciences, Oral Medicine Unit, Dental Institute, Barts and the London Queen Mary's School of Medicine and Dentistry, Turner Street, London E1 2AD, UK

Objectives for this chapter:

This chapter will attempt to:
- Teach/remind you of the basics of evidence-based medicine
- Provide you with further sources on how to keep this book updated
- Provide you with the criteria on which the book is written
- Provide a general further reading list on pain in general and evidence-based medicine

1. Introduction

This book aims to show you how evidence-based methodologies can be used to assess and manage patients with facial pain. In case you are not familiar with this methodology we are providing you with a short synopsis on evidence-based medicine and practise in this chapter. This will give you a better understanding of the methodologies we have used. You will find a definition of evidence-based medicine (EBM) in Table 1.

Until recently, medical and dental practise was based largely on intelligent guesswork and clinical experience and according to Archie Cochrane only 15–20% of medical practise was backed up by scientifically and statistically sound research. Go and ask three experts who do not practise evidence-based medicine how they manage a difficult problem. I guess you will get three different answers and find that you are really none the wiser about tackling your problem.

Evidence-based practise aims to move beyond anecdotal clinical experience by bridging the gap between research and the practice of medicine. The aim is to use diagnostic tests and interventions that are as accurate, as safe and as efficacious as possible. It should also provide a method for rigorous assessment of outcomes after different clinical actions. EBM shares many of the principles used in clinical audit:

- Uses rather than does research
- Aims at improving healthcare delivery and raising standards
- Considers the use of resources
- Focuses on a range of outcomes by insisting on explicit end points
- Is a tool for delivering education
- Is useful for standard setting

[*] Tel.: +44-20-7377-7053; Fax: +44-20-7377-7627;
E-mail j.m.zakrzewska@qmul.ac.uk

TABLE 1

KEY FACTS: definition of evidence-based medicine and resources

---

Evidence-based medicine is the conscientious and judicious use of current best evidence from clinical care research in the management of individual patients (Sackett et al., 1996)

The most up to date resources are to be found on the world wide web and there are many excellent sites that will get you started. The standard textbook is Evidenced-Based Medicine. 'How to Practice and Teach EBM' (Sackett et al., 2000)

In order to practise evidence-based medicine, we need both knowledge of evidence-based medicine and a mastery of clinical skills such has history taking, examination and ordering and interpretation of investigations so that an evidenced-based question can be generated. Once we have found the evidence we have to assess how to use it based on the patients' expectations and values as well as our own judgments. Evidenced-based clinical decisions therefore depend on a blend of clinical expertise, research evidence and patient preferences. It assumes that medical and dental education is a life-long process orientated towards problem solving and based on the principles that clinical experience is important but that observations must be recorded systematically and without bias, that regular reference must be made to the literature and that the results of studies must be critically examined using the rules of evidence. It is not cook book medicine as some suggest (Haynes et al., 1996). Qualitative and quantitative data are needed to ensure that we run evidence-based practice. (Greenhalgh, 1996).

This chapter may be heavy going so I suggest you may want to read it in small sections rather than plough through it all at once.

2. How do I acquire training in evidence-based medicine? What types of resources are available?

You can either go on a course or you can read material from textbooks, CD ROMs or the internet. Some of the courses are short, 2–5-day ones, while others lead to diplomas and postgraduate qualifications. When using books and CD ROMs, check whether explicit criteria have been used in retrieval and appraisal of the evidence and that these have been adhered to. It is also important to know something about the background of the authors and how the resource was developed.

You cannot go far wrong with reading or re-reading the classic textbook '*Evidenced Based Medicine, How to Practice and Teach Evidenced Based Medicine*' by Sackett, Richardson, Rosenberg and Haynes which is now in its second edition (2000). It keeps up to date by providing updated information on its web pages about new studies and methods of analysis. The book is small as it is intended for the white coat pocket and use at the bedside. You can further practise your skills by working through books such as '*The Evidence Based Medicine Workbook — Critical Appraisal for Clinical Problem Solving*' by Dixon, Munro and Silcocks, Butterworth-Heinemann (1997). You will need another small book to help you critically appraise what you are reading and an example is '*The Pocket Guide to Critical Appraisal: a Handbook for Health Professionals*' by Crombie (1996). This book is also very handy when refereeing articles as it provides you with an excellent structure on which to base your report. Other resources are listed in the references, which are not intended to be exhaustive, but rather an example of resources I have used.

CD ROMs include the Cochrane Library (published quarterly), which are also available on the world wide web and Best Evidence which is published yearly and incorporates the ACP Journal and Evidence-Based Medicine. Journals, which carry high quality material, and EBM journals are listed at the end of the chapter.

The most up to date material will be on the internet and many have downloadable programs. All the sites quoted in this chapter were last accessed in November 2000. When looking at internet-based material, check whether it:

- has an evidence-based medicine focus
- lists the developers of the site
- indicates when it was last updated
- lists any conflict of interest and if so, how it affects the material

More details on appraisal of web sites can be found in Chapter 9.

Some examples of sites I use to find further information are:

http://www.nettingtheevidence.org.uk/ which provides an index to many resources and has been recently revamped;

http://cebm.jr2.ox.ac.uk the NHS Research and Development Centre for evidence-based medicine;

http://www.york.ac.uk/inst/crd/welcome.htm the NHS York University web page;

http://www.cebm.utoronto.ca/ the University of Toronto web site from which most things began.

3. What are the four steps of evidence-based practise?

These are summarised in Table 2 key facts. It is important to evaluate the process you went through when trying to answer a clinical problem using evidence-based methodology as reflection on the process enables you to improve your skills when next applying the techniques to your patient.

3.1. How do I formulate an answerable clinical question?

The basis of evidenced-based practise is the well focused clinical question. This takes some practise which can be done by reading or practising with your colleagues. Not only must the question be directly relevant to your patient's problem, but it must also be phrased in such a way as to enable you to make an accurate search of the literature for the precisely relevant answer in a reasonable time frame. Sackett et al. (2000) suggest that a well-built question contains four elements shown below in Table 3 key facts.

An example of how this Patient Intervention Comparison Outcome (PICO) format is worked through can be found in an article in the first issue of Journal of Evidence-Based Dental Practise on what constitute the diagnostic features of trigeminal neuralgia (Drangsholt and Truelove, 2001). Now try formulating a question using the information shown in Table 4 Case study 2 learning box.

The Oxford Centre for Evidence-Based Medicine suggests accessing any of the following sites for help in formulating a well focused question:

- Anatomy of a Well-Built Clinical Question (Duke University Medical Center)
  http://www.mclibrary.duke.edu//respub/guides/questiontable.html
- BMA Finding the Evidence Course (Suzy Paisley, ScHARR)
  http://library.bma.org.uk/presentations/evidence1/index.htm
- CHENet — Introduction to Users' Guides to the Medical Literature
  *http://www.cche.net/principles/content_intro.asp#Asking_questions_that_are_pertinent_and_*
- Focusing Clinical Questions
  http://cebm.jr2.ox.ac.uk/docs/focusquest.html

TABLE 2

KEY FACTS: four steps of EBM

1. Asking a focused question
2. Carrying out the search
3. Evaluating the evidence
4. Applying it to the clinical situation

TABLE 3

KEY FACTS: elements of a well set question

	Patient problem	Intervention (cause, prognosis, therapy)	Comparison (if necessary)	Outcome, clinical
Generic question	Start with the patient or problem and ask How would I describe a group of patients who are similar to my patient?	Which main intervention am I considering? This must be specific	What other main alternatives/interventions are there? it is necessary to decide which they are	What effect would this therapy have/what would I achieve?
Example	In a newly diagnosed patient with trigeminal neuralgia	is carbamazepine	likely to be better than gabapentin	and lead to better pain relief with fewer side effects?

TABLE 4

Case study 1: framing a question

Mrs. Jones has come to you, her primary care doctor, with moderately severe throbbing pain over the left cheek. The pain is continuous and has been present for the last 3 days. It is made worse bending down and the use of decongestants has not helped. She has recently had a bad cold. The cheek is tender and tapping the upper teeth also provokes the pain. You suspect she has maxillary sinusitis and wonder what radiographs you need to take before treating her

Write down one question

Your best answer (without searching)

Initial evidence source you would look in

Please find the answer in Table 12 at the end of the chapter.

- Formulate a Focused Clinical Question
  http://abbc3.hsc.usc.edu/familymed/ evidencebased/questions.htm
- Formulating Patient-Centered Questions
  http://www.uic.edu/depts/lib/lhsp/resources/pico. shtml
- Instructional Model for Medical Informatics
  http://medweb.med.uci.edu/courses/informatics/ model/step3. html
- On Questions — Background and Foreground
  http://hiru.mcmaster.ca/ceb/newslett/ceb_17.htm
- Teaching/Learning Resources for EBP
  http://www.mdx.ac.uk/www/rctsh/ebp/ askquest.htm

There is also a useful article in Best Evidence on this topic entitled 'The well built clinical question; a key to evidence base decisions' (Richardson et al., 1995).

3.2. How do I find the evidence?

In this next stage not only do you need to know where to find the evidence but you also need to know how to search and filter the information you find. Try the exercise in Table 5 case study 2 before you read the next section.

You may have access to a wide variety of sources and so will need to make some decisions about the sources you will use and in which order. If you have limited resources, it is important to remember not to

TABLE 5

Case study 2: looking for evidence

You have just seen a patient you think has maxillary sinusitis. You want some foreground knowledge on this condition. List the possible sources you would use to search for your evidence as well as their strengths and weaknesses. Estimate how long it would take you to search the source

Please see the answer in Table 6.

rely on just one source, as the results are likely to be biased. In Table 6 key facts we list some major resources which may be useful.

You can read more on this in a generic article by McKibbon et al. (1999) in Best Evidence or in the series in '*Users Guide to the Medical Literature*' (Oxman et al., 1993).

The suggestions below have been compiled by the Oxford Centre for Evidence-Based Medicine. The majority of them utilise the research conducted by McMaster University and can be found on the centres web page together with their web addresses.

- Filters (Institute of Health Sciences, Oxford) *www.lib.jr2.ox.ac.uk/caspfew/filters*
- EBM Toolbox University of Alberta *www.med.ualberta.ca/edm/ebm.htm*
- Evidence-Based Medicine and MEDLINE (OVID) — North Thames
- Evidence-Based Filters for Ovid Medline
- PubMed: Clinical Queries using Research Methodology Filters
- Search Strategy to Identify Reviews and Meta-analyses in Medline and CINAHL
- Using Filters to Retrieve Valid Studies from the Primary Medical Literature

For example the evidence-based toolbox of the University of Alberta will provide you with search strategies for ovid/medline and pubMed for articles on causation/harm/aetiology/, diagnostic tests, therapy, prognosis, systematic reviews.

There are several specific journals and books that contain articles on facial pain which are prepared according to evidence-based methodology and some examples are:

- Evidence-Based Medicine, Evidence-Based Dentistry, Journal of Evidence-Based Dental Practise
- Clinical Evidence regularly updated and available on line *www.clinicalevidence.com* and its concise version
- Epidemiology of Pain published by the International Association of Pain

Further resources are listed at the end of the chapter.

3.3. How do I evaluate the evidence I have found?

You need to be able to critically appraise the data you have found as there is much published material that is of poor quality or irrelevant. Some of the sources mentioned above will help you. The evidence-based medicine toolboxes such as found at *http://www.cebm.utoronto.ca/teach/materials/cawor ksheets.htm* (worksheets with in built calculators) or *http://www.med.ualberta.ca/ebm/ebm.htm* provide downloadable tables that can be used in evaluating articles on diagnosis, causation, harm, therapy. Once you have done these it is useful to attach them to the article so you can refer to them in the future. A very basic grading of articles is shown in Table 7 below.

The systematic review is considered the 'gold standard' for evidence. A systematic review entails systematically locating, appraising and synthesising evidence from scientific studies in order to gain a reliable overview. Their advantage is that rather than being based on only a selection of the published work as chosen by the authors, they contain a comprehensive summary of the evidence which has been

TABLE 6

KEY FACTS: information sources for answering clinical questions

Resource	What it is and examples	Strengths	Weaknesses	Time to search
Textbooks/traditional paper based	1. Often written by a single or group of experts who have pooled their information 2. Every specialty has its examples	1. Information from many sources put together by experts 2. Relatively easy to use 3. Cheap 4. Excellent for 'facts' that do not change often, such as gross anatomy	1. Date quickly 2. Often based on opinion of expert rather than evidence 3. Often not all topics covered 4. Need a library or loan facility 5. Can take a long time to acquire	2–5 min once resource acquired
Computer based	1. Often multiple authors 2. Searchable and can be on CD ROM and/or Internet base 3. Excellent for 'facts' that do not change often	1. Prepared by experts 2. Easy to use	1. Can be expensive to keep current 2. Not all information is necessarily evidence based	2–5 min
Best evidence	Computer collection of all articles from Evidence-Based Medicine (1995–2000) and ACP Journal Club (1991–1999)	1. Clinical topics with strong methods and concise 2. Updated in a 5-year cycle 3. Commentaries by clinical experts 4. Very easy to search because of its small size	1. Limited topics (little on facial pain) 2. Provides a non-random sample or recent high-quality evidence 3. Not exhaustive	2–5 min using a search engine

Cochrane Library	Produced by the worldwide Cochrane Collaboration, computer collection includes completed systematic reviews; citations and abstracts to systematic review, largest citations and abstracts of controlled trials. Therapy and prevention only	1. Rigorous updated systematic reviews, peer reviewed 2. Of interest to all health care professionals and patient 3. Oral health section	1. Topics covered varied: not all are done 2. Very thorough, so take time to read 3. May not be easily accessible to all	2–5 min
MEDLINE	Citations and abstracts from more than 4000 journals	1. Comprehensive, constantly being updated 2. Low (or no) cost	1. Difficult and time-consuming to search because of its size	30 min per topic
Internet	Global network of computers	1. Can find something on almost any topic 2. Enormous	1. Difficult to search 2. Quality of content is uncertain and difficult to ascertain	10 min plus

---

TABLE 7

KEY FACTS: ranks of evidence — first is highest

1. Systematic reviews especially if meta analysis
2. Randomised controlled trials
3. Controlled trials without randomisation
4. Cohort or case-control studies
5. Descriptive studies (comparative or correlation)
6. Respected authorities, case reports, expert committees

---

screened using predefined criteria in order to reduce bias and so ensure reliability. Systematic reviews provide important data needed to formulate policies as they establish generalisibilty, increase the power and precision (if a meta-analysis has been possible) and limit bias. Systematic reviews therefore provide a way of managing large quantities of information and make it easier for the busy clinician to gather evidence. Systematic reviews differ from traditional reviews in that they attempt to answer a very specific question and track down all the literature and studies that are not selected just because they support the desired conclusion.

The randomised double-blind controlled trial attempts to reduce bias to a minimum by allocating participants in a random way to a group, accounting for all participants and assessing outcome in a blinded way. Further details are to be found in Chapter 9 on management. In the next level of evidence the trial is controlled but the participants have not been allocated randomly to the groups and so some selection bias could occur, e.g. patients with more severe disease could have been allocated to the active treatment group. In some areas there are no randomised controlled trials and observational studies must be used to provide the evidence. Within this area, the hierarchy adopted is the following: (a) well-designed cohort (prospective study) with concurrent controls; (b) well-designed cohort (prospective study) with historical controls; and (c) well-designed case-control (retrospective)

study (Anonymous 1996). When data are collected prospectively, the study is more likely to have been planned, is more reliable and complete, as the selection of participants is not based on outcome. At the bottom end of the evidence spectrum are descriptive studies by experts. They are the most likely to be heavily biased.

Having read the articles, you need to decide which level of evidence is being used and this can be done using Table 7 or if you are an expert in evidence-based medicine you can use the Oxford Centre for Evidence-Based Medicine levels of evidence which you can find in Table 10 in Appendix B of this chapter or look up on their web site. Within each of those sections, you then need to grade the strength of the evidence. An example of this is shown in the Table 11 in Appendix B and there is one that we have adopted to use in Chapter 9 on management (Chapter 9, Table 11). Recently a systematic review has been carried out by the US Agency for Healthcare Research and Quality and their study on 'Systems to rate the strengths of scientific evidence' is available on their web site *www.ahrq.gov/clinic/epcix.htm*.

3.4. How do I apply the evidence?

Now it is the time for your clinical expertise to be used and for you to practise evidence-based decision making. You need to assess your patients' values and expectations and see how they map on to your expertise and the research evidence you have found as shown in key facts in Table 8.

In some circumstances, your clinical expertise may dominate and dictate treatment, in others you may be treating a condition you rarely see and so you will rely on the research evidence. You may also find that there is new evidence available that should therefore modify your current clinical practise. In other cases the patient may be the driving force. Patients are increasingly knowledgeable about health matters, they seek second opinions, choose alternative therapies and can decide on adherence to treatment plans (Haynes et al., 1996).

TABLE 8

KEY FACTS: how to apply the evidence

You need to combine:

1. The best evidence found in the literature
2. Your patients values and expectations
3. Your own expertise
4. Your estimate of patient adherence
5. Your preparedness to change as new evidence becomes available

---

4. Conclusions

We hope that you are now convinced that this methodology:

- does improve confidence in decision making
- provides rules and rationale for problem-based case solving
- enables research findings to be applied quickly in clinical practise
- emphasises outcome as well as process
- can be used to involve patients in decision making

There remain limitations to the practise of EBM in that:

- finding and evaluating evidence is costly in terms of time
- not everyone is skilled yet in locating information and using computers
- resources are needed to maintain databases
- not all topics are covered

but it is hoped that these limitations will gradually change.

Throughout the book, we aim, as far as possible, to follow the principles I have outlined in this chapter. We hope to provide you with enough evidence to be able to find answers to practical problems you may face when seeing patients with orofacial pain. It should be stressed at the outset that there are many areas where evidence is missing or is of poor quality and we will highlight these. However, it is important that you continue to be on the look out for new evidence and so assess which sections of the book may become outdated. It is hoped that with your well honed skills in critical appraisal you will be aware of where new evidence can be found and will be better able to operate in the so-called 'grey zones' (where information is incomplete or of poor quality). For each chapter we performed literature searches using among others Medline, PubMed, Best Evidence and the Cochrane Library. We are attempting to use only the best quality evidence and to evaluate the data critically and so would hope to have been unbiased in our presentation of the data. We apologise in advance if we fail to keep to these standards in any sections.

5. Summary (Table 9)

TABLE 9

Summary of Chapter 1

1. Evidence-based medicine (EBM) and practice

- Improves confidence in decision making
- Provides rules and rationale for problem-based case solving
- Enables research findings to be applied quickly in clinical practise
- Emphasises outcome as well as process
- Can be used to involve patients in decision making

2. Practising EBM involves four stages

- Asking a focused question
- Carrying out a search
- Evaluating the literature
- Applying it to the clinical situation

EBM sources can be found on CD ROMs and the internet and all need to be critically evaluated

Major references to EBM and facial pain textbooks are to be found in this chapter's reference lists

---

Appendix A. Resources

A.1. A selection of journals with high quality EBM data

(1) ACP Journal Club
(2) Archives of Internal Medicine
(3) British Medical Journal
(4) Canadian Medical Association Journal
(5) Evidence-Based Medicine
(6) Journal of the American Medical Association
(7) Journal of Evidence-Based Health Care
(8) Lancet
(9) Evidence based dentistry
(10) Journal of Evidence-Based Dental Practice

A.2. CD ROM (often have a web site)

(1) Best Evidence
(2) Cochrane Library
(3) UpToDate — clinical reference for medical subspecialists and internists *www.uptodateinc.com/*

A.3. Books on EBM

See further reading.

A.4. Sample of World Wide Web sites containing evidence-based material

(1) UpToDate
(2) Audit, Clinical Governance and Evidence-Based Medicine Resources
(3) Bandolier
(4) Best BETS
(5) Centre for Clinical Effectiveness
(6) Centre for Evidence-Based Medicine
(7) Centre for Evidence-Based Mental Health
(8) Centres for Health Evidence
(9) Clinical Assessment of the Reliability of the Examination

(10) Clinical Decision Rules, The Samuel Bronfman Department of Medicine
(11) Clinical Evidence
(12) Clinical Examination Research Interest Group
(13) Clinical Resources, Clindx Update Listserv and Bibliography
(14) Critique et Pratique
(15) Evidence-Based Medicine
(16) Evidence-Based Mental Health
(17) McMaster Health Information Research Unit
(18) National Library of Medicine's Health Services/Technology Assessment Text (HSTAT)
(19) Netting the Evidence
(20) NHS Centre for Reviews and Dissemination
(21) Ovid EBM
(22) Pediatric Evidence-Based Medicine
(23) PubMed
(24) Resources for Practising Evidence-Based Medicine
(25) SumSearch (formerly SmartSearch)

Appendix B

See Tables 10 and 11 for Oxford Centre for Evidence-based Medicine levels of evidence and grades of recommendation, respectively.

Appendix C. Answers to case study

See Table 12 for the answers to case study 1.

Appendix D. Further background reading

More specific reading will be provided in other chapters and this is not an exhaustive list.

D.1. Pain

(1) Melzack R, Wall PD. The Challenge of Pain. Penguin, London, 1996: ISBN 0-14-025670-9. (A general book on pain for the lay man which

TABLE 10

Oxford Centre for Evidence-Based Medicine: levels of evidence (May 2001) produced by Bob Phillips, Chris Ball, Dave Sackett, Doug Badenoch, Sharon Straus, Brian Haynes, Martin Dawes since November 1998

Level	Therapy/prevention, aetiology/harm	Prognosis	Diagnosis	Differential diagnosis/symptom prevalence study	Economic and decision analyses
1a	SR (with homogeneity[a]) of RCTs	SR (with homogeneity[a]) of inception cohort studies; CDR[b] validated in different populations	SR (with homogeneity[a]) of level 1 diagnostic studies; CDR[b] with 1b studies from different clinical centres	SR (with homogeneity[a]) of prospective cohort studies	SR (with homogeneity[a]) of level 1 economic studies
1b	Individual RCT (with narrow confidence interval[c])	Individual inception cohort study with ≥80% follow-up; CDR[b] validated in a single population	Validating[k] cohort study with good[i] reference standards; or CDR[b] tested within one clinical centre	Prospective cohort study with good follow-up[m]	Analysis based on clinically sensible costs or alternatives; systematic review(s) of the evidence; and including multiway sensitivity analyses
1c	All or none[d]	All or none case series	Absolute SpPins and SnNouts[g]	All or none case-series	Absolute better-value or worse-value analyses[j]
2a	SR (with homogeneity[a]) of cohort studies	SR (with homogeneity[a]) of either retrospective cohort studies or untreated control groups in RCTs	SR (with homogeneity[a]) of level > 2 diagnostic studies	SR (with homogeneity[a]) of 2b and better studies	SR (with homogeneity[a]) of level > 2 economic studies
2b	Individual cohort study (including low quality RCT; e.g. <80% follow-up)	Retrospective cohort study or follow-up of untreated control patients in an RCT; Derivation of CDR[b] or validated on split-sample[f] only	Exploratory[k] cohort study with good[i] reference standards; CDR[b] after derivation, or validated only on split-sample[f] or databases	Retrospective cohort study, or poor follow-up	Analysis based on clinically sensible costs or alternatives; limited reviews(s) of the evidence or single studies; including multi-way sensitivity analyses
2c	'Outcomes' research; Ecological studies	'Outcomes' research		Ecological studies	Audit or outcomes research
3a	SR (with homogeneity[a]) of case-control studies		SR (with homogeneity[a]) of 3b and better studies	SR (with homogeneity[a]) of 3b and better studies	SR (with homogeneity[a]) of 3b and better studies
3b	Individual case-control study[h]		Non-consecutive study; or without consistently applied reference standards	Non-consecutive cohort study, or very limited population	Analysis based on limited alternatives or costs; poor quality estimates of data, but including sensitivity analyses incorporating clinically sensible variations
4	Case-series (and poor quality cohort and case-control studies[e])	Case-series (and poor quality prognostic cohort studies[l])	Case-control study, poor or non-independent reference standard	Case-series or superseded reference standards	Analysis with no sensitivity analysis

TABLE 10 *continued*

Level	Therapy/prevention, aetiology/harm	Prognosis	Diagnosis	Differential diagnosis/symptom prevalence study	Economic and decision analyses
5	Expert opinion without explicit critical appraisal, or based on physiology, bench research or 'first principles'	Expert opinion without explicit critical appraisal, or based on physiology, bench research or 'first principles'	Expert opinion without explicit critical appraisal, or based on physiology, bench research or 'first principles'	Expert opinion without explicit critical appraisal, or based on physiology, bench research or 'first principles'	Expert opinion without explicit critical appraisal, or based on economic theory or 'first principles'

Notes

Users can add a minus sign '–' to denote the level of failure to provide a conclusive answer because of:

- EITHER a single result with a wide confidence interval (such that, for example, an ARR in an RCT is not statistically significant but whose confidence intervals fail to exclude clinically important benefit or harm)
- OR a systematic review with troublesome (and statistically significant) heterogeneity
- Such evidence is inconclusive, and therefore can only generate grade D recommendations

[a] By homogeneity we mean a systematic review that is free of worrisome variations (heterogeneity) in the directions and degrees of results between individual studies. Not all systematic reviews with statistically significant heterogeneity need be worrisome, and not all worrisome heterogeneity need be statistically significant. As noted above, studies displaying worrisome heterogeneity should be tagged with a '–' at the end of their designated level.

[b] Clinical Decision Rule. (These are algorithms or scoring systems which lead to a prognostic estimation or a diagnostic category.)

[c] See note 2 for advice on how to understand, rate and use trials or other studies with wide confidence intervals.

[d] Met when *all* patients died before the treatment became available, but some now survive on it; or when some patients died before the treatment became available, but *none* now die on it.

[e] By poor quality *cohort* study we mean one that failed to clearly define comparison groups and/or failed to measure exposures and outcomes in the same (preferably blinded), objective way in both exposed and non-exposed individuals and/or failed to identify or appropriately control known confounders and/or failed to carry out a sufficiently long and complete follow-up of patients. By poor quality *case-control* study we mean one that failed to clearly define comparison groups and/or failed to measure exposures and outcomes in the same (preferably blinded), objective way in both cases and controls and/or failed to identify or appropriately control known confounders.

[f] Split-sample validation is achieved by collecting all the information in a single tranche, then artificially dividing this into 'derivation' and 'validation' samples.

[g] An 'Absolute SpPin' is a diagnostic finding whose specificity is so high that a positive result rules-in the diagnosis. An 'Absolute SnNout' is a diagnostic finding whose sensitivity is so high that a negative result rules-out the diagnosis.

[h] Good, better, bad and worse refer to the comparisons between treatments in terms of their clinical risks and benefits.

[i] *Good* reference standards are independent of the test, and applied blindly or objectively to all patients. *Poor* reference standards are haphazardly applied, but still independent of the test. Use of a non-independent reference standard (where the 'test' is included in the 'reference', or where the 'testing' affects the 'reference') implies a level 4 study.

[j] Better-value treatments are clearly as good, but cheaper, or better at the same or reduced cost. Worse-value treatments are as good and more expensive, or worse and the equally or more expensive.

[k] Validating studies test the quality of a specific diagnostic test, based on prior evidence. An exploratory study collects information and trawls the data (e.g. using a regression analysis) to find which factors are 'significant'.

[l] By poor quality prognostic cohort study we mean one in which sampling was biased in favour of patients who already had the target outcome, or the measurement of outcomes was accomplished in <80% of study patients, or outcomes were determined in an unblinded, non-objective way, or there was no correction for confounding factors.

[m] Good follow-up in a differential diagnosis study is >80%, with adequate time for alternative diagnoses to emerge (e.g. 1–6 months acute, 1–5 years chronic).

TABLE 11

Grades of recommendation from Oxford Centre of Evidence-Based Medicine

A	Consistent level 1 studies
B	Consistent level 2 or 3 studies or extrapolations from level 1 studies
C	Level 4 studies or extrapolations from level 2 or 3 studies
D	Level 5 evidence or troublingly inconsistent or inconclusive studies of any level

'Extrapolations' are where data are used in a situation which has potentially clinically important differences from the original study situation.

TABLE 12

Answer to case study 1 (Table 4)

Question	In patients with clinically suspected maxillary sinusitis will radiological investigations help me improve my chances of making the correct diagnosis so leading to more definitive treatment at an early stage?
Your best answer	I need to check I am not missing any other causes such as dental problems or cancer so it would be better to do a radiograph
Initial evidence	Best evidence 2001 has a section on diagnostic criteria of maxillary sinusitis which suggest that the presence of certain symptoms and signs make the possibility of diagnosis of maxillary sinusitis 92% probable. A radiograph may not be essential For further details please read Chapter 13

introduces the reader to the gate control theory of pain.)

(2) Wall P, Melzack R (eds). Textbook of Pain. Churchill Livingstone, London, 1999: ISBN 0-443-06252-8. (One of the classical textbooks recently updated and a handbook version of it is due in 2003.)

(3) Crombie IK, Croft PR, Linton SJ, LeResche L (eds). Epidemiology of Pain. IASP, Seattle, WA, 1999: ISBN 0-931092-25-6. (Contains two chapters on facial pain and other related chapters, systematic reviews.)

(4) Turk DC, Melzack R. Handbook of Pain Assessment, 2nd edn. Guilford Press, New York, 2001: ISBN 157230488X. (Describes a wide range of assessments that are used in pain, considerably updated.)

(5) Good MD, Brodwin PE, Good B, Kleinman A. Pain as Human Experience: an Anthropological Perspective. University of California Press, Berkeley, CA, 1994: ISBN 0-520-07512-9. (Provides a different perspective on pain.)

(6) Burrows GD, Elton D, Stanley GV. Handbook of Chronic Pain Management. Elsevier, Amsterdam, 1987: ISBN 0-444-80446-3. (Although it does not use evidence-based methodology it is worth glancing through this text.)

(7) Lund JP, Lavigne GJ, Dubner R, Sessle BJ (eds). Orofacial Pain, from Basic Science to Clinical Management. Quintessence Publishing, Chicago, 2001: ISBN 0-867-15-381-4. (This book from some of the leading basic science research workers brings together basic science and research and although primarily aimed at undergraduates there is much in it for the specialist.)

(8) Feinmann C (ed). The Mouth, the Face and the Mind. Oxford University Press, Oxford, 1999: ISBN 0-1926630628. (Written more from a psychiatric viewpoint it has input from a

multidisciplinary team that has vast experience of working with patients with facial pain. Not written in an evidence-based way.)

(9) McQuay H, Moore RA. An Evidence-Based Resource for Pain Relief, Oxford University Press, Oxford, 1998: ISBN 0-192630482. (Although it contains little on facial pain it provides insight on how good quality research work in the field of pain can be used.)

(10) Jensen TS, Turner JA, Wisenfeld-Hallin Z (eds). Proceedings of the 8th World Congress on Pain. Progress in Pain Research and Management. Vol. 8, IASP Press, Seattle, WA, 1997: ISBN 0-931-092-18-3. (This is a collection of research papers on a wide range of subjects judged to be some of the best presented at the 8th World Congress of Pain.)

(11) Devor M, Rowbotham MC, Wiesenfeld-Hallin Z (eds). Proceedings of the 9th World Congress on Pain. IASP Press, Seattle, WA, 2000: ISBN 0-931092-31-0. (This is a collection of research papers on a wide range of subjects judged to be some of the best presented at the 9th World Congress of Pain.)

(12) Diagnostic and Statistical Manual of Mental Disorders. American Psychiatric Association, Washington, DC, 1987. (This provides the classification system for psychiatric disorders.)

(13) Merskey H, Bogduk N (eds). Classification of chronic pain. Descriptors of Chronic Pain Syndromes and Definitions of Pain Terms. IASP Press, Seattle, WA, 1994: ISBN 0-931092-05-01. (This is one classification system for all pain.)

D.2. Evidence-based medicine: a selection of books and articles I have used

(1) Sackett DL, Straus SE, Scott Richardson W, Rosenberg W, Haynes RJ. Evidence-Based Medicine. How to Practice and Teach EBM. Churchill Livingstone, Edinburgh, 2000: ISBN 0-443-06240-4. (This small book is now in its second edition and includes a CD ROM and a web site to ensure it remains up to date.)

(2) Crombie IK. The Pocket Guide to Critical Appraisal. BMJ Publishing Group, London, 1996: ISBN 0-7279-1099-X. (Enables the reader to judge papers to preset criteria.)

(3) Dixon RA, Munro JF, Silcocks PB. The Evidence Based Medicine Workbook. A Critical Appraisal for Clinical Problem Solving. Butterworth-Heinemann, Oxford, 1997: ISBN 0-7506-2590-2. (An example of an interactive book with exercises and answers.)

(4) Greenhalgh T. How to Read a Paper: the Basics of Evidence Based Medicine, 2nd edn. BMJ, London, 2000: ISBN 0727915789. (This is based on the series of articles that appeared in the Br Med J. It is very useful.)

(5) Evans D, Haines A. Implementing Evidence-Based Changes in Healthcare. Radcliffe Medical, Abingdon, 2000: ISBN 18577-53828. (Helps to show how to ensure that recent research enters practice rapidly.)

(6) Br Med J series 'How to Read a Paper' 1996–1997 a series of papers that appeared over a period of time and can be downloaded from the Br Med J web site or buy the book (see above).

(7) J Am Med Assoc series 'Users Guides to the Medical Literature 1993 Onwards'. (These articles appear regularly in the J Am Med Assoc on a very wide range of topics always illustrated with a case study.)

(8) Forrest JL, Miller SA. Enhancing Your Practice Through Evidence Based Decision Making. J. Evid-Based Dent Pract 2001; 1: 51–57. (A useful paper.)

(9) The Cochrane Library as well as having the largest databases of clinical trials also contains useful data on evidence-based methodology.

References

Anonymous. CRD Report Number 4. 4. 1996. NHS Centre for reviews and dissemination.

Drangsholt M, Truelove EL. Trigeminal neuralgia mistaken as temporomandibular disorder. J Evid Base Dent Pract 2001; 1: 41–50.

Greenhalgh T. Is my practice evidence-based? Br Med J 1996; 313: 957–958.

Haynes RB, Sackett DL, Gray JA, Cook DJ, Guyatt GH. Transferring evidence from research into practice: 1. The role of clinical care research evidence in clinical decisions. Evid-Based Med 1996; 1: 196.

McKibbon KA, Richardson WS, Walker-Dilks C. Finding answers to well built questions. Evid-Based Med 1999; 4: 164–167.

Oxman AD, Sackett DL, Guyatt GH. Users' Guides to the Medical Literature. I. How to Get Started. The Evidence-Based Medicine Working Group. J Am Med Assoc 1993; 270: 2093–2095.

Richardson WS, Wilson MC, Nishikawa J, Hayward RS. The well built clinical question: a key to evidence-based decisions. ACP J Club 1995; 123: a12.

Sackett DL, Rosenberg WM, Gray JA, Haynes RB, Richardson WS. Evidence based medicine: what it is and what it isn't. Br Med J 1996; 312: 71–72.

Assessment and Management of Orofacial Pain
Pain Research and Clinical Management, Vol. 14
Edited by J.M. Zakrzewska and S.D. Harrison
© *2002 Elsevier Science B.V. All rights reserved*

CHAPTER 2

Background: neurobiology of pain

Behnam Aghabeigi [*]

Department of Oral and Maxillofacial Surgery, Eastman Dental Institute, 256 Gray's Inn Road, London WC1X 8LD, UK

Objectives for this chapter:

This chapter will attempt to:
- Define pain and explain the difference between nociception and pain; acute and chronic pain
- Explain peripheral pain mechanisms and demonstrate the chemical basis of nociception and peripheral sensitisation
- Recognise the role of ascending neural pathways and their mechanisms of action through nociceptive fibres, second order neurones, convergence and divergence, pain referral and radiation
- Evaluate the theories of pain perception especially those of the Specificity theory, Pattern theory and the Gate control theory
- Explain how 'gate' activation by primary afferents and by descending pathways can occur
- Describe the role of wind up and central sensitisation
- Demonstrate the clinical implications of central sensitisation
- Propose some mechanisms of neuropathic pain
- Explain neurobiology of dental pain, innervation of dentine and pulp and mechanisms of dentine sensitivity

1. Introduction

An effective evidence-based management of orofacial pain requires appreciation of the underlying pain mechanisms. Over the recent years, the field of pain research has changed rapidly, and understanding of the pathophysiology of orofacial pain has expanded concomitantly. This chapter will describe some of our current understanding of these mechanisms and how this knowledge may be used in controlling pain. The reader may wish to refer to comprehensive reviews on the subject found at the end of the chapter in Further reading (Sessle, 2000).

————————
[*] Tel.: +44-20-7915-1275; Fax: +44-20-7915-1259;
E-mail: b.aghabeigi@eastman.ucl.ac.uk

2. Definitions

The words pain and nociception are not synonymous. The term nociception is defined as pain sensation (L. *nocere*: to injure) and refers to the mechanisms that provides for reception and conversion of noxious or potentially noxious stimuli into neural impulses and the transmission of such impulses by nerve fibres to the central nervous system where they are modulated and acted on (Okeson, 1996). Much of our understanding of pain mechanisms comes from studies of nociception in anaesthetised animals.

Pain is often referred to as a sensation and there are certain qualities of somatic sensations that are almost exclusively associated with pain such as stinging and burning. However, the newer concepts regard

TABLE 1

KEY FACTS: definitions of pain — International Association for Study of Pain (IASP)

- Pain: an unpleasant sensory and emotional experience associated with actual or potential tissue damage
- Nociception: the mechanism for reception and conversion of noxious or potentially noxious stimuli into neural impulses and their transmission to CNS
- Nociceptor: a receptor preferentially sensitive to a noxious stimulus or to a stimulus which would become noxious if prolonged
- Noxious stimulus: a noxious stimulus is one which is damaging to normal tissues
- Acute pain: short lasting, warns the body of danger, protective
- Chronic pain: outlived its apparent biological function

pain as a subjective psychological state rather than an unpleasant sensory activity that is induced solely by noxious stimulation. The definition of pain adopted by the International Association for the Study of Pain (IASP) (Merskey and Bogduk, 1994) defines pain as "an unpleasant sensory and emotional experience associated with actual or potential tissue damage or described in terms of such damage" (Table 1). This definition avoids linking pain to a stimulus and regards pain always as an affective state, that is, an emotional experience and not merely the perception of a pure sensation. However, the affective state of pain differs from other affective states in that it is always referred or projected to some part of the body with varying degrees of precision. Unlike elation or sorrow, pain is always 'felt' in some part of the body, even when that part is no longer present, as in the case when pain is felt in a 'phantom limb' after its amputation and possibly also after an extracted tooth. As pain is a totally subjective experience which cannot be simultaneously shared and reported by another individual, it is clinically important to accept the subject's description of the pain experience. Conversely, it is unhelpful to question or reject

it. The term 'idiopathic pain' may be preferable to 'psychogenic' pain where there is no identifiable organic disease. No pain problem is conceived of as either solely in the body, hence 'real' or in the mind, hence 'imagined'.

A distinction between acute and chronic or recurrent pain is important as the management and to some extent the pathophysiology is different. Acute pain may be considered to be a protective mechanism for the body, which by stimulating the sympathetic nervous system, is often accompanied by the autonomic signs of stress and anxiety. It is also of considerable diagnostic value to the clinician in determining the nature and site of the disturbance. It also warns of outside danger. In managing patients with chronic pain, the fact that pain is also beneficial is important when trying to change patients' negative attitude to pain into something more positive. On the other hand, chronic pain does not serve any apparent biological function and is socially and psychologically destructive. The sympathetic response becomes less apparent and signs and symptoms similar to those seen in depressive syndromes emerge.

3. Peripheral mechanisms of orofacial pain

Most knowledge of peripheral pain mechanisms is derived from studies of the limbs rather than the orofacial region. However, there is adequate evidence to believe that spinal cord mechanisms also apply to the trigeminal system (Sessle, 2000). This knowledge has led to development of new analgesics, which are more effective and have fewer side effects.

3.1. Chemical basis of nociception

Pain is provoked when a variety of substances are released or injected into the tissues. These algogenic (pain producing) substances can be released from the cell membranes, mast cells and nerve endings by trauma, infection, allergenic reactions, neurogenic reflexes and central emotional changes. There is evidence that some of these agents are present in inflamed oral tissues, such as tooth extraction sockets

(Hargreaves et al., 1994), temporomandibular joint (TMJ) (Appelgren et al., 1991) and the periodontium (Linden et al., 1997).

The exact process by which noxious stimuli lead to electrical activity in the appropriate sensory endings (*transduction*) is not known, but because of the short response latency it is assumed that nociceptive stimuli can directly activate the receptors. However, because it has been shown that certain chemicals can activate nociceptors, it has been hypothesised that tissue damage leads to release of these chemicals and stimulates the nociceptive endings. Regardless of whether a direct or indirect mechanism is involved, one can assume that the activation will involve an increase in the membrane permeability of the nerve ending resulting in a depolarisation, which if large enough, will generate action potential in the nerve fibre.

Damaged tissues release a cocktail of chemicals which can either directly or indirectly affect nociceptive nerves. Some chemicals such as potassium and hydrogen ions can activate or sensitise the endings depending on whether they are in high or low concentrations, respectively. Other mediators such as serotonin and histamine can only activate the nerve endings. One of the most important pain-producing substances that appear in the injured tissue is bradykinin which is a 9 amino acid peptide created by enzymatic breakdown of large plasma proteins and is a potent pain producing substance. It activates neighbouring C polymodal neurones contributing to expansion of the area of pain.

Another group of compounds that are synthesised in the region of tissue damage are the metabolic products of arachidonic acid. The cyclooxygenase enzyme results in the production of prostaglandins. There are two identified isomers of cyclooxygenase (COX): Cyclooxygenase-1 (COX-1): which is the constitutive (constantly present) form of the enzyme and is associated with the physiological 'protective' role of prostaglandins. Prostaglandins play a housekeeping role in renal parenchyma, gastric mucosa, platelets and other tissues. Inhibition of COX-1 by non-steroidal anti-inflammatory drugs is responsible for the commonly known side effects of these drugs such as renal and gastrointestinal toxicity and defects of platelet function. COX-2 is the inducible form of the enzyme, which has a limited constitutive role in some normal tissues but is expressed primarily in sites of tissue damage and inflammation (Kam and Power, 2000). COX-2 produces the same prostaglandins as does COX-1, but in greater amounts. Thus, the effects of prostaglandins in inflamed tissues are due principally to their increased concentration rather than to the actual prostaglandins present. Novel inhibitors of COX-2 have been developed for pain management as they lack the serious side effects of the COX-1 inhibitors. Prostaglandins do not seem to be allogenic substances per se. They sensitise nociceptive nerve endings to different types of stimuli, thus lowering their pain threshold to all kinds of stimulation. The peripheral sensitisation that occurs as a result of injury is known as primary hyperalgesia and accounts for part of the increase and expansion of the area of sensitivity around the site of injury.

Another important metabolic pathway of arachidonic acid is the lipoxygenase pathway which produces the leukotrienes. This is not inhibited by non-steroidal anti-inflammatory analgesics. Leukotriene B4 is a hyperalgesic substance, which is derived from the 5-lipoxygenation of arachidonic acid. This is the result of the action of the lipoxygenase enzyme on the fifth carbon atom of arachidonic acid. LTB4 has been identified in the saline aspirates of painful TMJs (Quinn and Bazan, 1990). This may explain why the non-steroidal anti-inflammatory analgesics are not fully successful in relief of chronic temporomandibular joint pain.

Substance P is the neurotransmitter at the primary sensory synapse. This neuropeptide is synthesised by the nerve cell body and can be released antidromically (against the normal flow of activity) to the periphery which further mediates the inflammatory response. Substance P causes the mast cells to release histamine and the platelets to release serotonin. Both these mediate inflammation and increased peripheral sensitivity to pain. Capsaicin is the irritant compound found in the fruits of the capsium plant (red pepper chilli). When administered to animals subcutaneously, it causes depletion of substance P

TABLE 2

KEY FACTS: effect of inflammatory mediators on nociceptors

Mediator	Effect
Potassium ion	Activate/sensitise
Hydrogen ion	Activate/sensitise
Histamine	Activate
Serotonin	Activate
Bradykinin	Activate ++
Substance P	Sensitise
Arachidonic acid metabolites:	
Prostaglandin	Sensitise
Leukotriene	Sensitise

TABLE 3

KEY FACTS: types and examples of peripheral sensitisation

Allodynia	Pain due to a stimulus which does not normally provoke pain, e.g. pain provoked by clothes rubbing on skin in sunburn, tenderness to percussion in apical periodontitis
Hyperalgesia	An increased response to a stimulus which is normally painful — as seen in sites of tissue injury and inflammation
Hyperaesthesia	Increased sensitivity to stimulation and includes both allodynia and hyperalgesia but the more specific terms should be used wherever they are applicable

and then insensitivity to noxious stimuli. Desensitisation of nociceptors has therapeutic value and capsaicin has been used in the management of neuropathic pains (Ellison et al., 1997). The effect of these mediators is summarised in key facts Table 2.

3.2. Peripheral sensitisation

Tissue damage results in an increased sensitivity of nociceptors at the site of injury. This is called peripheral sensitisation. Peripheral sensitisation may occur following the presence of chronic dental or other intraoral irritation or inflammation. The nociceptors exhibit spontaneous activity, lowered threshold and increased responsiveness to subsequent noxious stimuli. This increased responsiveness appears to be a major factor in the production of hyperalgesia or allodynia. From personal experience we know that damaged tissue displays increased sensitivity. The term hyperalgesia refers to an increased response to a stimulus that is normally painful. Pain due to a stimulus that does not normally provoke pain is called allodynia. For example the perception of pain produced by light touch after a sunburn is an example of touch allodynia. Testing for allodynia and hyperalgesia are essential in dental examination. For example, percussing a tooth is not painful in normal teeth but produces a pain sensation in apical periodontitis when nociceptors innervating the apical periodontal ligament are sensitised. Similarly

pulpal nociceptors can be sensitised and may exhibit a prolonged discharge after pulp vitality testing. Additional properties of sensitised pulpal nociceptors include a reduced mechanical threshold (e.g. throbbing pain may be due to the pulsatile systolic increase in blood pressure).

See Table 3 for key facts of types and examples of peripheral sensitisation.

4. Ascending neural pathways transmitting nociceptive information

Nociceptive stimuli from the orofacial region result in generation of electrical impulses, which travel mainly via the trigeminal nerve but also by the sensory roots of facial, glossopharyngeal, vagus and upper cervical nerves. The peripheral basis for coding the intensity and duration of the noxious stimulus is the frequency of nerve impulses and the duration of the nerve impulse discharge of the nociceptive afferent fibre.

As pain is a perception, not a stimulus, the term 'pain receptor' is not appropriate. The term nociceptor is used to refer to the receptors that respond to harmful or potentially harmful (noxious) stimuli. From a morphological point of view, most or

TABLE 4

KEY FACTS: mechanisms for transmitting nociceptive information

1. Nociceptive fibres

- A-δ fibres responding to noxious mechanical stimuli
- C-polymodal neurones responding to mechanical, thermal and chemical stimuli
- Silent or sleeping nociceptors

2. Second-order neurones

- Nociceptive specific (NS) responding to nociceptive mechanical or thermal stimulation
- Wide dynamic range (WDR) responding to both non-noxious and noxious stimuli (nociceptive non-specific)

all nociceptors are believed to be free nerve endings. Because the nociceptive endings of pain fibres lack specialised terminals, they are named after their afferent fibres and the stimulus that activates them.

4.1. Nociceptive fibres

The nociceptive fibres are divided into three types as shown in Table 4 key facts.

4.1.1. A-δ nociceptors

Except for the A-β nerves supplying tooth pulp (Orchardson and Cadden, 2001) all myelinated nociceptors may be categorised as A-δ fibres. Myelinated fibres convey impulses more rapidly than unmyelinated fibres (salutatory conduction). The A-δ fibres transmit the initial wave of afferent nociceptive activity going to the CNS signalling sharp acute pain. These are small diameter (2–5 μm) myelinated fast conducting (5–30 m/s) fibres. In humans, most A-δ fibre nociceptors respond only to noxious mechanical stimuli (Lynn, 1994) and are known as A-mechanical nociceptors. Some larger A-δ fibres respond to all types of noxious stimuli (mechanical, thermal, chemical) and are referred to as A-δ polymodal nociceptors.

4.1.2. C-fibre nociceptors

These are the most numerous (Lynn, 1994) and arguably the most important nociceptors in the human body (Le Bars and Willer, 1991). These fibres have a diameter of 0.3–3 μm and are unmyelinated with a conduction velocity of 0.5–2 m/s. These are also polymodal, responding to strong mechanical stimuli, intense heat, or cold and various pain-producing chemicals.

4.1.3. Silent nociceptors

These are mechanically insensitive and become active when tissue is injured and add to the nociceptive input to the CNS (Schmidt et al., 1994). Silent nociceptors can undergo a process of peripheral sensitisation.

In some parts of the body, a brief strong (e.g. electrical) stimulus can evoke two distinct painful sensations: first (fast) and second (slow) pain due to the very different speeds of impulse conduction in A-δ and C-fibres, respectively. However, these two components cannot easily be distinguished in the orofacial region because of the short conduction distances to the brain.

4.2. Second-order neurones

The cell bodies of most orofacial nociceptive neurons are in the trigeminal (Gasserian) ganglion. The central processes of these neurones enter the brainstem, branch and synapse on the second-order neurones at various levels of the trigeminal brainstem sensory nuclear complex. Second-order neurones are of two types:

(1) Nociceptive specific (NS): exclusively activated by nociceptive cutaneous mechanical or thermal stimulation. The receptive fields of these neurones is small (one to several square mm).
(2) Wide dynamic range neurones (WDR): named so because they respond to stimulus intensities in both the non-noxious and noxious ranges, although other terms such as polymodal, multimodal and multireceptive neurones have also been used. Cutaneous receptive fields of WDR

are variable and are frequently much larger than receptive fields of primary afferent neurones. These neurones receive convergent input from large and small diameter fibres and are a critical component of the gate control hypothesis in which they fulfil the role of the central transmission or T cells (see below).

It seems that these neurones serve different but complementary functions: nociceptive specific neurones may signal the presence and location of a noxious stimulus, while the wide dynamic range cells may grade its overall severity (Cadden and Orchardson, 2001).

The trigeminal brainstem sensory nuclear complex is divided into three parts:

(1) The uppermost part: subnucleus oralis
(2) The middle part: subnucleus interpolaris
(3) The most inferior part: subnucleus caudalis

The subnucleus caudalis extends into the cervical spinal cord and merges with the spinal dorsal horn. Most textbooks of pain talk about dorsal horn mechanisms when referring to the central nervous system. For orofacial pain, the trigeminal correlate of the dorsal horn is the trigeminal nucleus within the brainstem pons. Evidence suggests that subnucleus caudalis is the principal relay site of orofacial nociceptive information and is homologous to the substantia gelatinosa of the spinal dorsal horn and acts as a gating mechanism capable of modulating sensory information. Because of the close structural and functional relationship between spinal and trigeminal regions, the term medullary dorsal horn is used by some instead of subnucleus caudalis for the caudal end of trigeminal sensory complex.

It is appropriate here to consider the phenomena of convergence and divergence, which help to understand pain radiation and referred pain.

4.3. Convergence and divergence

Divergence and convergence in nociceptive pathways are shown in Fig. 1.

4.3.1. Convergence

It has been known for many years that there are more primary afferent neurones entering the central nervous system than there are second-order neurones to carry impulses to the higher centres. It therefore follows that several primary sensory neurones must synapse with a single second-order neurone. The synapsing of several primary afferent neurones with one second-order neurone is known as 'convergence'. It has been shown that while primary trigeminal neurones normally respond only to stimuli located within their receptive fields, at least half the second-order WDR and nociceptive specific neurones are activated by electric stimulation applied outside the normal receptive fields of corresponding primary neurones. Furthermore, the trigeminal spinal tract nucleus receives converging input from nerves other that the trigeminal. Cranial nerves VII, IX, X and the upper cervical nerves supply input to this tract. This explains the referral of pain from cervical region to the trigeminal region as seen in patients with cervical spondylosis.

4.3.2. Divergence

The primary afferent neurones branch and synapse with several second-order neurones. This phenomenon explains why pain often radiates and appears to arise from a larger area than that which has been injured or is diseased.

From the brainstem, second-order neurones project to the contralateral thalamus and from there via third order neurones to cerebral cortex. There is some reason to believe that the sensory and affective aspects of pain are subserved in part by separate neural mechanisms. The spinothalamic projection to ventrobasal thalamus and its projection to the somatosensory cortex is required for the discriminative sensory aspect of pain. This is the means whereby the nature and source of pain are determined. However, projection to the medial thalamus and from there to the frontal cortex seems to be concerned with the affective aspects of pain. This view is supported by the observation of patients who underwent frontal lobotomy. Interestingly, these patients usually obtained striking relief of their pain problem

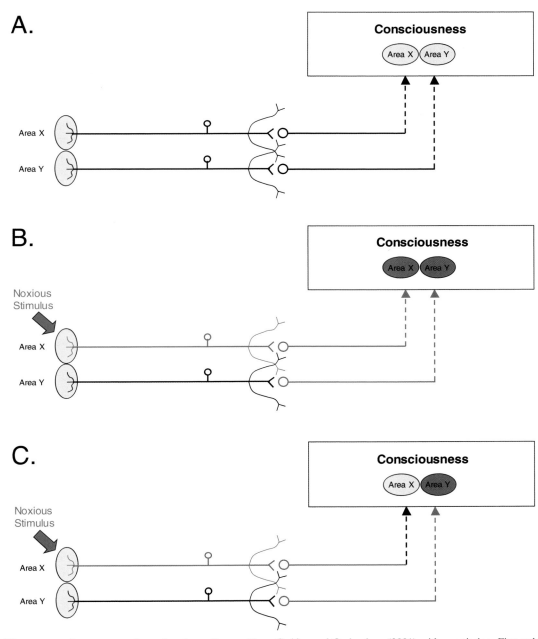

Fig. 1. Divergence and convergence in nociceptive pathways. From Cadden and Orchardson (2001) with permission. First published in Dental Update, Goerge Warman Publications. (A) Peripheral nociceptive nerves, before synapsing in the CNS, branch and diverge to make contact with more than one second-order neurone. In this way, information may 'converge' onto these second-order neurones. (B) Radiating pain. If one of these nociceptive nerves is activated, it may result in activation not only of its 'own' second-order neurone but also of neighbouring ones. This can result in a conscious perception that the pain is originating from a larger area ($X + Y$) than it actually is (X). (C) Referred pain. Under certain circumstances, the signal in the 'straight-through' pathway may not reach, or not be recognised by, the conscious centres — the pain is then ascribed to the uninjured area (Y) rather than the injured area. Activated neurones are shown in red.

but with no impairment in their ability to detect and identify noxious stimuli as painful. The suffering was thus eliminated with no effect on the purely sensory aspect of their pain. Functional imaging studies of regional cerebral responses to painful and non-painful stimuli in patients with atypical facial pain and control subjects have shown that in the patient group there were substantial responses to pain in areas of brain relating to affective aspects of pain including the medial pain system and its connection to wide areas of cortex (Derbyshire et al., 1994).

5. Theories of pain perception

5.1. Specificity theory

Descartes in 1664 (Melzack and Wall, 1996) described the pain system as a straight through channel from skin to brain. Others carried on and sought specific fibres from the receptors to the central nervous system and then specific pathways in the central nervous system itself. The modern day specificity theory is essentially similar to Descartes' concept of pain proposed 300 years earlier. It proposes a conceptual model of nervous system as a fixed direct line of communication from skin to the brain. The system consists of distinct nerves and pathways of different qualities to specific receivers in the brain. The theory proposes a direct, invariant relationship between pain perception and intensity of the stimulus and is reflected in definitions of pain such as that of the Butterworths Medical Dictionary: "the distressing sensation excited by noxious stimuli of sufficient intensity acting on nerve endings." This concept has dominated the medical and particularly dental teaching where it is usually possible to relate the severity of the pain to the noxious stimuli.

5.1.1. Shortcoming of the specificity theory
Although much pain results from noxious stimulation, it can also occur from non-noxious stimuli, as well as spontaneously when there is no stimulus at all. Phantom limb pain, causalgia, and the neuralgias provide a dramatic refutation of the concept

of a fixed direct line nervous system. Consider the following examples:

(1) Surgical lesions of the peripheral and central nervous system have been unsuccessful in abolishing idiopathic pain.
(2) Gentle touch, vibration and other non-noxious stimuli can trigger excruciating pain in neuralgia and sometimes pain occurs spontaneously for long period without any apparent stimulus.
(3) Pain from hyperalgesic skin areas often occurs after a long delay and continues long after removal of the stimulus which implies a remarkable temporal and spatial summation of inputs in the production of these pain states.

5.2. Pattern (summation) theory

Goldscheider's (1894, cited in Melzack and Wall, 1996) pattern or summation theory proposed that particular patterns of nerve impulses that evoke pain are produced by the summation of skin sensory input at the dorsal horn cells. Goldscheider was profoundly influenced by studies of pathological pain in patients with tabes dorsalis. Tabes dorsalis occurs in patients suffering the late stages of syphilis and is characterised by degeneration in the dorsal spinal cord and dorsal root, and one of its major symptoms is the temporal and spatial summation of somatic input in producing pain. Successive brief application of a warm test tube to the skin of a tabetic patient are first felt only as warm, but then feel increasingly hot until the patient cries out in pain as though his skin is being burned. Such summation never occurs in normal persons who simply report successive applications of warmth.

The fundamental assumption of pattern theory is that all cutaneous qualities are produced by spatial and temporal pattern of nerve impulses rather than separate modality specific transmission proposed by 'specificity theory'. The pattern theory proposes that all nerve endings are similar, so that pattern for pain is introduced by intense stimulation of non-specific receptors. The coding of information in the form of nerve impulse pattern is a fundamental concept in contemporary neurophysiology. However, the pattern theory fails to recognise that fact of physiological specialisation of nerve endings.

5.3. Gate control theory

The Gate control theory of pain is shown in Fig. 2.

More than 35 years ago when the specificity theory had little neurobiological basis and because of its inability to account for some clinical observations such as lack of a direct pain–injury relationship, Melzack and Wall (1965) proposed an alternative theory known as 'the gate control hypothesis'. They suggested:

(1) The transmission of nerve impulses from primary afferent nociceptive nerves to second-order cells (in the spinal cord or the trigeminal system) have to pass through a 'gate', which may be wide open (in which case the resulting pain may be severe), closed (in which case no pain will be felt) or, most commonly, partly open.
(2) The spinal gating mechanism is influenced by the relative amount of activity in large diameter (L) and small diameter fibres; activity in large diameter fibres tends to close the gate, whereas activity in small fibres tends to facilitate transmission (open the gate).
(3) The spinal gating mechanism is also influenced by nerve impulses that descend from the brain.
(4) When the output of the spinal cord transmission cell (second-order neurone) exceeds a critical level it activates the action system. The action system refers to those neural areas that underlie the complex sequential pattern of behaviour and experience, that are characteristic of pain.

Although many of the details of the original model have been modified as knowledge has increased, the concept has endured because it is consistent with both clinical observations of pain and laboratory findings regarding nociceptive mechanisms. It seems that the 'gate' consists of interneurones, which can inhibit activity beyond the first synapse, either by decreasing the release of the excitatory transmitters (presynaptic inhibition) or by inhibiting the second-order cells (postsynaptic inhibition). These inhibitory effects are mediated by a variety of agents, including γ-aminobutyric acid (GABA), glycine and endogenous opioid peptides. The interneurones themselves may be activated either by signals in other afferent nerves or by signals descending from the brain. In Chapter 9 you will find a diagram of how this theory has been used to explain the development of orofacial pain to patients.

5.3.1. Gate activation by other primary afferents

At a clinical level, the modulating effect of cutaneous stimulation has been known throughout the ages. The almost instinctive act of grabbing, holding, pressing or rubbing a painful site exemplifies this effect. Many useful pain-reducing remedies are of this category. Massage, counter-irritants, hot and cold compresses are examples.

Neurophysiological studies have shown that activity in large diameter (A-β) afferent nerves from the same neural segment of the body can inhibit activity in second-order nociceptive neurones. Since the vast majority of A-β nerves are mechanosensitive, these segmental inhibitory controls can be activated naturally by rubbing close to an injury. Under normal circumstances, these fibres will almost always be active to a limited extent (given that mechanoreceptors are constantly being excited by our movements). Thus anything that reduces mechanoreceptive activity from part of the body is likely to increase the sensitivity of that area for pain by 'opening the gate'. For example, this might occur after pressure damage to a nerve (A-β fibres are amongst the most easily damaged by physical insult) or when a patient reduces movement of a chronically painful region. This may explain why re-establishing normal mobility can contribute to the successful treatment of some chronic pains.

One of the chief products of the gate control theory was the introduction of transcutaneous electrical nerve stimulation (TENS) as a therapeutic modality. An interrupted current of very low intensity at a frequency of 50–100 Hz is used. The stimulation is usually below that required to activate A-δ and C nociceptive fibres. Stimulation of the thick A-β fibres

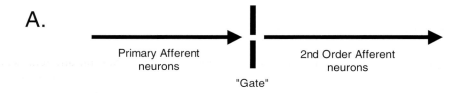

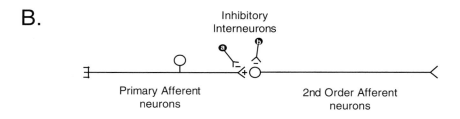

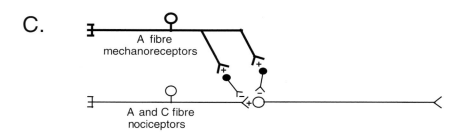

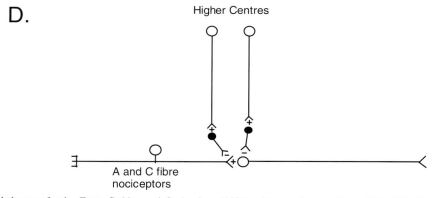

Fig. 2. Gate control theory of pain. From Cadden and Orchardson (2001) with permission. First published in Dental Update, Goerge Warman Publications. (A) The concept. Signals carried by primary afferent nociceptive nerves must pass through a 'gate' before being passed on by second-order afferents in the CNS. (B) The same scheme using the conventional shorthands for nerves. The primary afferent nerves excite (+) the second-order neurones. The 'gate' is made up of small inhibitory interneurones, which can either reduce the amount of excitatory transmitter released by the primary afferents or directly inhibit the second-order neurones. The inhibitory interneurones themselves may be excited: by activity in the adjacent large diameter mechanoreceptive nerves ('segmental inhibition') (C); or by activity originating in higher centres in the CNS ('descending inhibition') (D).

results in the anti-nociceptive effect. Kane and Taub (1975) reviewed the history of local electrical analgesia from the time the early Egyptians used electric fish to minimise pain. They reported that in 1858, Francis used forceps charged with electricity to extract teeth with less pain and more recently in various forms of so-called electronic dental analgesia, although these are not always successful (Cameron et al., 1993). It should be noted that not all forms of TENS work via A-β fibres acting segmentally. In particular, when TENS is used at relatively high intensities it may exert its effect via descending pathways.

5.3.2. Gate activation by descending pathways

In 1983, while studying nerve injuries in rats, Wall and Devor (1983) showed that peripheral nociceptors are not the only source of afferent impulses. The dorsal root ganglion cells also initiate sensory impulses. This source of afferent input may account for nociceptive impulses persisting after peripheral anaesthesia.

The neural mechanism in the brainstem that appears to balance this continuous barrage of sensory impulses is called the 'descending inhibitory system'. This inhibitory system is generally thought to affect all sensory input ascending into the central nervous system. The portion of this system that affects the nociceptive input has been referred to as the 'analgesic system'.

It is not entirely clear how these pathways are activated naturally but there is evidence that this may occur under at least two different circumstances: conditions of stress or anxiety; this explains the reduced levels of pain felt in battle or on the sports field and the presence of noxious/painful stimulus in another part of the body: this is the basis for counter-irritation phenomena whereby 'one pain masks another'. It is possible that some traditional methods for pain control, such as acupuncture, may be forms of counter-irritation (Cadden and Orchardson, 2001).

The analgesic system consists of three major components: periaqueductal or periventricular grey matter (PAG), nucleus raphe magnus (NRM) and a group of descending neurones that terminate in the substantial gelatinosa of the dorsal horn. Electrical stimulation either in the PAG or in NRM can almost completely suppress strong nociceptive impulses or inhibit the responses of second-order nociceptive neurones. Several different neurotransmitter substances are involved in the analgesia system especially serotonin (5-HT) and endorphins. In the CNS, serotonin is synthesised from L-tryptophan, a dietary essential amino acid when the nucleus raphe magnus is stimulated by sensory input. In the periphery, 5-HT is released by the blood platelets and is an algogenic substance and is thought to relate especially to vascular pain syndromes. In the CNS, 5-HT is an important chemical in the endogenous anti-nociceptive mechanism and is thought to potentiate endorphin analgesia. Pharmacological manipulation of serotonin and monoamines in the CNS raises the possibility of new centrally acting analgesic agents. In fact there is evidence that the value of tricyclic antidepressants in chronic pain management relates to their potency as blockers of the re-uptake of monoamines such as serotonin. The use of antidepressants as analgesics opens up a new approach to drug treatment for chronic pain.

6. Wind-up and central sensitisation

Although there has been much emphasis on the pain suppressing effect of the modulation system, the brainstem modulating neurones have a bi-directional control of transmission in that the network has both excitatory and inhibitory actions on pain conduction. Therefore pain can result from either the loss of inhibitory control or the activation of excitatory modulating neurones.

In recent years, significant insight has been achieved that helps us better understand chronic pain and persistence of pain in the absence of any identifiable organic abnormality. Clinicians have observed that with the passage of time painful peripheral neuropathies become increasingly refractory to any treatment indicating a more centralised process. It has been shown that if the nociceptive activity from the periphery has been of sufficient intensity, changes occurs in the central nervous system that

TABLE 5
KEY FACTS: the underlying mechanisms of central sensitisation
• Increased release of neurotransmitters and excitatory amino acids from C-fibres
• Increased expression of receptors on the post-synaptic neurones
• Genetic changes in post-synaptic neurones

TABLE 6
KEY FACTS: clinical implications of central sensitisation
• Pain with no obvious 'organic' cause
• Pre-emptive analgesia
• Immediate management of acute pain
• Novel centrally acting analgesics

significantly alter the central response to subsequent peripheral stimulation. In other words, with continued nociceptive input, the second-order neurones become increasingly sensitised, allowing the next impulses to depolarise the neurone even quicker. This change in the processing of second-order neurones is called *central sensitisation or neuroplasticity*. The underlying mechanisms of neuroplastic changes are as follows and are summarised in key facts Table 5.

There is an increased release of neurotransmitters and excitatory amino acids from presynaptic neurone (C-fibre). Furthermore there is an associated increased responsiveness of post-synaptic receptors for substance P (NK 1 receptor) and excitatory amino acids receptor (NMDA receptor). Activation of the NMDA receptor leads to production of nitric oxide is the WDR neurones. Nitric oxide is thought to be one of the agents that causes 'wind up' because pretreatment with an NMDA antagonist or a non-active substrate of nitric oxide prevents it. It is thought that part of the mechanisms that lead to chronic ongoing pain is the loss of segmental inhibition interneurones which may be particularly susceptible to the neurotoxic effects of nitric oxide and lose their ability to function. There is also evidence that painful stimulus can lead to long lived genetic alterations in the postsynaptic neurone.

7. Clinical implication of central sensitisation

The clinical implications of central sensitisation are summarised in Table 6 key facts.

(1) Once neuroplasticity has occurred the original source of pain can resolve leaving a neuropathic pain disorder that seems to have no apparent clinical source. This can be extremely frustrating to the clinician who may not be aware of this condition.

(2) If any tissue damage produces neuroplasticity that lasts far longer than the stimulus itself, then the potential for permanent neuroplastic changes is always a risk. If this is true then one could certainly appreciate the need for local anaesthetic each and every time tissue is to be surgically injured. When a patient is placed under general anaesthesia, the nociceptive impulses created at the surgical site are blocked from reaching the cortex at the brainstem level. Therefore, the C-fibres stimulated at the site of the surgical trauma carry the nociceptive impulses into the dorsal horn (or spinal tract nucleus) and excite the second-order neurones. This nociceptive input will sensitise these neurones, creating central sensitisation even though the anaesthetised patient feels no pain. Upon awaking, the patient will often feel postoperative pain secondary to the sensitised second-order neurones. This may be avoided in clinical practice by the infiltration of a local analgesic prior to surgery even when carried under a general anaesthetic.

(3) Even a protracted toothache risks a chance of becoming an ongoing pain condition even after the tooth is extracted. With this in mind, the importance of immediate management of acute pain becomes obvious.

(4) The possibility of development of novel centrally acting analgesics blocking NMDA receptors, potentiating inhibitory interneurones or neutralising the allogenic action of nitric oxide.

8. Mechanisms of neuropathic pain

Neuropathic pain is defined by the International Association for the Study of Pain as "pain initiated or caused by a primary lesion or dysfunction in the nervous system". Several neuropathic pain conditions affect the orofacial region as shown in Table 7 key facts.

8.1. Post-traumatic neuropathic pain

Trauma to the nerves in the orofacial region is a common cause of orofacial pain. It has been reported that up to 5% of patients undergoing endodontic therapy and apicectomy have persistent pain (Holland, 2001). Other possible examples of this mechanism include inferior alveolar nerve trauma following extraction of a wisdom tooth, placement of dental implants and orthognathic surgery. Within hours or days, numerous fine processes start to grow out from the proximal cut end of the axon. Under optimal conditions, one of these regenerating 'sprouts' reaches peripheral target tissue and establishes a functional receptor ending. When forward growth is blocked, terminal endbulbs persist, and sprouts either turn back on themselves or form a tangled mass. This structure is a 'neuroma'. In the neuroma, both myelinated and unmyelinated nerve fibres develop abnormal spontaneous and provoked activity (so-called ectopic), particularly following light tactile stimulation. Nerve compression may also cause a loss of large afferent fibres leading to decreased activity in the inhibitory pain system.

8.2. Involvement of the sympathetic nervous system

Normal pain sensation is not dependent upon the sympathetic nervous system. In some patients, the pain may be sustained by efferent activity in the sympathetic nervous system; this pain is referred to as sympathetically maintained pain. It has been shown that C-fibre nociceptors that survive a partial nerve injury acquire an excitatory response to noradrenaline and sympathetic stimulation and are more easily sensitised by the normal tissue injury. They fire spontaneously and develop abnormal sensitivity to noradrenaline, cold and mechanical stimulation. Additionally it has been shown that injured C-fibres express or up-regulate α_1-adrenoreceptors. Presence of this receptor would cause the pain fibre to discharge when it is activated by sympathetic fibre release of noradrenaline. α_2-Receptors on the other hand act as auto-receptors on terminal endings of sympathetic fibres. The receptor functions as a feedback mechanism to stop release of noradrenaline when the receptor is activated. α_2-Agonists such as clonidine would turn off terminal release of noradrenaline and reduce the pain. α_1-Antagonists such as phentolamine are used to aid in diagnosis and treatment of sympathetically maintained pain.

8.3. Trigeminal neuralgia

There is now persuasive evidence that trigeminal neuralgia is usually caused by demyelination of trigeminal sensory fibres within either the nerve root or, less commonly, the brainstem (Love and Coakham, 2001). There are likely to be several reasons for demyelination of these nerve fibres:

(1) An aberrant loop of superior cerebellar artery that may lie on the nerve root and produce

---

TABLE 7

KEY FACTS: examples of neuropathic pain

- Post-traumatic neuropathic pain
- Sympathetically maintained pains
- Trigeminal neuralgia
- Post-herpetic neuralgia

a significant microvascular compression. This compression is thought to cause the demyelination of the nerve.

(2) Space-occupying lesions such as cerebellopontine angle tumours.
(3) Systemic conditions such as multiple sclerosis.

Clinical observations and electrophysiological studies support the concept that demyelination and ephaptic (non-synaptic) spread of nerve impulses underlie most, if not all, of these conditions. Ephaptic cross talk between fibres mediating light touch and those involved in the generation of pain may account for the precipitation of attacks of neuralgia by light tactile stimulation of facial trigger zones. The frequency of involvement of the trigeminal nerve root entry zone in multiple sclerosis patients with trigeminal neuralgia as well as in patients with vascular compression probably reflects the fact that fibres subserving light touch and those involved in the generation of pain are in closest proximity in this region, so that ephaptic cross talk between the two pathways is most likely to occur when the demyelination is in this region (Love et al., 2001).

Decompression of the nerve root produces rapid relief of symptoms in most patients with vessel-associated trigeminal neuralgia, probably because the resulting separation of demyelinated axons and their release from focal distortion reduce the spontaneous generation of impulses and prevent their ephaptic spread. The role of remyelination in initial symptomatic recovery after decompression is unclear.

8.4. Post-herpetic neuralgia

Post-herpetic neuralgia (PHN) is one of the commonest intractable conditions seen in pain clinics. Acute herpes zoster is a viral inflammation of the dorsal root and ganglion that seems to destroy large myelinated fibres preferentially (Scadding, 1999). It also leads to atrophy of the dorsal horn and sometimes to persistent and widely spreading inflammatory changes. It has been proposed that post-herpetic neuralgia does not involve a single mechanism but instead that different clinical presentations parallel different mechanisms. Central sensitisation related to nociceptor hyperactivation that may or may not be maintained by the sympathetic system occurs in the initial form of the condition. Alteration of segmental or descending inhibitory control could occur in other forms of the disease.

9. Neurobiology of dental pain

9.1. Innervation of dentine and pulp

Dental pulp is a highly vascular and richly innervated connective tissue that forms the soft tissue core of a tooth. The mean number of axons entering one human premolar tooth is close to a thousand. In many respects, the pulp of a fully formed tooth has physiological properties that are similar to those of loose connective tissue elsewhere in the body but it is different in at least two important aspects: it is exquisitely sensitive, so much so that just touching exposed pulp with a wisp of cotton wool can cause severe pain, and in a fully formed, intact tooth it has a very low compliance, probably the lowest compliance of any tissue in the body. This low compliance is due to the surrounding calcified dentine, which prevents any significant volume change when the pressures within the tissue change. As a result of this low compliance, the equilibrium between the various factors that affect blood flow and the circulation of the tissue fluid in pulp are different from those in most other tissues. Dentine is a non-vascular tissue, but it also can be very sensitive despite its sparse innervation.

The nerve fibres that innervate the pulp branch extensively in the coronal part of the tooth and form a subodontoblastic plexus. The branches of the trigeminal nerve that innervate teeth contain both afferent and postganglionic sympathetic fibres. The trigeminal primary afferent neurons have their cell bodies in the trigeminal ganglion and are primarily sensory in function, although some produce vasodilatation when stimulated. This vasodilatation is part of the axon reflex. The sympathetic fibres supply pulp vessels and are vasoconstrictor. Their cell bodies are in the superior cervical ganglion from which the axons pass to the trigeminal ganglion and then on to the tooth in the branches of the trigeminal nerve. Unlike other orofacial tissues, the pulp does not receive a parasympathetic innervation.

The pulp is innervated by myelinated A-β and A-δ fibres and non-myelinated C-fibres. About 50% of the myelinated axons are of the fast conducting A-β class, which is surprising for a tissue whose innervation supports in the main only pain sensation. It appears that all afferents that innervate pulp seem to be capable of producing pain. However, under certain conditions, other sensations than pain can be evoked by stimulation of the tooth pulp (Sessle, 1979). It has been suggested that the low intensity stimulation of A-β fibres gives rise to the sensation of pre-pain (Narhi, 1985).

The dentinal tubules taper from a diameter of about 2 μm at their pulpal end to 0.5 μm or less peripherally. Each tubule contains the process of an odontoblast whose cell body is situated at the pulpal end of the tubule. The odontoblast processes extend no more than half the length of the tubules, and under the tip of the cusp they are much shorter than this. Some dentinal tubules also contain one or more fine nerve terminals. These are unmyelinated (diameter approximately 0.1 μm) and penetrate up to 100 μm into the dentinal tubules. The highest density of innervation is under the tip of the cusp, where almost every tubule contains a nerve terminal. There are no myelinated axons in the ondontoblast cell layer. Some of the dental nerve endings contain neuropeptides, including substance P and calcitonin gene-related peptide (CGRP), which have been implicated in the responses of pulp afferent fibres to injury and inflammation.

9.2. Mechanisms of dentine sensitivity

Three major theories of dentine sensitivity are shown in Table 8 key facts.

The neural theory has largely been abandoned, as there is no satisfactory evidence to show that there are nerves in the outer dentine, which is the

---

TABLE 8
KEY FACTS: mechanisms of dentine sensitivity

- Activation of intradentinal extensions of pulpal nerves
- A transduction mechanism involving the odontoblast or its dentinal process
- A hydrodynamic mechanism within the dentinal tubules and pulp

---

most sensitive. Furthermore, agents that cause pain when applied to the skin do not do so when applied to dentine (Torneck, 1989). It has also been shown that the existence of nerve fibres in dentine is not a necessary prerequisite for its sensitivity (Narhi, 1990).

The second theory considers odontoblast to be a receptor coupled to the nerves in the pulp. It used to be argued that because the odontoblast was of neural crest origin it could have retained an ability to transducer and propagate an impulse. However, the dentine remains sensitive despite the destruction of not only the intradentinal nerve fibres but also the odontoblast layer (Narhi, 1990). This gives support to the concept that transmission of external irritation from the dentine surface to the pulp nerves must be indirect.

The hydrodynamic theory of dentine sensitivity fits much of experimental and morphologic data. It proposes that the fluid movement through the dentinal tubules distorts the adjacent pulp and is sensed by its free nerve endings. This theory explains why topical anaesthetics fail to block dentine sensitivity and why pain is produced by dehydration, hypertonic solutions, thermal change and mechanical probing. The increased sensitivity at the dentino-enamel junction is explained by the profuse branching of the tubules in this region. A rather surprising finding (Holland, 2001) has been that the pulpal sensory receptors are much more sensitive to outward than inward flow through the dentinal tubules.

TABLE 9
Summary of Chapter 2

- Pain is an unpleasant sensory and emotional experience associated with actual or potential tissue damage

- The key inflammatory mediators on nociception are potassium ion, hydrogen ion, histamine, serotonin, bradykinin, substance P, arachidonic acid metabolites

- Nociceptive information is transmitted by nociceptive fibres, second order neurones which include nociceptive specific and wide dynamic range neurones

- Central sensitisation results in pain with no obvious 'organic cause', explains the mechanisms underlying pre-emptive analgesia, immediate management of acute pain and the centrally acting mechanisms of some drugs

- The gate control theory of pain explains how pain is perceived and modified by a variety of mechanisms

- Wind up and central sensitisation are responsible for the continuation of pain after the initial stimulus has been lost

- Examples of neuropathic pain in the facial region are trigeminal neuralgia, post-herpetic neuralgia and post-traumatic neuropathic pain

- A variety of theories have been put forward to explain dental pain

10. Summary

See Table 9 for a summary of this chapter.

11. Further reading

(1) Lund JP, Lavigne GJ, Dubner R, Sessle BJ (eds). Orofacial pain, from basic science to clinical management. Quintessence Publishing, Chicago, 2001. (This book, from some of the leading basic science research workers, brings together basic science, research and their clinical applications.)

(2) Melzack R, Wall PD. The Challenge of Pain. Penguin, London, 1996. (A general book which introduces the reader to evolution of different pain theories.)

(3) Sessle BJ. Acute and chronic craniofacial pain: brainstem mechanisms of nociceptive transmission and neuroplasticity, and their clinical correlates. Crit Rev Oral Biol Med 2000; 11: 57–91. (This review paper describes the recent advances in knowledge of brainstem mechanisms related to craniofacial pain, draws attention to their clinical implications and suggests directions for future research.)

(4) Wall PD, Melzack R (eds). Textbook of Pain. Churchill Livingstone, London, 1999. (A classic textbook of pain.)

References

Marked as regards quality according to criteria set by author.
* Case studies, no controls, only evidence.
*** Randomised controlled trials, high quality original studies.

* Appelgren A, Appelgren B, Eriksson S et al. Neuropeptides in temporomandibular joints with rheumatoid arthritis: a clinical study. Scand J Dent Res 1991; 99: 519–521.

* Cadden SW, Orchardson R. The neural mechanisms of oral and facial pain. Dental Update 2001; 28: 359–367.

* Cameron WA, Pairman JS, Orchardson R. The effect of an electronic analgesia device on dental pain thresholds. Anesth Pain Control Dent 1993; 2: 171–175.

* Derbyshire SW, Jones AK, Devani P et al. Cerebral responses to pain in patients with atypical facial pain measured by positron emission tomography. J Neurol Neurosug Psychiatry 1994; 57: 1166–1172.

*** Ellison N, Loprinzi CL, Kugler J et al. Phase III placebo-controlled trial of capsaicin cream in the management of surgical neuropathic pain in cancer patients. J Clin Oncol 1997; 15: 2974–2980.

* Hargreaves KN, Swift JQ, Bozkowski MT, Garry MG, Jackson DL. Pharmacology of peripheral neuropeptide and inflammatory mediator release. Oral Surg Oral Med Oral Pathol 1994; 78: 503–510.

* Holland GR. Management of Dental Pain. In: Lund JP et al (eds) Orofacial Pain: From Basic Science to Clinical Management. Quintessence Publishing, London, 2001: 211–221.

* Kam PCA, Power I. New Selective COX-2 inhibitors. Pain Rev 2000; 7: 3–13.

* Kane K, Taub A. A history of local electrical analgesia. Pain 1975; 1: 125–138.

* Le Bars D, Willer JC. Physiology of pain. In: Bonnet F (ed)

Pain in the perioperative period. Librairie Arnette, Paris, 1991: 3–51.

* Linden GL, McKinnell J, Shaw C, Lundy FT. Substance P and neurokinin A in gingival crevicular fluid in periodontal health and disease. J Clin Periodontol 1997; 24: 799–803.

* Love S, Coakham HB. Trigeminal neuralgia, pathology and pathogenesis. Brain 2001; 124: 2347–2360.

* Love S, Gradidge T, Coakham HB. Trigeminal neuralgia due to multiple sclerosis: ultrastructural findings in trigeminal rhizotomy specimens. Neuropathol Appl Neurobiol 2001; 27: 238–244.

* Lynn B. The fibre composition of cutaneous nerves and the classification and response properties of cutaneous afferents, with particular reference to nociception. Physiol Rev 1994; 1: 172–183.

* Melzack R, Wall PD. Pain mechanisms: a new theory. Science 1965; 150: 971–979.

* Merskey H, Bogduk N (eds). In: Classification of Chronic Pain, 2nd edn. IASP Task Force on Taxonomy. IASP Press, Seattle, WA, 1994: 209–214.

* Narhi M. The characteristics of intradental sensory units and their response to stimulation. J Dent Res 1985; 64: 564–571.

* Narhi MVO. Intradental sensory units. In: Inoki R (ed) Dynamic Aspects of Dental Pulp. Molecular Biology, Pharmacology and Pathophysiology. Chapman and Hall, London, 1990: 144–145.

* Okeson JP (ed). Bell's orofacial Pains, 5th edn. Quintessence Publishing, London, 1996, pp xviii.

* Orchardson R, Cadden SW. The physiology of the dentine–pulp complex. Dent Update 2001; 28: 200–209.

* Quinn JH, Bazan NG. Identification of prostaglandin E2 and leukotriene B4 in the synovial fluid of painful, dysfunctional temporomandibular joints. J Oral Maxillofac Surg 1990; 48: 968–971.

* Scadding JW. Peripheral neuropathies. In: Wall PD, Melzack R (eds) Textbook of Pain. Churchill Livingstone, New York, 1999: 815–834.

* Schmidt RF, Schable HG, Messlinger K, Heppelmann B et al. Silent and active nociceptors: structure, functions and clinical implications. In: Gebhart GF, Hammond DL, Jensen TS (eds) Progress in Pain Research and Management, Vol. 2. IASP Press, Seattle, WA, 1994: 213–250.

* Sessle B. Is the tooth pulp a 'pure' source of noxious input? Adv Pain Res Ther 1979; 3: 245.

* Sessle BJ. Acute and chronic craniofacial pain: brainstem mechanisms of nociceptive transmission and neuroplasticity, and their clinical correlates. Crit Rev Oral Biol Med 2000; 11: 57–91.

* Torneck CD. Dentine–pulp complex. In: Ten Cate AR (ed) Oral histology, development, structure and function. Mosby, St. Louis, MO, 1989: 188.

* Wall PD, Devor M. Sensory afferent impulses originate from dorsal root ganglia as well as from periphery in normal and nerve injured rats. Pain 1983; 17: 321–329.

Assessment and Management of Orofacial Pain
Pain Research and Clinical Management, Vol. 14
Edited by J.M. Zakrzewska and S.D. Harrison

CHAPTER 3

Psychology of pain

Toby Newton-John [*]

Department of Clinical Psychology, Eastman Dental Hospital, Gray's Inn Road, London WC1X 8LD, and Sub-Department of Clinical Health Psychology, University College London, Gower Street, London WC1E 6BT, UK

Objectives for this chapter:

This chapter will attempt to:
- Present a historical overview of pain theories and models, highlighting the change in thinking about psychological processes in pain
- Offer empirical evidence to demonstrate the importance of psychological factors in determining how pain is experienced
- Review the evidence for psychological predictors of the transition from acute pain to chronic pain
- Provide an overview of psychological pain management techniques, and discuss the evidence evaluating their efficacy

1. Introduction

Although there has been an awareness of the role of psychological processes in pain for millennia, it is only in more recent times that an experimental approach has been adopted in order to quantify them. The aim of this chapter is firstly to present an historical overview of how theories about the nature of pain have changed. Secondly, the research literature as it pertains to psychological variables and pain experience will be discussed, both in experimental and in clinical settings. Studies that have explored psychological factors in facial pain will be a particular focus, although much of the work has been done with more common pain disorders such as chronic low back pain. The role that psychological variables

play in the transition from acute pain to chronic pain will also be discussed. Finally, the literature that pertains to the psychological management of pain will be reviewed.

2. Pain theories

Whether you are aware of it or not, you are already likely to have a theory about pain which you hold to be true. Because of its universality (congenital analgesia, or the inability to experience pain, is an extremely rare condition), you are likely to have experienced the internal sensations which are commonly labelled as 'painful' on quite a number of occasions. Falling over as a child, normal biological processes such as menstruation or 'growing pains', later sporting injuries, surgical operations and so on all constitute everyday life experience of pain. You will have therefore built up a series of thoughts,

[*] Tel.: +44-20-7915-2351; Fax: +44-20-7915-1194;
E-mail: toby.newton-john@uclh.org

beliefs, expectations and predictions about pain — based on your own experience and those around you — which will influence the ways in which you assess and treat pain in your patients.

It is also likely then that your model of pain is more or less consistent with a pain theory which was developed as far back as the 17th century. In 1664, the French philosopher Rene Descarte proposed that there was a linear relationship between the intensity of a painful stimulus and the amount of observable tissue damage. Massive damage would result in great pain, and minor trauma would lead to minimal discomfort. A report of pain in the absence of tissue damage was not considered to be genuine pain, but a function of psychic disturbance in a biologically normal individual (now termed 'functional' or 'psychogenic' pain). Individuals complaining of pain when no pathological process has been identified are often considered at best to be deriving some benefit from their complaint (termed secondary gain, such as attention from loved ones, or the avoidance of undesirable activities, such as work). At worst, they are considered to be malingering. Our pain terminology reflects such beliefs, in the pejorative terms 'low back loser', 'Mediterranean back' and 'kangaroo paw', which was used to describe the repetitive strain injury (RSI) phenomenon in Australia in the 1980s (Reilly, 1995).

Unfortunately, this dualistic view of pain has persisted into the 21st century despite the accumulation of overwhelming evidence to the contrary. For example, there are many instances of significant tissue damage in the absence of pain, such as that reported by athletes on the playing field or soldiers on the battlefield; painful conditions such as 'tension' headache or trigeminal neuralgia which are not associated with tissue trauma; and phantom limb pains, in which pain is reported in an area which no longer exists (see Melzack and Wall, 1988 for a fuller account of pain anomalies). You may also have had the experience of observing a bruise or scratch on your body, and not being aware of how or when it occurred. It would seem that although you sustained an injury which *should* have hurt, you did not perceive pain at the time. It is difficult to reconcile this everyday event with the pain model described above.

3. The gate control theory

The publication of the gate control theory of pain (Melzack and Wall, 1965) revolutionised pain theory by stating that psychological processes are an inextricable part of all pain experience — irrespective of the extent of tissue damage. Melzack and Wall said that variables such as mood state, attention, past experience of pain, and the meaning of the pain to the individual, would all influence the response to pain. The limits of medical science in being able to detect 'all forms of pathology' given the technology available at any one time were also acknowledged. Pain was now a much broader and more complex construct than a correlate of the amount of tissue damage that could be observed.

Largely as a consequence of the gate control theory and the research evidence that has accrued to support it, the International Association for the Study of Pain published the following definition of pain: "an unpleasant sensory and emotional experience associated with actual or potential tissue damage, or described in terms of such damage" (IASP, 1979). This definition explicitly recognises that all pain, whether an organic basis can be observed or not, necessarily involves psychological processing. It also recognises the loose association between injury and the experience of pain, and ultimately rejects notions such as psychogenic as being unscientific and invalid. In our example above, you did not experience any pain associated with the bruise because of distraction. Although your pain receptors and afferent nerve fibres are in perfect working order, your cognitive resources were being strongly deployed elsewhere. Hence the gating mechanism was brought into play, and the pain messages were blocked.

The contemporary term 'biopsychosocial' refers to the integration of biological, psychological and social factors within the experience of health or illness (Skevington, 1995). When applied to the issue of pain, this model is theoretically consistent with the tenets of the gate control theory. It suggests that biological factors represent only one element of a multifactorial phenomenon termed pain, and that pain should be seen as a dynamic, fluid process rather

TABLE 1

Pain models

1. Biomedical model

- Pain is always a sign of tissue damage or compromise

- Pain and tissue damage have a linear relationship, such that greater tissue damage (observable pathology) should always result in greater levels of pain, and vice versa

2. Psychiatric model

- Pain in the absence of observable pathology is 'psychogenic' i.e. the somatic expression of unresolved emotional conflicts

- Certain personality types are more prone to developing pain than others

3. Biopsychosocial model

- Pain is a multifactorial phenomenon, involving a fluid interaction of biological, psychological and social factors

- It is not possible to separate out the 'physical' elements of pain from the 'psychological', as both operate at all levels of the pain experience

than an endpoint of nociception, transmission and perception. It is on a biopsychosocial understanding of pain that the remainder of this article is based. Differences in these conceptualisations of pain are illustrated in Table 1. The table shows the move from dichotomised models of pain and psychology to the integrated biopsychosocial perspective.

4. Psychological aspects of the gate control theory

The gate control theory posited a number of dimensions of 'descending influence' on pain experience, which may be considered as the precursors to the systematic investigation of psychological influences on pain. There is now an enormous literature documenting these influences, and the interested reader is referred to texts by Skevington (1995), Gatchel and Turk (1996) and the reviews by Gamsa (1994a,b). The present chapter gives merely a brief overview of this extensive body of research.

4.1. Culture

Cultural factors are known to significantly influence pain behaviour (Rollman, 1998), and the differences between cultures can be startling. For example, there is evidence that headache, which affects as many as 70% of the Western population at least once per month, is almost non-existent in Oriental and African countries (Ziegler, 1990). An analysis of cross-cultural nursing assessments revealed significant differences between Mexican Americans and white Americans of Northern European descent in their expression of pain. Stoicism and tolerance of pain are seen as desirable pain responses amongst white Americans, whereas the Mexican culture accepts crying out and the expression of strong emotions when in pain (Calvillo and Flaskerud, 1991).

However, there are numerous problems with cross-cultural methodologies when exploring pain differences, not the least of which is the reliance on language to provide the dependent variable. Pain cannot be directly measured, only described, and linguistic nuances represent a major source of error variance. As is stated in Chapter 6, reliance on self-report questionnaires to compare pain characteristics between patient groups must be done very carefully. For example, it is never clear whether subjects with different cultural or linguistic backgrounds interpret the same instructions in exactly the same way, and whether they intend their responses to the same items to be interpreted by the experimenters in exactly the same way. Despite this range of variability, pain report can be remarkably consistent across cultures. For example, Dahlstrom et al. (1997) were able to replicate the patient profiles found in a US sample of TMD patients with their sample of Swedish TMD sufferers.

4.2. Past experience of pain

An individual's past experience of pain can also greatly affect future responses to painful stimuli. Social learning theory has offered a number of theoretical perspectives on classical and operant conditioning factors in pain, particularly in relation to childhood experiences of injury or disease (Osborne et al., 1989). It is estimated that 70–90% of all sickness episodes are handled outside the formal health care system, and that self-treatment within the family provides a substantial proportion of health care (Turk et al., 1985). Hence, the influence of the family on pain is significant. In particular, the modelling of parental responses to injury (and hence vicarious learning from parental attitudes towards pain), has been shown to be an important predictor of later pain experience (Fillingim et al., 2000). For example, Fillingim and colleagues showed that individuals with a family history of chronic pain were significantly more likely to have experienced pain themselves in the past month and to report poorer health, than a matched sample of individuals with no family pain history. Whether for genetic, social learning or some other reason, pain does appear to 'run in families', although not all evidence has supported this association (Raphael et al., 1999).

Conditioning is another psychological phenomenon which can powerfully influence pain experience. An aversive experience at the dentist can result in the conditioned association of pain and fear with the sound of the drill, the smell of the dental surgery, and the sight of white coats and masks. The fact that 45% of dentate adults in the UK report fear as being their most important barrier to dental care attests to the strength of classical conditioning to pain (Naini et al., 1999). Operant conditioning is also an important social learning influence on pain and disability, at both acute and chronic ends of the pain spectrum. You may have witnessed the situation in which a child who falls and scrapes a knee immediately looks up to see if his or her mother is watching — before bursting into tears. The promise of a sympathetic maternal reaction can powerfully shape the pain response. Similarly, chronic pain patients with solicitous (overprotective) spouses tend to be significantly more disabled and to report greater pain intensity than patients whose spouses are less overtly sympathetic (Newton-John and Williams, 2000). This in no way suggests that patients consciously seek the solicitous responses from their spouses; in fact they invariably report wishing the spouse responded differently. But the fact is that the provision of help and assistance for pain behaviour tends to generate more pain behaviour.

4.3. Mood

The gate theory hypothesised mood state as an important psychological variable in the response to pain, and this has been reliably shown to be the case. In the classical laboratory experiment, a sample of normal healthy subjects (usually university students) undergo a mood induction procedure, such as completing a bogus exam. Half the sample are given false feedback that they have scored in the bottom 10% for their year; the other half are told that they are in the top 10%. Both groups then rate their current mood state to confirm that the induction has produced an appropriately dichotomised sample ('high mood' vs. 'low mood', and they are then exposed to an identical noxious stimulus. The 'low mood' groups reliably rate the stimulus as significantly more painful than the 'high mood' group.

It is hardly surprising that many chronic pain patients experience difficulties with mood as their disorder continues without respite. Ongoing pain can herald many losses — of work, of role within the family, of financial security, of future plans, of leisure and sporting interests — virtually any area of life activity can be affected. Ultimately, many patients who have unsuccessfully tried the wide range of different pain treatments and procedures come to experience a loss of hope that their situation can improve at all, a phenomenon known as 'learned helplessness' in the psychological literature (Overmier and LoLordo, 1998). The sum of all these experiences in the context of unremitting pain helps to explain prevalence rates of major depression of up to 50% of chronic pain patients (Banks and Kerns, 1996).

Within chronic facial pain patients, depression is consistently found to influence coping and adjustment to illness (Madland et al., 2000). However, there are a number of mechanisms by which this association may be mediated, and the contribution of each to the final outcome is not clear. Biochemical changes related to depression may directly influence the perception of pain, or lethargy and hopelessness may lead to a failure to employ effective coping strategies, or the 'depressogenic' thinking style which is characteristic of low mood may systematically bias patient self-report when questioned about coping with pain (Williams, 1998). Each of these factors may operate independently or synergistically

Anxiety also figures strongly in terms of influencing pain experience, as the previously cited data regarding the prevalence of dental fears would attest. Preoperative anxiety levels have also been shown to predict outcome from cardiac surgery better than a host of clinical variables including medical status, type of surgical procedure, preoperative length of stay, priority of surgery, gender and age (Stengrevics et al., 1996). McCraken et al. (1992) showed that chronic pain patients reporting higher levels of anxiety specifically in relation to their pain also reported higher pain intensity scores, greater self-reported disability and more use of anxiolytic medication.

4.4. Cognitions and interpretations of pain

The chapter on psychosocial assessment in chronic pain (Chapter 6) referred to the notion of self-efficacy as an important aspect of pain evaluation. The success of the patient-controlled analgesia (PCA) system is evidence of the influence that beliefs about pain control can have upon the experience of pain itself. A comparison of PCA versus the continuous infusion method for administering spinal epidurals found that the level of analgesia was equivalent across the two conditions, but the PCA group required less local anaesthesia and reported higher satisfaction (Curry et al., 1994). Ultimately, how one construes pain — the meaning that is attributed to the sensation labelled as 'painful' — determines the behavioural and affective reaction to it. The interpretation of clicking and popping noises in the temporomandibular joint as evidence of impending degeneration and/or sudden dislocation, will result in a quite different set of behaviours and emotions to an interpretation which normalises joint noises. Beliefs about the predictability and controllability of the pain, about the potential threat posed by the pain, and about the individual's resources to respond effectively to the pain, all impact upon the pain experience.

A factor analysis of the McGill Pain Questionnaire (see Chapter 6), revealed that the questionnaire items clustered into three categories, termed sensory-discriminative, cognitive-evaluative and motivational-affective domains. These three dimensions in many ways encompass the broad spectrum of psychological variables which are relevant to the experience of pain. The individual locates and discriminates the stimulus as painful, the stimulus is actively processed and evaluated against past experience and for current meaning, and these in turn lead to emotional and behavioural reactions to the pain. This chain then becomes cyclical rather than linear, as beliefs and interpretations about the pain influence mood and behaviour, which in turn affect how the individual thinks about the pain.

The overview given above offers something of the complexity and diversity of influences upon pain, and reinforces the importance of the biopsychosocial model when considering pain in any context.

TABLE 2

KEY FACTS: psychological influences on the perception and experience of pain

1. Cultural factors — social modelling, family norms, societal norms, cultural norms

2. Past experiences of pain — previous injuries, experiences of treatment

3. Mood — fear, anger, depression, worry

4. Beliefs about pain — the meaning of the pain, the ways in which it is interpreted, the expectations about its course and treatment, beliefs about personal control over it

5. Gender

6. Context in which it occurs — the sporting field versus a dental/medical surgery

7. For clinical pain — the relationship with the treating clinician

Table 2 gives an overview of the direct psychological influences on pain experience.

5. Pain: acute versus chronic

In the majority of cases, pain is a (fortunately) relatively short-lived experience. The injury heals, or the precipitant of the pain is removed from the environment, and the central nervous system returns to normal. However, for a significant minority of pain sufferers, the pain does not ameliorate over time. Acute pain in the temporomandibular joint, which is extremely common, will become chronic pain in approximately 12% of cases (Epker and Gatchel, 2000). Chronicity is defined here as pain experienced on a daily basis for a period of 6 months or longer (Turk, 1997). Chronic pain is the term used to describe long-term, intractable, non-malignant pain conditions such as complex regional pain syndrome, fibromyalgia and chronic low back pain. There has been a great deal of debate within the dental literature about the nomenclature for long-term benign pains in the face, and terms have included myofascial pain, facial arthromyalgia, atypical facial pain and chronic orofacial pain. None of these labels is without its deficiencies, but chronic facial pain appears to be the most parsimonious and is therefore used throughout this chapter.

Chronic pain conditions constitute an enormous drain on social, economic and personal resources. Often sufferers are unable to remain in paid employment, are frequent users of health care services, take high levels of medication, both prescription and over the counter, and experience a great deal of stress within their families and social networks. In this country, it is estimated that when work and production losses are included along with assessment and treatment costs, the total cost of back pain alone approaches £10.6 billion per annum (Manaidakis and Gray, 2000). Attempts have therefore been made to try to identify which acute pain sufferers are at risk of developing a chronic, disabling pain problem — and psychological factors have also been shown to play an important role in this transition.

TABLE 3
KEY FACTS: psychological predictors of chronic pain
1. History of depression or anxiety
2. Fear avoidant behaviours (resisting attempts to move the affected area for fear of damaging it/exacerbating the pain)
3. Current depression
4. Historical or current alcohol and/or substance abuse
5. Poor pain coping skills (passivity regarding self-management, tendency to catastrophise about pain, overuse of analgesia and rest, low self-efficacy regarding control over pain)
6. Perceived life stress
7. Heightened somatic concern/disease conviction/perception of poor health

6. Psychological predictors of chronic pain

Most of the research exploring predictive factors in chronic pain has been done with chronic low back pain problems. The review of this literature by Turk (1997) simply states, "Many studies have demonstrated that demographic and psychosocial factors are better predictors of chronicity than are clinical or physical factors" (Turk, 1997, p. 205). The psychosocial characteristics that have been identified as predictive of chronicity include a premorbid history of psychological problems (particularly depression or anxiety), current depressive disorder, a past history or current alcohol or substance abuse, and high levels of anxiety or fear avoidance behaviour (Croft et al., 1998; Klenerman et al., 1995; Thomas et al., 1999 — see Table 3). Specific health beliefs have also been identified as crucial predictive factors at this early stage of pain. Heightened concern about bodily processes, strongly held beliefs about pain being a sign of disease, and perceptions of poor health premorbidly are also suggestive that a chronic pain problem may develop (Turk, 1997).

Much less work has been done to examine the factors associated with the transition of acute facial pain into a chronic pain state, however Epker et al. (1999) did follow 204 patients with acute TMD over a 6-month period to determine which of those developed chronic TMD problems. Their two-variable regression model accurately predicted 91% of those with chronic TMD at follow-up. The significant predictor variables were higher reported pain intensity over the previous 3 months, and the presence of muscle pain on palpation. However numerous psychosocial variables also distinguished the chronic and non-chronic groups, including current anxiety and depression levels, history of psychological disturbance and dysfunctional pain coping styles.

Once again, psychological factors have been shown to be an integral part of the pain experience.

7. Sex and gender differences in pain

It is important to differentiate between the terms sex difference and gender difference. Sex differences exclusively refer to biological differences between males and females, whereas gender differences refer to the wider issues of how men and women are expected to behave within their cultural and societal contexts. Making a theoretical distinction between sex and gender is straightforward enough, however in research contexts the two are often difficult to disentangle. For example, it has been found in laboratory studies that when a noxious stimulus is applied and subjects are asked to rate at what point that stimulus becomes 'painful', women tend to report a lower pain threshold than men (Robinson et al., 1998; Unruh, 1996). However, it has also been found the sex of the experimenter affects such ratings: men will give significantly lower pain ratings (i.e. stimulus is 'not painful') to a female experimenter than to a male, whereas female subjects do not discriminate on this basis (Levine and De Simone, 1991; see Chapter 6). Are the findings demonstrating a difference in pain threshold between males and females therefore reflecting a biological or sex difference,

or presenting an example of gender stereotyping in which men must appear 'macho' and stoical in front of women? Whatever the case, gender is an influential variable in pain experience.

7.1. Women's pain

It is also important to recognise that irrespective of how the experimental variables are manipulated in research settings, women's experiences of pain are fundamentally different from those of men. For women, pain is often a 'normal' aspect of biological functioning as it relates to reproductive cycles. Pain may also be indicative of pathological processes such as endometriosis or ectopic pregnancy which are sex-specific. As Skevington has said "Intermittent periodic pain is a potentially regular life event for half of the population. Where such pains occur, they create schematic markers, being carefully monitored for a host of social and cultural reasons, as well as those connected with health and well-being" (Skevington, 1995, p. 275). By contrast, men are more likely than women to experience pain from injury, and from acute and chronic life-threatening diseases (Unruh, 1996). Thus for women pain conceivably may be a recurrent, benign and non-pathological phenomenon, whereas this is not the case for men.

8. Psychological treatment of chronic pain: the pain management programme

In chronic pain conditions where medical and surgical treatments have little to offer, pain management programmes have been developed in order to combat the effects of living with pain. The essential difference between the pain management approach and the biomedical approach to pain is that the goal of pain management is not to cure or necessarily even to relieve pain. Rather, the aims are to improve fitness, to restore meaningful activity within the patient's daily life, and to improve psychological function. Patients are helped to move towards a model in which improved quality of life is possible despite there being no resolution of their pain.

Pain management is ideally delivered as a multidisciplinary package, involving physical therapists, occupational therapists, nurses, medical personnel (typically Consultant Anaesthetists or Rheumatologists), and clinical psychologists. However, irrespective of the specialty, the various components of this kind of intervention are based on established psychological principles of reinforcement, learning theory and cognitive theory. Detailed guidelines of cognitive behavioural pain management programmes are available (Turk and Meichenbaum, 1994; Williams and Erskine, 1995), however a brief overview of the approach will be given here.

8.1. Exercise and stretch programme

Physiotherapy in the context of managing chronic pain involves a different approach than that offered for acute injuries and disorders. Rather than applying passive treatments such as mobilisation or ultrasound for the purpose of relieving pain, physiotherapy for the chronic pain patient is a 'hands off' intervention. Here, the physiotherapist's aims are to help the patient to regain strength, fitness and flexibility *despite* the presence of ongoing pain. The patient is given a specific set of stretches and exercises to perform, having firstly established a baseline level which they can manage without causing a sustained increase in pain. By systematically monitoring the amount that is performed and setting a realistic quota to be achieved each week, the patient can gradually increase his or her exercise capacity. The efficacy of this approach for chronic musculoskeletal pain problems has been well established (Frost et al., 1998).

The notion of pacing activity has much in common with this approach. The approach involves the patient timing how long he or she can engage in a specific activity (e.g. walking, sitting, standing, lying) before the pain is increased. By using this baseline time period as a starting point, the patient is encouraged to change position before the time period is up, thereby avoiding a provocation of the pain. Over time, the tolerance can be gradually extended out, so that the amount of time the patient engages in the activity systematically increases.

Physiotherapeutic approaches for facial pain have tended to be limited to acute pain conditions, such as following trauma to the TM joint or for post-surgical mobilisation (Gray and Davies, 1997). However, many of the same difficulties that the chronic low back pain patient experiences have their parallels in chronic TMD. For example, patients suffering from chronic TMD will also experience muscle spasm, limitations in movement (mouth opening), a fear of provoking pain (from chewing hard foods or laughing), and even anxiety about eating or laughing in public for fear of their TM joint locking in place. Molin (1999) has argued that physiotherapy has a role to play in the management of chronic facial pain, and there is emerging evidence that chronic TMD sufferers may benefit from this approach (Di Fabio, 1998; Yuasa and Kurita, 2001).

8.2. Cognitive therapy

This chapter has already highlighted several kinds of psychological distress, such as fear, anger and low mood, which often impact negatively upon coping with chronic pain. Cognitive therapy firstly aims to identify the beliefs, assumptions, interpretations and predictions which generate these kinds of affective disturbances. Having determined the idiosyncratic cognitive processes which give rise to the emotions, patients are taught methods of modifying their beliefs in order to reduce the associated distress.

Cognitive therapy is often described in a rather simplistic fashion as being a matter of teaching patients to 'think positively' about their situation. Apart from being inaccurate, this notion does the patient an enormous disservice: surely they would already be doing that if they possibly could! A recent study has also demonstrated that practising cognitive therapy effectively is not so simple either (King et al., 2002). In this study, 84 general practitioners were given four half-day intensive training in cognitive theory and practice, and then treated 272 mild to moderately depressed patients using these techniques. The outcomes for GPs given the cognitive therapy training were not significantly different from those who did not receive the training.

In relation to chronic pain, cognitive theory has highlighted a number of variables which influence adjustment and coping. As was described in Chapter 6, catastrophising has become a key concept in the pain field (Sullivan et al., 2001). It is a 'cognitive error', in that it refers to the expectation of the worst possible outcome from an event based on minimal evidence. A flare-up of pain might provoke such beliefs, and patients report thinking "I won't be able to manage this at all", "This pain will overwhelm me", "The pain will never subside". Such catastrophic thoughts will generate significant levels of anxiety which further erode coping with the pain. Therefore, catastrophising is often a target in treatment and evidence shows that patients who learn to reduce the frequency of their catastrophic cognitions benefit the most from treatment (Jensen et al., 2001).

Attention diversion exercises are another cognitive strategy that may form part of a psychological pain management package. These might be in the form of mental exercises (e.g. counting backwards from 1000 by 7s, reading), intentional recall of pleasant memories (holidays taken, books or movies seen), concentrated awareness of surroundings (describing objects in room or sounds heard in detail), or carrying out routine tasks (light household chores, self-care such as washing or dressing). The more pain the patient is experiencing, the less concentration he or she will have, so it is important not to suggest patients attempt strategies that are beyond them at these difficult times. This will only increase their frustration and despair.

8.3. Relaxation

Based on the principle that pain evokes muscle tension, and muscle tension in turn exacerbates pain, relaxation methods are commonly used with chronic pain patients. Generally patients are instructed to make themselves as comfortable as possible (sitting is preferable to lying in order to avoid falling asleep), to close their eyes, and to concentrate on slowing and deepening their breathing. Once this has been achieved, patients' attention may be drawn to each of the major muscle groups, and various

forms of imagery used to produce a feeling of relaxation (muscles warming up, becoming heavier etc.). Or patients may be asked to generate pleasant and relaxing images directly, which can serve as both relaxation-inducing and an attention diversion exercise.

To be optimally effective, relaxation training should eventually be carried out in an applied fashion, such that patients are taught to use their relaxation skills during active movement (walking, standing, writing), as well as during non-physically active periods. Relaxation is often included as a component of cognitive behavioural pain management programmes rather than being an independent treatment (Morley et al., 1999). However, all the evidence points towards it being a safe, inexpensive and moderately effective intervention (Skevington, 1995).

8.4. Biofeedback

Electromyographic (EMG) biofeedback has been used extensively with chronic TMD, based upon the rationale that increases in muscle tension will result in increased pain. Furthermore, higher levels of worry and stress will provoke muscle tension, which in turn can precipitate more pain. Patients undergoing the treatment have silver chloride electrodes taped to their masseter or frontalis muscles which detect and 'feed back' the electrical activity within the muscle to the patient. The feedback is usually in the form of an audible signal, where increases in tension cause the pitch to rise. Using relaxation or attentional control procedures, the patient learns to reduce muscle tension by lowering the pitch of the audio signal. The feed back is instantaneous, and the sensitivity can be altered to indicate very minor changes in muscle tension levels. Thermal biofeedback offers temperature variation as the goal of intervention, and tends to be used with circulatory disorders or migraine.

Like much of the literature on psychological approaches to pain management, the efficacy of EMG biofeedback has been extensively investigated. A recent meta-analytic review of 13 studies evaluating

EMG biofeedback for TMD found the intervention to be successful in the majority of cases (Crider and Glaros, 1999). The meta-analysis demonstrated a two-fold superiority for the active treatment over no treatment or placebo controls.

8.5. Hypnosis

Part of the broader family of relaxation approaches is that of hypnosis. There is an ongoing debate about the true nature of hypnotic induction — does it produce an altered state of consciousness or trance, or does it represent the manipulation of social influence between a charismatic practitioner and a receptive patient?

There is considerable overlap between the relaxation training outlined above and the use of hypnosis for chronic pain. Both involve attempts to decrease sensory and proprioceptive input, to lower arousal, and to increase feelings of calm and well-being. However, hypnosis involves a specific induction (telling the patient that they will or are likely to experience certain things) and the narrowing of attention. The literature exploring the utility of hypnosis for pain has been broadly supportive (Eimer, 2000), despite the problems concerning the mechanism of action. However, most of this work has been done with experimental pain rather than with clinical subjects; and within the clinical populations, most have been acute pain procedures such as catheterisation or wound dressing rather than chronic pain disorders (Eimer, 2000).

Most of the research examining the use of hypnotic inductions with facial pain has also been in the context of non-chronic disorders, such as treating dental phobia or tooth extraction (Patel et al., 2000). Recently, however, Simon and Lewis (2000) carried out an uncontrolled trial of hypnosis for chronic TMD, and obtained positive results both at post-treatment and at 6 months follow-up. Although the trial contained only 28 subjects and did not include a control group, the long-term nature of the condition gives some cause for optimism.

8.6. Couples-based pain management

Given that chronic pain is by definition a lengthy disorder, it is not surprising that the effects of the pain can be far-reaching. We noted in Section 4.3 that many areas of life can be affected by pain, including work, social life, leisure activities, and domestic roles, and changes in these areas for the patient will in turn impact upon the patient's spouse. Although it is rare for the spouse to be included in the pain assessment in the first instance, despite the evidence indicating the importance of the spouse in terms of patient adjustment to pain (Schwartz and Ehde, 2000), it is even rarer to consider the couple as the target for treatment. Nevertheless, there is some evidence in the musculoskeletal pain field that the inclusion of the spouse in treatment can enhance treatment efficacy (Keefe et al., 1996). Spouses are taught how to respond to pain behaviours appropriately, how to reinforce the patient's attempts to regain functional activity, and to improve the communication within the couple about pain in general.

This is an area that warrants more investigation, particularly in relation to chronic facial pain.

8.7. Dealing with flare-ups of pain

Every chronic pain sufferer, whether their pain is constant or intermittent in nature, will occasionally experience major exacerbations of the pain. This may be the precipitating factor in the patient contacting you in a great deal of distress and anxiety, struggling to cope with the intensity of the pain that they are experiencing. Managing these flare-ups of chronic pain is one of the most difficult tasks for the chronic pain sufferer, as it tends to draw on most if not all of the skills and strategies outlined above. However, patients who manage their flare-ups well, tend to also cope with the pain well in general.

The first task for the patient (and perhaps then you as their clinician) is to confirm that the pain that they are experiencing is indeed a flare-up of their chronic, and not a new or different pain. This differentiation is not always a straightforward matter, and can cause a great deal of anxiety in itself. However, once it has been established that the pain does not require any different approach to management, the use of a Flare-Up Plan is advised. The Appendix A gives an example of a Flare-Up Plan for chronic facial pain, in this case trigeminal neuralgia, which can serve as a model. The central aim of carrying out these strategies is to try and maintain a sense of control over the pain as far as possible. This will prevent the patient's anxiety levels rising, which is known to worsen the pain experience (McCraken et al., 1992).

9. Case study

Now see if you can design a pain management intervention for Mrs. L. described in Table 4. Consult Table 7 in Appendix B for a description of the actual intervention carried out.

10. The evidence base for psychological approaches to pain management

The evidence clearly supports the utility of these approaches. The most recent meta-analysis of cognitive behavioural pain management interventions showed significant improvements in most areas of assessment, including positive coping measures, reducing behavioural expressions of pain, and pain intensity (Morley et al., 1999). These programmes were compared with waiting list control groups or alternative treatments such as pharmacotherapy. However, these studies do not examine the individual components

TABLE 4

Case study

Mrs. L. is a 47-year-old married woman with chronic facial pain and burning mouth syndrome referred for psychological pain management. She was referred by an Oral Surgeon who had been treating her for the past year without much success. Mrs. L.'s pain began 18 months previously following an extended period of dental work in which she underwent an extraction and several root fillings. The pain began almost immediately that this dental treatment finished, while the burning mouth syndrome had a more insidious onset. At the time of assessment, she was taking amitriptyline 125 mg, clobazam 20 mg daily, and up to six co-proxamol per day.

Prior to developing the pain Mrs. L. was a successful health care professional, who worked long hours in her job but found it highly rewarding. She was very socially active with friends and attending the theatre in her leisure time, and also enjoyed jogging in her local park

Over a period of 6 months following the onset of the pain, she gradually reduced her work commitments until she finally stopped altogether. At the time of assessment, she spent much of her day lying down or sitting still in order to avoid moving her head and aggravating the pain. She was especially fearful of having 'an attack' of the pain while out and away from the security of her home. She therefore did not venture further than her local shops alone, and would not travel much further when accompanied. Her husband, also a health care professional, was extremely concerned about her as he regularly witnessed her in great distress with the pain. He encouraged her to rest as much as possible, and took over many of the household chores such as shopping and cooking. Although she was taking a significant amount of medication, she continued to experience high levels of pain without any obvious benefit from her drugs. Below are the results of her assessment measures. Based on the information given in the treatment outline above, how would you design a pain management intervention for Mrs. L.? Consult Table 7 in the Appendix B for a description of the actual intervention carried out.

Measure	Pre-treatment	Post-treatment
Pain intensity rating (VAS 0–100)	80	50
Pain distress (VAS 0–100)	95	20
Pain self-efficacy questionnaire	13/60	34/60
Pain disability index	49/70	25/70
Beck depression inventory	28/63	12/63

TABLE 5

KEY FACTS: evidence base for psychological approaches to pain management

Treatment component	Evidence for chronic back pain	Evidence for chronic facial pain
Cognitive therapy	Strong	Minimal
Operant behaviour therapy	Strong	Minimal
Relaxation training	Strong	Moderate
Graded exercise	Strong	Non-existent
Pacing	Minimal	Non-existent
Supportive group	Moderate	Moderate
Hypnosis	Moderate	Moderate
EMG biofeedback	Strong	Strong

of the cognitive behavioural treatments and none of the studies explicitly included chronic facial pain patients.

It can be seen from Table 5 that the evidence to support psychological pain management strategies for chronic pain generally is strong, but there has been limited application of these techniques for chronic facial pain.

11. Clinician factors: the 'non-specific effects'

The risk in detailing a host of specific treatment strategies and summarising their known efficacy is that the importance of the interaction between clinician and patient can be overlooked. This issue is discussed in some detail in Chapter 9, however the message underpinning much of the health services research is: "the way in which you deliver the treatment is as important as the treatment itself".

Gracely (2000) summarises a large literature on this subject, and arrives at the conclusion that the behaviour of the clinician alone is sufficient to evoke responses that can result in therapeutic success. The therapeutic success is independent of the treatment being instigated. While this may be somewhat startling, there are several caveats which put this into perspective. Firstly, it does not mean that certain doctors have mystical powers by which they can manipulate patients into 'feeling' that they are well when they are not. Nor does it mean that only highly charismatic practitioners are capable of exerting this influence on patients. This literature does, however, refer to the active and deliberate use of basic principles of human interaction in order to maximise the likelihood of a positive outcome from treatment. For example, Gracely (2000) cites several studies in which a brief preoperative discussion with patients, and an equally brief post-surgical interaction between surgeon and patient, resulted in massive reductions in opiate usage when compared to control patient groups who did not 'chat with the doctor' before and after their operation.

Consistent with the notion that good communication and genuine empathy will enhance your treatment effectiveness is the view that the assessment should be conceptualised as an important part of the treatment process. As Price (2000) has cogently argued, the assessment is far more important than just being a data-gathering exercise that is seen as being separate from the delivery of the treatment. From the first patient contact, the way in which you ask questions and the way in which you respond to the replies will establish whether your intervention is going to be more or less effective. A friendly, warm approach, genuine concern, active listening (following up on patient statements to indicate that you have listened and understood, such as "That must have been difficult. What did you do then?" or "What did you think was happening at the time?") and humour when it is appropriate will all convey these important apparently non-specific factors.

12. Conclusion

It has been suggested in this chapter that although psychological factors have been acknowledged as an intrinsic part of the pain experience since ancient times, their role has been often been misconstrued. The false dichotomy between physical and psychological domains that was established in early theories of pain has persisted in many ways until the present day, in both medical and lay circles. And yet, there is a large body of evidence which clearly shows that mind and body are not independently functioning entities, but closely interrelated in all aspects of pain detection, transmission and perception. Cognition, affect and behaviour are known to share a reciprocal relationship with noxious stimuli, in such a way that each exerts some influence upon the other. This was seen to be the case when discussing examples of acute pain, both laboratory based and naturally occurring, in relation to the transition of acute injury to chronic pain disorder, and in relation to the management of chronic pain itself. In each facet of pain, psychological variables were found to be salient.

It is hoped that you now have some appreciation of the diversity of factors which influence the perception and experience of pain. For those unfortunate patients whose pain is not successfully treated by the various pain-relieving approaches, there are now a range of psychologically based interventions which are demonstrably useful in reducing the suffering which is at the core of chronic pain states.

13. Summary

See Table 6 for a summary of this chapter.

Appendix A. Strategies for coping with pain

These strategies are taken from the Trigeminal Neuralgia Association UK Newsletter of June, 2002.

At the risk of stating the obvious, coping with pain — and in particular, trigeminal neuralgia pain

TABLE 6

Summary of Chapter 3

This chapter has attempted to highlight the following:

1. All pains (acute or chronic) represent an interaction of both physical and psychological processes. Notions of 'physical pain' and 'psychogenic pain' are a false dichotomy, and should be abandoned

2. Cultural factors, emotional states, past experiences of pain, and current beliefs and expectations about pain all strongly influence how pain is experienced and responded to

3. Psychological factors tend to be stronger predictors of the development of chronic pain than physical findings

4. Chronic pain management is a multidisciplinary intervention involving physical therapy, cognitive therapy, relaxation training and other coping skill techniques

5. The available evidence supports the use of cognitive behavioural therapy for chronic pain in general, but there is little specific application of these techniques to chronic facial pain

6. Clinicians should be aware of the importance of the relationship that they develop with their patients, as evidence indicates that such 'non-specific factors' contribute substantially to the outcome of treatment

— is one of the more difficult tasks in life. Pain is often conceptualised as a 'warning signal', alerting us to the fact that there is something wrong in our bodies. Severe pain therefore is an alert of something very wrong, which needs urgent attention in order to be put right. This is of some value when the pain is telling us we have broken a limb, or have a appendicitis, or are about to give birth. We have some idea of how to use the information that the pain is giving us in these situations — we know what to do, or at least what we should be doing.

Chronic neuropathic pains such as TN defy such rational explanations — what is the pain telling us to do in these cases? This urgent, insistent message from our bodies alerting us to the fact that something is very wrong does not convey the same information about how to respond. After all, other than taking medication, there does not appear to be very much that we can do to stop the pain. One of the most upsetting aspects of chronic pain can be the sense of helplessness that accompanies it. You feel as though you must do something to make it better, but there is no obvious resolution to the pain that you can apply.

Pain psychologists and physicians have put together a list of potential 'coping strategies' for managing these flare-ups of pain. The value of these strategies lies mainly in how realistically they are used. The first thing to remember is this: once your pain has flared-up, it is virtually impossible to shut it down rapidly (unless you get good relief from your pain medications). Although it is quite natural to want the pain to stop immediately, when it does not stop you can feel even more distressed and panicky. So, it is perhaps better to change your expectations from the outset.

One of the ways in which you might think about changing your approach to the pain is to think of a flare-up of pain not as a disaster, but as a challenge. How are you going to respond to this — with an increase in anxiety and frustration and distress, which will inevitably worsen the pain; or with as much calmness and rational thought as you can muster? Coping well with a flare-up of pain is a bit like riding a wave: you cannot stop it, but you can stay on your feet and flow along with it until it eventually subsides (which it *always* does, even though it often does not feel like it at the time!).

Having made a decision that this flare-up is a challenge that you are going to attempt to meet, the following strategies can be useful. They are not presented in any particular order, you can try them in any sequence that you like. The main idea is to keep yourself occupied by moving from one strategy to another, alternating between rest and activity. You need to be aware that overdoing things when you are in pain is tiring, and will reduce your resources for coping, whereas doing very little at these times will not leave your brain sufficiently distracted and you become at risk of focusing more on your discomfort.

Try out the following ideas for coping with flare-ups of pain:

- Do not panic: try to think of the pain as a challenge, and you are going to experiment with different ways of coping with it.
- Prioritise: coping with this pain is going to mean that you do not necessarily do all the things that you were planning to do in the next hour or two (or even longer). What can you leave until later, or ask someone else to do, or cancel completely? For example, is it really so important that you do the vacuuming today, or can it wait until tomorrow?
- Communication: although coping with pain is a personal event, it may be useful to let those close to you know what is happening at this time. This is especially important if you prefer to be alone, or if you tend to become quieter so that you can concentrate on dealing with the pain. It is easy to misinterpret someone leaving the room or 'going quiet' — family members will often think they have done something to upset you. Communicating about pain does not mean endlessly complaining about it: something like this can be useful — "Listen, I am just going upstairs to manage this pain for an hour. You (husband, wife, kids) keep doing what you are doing, I am OK but I just need to concentrate on this for a bit. I'll ask you if I need any help".
- Relaxation (5–10 min): doing some deep, controlled breathing can help to keep you feeling reasonably calm and in control. There are many techniques for relaxation, from yoga to meditation to hypnosis. They all share a common element, which is that you are doing something quite active even though you may not be moving at all. Relaxation is not the same as doing nothing, you do have to concentrate. But be realistic — being in pain is about the least 'relaxing' state you can be in, and very few people are able to drift off into a completely comfortable state. Whenever the pain intrudes on your thoughts, just gently bring your mind back to your controlled, regular breathing. Your aim is to try and keep as calm as possible, rather than to go to sleep. Sleeping during the day

can seriously interfere with your sleep at night, and that can compound the situation.

- Light activity (10–15 min): even though you are in pain, you should still attempt to do some non-vigorous activity. Things like watering the plants, paying a bill, simple cooking, polishing shoes, gentle ironing, and so on. The activities must be physically and mentally undemanding, and you should not attempt to do them for any longer than about 15 min. However, you will discover that even when in a bad way with the pain, you can still achieve things that need doing — and that can bring some satisfaction.

- Rest (any time up to 20 min): this is complete time out, where you do not need to concentrate on anything other than giving your body a chance to recoup some energy. You might lie down on the bed or floor, or sit in a comfortable chair. Having a cup of tea, listening to music or watching TV can all be restful activities, but remember not to 'do nothing' for too long because the pain will begin to dominate your thinking if you are not sufficiently distracted.

- Gentle stretching (10–15 min): pain can often result in increased muscle tension, which will then make the pain worse. Simple, gentle stretching of the neck, upper back, shoulders, arms and lower back can all help to keep you from getting too tight during a flare-up. Going for a slow, gentle walk can also be helpful. As long as you do the stretches slowly and gently, and do not try to overstretch, you will not do yourself any harm.

- Distraction (5–10 min): all of the activities above have a distracting element to them, but you might also try and divert your mind away from the pain as an activity in itself. Distraction requires concentration, so think of an activity that you get really absorbed in such as sewing, or model making, or painting. Have these activities at the ready, so that you can just pick them up when the flare-up requires them. Talking to someone can also be excellent distraction — provided that you do not talk too much about the pain! You might say: "Hi, I am in a pain flare-up at the moment. No need to worry, I'm OK, but I need you to take my mind off it for a while. Tell me what you did today/movie you saw recently/holiday you are next going on etc.". Try and involve yourself in the conversation as much as possible.

- Reflection and reinforcer: once you have got through the flare-up, having tried out these various strategies, have a think about how it went. Did the pain last as long as it usually does? Did you feel more in control of the pain? Were you still able to achieve a few things, even though you were in pain? Is there anything that you could do differently next time — change the order in which you do things, do certain activities for longer or shorter, get partner/friend involved more? Whatever you decide, it is very important that you give yourself a 'reinforcer' for having tried to cope with the pain in this way. A reinforcer is a small treat that you give yourself for your own hard work in coping with pain, such as a magazine, pot plant, makeup, special food (chocolate is often used!) or video. It is a small pat on the back that you give yourself for your efforts, because only you really know how tough it is to cope with the pain.

This is a brief run through of different ways in which you might cope with a flare-up of pain. It is by no means an exhaustive list and there are no absolute rules, so be creative and experiment with different ideas. Each flare-up gives you the opportunity of learning something more about the pain, and something more about your capacity to cope with it, so good luck!

Appendix B

The answer to the case study shown in Table 4 is given in Table 7.

TABLE 7

Answer to case study: pain management intervention

Assessment	Explanation of gate control model, and the role of psychological factors in pain. Identification of treatment goals: reduce pain medication, increase functional activity (specifically return to work, socialising with friends, exercise), decrease distress around pain.
Sessions 1–4	Begin on gentle stretch programme for upper back, shoulders, neck and jaws. Once per day, 15–20 min only. Begin pacing programme, starting with walking outside. Introduction to cognitive therapy principles. Begin relaxation training, twice per day 15 min only. Begin reducing antidepressant — patient's choice as side effects outweighing benefit.
Sessions 5–10	Continuing stretch programme and twice daily relaxation practise. Increase tolerance for walking. Consolidating cognitive therapy skills — increasing ability to challenge catastrophic thoughts about pain. Communication skills training regarding explaining pain to others, advising husband regarding supportive responses to pain behaviours. Begin reducing benzodiazepine.
Sessions 11–16	Continuing stretch programme, reduce relaxation practise to once daily. Begin gentle swimming once per week, 20 min only. Walking tolerance extended to lunch in local restaurant and brief dinner with friends, using communication skills discussed previously. Further cognitive therapy, husband attending session to discuss delivery of appropriate support. Begin reducing analgesic.
Sessions 17–23	Continuing stretch programme, change from swimming to gentle jogging as preferred exercise. Three times per week, 20 min only. Begin return to work programme, initially 1 day per week. Begin driving independently to shopping centre. Continued cognitive therapy, specifically targeting relapse prevention issues.
Three month follow-up	By this point, Mrs. L. had made a return to work on a 3-day per week basis and was managing this successfully. She had been on a short holiday with her husband, the first in nearly 2 years. She had stopped all her medication other than the occasional co-proxamol as part of her management of pain flare-ups.
	Mrs. L. made significant progress over the course of this intervention, despite the ongoing presence of her facial pain. This is not to suggest that progress was smooth and linear; on the contrary, there was a period around session 16 where she was unable to increase her activity levels because of pain and became despondent about her ability to regain a semblance of normal life. By accepting and validating her concerns, rather than becoming equally annoyed with her slowness of progress, we were able to problem-solve ways in which she might overcome her sense of inertia. It was decided to change her exercise routine, help her to apply the cognitive therapy strategies more frequently, and spend more time working on improving her communication with her husband when in pain. These strategic moves allowed to regain her momentum in treatment.
	Mrs. L. completed treatment with an expectation that her facial pain may always be a part of her life. But by following the guidelines described above, she was able to accept responsibility for making changes in her management of the pain. Rather than continuing to seek further medical or dental care for the problem ('doctor shopping'), she recognised that she needed to take a different stance. Over a period of time, she systematically increased her exercise and movement as well as increased her sense of control over her emotional response to the pain. By including her husband in the intervention, they were able to develop better communication skills and overcome the potential difficulty of the partner inadvertently making the situation worse by being overprotective.

Appendix C. Further reading on the psychology of pain

(1) Gamsa A. The role of psychological factors in chronic pain. I. A half century of study. Pain, 1994a; 57: 5—15.

(2) Gamsa A. The role of psychological factors in chronic pain. II. A critical appraisal. Pain, 1994b; 57: 17—29.

(3) Gatchel RJ, Turk DC. Psychological Approaches to Pain Management: A Practitioner's Handbook. Guilford Press, New York, 1996.

(4) Hanson RW, Gerber KE. Coping With Chronic Pain: A Guide to Patient Self-Management. Guilford Press, New York, 1990.

(5) Skevington SM. Psychology of Pain. John Wiley and Sons, Chichester, 1995.

References

Marked as regards quality according to criteria set by author.

SR = systematic review or high quality review with methodology.

*Poorer quality studies but only ones in the field, old style reviews.

***Randomised controlled trials, high quality original studies.

Banks SM, Kerns RD. Explaining high rates of depression in chronic pain: a diathesis-stress framework. Psychol Bull 1996; 119: 95–110.

Calvillo ER, Flaskerud JH. Review of literature on culture and pain of adults with focus on Mexican Americans. J Transcult Nurs 1991; 2: 81–91.

SR Crider AB, Glaros AG. A meta-analysis of EMG biofeedback treatment of temporomandibular disorders. J Orofac Pain 1999; 13: 29–37.

***Croft PR, Macfarlane GJ, Papageorgiou AC, Thomas E, Silman AJ. Outcome of low back pain in general practice: a prospective study. Br Med J 1998; 316: 1356–1359.

Curry PD, Pacsoo C, Heap DG. Patient controlled epidural analgesia in obstetric anaesthetic practice. Pain 1994; 57: 125–128.

Dahlstrom L, Widmark G, Carlsson SG. Cognitive-behavioral profiles among different categories of orofacial pain patients: diagnostic and treatment implications. Eur J Oral Sci 1997; 105: 377–383.

*Di Fabio RP. Physical therapy for patients with TMD: a descriptive study of treatment, disability, and health status. J Orofac Pain 1998; 12: 124–135.

Eimer BN. Clinical applications of hypnosis for brief and efficient pain management psychotherapy. Am J Clin Hypn 2000; 43: 17–40.

***Epker J, Gatchel RJ. Prediction of treatment-seeking behavior in acute TMD patients: practical application in clinical settings. J Orofac Pain 2000; 14: 303–309.

***Epker J, Gatchel RJ, Ellis E. A model for predicting chronic TMD: practical application in clinical settings. J Am Dent Assoc 1999; 130: 1470–1475.

Fillingam RB, Edwards RR, Powell, T. Sex-dependent effects of reported familial pain history on recent pain complaints and experimental pain responses. Pain 2000; 86: 87–94.

***Frost H, Lamb SE, Klaber Moffett JA, Fairbank JC, Moser JS. A fitness programme for patients with chronic low back pain: 2-year follow-up of a randomised controlled trial. Pain 1998; 75: 273–279.

Gamsa A. The role of psychological factors in chronic pain. I. A half century of study. Pain 1994a; 57: 5–15.

Gamsa A. The role of psychological factors in chronic pain. II. A critical appraisal. Pain 1994b; 57: 17–29.

Gatchel RJ, Turk DC. Psychological Approaches to Pain Management: A Practitioner's Handbook. Guilford Press, New York, 1996.

Gracely R. Charisma and the art of healing: can nonspecific factors be enough? In: Devor M, Rowbotham M, Wiesenfeld-Hallin Z (eds) Proceedings of the 9th World Congress on Pain. Progress in Pain Research and Management. IASP Press, Seattle, WA, 2000: 1045–1067.

Gray RJ, Davies SJ. Emergency treatment of acute temporomandibular disorders: Part 1. Dental Update 1997; 24: 170–173.

Hanson RW, Gerber KE. Coping With Chronic Pain: A Guide to Patient Self-Management. Guilford Press, New York, 1990.

International Association for the Study of Pain. Pain terms: a list with definitions and notes on usage. Pain 1979; 6: 249.

***Jensen MP, Turner JA, Romano JM. Changes in beliefs, catastrophizing, and coping are associated with improvement in multidisciplinary pain treatment. J Consult Clin Psychol 2001; 69: 655–662.

***Keefe FJ, Caldwell DS, Baucom DH, Salley A, Robinson E, Timmons K, Beaupre P, Weisberg J, Kelms M. Spouse-assisted coping skills training in the management of osteoarthritic knee pain. Arthr Care Res 1996; 9: 279–291.

***King M, Davidson O, Taylor F, Haines A, Sharp D, Turner R. Effectiveness of teaching general practitioners skills in brief cognitive behaviour therapy to treat patients with depression: randomised controlled trial. Br Med J 2002; 324: 947–950.

***Klenerman L, Slade P, Stanley IM, Pennie B, Reilly JP, Atchison LE. The prediction of chronicity in patients with an acute attack of low back pain in a General Practice setting. Spine 1995; 20: 478–484.

***Levine FM, De Simone LL. The effects of experimenter gender on pain report in male and female subjects. Pain 1991; 44: 69–72.

Madland G, Feinmann C, Newman S. Factors associated with anxiety and depression in facial arthromyalgia. Pain 2000; 84: 225–232.

Manaidakis N, Gray A. The economic burden of back pain in the UK. Pain 2000; 84: 95–103.

McCraken LM, Zayfert C, Gross RT. The Pain Anxiety Symptoms Scale: development and validation of a scale to measure fear of pain. Pain 1992; 50: 67–73.

Melzack R, Wall PD. Pain mechanisms: a new theory. Science 1965; 150: 971–979.

Melzack R, Wall PD. The Challenge of Pain, 2nd edn. Penguin, Harmondsworth, 1988.

Molin C. From bite to mind: TMD — a personal and literature review. Int J Prosthodont 1999; 12: 279–288.

SR Morley S, Eccleston C, Williams, ACdeC. Systematic review and meta-analysis of randomized controlled trials of cognitive behaviour therapy and behaviour therapy for chronic pain in adults, excluding headache. Pain 1999; 80: 1–13.

Naini FB, Mellor AC, Getz T. Treatment of dental fears: pharmacology or psychology? Dental Update 1999; September: 270–276.

Newton-John TRO, Williams ACdeC. Solicitousness revisited: a qualitative analysis of patient–spouse interactions in chronic pain. In: Devor M, Rowbotham M, Wiesenfeld-Hallin Z (eds) Proceedings of the 9th World Congress on Pain. Progress in Pain Research and Management. IASP Press, Seattle, WA, 2000: 1113–1122.

*** Newton-John TRO, Spence SH, Schotte D. Cognitive–behavioural therapy versus EMG biofeedback in the treatment of chronic low back pain. Behav Res Ther 1995; 33: 691–697.

Osborne RB, Hatcher JW, Richtsmeier AJ. The role of social modeling in unexplained pediatric pain. J Pediatr Psych 1989; 14: 43–61.

Overmier JB, LoLordo VM. Learned helplessness. In: William T (ed) Learning and Behavior Therapy. Allyn and Bacon, Needham Heights, MA, 1998: 352–373.

Patel B, Potter C, Mellor AC. The use of hypnosis in dentistry: a review. Dental Update 2000; 27: 198–202.

Price JR. Managing physical symptoms: the clinical assessment as treatment. J Psychosom Res 2000; 48: 1–10.

Protas EJ. Physical activity and low back pain. In: Max M (ed) Pain 1999 — An Updated Review. IASP Press, Seattle, WA, 1999: 145–152.

Raphael KG, Marbach JJ, Gallagher RM, Dohrenwend BP. Myofascial TMD does not run in families. Pain 1999; 80: 15–22.

Reid J, Ewan C, Lowy E. Pilgrimage of pain: the illness experiences of women with repetitive strain injury and the search for credibility. Soc Sci Med 1991; 32: 601–612.

Reilly PA. Repetitive strain injury: from Australia to the UK. J Psychosom Res 1995; 39: 783–788.

Robinson ME, Wise E, Riley J, Atchison JW. Sex differences in clinical pain: a multisample study. J Clin Psychol Med Sett 1998; 5: 413–424.

Rollman GB. Culture and pain. In: Kazarian J, Evans P (eds) Cultural Clinical Psychology. Oxford University Press, Oxford, 1998: 267–286.

Schwartz L, Ehde DM. Couples and chronic pain. In: Schmaling K, Goldman Sher T (eds) The Psychology of Couples and Illness. American Psychological Association, Washington, DC, 2000: 191–216.

Simon EP, Lewis DM. Medical hypnosis for temporomandibular disorders: treatment efficacy and medical utilization outcome. Oral Surg Oral Med Oral Pathol Oral Radiol Endodont 2000; 90: 54–63.

Skevington SM. Psychology of Pain. John Wiley and Sons, Chichester, 1995.

*** Stengrevics S, Sirois C, Schwartz CE, Friedman, R. The prediction of cardiac surgery outcome based upon preoperative psychological factors. Psychol Health 1996; 11: 471–477.

Stewart DE, Reicher AE, Gerulath AH, Boydell KM. Vulvodynia and psychological distress. Obstet Gynecol 1994; 84: 587–590.

Sullivan MJ, Thorn B, Haythornthwaite J, Keefe FJ, Martin M, Bradley L, Lefebvre JC. Theoretical perspectives on the relation between catastrophizing and pain. Clin J Pain 2001; 17: 52–64.

*** Thomas E, Silman AJ, Croft P, Papageorgiou AC, Jayson MIV, McFarlane GJ. Predicting who develops chronic low back pain in primary care: a prospective study. Br Med J 1999; 318: 1662–1667.

Turk DC. The role of demographic and psychosocial factors in transition from acute to chronic pain. In: Jensen TS, Turner JA, Wiesenfeld-Hallin Z (eds) Proceedings of the 8th World Congress on Pain. IASP Press, Seattle, WA, 1997: 185–213.

Turk DC, Meichenbaum D. A cognitive–behavioural approach to pain management. In: Wall PD, Melzack RM (eds) Textbook of Pain, 3rd edn. Churchill Livingstone, Edinburgh, 1994: 1337–1348.

Turk DC, Rudyy TE, Flor H. Why a family perspective for pain? Int J Fam Ther 1985; 7: 223–234.

Unruh A. Review Article: Gender variations in clinical pain experience. Pain 1996; 65: 123–167.

Williams ACdeC. Depression in chronic pain: mistaken models, missed opportunities. Scand J Behav Ther 1998; 27: 61–80.

Williams ACdeC, Erskine, A. Chronic pain. In: Broome A, Llewelyn S (eds) Health Psychology: Processes and Applications. Chapman and Hall, London, 1995: 353–376.

*** Yuasa H, Kurita K. Randomized clinical trial of primary treatment for temporomandibular joint disk displacement without reduction and without osseous changes: a combination of NSAIDs and mouth-opening exercise versus no treatment. Oral Surg Oral Med Oral Pathol Oral Radiol Endodont. 2001; 91: 671–675.

Ziegler DK. Headache: public health problem. Neurol Clin 1990; 8: 781–791.

Assessment and Management of Orofacial Pain
Pain Research and Clinical Management, Vol. 14
Edited by J.M. Zakrzewska and S.D. Harrison
© *2002 Elsevier Science B.V. All rights reserved*

CHAPTER 4

History taking

Joanna M. Zakrzewska [*]

Department of Clinical and Diagnostic Oral Sciences, Oral Medicine Unit, Dental Institute, Barts and the London Queen Mary's School of Medicine and Dentistry, Turner Street, London E1 2AD, UK

Objectives for this chapter:

This chapter will attempt to:
- Illustrate the vital importance of a thorough history in patients with pain
- Highlight the communication skills required to take an adequate history
- Stress the various elements of the history that need to be included in all patients with facial pain
- Provide key questions that may be diagnostically useful
- Provide key details on how to take a psychiatric history
- Illustrate the need for a psychosocial assessment including quality of life issues and health beliefs
- Provide some pointers on transcultural history taking
- Stress the role of history taking in the overall management of patients with chronic facial pain

1. Introduction

A history is essential for determining the severity of the symptoms, the diagnosis and the prognosis of a condition as well as in monitoring the symptoms over time. A thorough history enables the clinician to tailor the investigations more accurately, interpret results with increased precision and so lead to potential cost savings (McAlister et al., 1999).

There are many instances especially in primary care where the greatest contribution to the making of a medical diagnosis is the history (over 82%) with physical examination and investigations contributing 9% each (Hampton et al., 1975). Clinicians' confidence, however, in making the diagnosis is markedly increased after completion of examination and investigations even though these contribute relatively few new facts (Peterson et al., 1992; Roshan and Rao, 2000). The increased emphasis of medical technology in diagnosis has shifted interest from the bedside and in some areas the history has come to play a much lower role in the whole diagnostic process. Sandler (1984) showed that he could diagnose 69% of cardiovascular problems but only 29% of gastrointestinal problems from the history. The increasing number of diagnostic tests with high specificity and sensitivity has also diverted attention from careful history taking. Unfortunately, there are relatively few studies that have assessed the importance of clinical manifestations in the making of a differential diagnosis and checked their validity (McAlister et al., 1999). In the field of facial pain, history taking continues to make a large contribution to the diagnosis, as there are few objective signs and investigations to

[*] Tel.: +44-20-7377-7053; Fax: +44-20-7377-7627;
E-mail j.m.zakrzewska@qmul.ac.uk

TABLE 1

KEY FACTS: evidenced-based approach to history taking

Patient/problem	In patients with ...
Intervention	Do specific questions in the history or specific examination findings
Comparison /intervention	Do better than a standard dental or medical history or examination
Outcomes	To increase the likelihood of a correct diagnosis?

aid in the diagnosis or to judge the severity of the symptoms. Hampton et al. (1975) argue that extra time spent on history taking is more profitable than time spent on examination. For the history to be of value in making an accurate diagnosis it is essential to know how relevant each piece of information is to the process and how reliable it is.

The evidence-based approach to taking a history and evaluating its usefulness involves the use of a PICO (see Table 1 key facts and Chapter 1 for an explanation).

This approach has been reported with regard to taking a history of trigeminal neuralgia (Drangsholt and Truelove, 2001). Despite our apparent assumption that the diagnostic criteria of this condition are clear, the use of this approach revealed a deficiency. The level of evidence is low, based on case series or simulated cross sectional studies and not on case control studies. This question could be asked for each of the conditions that we will describe in subsequent chapters and we challenge you, the reader, to develop some of these by becoming involved in the CARE project which aims to improve clinicians' skills by the use of internet reporting of data (McAlister et al., 1999) *http://www.carestudy.com*. It is important, however, for you to remember that pain, as compared to other conditions does not and never will conform to the biomedical model of disease as it is inseparable from personal perception and social influences and hence will never be measured totally objectively. Even though you may be able to make

an accurate diagnosis the same diagnosis may have widely differing effects on different patients. It is this aspect that will often affect management.

2. Communication skills

Pain is a subjective symptom and is reported by patients in a wide range of ways both in terms of its physical and psychosocial effects. It remains an inner experience that cannot be totally shared with anyone. Patients with facial pain who come to the secondary care sector often feel that they are disbelieved and misunderstood both by the medical profession and also by their family and friends. This can make history taking even more difficult and time needs to be spent listening to the patients in order to elicit all relevant data and then educating them. Your communication skills may be tested to the full with certain types of patients, e.g. hysterical, obsessive–compulsive, paranoid, narcissistic, dependant, impulsive. Craig and Boardman (1997) suggest that doctors with good interviewing skills are much more likely to identify a mental health problem than a doctor who suppresses the patient's expressions of emotion. Remember that communication occurs at several levels:

- linguistic
- grammatical
- gestural
- postural
- attitudinal
- conceptual

Bird and Cohen-Cole (1990) writing in a book on 'Methods in teaching consultation–liaison psychiatry' provide evidence that physicians communication skills are poor and they therefore fail to elicit an adequate history. They suggest that training is essential and involves not just ensuring that the physicians know how to take a history but that they need to change their attitudes and beliefs in order to effect a permanent behavioural change. There is now a considerable body of material on this topic and a few references are provided at the end of the chapter.

TABLE 2

KEY FACTS: communications with patients are improved if

- Patients are allowed to express their major concerns without interruption

- Patients' specific requests are sought, e.g how do you hope I might be able to help you? This can be very different from the presenting complaint

- Patients' explanations of their illnesses are elicited

- Facilitation of patients' emotions is encouraged

- Patients are given information

- Patients are involved in developing treatment plans

TABLE 3

Case study 1

If you are to improve patient disclosure and develop a personal partnership with your patient you need to have a personal approach to history taking. List the factors that could help you achieve this goal.

What questioning techniques would you employ to increase the quality and quantity of the data you collect from a patient with chronic facial pain?

Please see Table 15 at the end of the chapter for the answers.

There are also a considerable number of books on communication skills and breaking bad news, some of which provide you with exercises to improve your skills. Courses may also be of benefit and you can attend e.g. Medical Interview Teaching Association courses held in the UK which enable you to practise these skills in a safe environment with actors (Bird et al., 1993). Communication skills can be taught (Maguire, 1990) and teaching these skills has now become an essential element of undergraduate curricula (Davis and Nicholaou, 1992; Novack et al., 1992; Miall and Davies, 1992) as it results in marked improvement in several areas (Table 2 key facts).

It is therefore essential when you take a pain history to place special emphasis on communication skills. You should respond to mood cues and explore mood. If you listen carefully your patient will come to trust you and this will improve disclosure and subsequent adherence to treatment. Remember that listening is doing something, it is not a passive activity. Resist the temptation to interrupt the patient at the start of the history taking as you will decrease both the satisfaction and efficacy of the consultation. This general discussion of the patient's main concerns at the beginning may take only 2.5 min although on average only 90 s are needed (Simpson et al., 1991, Blau, 1989). Interestingly research on communication tells us that we tend to interrupt patients within a few seconds. Marvel et al. (2000) have shown that physicians redirect a patient's statement in a mean of 23.1 s and yet patients who are allowed to complete only take a further 6 s on average to finish. Another study (Beckman and Frankel, 1984) showed that in 74 consultations only 17 (23%) of patients were allowed to complete their opening statement. Try it yourself. Ask a colleague/nurse to time the period between the patient beginning his/her history and your first interruption. Remember that you can show the patient that you are actively listening, not only by your words and use of silence, but also by your non-verbal behaviour. Putting away papers or writing in notes will not give the patient the message that you are listening. You need to listen at a variety of levels, which will include noting not only the words but also aspects such as the choice of words, the syntax, the tense, the affective expression, the missing information and the non-verbal behaviour. When patients use technical words such as depression, neuralgia check that their meaning is the same as yours.

We will now briefly look at ways of improving our communication skills and you may like to start with the exercise in Table 3 case study 1, to assess how you may develop a positive partnership with your patient.

2.1. Positive partnership

If you establish a positive partnership with your patient you will find your patient will be more co-operative, satisfied and trusting. To achieve this you must be empathic and take a personal approach to the collection of data for diagnosis, taking a history is an interview not an interrogation.

Bird and Cohen-Cole (1990) suggest the following strategies for establishing this:

- **Presentation**: create the right environment, introduce yourself with a handshake, make the patient feel comfortable both physically and psychologically, e.g. *"How was your journey here"*, *I hope all is well with you"* ensure the patient knows that you will safeguard their confidentiality, give them the impression that you have plenty of time or tell them up front how much time you have, prevent interruptions, explain the role/purpose of the meeting
- **Empathy**: patients need to feel that you understand them and that you too have emotions, *"I can see how distressing this is to you"*, *"I have felt like this sometimes"*
- **Respect** your patient's behaviour: *"I can see that you have been doing your best to cope"*
- **Support** the patient's emotions, feelings: *"Let us talk about ways we could help you to cope"*
- **Organise** your time and agenda: *"we may have to discuss some of these issues another time"*
- **Non-judgmental** — you need to accept the person not necessarily the behaviour, remain neutral: *"I am trying to understand you"*, beware of your non-verbal behaviour
- **Alliance and partnership** you need to ensure that it occurs on an equal basis: *"Let us try and do this together"*
- **Leave taking** ensure that you make it clear that there is a commitment on both sides to further management: *"It has been good to talk. Let us arrange another time to meet"*

2.2. Data collection

The data you collect needs to be comprehensive, reliable and relevant to the problem being explored. Try to create a narrative thread and organise the patient's story by asking questions such as *"when did you last have no pain"*, or*"how has the pain changed over the months?"* All patients know how stories are organised and so will naturally fall into this pattern. You may, however need to train the patient to give you precise details so that they know what level of information you need. *"Tell me precisely how long each pain episode lasts?"* is a crucial detail you need to elicit when trying to establish a diagnosis of trigeminal neuralgia. If the narrative is flowing well you can then digress from the path at times but have a way of returning to the story which both of you know. Using exploratory questioning will enable you to supplement the patient's narrative and ensure that you have collected all the required data. Examples of questions and comments that are likely to yield good quality information include:

- Simple questions: *"Tell me what is troubling you"*
- Open questions: *"What happened to you next?"* *"How was that for you?"*
- Unbiased questions: *"What effects good or bad did the medicine have?"*
- Responsive questions: *"You mentioned your toothache let's hear more about that"*
- Clarification: *"Tell me what you mean by neuralgia"*
- Encouragement: *"This is very helpful information, tell me more"*
- Summarising: *"Let's go over the main points again so we can be sure we've got it straight"*

The last phase of the consultation is educating and managing the patient and will be discussed in Chapter 9 on management.

3. The general medico-dental and pain history

A wide range of material needs to be collected and this is summarised in Table 4 key facts.

Before you move on to the next section, you may like to try the exercise in Table 5 case study 2 to see if you can pick up key pain features.

TABLE 4

KEY FACTS: the history should include the following areas

- General pain history
- Specific pain history and review of facial structures
- Medical and dental history including review of systems and drug history
- Short psychiatric history
- Social and family histories
- Quality of life including effect of pain on their environment
- Health beliefs and expectations

TABLE 5

Case study 2

Mrs. Daly has had pain in her left jaw joint for 6 months. It was initially localized to the left pre-auricular area but is now also felt in the post-auricular area and may radiate up into the left temporal region. It has gradually become more severe and now measures 7 out of 10 on a scale of 1–10. Mrs. Daly describes the pain as being a dull, aching pain with some sharp exacerbations which is present continuously but often becomes worse in the afternoon. Eating hard foods makes it worse, whereas warming the area gives her relief. When she opens her mouth wide she hears a click in her joint and thinks that she cannot open her mouth as wide as previously.

Under what generic headings would you describe her pain which would be useful to use whenever you take a pain history.

Please see Table 16 at the end of the chapter for the answer.

TABLE 6

KEY FACTS: the following pain details need to be ascertained

Character of the pain	What sort of a pain is it?
Duration/onset time	When did it start, did it start suddenly?
Periodicity	Is there a pattern to the pain?
Severity	How severe is the pain, how does it vary?
Site	Where do you feel the pain?
Radiation	Where does the pain spread?
Provoking factors	Does anything make the pain worse?
Relieving factors	Does anything make the pain better?
Associated factors	Do you notice anything thing else when you have pain?

or facial pain history which you may find useful. You should also use more objective measures of pain, which are described in Chapter 6 on measurements.

Woolf and Mannion (1999) suggest that the mechanism by which the symptoms are produced is more important than the symptom itself when it comes to treatment. This means particular care needs to be taken to elicit which types of stimuli induce the pain — noxious or non-noxious such as mechanical, thermal or chemical. Mechanical hyperalgesia can be further divided into brush evoked/pressure or punctate evoked. These can help to differentiate trigeminal neuralgia from post-herpetic neuralgia.

3.2. What specific facial pain data to collect

In order to improve the specificity and sensitivity of the history as a diagnostic tool you need to ascertain more specific symptoms in relation to certain anatomical structures found in the mouth or around the face. Ideally, you should ask all the questions but

3.1. General pain history

You need to supplement the standard medical history with a pain history as suggested by Ryle (1936) in 1936 and summarised in Table 6 key facts. Blau (1982) has also suggested schemata for taking a head

the patient's description of the complaint may lead you to concentrate on more specific questions which have a high diagnostic yield, for example if a patient gives you a history suggestive of a cluster headache it is important to ask about tearing of the eye, but this will be less important if a patient describes a pain in a lower molar tooth. The value of each symptom or group of symptoms in all conditions causing facial pain have not yet been determined. An example of how useful this approach can be is shown in the diagnosis of maxillary sinusitis where it is argued that the medical history and examination is 92% diagnostic and that other investigations should be reserved for special circumstances (Chodosh, 1999). The challenge to do this is open to you! Join the CARE group.

You may also like to join some national audit group which is collecting data. One such group is the patient audit collection system, a voluntary database that clinicians can join through the UK Pain Society special interest group, *http://www.painsociety. org/sig_clinical_info.html*. The following is an extract from the site which sets out the aims and objectives of the group:

- To promote the collection of clinical information in chronic pain management for the purpose of audit, research and resource management.
- To provide reliable information to facilitate the measurement of clinical effectiveness and the assessment of chronic pain services.
- To promote regional and national audit and research in chronic pain relief.
- To establish agreed clinical terms and common datasets.
- To establish links with other speciality groups with similar interests.
- To facilitate the collection of data, the Pain Audit Collection System (PACS) database has been designed and has been distributed free of charge to many pain clinics throughout the UK.

The PACS system is sponsored by an unrestricted educational grant from Pharmacia Ltd. This is also discussed in Chapter 6.

The following is a list of questions that may be asked.

3.2.1. Eyes

- Do you have any visual disturbances either before, during or after a pain episode?
- Do you ever see double images?
- Do your eyes appear red at any time?
- Do you notice increased or decreased tearing at any time?
- Do your eyes feel dry, sandy or gritty?
- Do you notice any swelling of the eye?
- Do you feel any pain deep inside the eye?
- Have you noticed any impairment in your visual acuity?
- Do you notice floaters in your field of vision?
- Do you avoid bright lights?

3.2.2. Nasal

- Do you have a runny or stuffed up nose in association with the pain, is it unilateral?
- Are you aware of something running down the back of you throat?
- Do you have a coloured discharge from your nose?
- Have you recently had dental treatment done on your top teeth?
- Have your symptoms failed to respond to decongestants?

3.2.3. Face in general

- Does any part of your face feel swollen?
- Do you notice any swellings under your jaw or in front of your ear and are they unilateral or bilateral?
- Does any part of your face feel and/or look red?
- Have you noticed any prominent veins on your face especially round the temple region?
- Do you notice any change in the sensation of your face, e.g pins and needles, tingling, numbness, coldness, burning and over how large an area do you notice this?
- Are there any areas of your face that are exquisitely sensitive to touch?

- Does touching a specific spot on your face start up the pain?
- Do any of your facial muscles feel painful?

3.2.4. Ear

- Do you have ringing, buzzing or hissing noises in your ears?
- If tinnitus is present, ask as to its timing, character, alleviating factors, location times when at its worse, history of head injury?
- Have you noticed any hearing loss?
- Do you feel any pain deep inside your ear?
- Do you have any discharge from your ears?
- Do you feel dizzy?
- Do you feel your jaw is sore?
- Do you have noises in your jaw when you open and close your mouth?

3.2.5. Intraorally

- Can you open your mouth as widely as usual?
- Do you notice any clicking of your jaws when you open widely?
- Do you feel your bite is not right?
- Does your jaw ever lock, in which position?
- Do you find it difficult to bite into large pieces of food with your front teeth?
- Do you clench or grind your teeth?
- Do you have pain while chewing?
- Have you seen any ulcers, white or red patches on the lining of your mouth?
- Have you noticed any swelling/s inside your mouth either related to a tooth or in other parts such as the floor of mouth?
- Does any part of your mouth burn?
- Do you have difficulty swallowing?
- Do you have any pain swallowing?
- Do any of your teeth or gums feel painful?
- If wearing dentures:

  - do they feel comfortable?
  - is the pain affected by the wearing of the dentures?
  - do you find your tongue playing with the dentures?
  - does your bite feel wrong?
  - how long have you had dentures for?
  - how old is the present set and were they made at the same time?
  - what do you do with your dentures at night?

3.3. Medical and dental history including systems review

You need to take a standard medical and dental history. A dental history is important as the commonest causes of orofacial pain are dental causes. This history should include:

- Frequency of attendance at the dentist — regular, irregular, rare
- Types of procedures done at the dentist, e.g. restorative including root fillings, periodontal, prosthetic, oral surgical
- Attitude towards dental treatment

Evidence has shown that a systems review can provide additional data even when done in the form of a structured questionnaire (Verdon and Siemens, 1997). These questions are also used to gauge patients' perception of illness and identify patients who somatise their psychological problems.

Questions would include:

- Do you have pain in any other parts of the body including headache
- Do you ever feel sick or vomit?
- Have you lost weight?
- Do you have irritable bowel syndrome or upset stomach?
- Does your skin itch?
- Do your joints feel stiff?
- Do you feel breathless?
- Do you feel you have no strength and get tried easily?
- Do you sleep well?
- Do you suffer from dizziness?
- Do you get headaches?
- Do you have ME?

If a patient is depressed you may need to ask for other symptoms of hypothyroidism. It is also important to enquire about smoking habits and alcohol use.

3.3.1. Drug history

A history of past and present drug and therapy history will provide you with useful insight into the patients' behaviour in relation to their pain. You especially need to note the following:

- dose size, frequency, duration of prescription and side effects of each drug used
- the patient's perception of the efficacy of the individual drugs
- the list of drugs that have proven to be ineffective
- any other drugs the patient may be using for other conditions
- any patient's idiosyncrasies about drug therapy
- use of homeopathic drugs
- use of over the counter preparations
- any surgical procedures
- alternative forms of treatment

The following case study 3 in Table 7 illustrates a problem I often encounter in patients who have been referred to many physicians over a period of time.

TABLE 7

Case study 3

A 56-year-old patient attended a secondary care pain clinic with a long history of facial pain. When asked about the drugs she was currently taking for her facial pain she produced the following list saying she took all these daily in divided doses: amitriptyline 50 mg, dihydrocodeine 60 mg, gabapentin 600 mg, diazepam 5 mg, clonazepam 5 mg and buprenorphine 400 μg.

What is your differential diagnosis and why is this an inappropriate regimen? What does it tell you about the patient and her doctors?

See Table 17 the end of the chapter for the answer.

---

4. Short psychiatric history

In some patients, it may be important to take a psychiatric history and this section aims to remind you of the key elements of a psychiatric history. You need to remember that a psychiatric interview involves not only a history but also examines mental state and cognition and is briefly described in Chapter 5 on examination and it can be difficult to separate the two. The series 'ABC of mental health' edited by T. Davies (1997) which ran in the British Medical Journal in 1997 is a very useful starting point as it is aimed at primary care physicians and Carlat's article on psychiatric review of symptoms (Carlat, 1998): a screening tool for family physicians gives some very useful tips on how this can be done in a non-psychiatric setting (Hale, 1997a,b).

When taking a history in a patient with psychiatric symptoms you need to ensure that you use all the skills described earlier in this chapter. You are essentially screening for psychiatric disorders but often not making a full diagnosis of a psychiatric condition. Additionally you should be aware that you may need to allow time for emotions to calm and offer reassurance whenever possible. You must enquire about thoughts of suicide or violence and must not avoid sensitive or embarrassing topics if you feel they may be relevant. A risk assessment of suicidal thoughts needs to be made. A major component of a psychiatric history is to put the patient's present complaint within the context of the patient's psychosocial development, premorbid personality, and current circumstances. This can sometimes take a long time and may not be achieved at the first visit.

Feinmann and Harris (1984) suggest that psychiatric disorders detected in facial pain patients are likely to be mild and of relatively short duration but you need to be prepared to face a psychiatric emergency. This is more likely in the secondary care system. You will need to know how to recognise it and refer it. Table 8 lists the mostly likely conditions you may encounter in facial pain patients and their manifestations.

If you want to read more on the connection between psychiatry and the face then we recommend

TABLE 8

KEY FACTS: psychiatric disorders in oro-facial pain

Disorder	Symptoms	Signs
Adjustment disorder	Depressed mood, anxious, worry, unable to cope	Liable to display dramatic behaviour emotion, violence
Anxiety, acute/chronic	Apprehension, tension headaches, autonomic overactivity, breathless, choking, palpitations, dizzy, tingling hands or feet, flushes hot or cold, sweaty, faintness panic attacks	Motor tension, tremor, fidgeting, nail biting, squirming in the chair, sitting on the edge of the chair, shuffling feet
Depressive, mild, moderate or severe	Depressed mood or lack of pleasure, anhedonia, for 2–4 weeks, must then have four or more of the following: feeling worthless; lack of energy; change in sleep pattern; inability to concentrate; suicidal thoughts; diurnal mood variation; change in appetite and weight	Slowed down or agitated, little eye contact, tears, hunched self-hugging posture, change in weight
Obsessional compulsive	Persistent concern about some aspect of bodily function which could be in the mouth or face, have insight	Rituals
Post-traumatic stress	Intrusive thoughts, insomnia, depression, preoccupation with trivia, history of some psychological trauma	Dyspepsia, nausea, fainting, palpitations, hyperventilation
Somatisation, somatoform, conversion	Repeated reporting of symptoms for which no signs can be found, long history, changing symptoms, depression and/or anxiety may be present, little insight	Nil
Psychosis	Loss of contact with reality, delusions, hallucinations and thought disorder, no insight, e.g. mania, schizophrenia, paranoid illness	Unable to communicate, inexplicable laughter, silent and distracted, random meaningless gestures. In cases of mania, excessive activity
Personality	Features of anxiety, wide variety which include psychopath, paranoid, schizoid, histrionic	

the book 'The mouth, the face and the mind' (see the end of the chapter for further details). For further details on diagnostic criteria you are referred to two systems: the WHO International classification of disease (1992) or the Diagnostic and Statistical Manual of Mental Disorders of the American Psychiatric Association (1994) (Weissman et al., 1998).

Depression is common and may be minor (now termed dysthymia), moderate or severe. Hale (1997b) estimates that one in 20 visits to a doctor are due to depression, half go unrecognised and 20% develop into chronic depression (Hale, 1997b). A study has shown that the two simple questions "during the past month have often been bothered by feeling down, depressed or hopeless?" and "during the past month have you often been bothered by having little interest or pleasure in doing things?" are highly effective in detecting depression (Whooley et al., 1997). Carlat then suggests some sensitive ways of asking further questions to ascertain the neurovegative symptoms of depression which could begin with such simple questions as "do you have any problems sleeping?" or "how has the depression affected your life over the last few weeks?" (Carlat, 1998).

Patients will avoid mentioning that they are depressed as they do not want to annoy or embarrass their doctor, because of the stigma attached to such a diagnosis and the fear that they will not be dealt with sympathetically. Some patients overcome this by somatising their depression. Patients who somatise are often called "heart sink", "fat file", patients as they consult very frequently and often see a variety of healthcare professionals. They account for a disproportionately high proportion of the budget as they are often also extensively investigated.

Patients may have varying degrees of depression ranging from minor (2–4 depressive symptoms for more than 2 weeks) to major depression (5 or more depressive symptoms including depressed mood or anhedonia).

5. Family history

In addition to finding out whether the parents and siblings are alive and well you should enquire whether there is any history of facial pain or psychiatric problems. There is research to suggest that chronic pain patients' families are more likely to have had pain complaints than control families with no pain complaints (Mohamed et al., 1978). It is also important that you ascertain how the family cope with pain and the type of support that has been offered to the patient by them both in the past and recently. Brodwin and Kleinman (1987) argue that the family and close friends provide a crucial context for chronic pain. You need to explore this area in a sensitive way.

6. Social history

There is an increasing awareness that physical or psychological stress or well-being will affect the immune system. A search on Medline in 2001 using psychoneuroimmunology as a Mesh heading yielded 605 articles and there is a journal devoted to the subject 'Brain Behaviour and Immunity'.

Stress can be viewed as either an event that requires adaptation or as the response of the individual such as change on heart rate. Psychological stress has been defined by Lazarus and Folkman (1984) as "a particular relationship between the person and environment that is appraised by the person as taxing or exceeding his or her resources and endangering his or her well being." Stress may alter or intensify existing physical symptoms or may induce emotional responses. Details of the social history will enable you to identify the presence of stress factors such as:

- chronic difficulties — social, financial
- psychological factors — low self esteem, anxiety, lack of control over life, lack of confiding relationship
- environmental factors — housing, job
- specific life events — bereavement, moving house, job loss, divorce

All or any of these factors may impinge on both the reporting of the pain and its subsequent management.

Hotopf et al. (2000) have shown that patients who have unexplained hospital admissions are likely to have had childhood experiences of illnesses. These are not necessarily illnesses in themselves but in close family members especially in the father. You need to look for these factors in your patients' social history.

The social history will put the patient into context for you and is essential if you are to manage the patient using the biopsychosocial model of care. It may dictate the treatment you will consider, e.g. you may avoid the use of drugs that cause ataxia in an elderly patient living on their own.

You can explore these social issues under the headings listed in Table 9 key facts. Further details of how this can be achieved in a sensitive manner can be found in books on communication skills. Please also see Chapter 3.

TABLE 9
KEY FACTS: social history

- School and childhood: happy, unhappy, lonely, history of bullying, truant, illness
- Education: level of education, satisfaction
- Work and satisfaction: previous posts, present job, stress factors
- Leisure activity: how relax — physical, cognitive, alone, team activities
- Marital status: past and present, stress factors
- Children: number, ages, problems, worries
- Finance: worries
- Housing: type, quality, satisfaction

7. Quality of life including effect of pain on patient's environment

Some general question relating to the patient's own perception of how life has been affected by the pain, e.g. time off work, inability to do usual household activities, restriction of leisure activities and the effect of pain on personal relationships, will give you some idea of the extent to which the pain is affecting your patients' lives. This can often be done effectively using questionnaires, some of which are described in Chapter 6.

Chronic pain can result in secondary 'gains' for the patient such as sympathy, increased attention, or ability to avoid unpleasant tasks or situations e.g. housework, sexual intercourse, and it is therefore important to ascertain this (Brodwin and Kleinman, 1987; Kleinman et al., 1992).

8. Health beliefs and expectations

Beliefs are defined as the thoughts (cognitions) patients have regarding their pain problem. Peoples' cognitions (beliefs, appraisals or expectations) regarding the consequences of the pain and their ability to cope with the pain can impact on patients in two ways. They may have a direct effect on mood and negative thoughts that emphasise the catastrophic consequences of the pain or the patient's inability to control these consequences can lead to depression. Appraisals such as thoughts about controllability of pain can impact upon coping mechanisms and adaptation. It can be argued that in most acute medicine and dentistry, the patients' belief about their condition is given little attention, as it does not impact heavily on treatment. In patients with chronic pain the pain beliefs of the patient are crucial, as they will determine the patient's actions and intensity of emotions. Patients who believe their pain is due to a tumour rather than muscle tension will react very differently and have differing levels of distress although the pain intensity may be the same.

Please read through the case history in Table 10 case study 4 before reading the next section.

Kleinman et al. (1978) and Brodwin and Kleinman (1987) propose that chronic pain takes two forms: the pain disease and the pain illness. Pain disease refers to the doctors' perspective of the patient's suffering using a biomedical model, which aims to define the cause of the pain and then look for ways of treating. The patient's illness, on the other hand, is the patient's accounts of their illness and how it results in disability, life style changes and associated feelings. It is extremely complex and influenced by the patient's family, ethnic/cultural community, work site and health care organisations. It also includes the patient's perception of the meaning of pain as a threat, gain or loss and the response it will elicit from others around them. We need to remember that pain behaviour is not just restricted to the individual patient, but is always embedded in the patient's immediate family group. Knowledge of the patient's illness will enable you to determine whether there is a discrepancy between these two models. If discrepancies exist it is possible for patient compliance and satisfaction to be affected. This biopsychosocial model is further expanded on by Misselbrook, a London general medical practitioner, in his book 'Thinking about patients' where he stresses that medicine "does not occur in a vacuum but has social and cultural context".

TABLE 10

Case study 4

Mrs. B, now 57 years old has had continuous facial pain for 30 years beginning when she was a teenager. She relates the start of her pain to an injury to her front teeth in the swimming pool. Mrs. B admits to anhedonia, occasional depression and has had suicidal thoughts and this is substantiated on the Hospital, Anxiety and Depression scale and the Brief Pain Inventory shows that this pain has a considerable effect on her life (see Chapter 6 for details of these measures).

Further questioning elicits the following social history. Her father frequently struck her in the face when she was disobedient and her mother gave her no support. Her parents died some time ago but due to their poor relationship she had no regrets about their death. She left school at 15 years and went to work in a shop. She soon became pregnant, married and left home. She had two children who are now grown up and have their own children. She says the pain has not allowed her to keep any long-term job. Her husband of 41 years was a coach maker until he was made redundant 5 years ago at the age of 60 years. Mrs. B says she cannot cope with socialising with her friends because of her pain which is made worse by talking. When her husband retired she suggested they move away from their friends. They now live in a remote part of the country to which there is no regular transport and where they have few friends.

She feels that people, on the whole, do not understand her pain and although initially she said her husband was supportive of her pain during the consultation it became obvious that there was considerable tension about the way support was given for this pain on both sides.

Although until recently she was prepared to accept that her pain was a psychological one, she now thinks that it could be due to nerve damage and that she would like a new approach for this treatment. She was hoping a new consultant could offer some surgical treatment. How would you approach this?

See Table 18 at the end of the chapter for a possible answer.

In Chapter 6, you will find some useful measures that have been developed to try and elicit these factors. Some of these measures may be completed before the interview with someone who has been trained e.g. nurse, others may be completed with the clinician during the consultation. These issues are also discussed in Chapter 3. In Table 11, key facts below you will find some questions that Brodwin and Kleinman (1987) suggest you may ask.

It is also useful to elicit some information on how the patient is coping. Patients can develop coping strategies to solve or relieve the pain or they may be directing their strategies towards managing the negative emotions associated with stress and pain.

TABLE 11

KEY FACTS: questions to determine a patient's illness (Brodwin and Kleinman, 1987)

1. What do you think caused your pain?

2. Why do you think it started when it did? What else was happening in your life at the time?

3. What do you think your chronic pain does to you (your body, your emotional reactions)? How do you think this pain works?

4. How severe is your pain? Will it have a short or long course?

5. What type of treatment do you think you should receive?

6. What results do you hope to receive from this treatment?

7. What are the chief problems (at work, at home, with friends) your continued pain has caused you?

Adjustment to chronic pain can be assessed by determining the level of activity the patient can undergo, their psychological functioning and their utilisation of both medication and professional services.

9. Transcultural issues of history taking

Just as we adapt our consultation to the patient's intellectual, social and emotional needs, so we must do when communicating in a cross cultural setting. For additional details please see further reading. For a further discussion of the effect of ethnicity on pain please see Chapter 3.

It is essential that you look beyond cultural differences and establish a meaningful and respectful relationship as people from different cultures have different ways of sending and receiving information, expressing their wishes and commands and demonstrating feeling.

Some of the problems you may encounter during a consultation include:

- Cultural boundaries, e.g. time-keeping
- Transference of our own prejudices, racial stereotypes, fears, areas of ignorance
- Possible misuse of power — if you consider yourself to be a high status expert you may disempower and distance yourself from your patient
- Communication problems both verbal and nonverbal — use of eye contact/facial expression/body posture and gestures all vary significantly according to race and culture

Many of us encounter patients whose first language is not the same as ours and in order to have an effective consultation we need to observe some simple rules as summarised in Table 12.

Remember that cultures get masked when you share the same language, e.g. an American, Afro Caribbean and Englishman may think they are using the same language but misunderstandings can easily arise. It is also easy to assume that if their English is not the same as yours, that they are intellectually slow or uneducated. Class and education are also

---

TABLE 12

KEY FACTS: improving transcultural communication

- Communicate to the patient that they are understood
- Show warmth and respect for the patients' values
- Do not impose your own values on the patient
- Be aware of the patient's cultural norms and values
- Listen attentively, show empathy and reflect accurately
- Communicate effectively especially attempting to clarify any differences

---

likely to produce alternative forms of English. When communicating distressing or personal material or when stressed, angry or fatigued it is often difficult to communicate effectively even in your own first language, never mind trying to do this in another language. If patients cannot communicate effectively you will lose access to important familial and cultural experiences.

Although English is a very rich language in terms of mood or feeling, it may not be as effective for other factors e.g. the range of words used to describe family relationships is much broader and explicit in Bengali, but, on the other hand, the word 'depression' does not exist in that language.

If you consult in a multicultural society, you will need to know how and when to use interpreters or advocates with your patients. Patients have '*a right*' to be understood and this means a consultation should be offered in the language of their choice.

It is very common for us to use children, neighbours or other healthcare professionals who may be around to act as interpreters, however, there are real dangers using untrained people for this task. Unofficial translators may:

- provide inaccurate translations due to their lack of understanding of the subtleties of different words
- introduce bias and distortion
- not maintain confidentiality

TABLE 13

KEY FACTS: check list when using an interpreter

- Check that interpreter and patient speak same language/dialect
- Check that the interpreter is acceptable to the patient and trusted
- Discuss before the consultation the content of the interview and how you want to work
- Encourage the interpreter to interject if necessary
- Use easy language
- Observe interpreter and patient to pick up non-verbal behaviours
- Check that patient has understood
- Leave yourself extra time
- Ensure patient has time to raise questions
- After the consultation check with interpreter how the interview went

- not fully understand their role in a consultation
- not explain significant cultural differences
- be personally unsuitable

When using an interpreter or advocate it is useful to check some of the items mentioned in Table 12 key facts and for you to remember that you as the doctor remain responsible for everything during the consultation. Table 13 is a check list for use when an interpreter is required.

10. Structured history taking sheet

It takes a considerable amount of time to record all the data you have gathered and its recording during an interview can affect your relationship with the patient. We have found the use of semi-structured histories to be not only useful for speeding up the process for recording, but it also acts as a memory aid ensuring that the most essential details are recorded. Everybody using the structured history sheets should feel that they have had their say in

their design and structure as ownership improves their use. If using such a tool, it is useful if you can audit from time to time the completeness of the notes and their value in making the diagnosis, recording data and influencing management. In Appendix A, a history sheet that has been developed on the most commonly reported symptoms of patients with facial pain in our department is shown. The history sheets will also include any other completed questionnaires. Too often we record our history in the biomedical model and omit the social and psychological factors we have gathered. It is important to record these, as often these are the factors that determine our management of the patient.

11. Summary

See Table 14 for a summary of this chapter.

TABLE 14

Summary of Chapter 4

1. Improved communication skills which ensures time to listen to the patient will markedly improve the value of the history

2. Standard questions that must be put to all pain patients and more specific ones that relate to the different structures of the face are provided

3. Techniques for taking a mini psychiatric history are suggested

4. Methods to determine patient's pain disease and illness are suggested

5. Details of family and social history that are required for patients with facial pain are discussed

6. Hints on consulting in a multicultural setting are provided

7. An example of a structured history sheet is supplied

Appendix A

Example of structured facial pain histories. Please also see Appendix A in Chapter 5 for the rest of the examination.

FACIAL PAIN   FIRST VISIT

DATE: **CONSULTANT:** **REFERRED BY:** Medical practitioner dentist specialist **C/O:**	**SURNAME:** **OTHER NAME:** **HOSPITAL NO:** **DOB:** **M/F**

Date first attack :

Circumstances around first attack: *acute*   *slow to develop*

Dental treatment: extraction endodontic restorative periodontal;

trauma, infection, stress, other

Date present attack if remission:

Current Status: *better   /   worse   /   no change*

Character: *aching dull sharp stabbing shooting throbbing drawing nagging electric fearful*

burning, gnawing, annoying, tender, other

Deep   superficial   mixture   intense   light   diffuse   focused

---

Types of measures : McGill, Hospital Anxiety & Depression, Brief Pain Inventory, Beliefs, Coping

---

severity <u>average</u>:   *none mild moderate severe   most severe VAS:*

       <u>Least and worse</u>: *none mild moderate severe most severe VAS: VAS:*

Does it vary in severity: daily/ weekly/ monthly, does it build up gradually

---

Site of pain: *I supraorbital, eye, temporal   frontal - intra-oral/ extra-oral*

II infraorbital palatine PSD nasolabial, nasal pre-auricular post-auricular –intra-oral/extra

III mental mandibular long buccal lingual - intraoral/ extraoral

Outside trigeminal area   complete details on a picture together with patient

Side: *R / L / Bilateral*

Referred to*: nowhere   I   II   III   outside V   neck   head   R   L*

Timing of pain: *Intermittent: regular/ irregular   Continuous   timing of worse pain : am/ pm*

Length of each bout of pain*: secs   mins   hours   days   weeks*

Frequency of bouts*:   minutes   hourly   daily   weekly*

Periods of no pain: *No / Yes   days   weeks   months   years*

                    Stops sleep   affects quality of sleep   pain at night

Mode of onset *: spontaneous   stimulus induced – noxious   innocuous   light touch   functional activity*

Tick as appropriate

Provoking	Factor	Relieving
	Talking	
	Eating	
	Brushing teeth	
	Shaving/washing	
	Brushing hair/touching temples	
	Cold /wind	
	Warmth	
	Foods cold or hot	
	Pressure on teeth/biting	
	Opening wide	
	Stooping/bending	
	Stress/tension/ relaxing	
	Sleep/rest	
	Lying down	
	Fatigue	
	Distraction	
	Working	
	Alcohol	

**Associated factors*: tick if present*

Presence	Factor	Presence	Factor
	Altered /poor taste		Clicking joint
	Disturbed salivation		Bruxism
	Altered sensation/numbness		Cheek clenching
	Sleep disturbance		Unable to open wide
	Waking due to pain		Ringing in the ears
	Colour change tissues/ redness		Deafness
	Swelling of face		Headaches
	Nasal stuffiness/post nasal drip		Dizziness
	Double or blurred vision		Migraine
	Excessive tearing of eyes		Neck pain
	Excessive dryness of eyes		Back pain
	Visual disturbances		Irritable bowel
	Eye redness		Nausea
	Fatigue/loss strength		Abdominal pain/ menstrual
	Stiffness of joints		Impaired concentration
	Reduced appetite		Other specify

PAST TREATMENTS:

Drugs	Daily Dosage/ time used	Side effects	Efficacy

Previous surgery

Other treatments: *splints   dental – conservation endodontics, periodontics, dentures, extraction, alternative medicine, acupuncture / low intensity laser/ TENS*

Previous consultations/ number *: GP   dentist   oral surgeon   neurologist   psychiatrist   ENT surgeon   neurosurgeon   psychologist   pain specialist   counsellor   other*

EFFECT OF PAIN AND COPING:

Measures completed: coping strategies, family impact, treatment goals
Effect of pain on quality of life : *none   mild   moderate   considerable*
What changes have occurred in your life as a result of the pain:
Have you taken time of work: *No/ Yes how much:*
Do people respond to your pain / how and is it appropriate:

In the last month have you felt a lack of pleasure in life*: no   yes*
In the last month have you felt depressed*: no   yes*

Do you have: *feeling of worthlessness / guilt/   disturbed sleep / early am wakening /   appetite changes*
Do you feel anxious *: no   yes*
What do you think has caused the pain and what do you think I can do *:*

F.H.: (age, health status)	
Father:	**Mother:**
Sibs:	

Any FH of facial pain:
Social History and the effect the pain has on it
School & childhood: Relationship with parents, siblings, other family :Work and satisfaction
Leisure activity: Marital status: Children:Finance:Housing: Other life events

FACIAL PAIN- FOLLOW-UP

DATE: **CONSULTANT:**	**SURNAME:** **M/F**
GLOBAL OUTCOME (patient) Worse / No Change / Little Better/ Better / No Symptoms **Or % improvement**	**OTHER NAME:** **DOB:**
History since last visit:	**HOSPITAL NO:**

Surgery since last visit:
Pain diary returned: Yes   Not given   No (reason):

HAD Scale   McGill (short/long)   Brief Pain Inventory

Character: **Aching   Dull   Sharp   Stabbing   Shooting   Electric   Throbbing   Drawing**
          Nagging   Burning   Other:

Frequency: more   /   same   /   less

Periods of complete pain remission: No   Yes   How long?

Severity: worse   /   same   /   better
VAS since last visit: Average   Worse   Best

Site: Same/different
Side: R   L   Bilateral

Medication: able to take   took regularly   took for :   irregular
Did not take (reasons)

DRUGS SINCE LAST VISIT	**DOSE or total DAILY DOSE**	**FREQUENCY**

Side effects from drugs: NONE   Rash   Dry mouth   Dizzy   Drowsy/tired   Disturbed vision   Ataxia
      Unable to concentrate   Feel like zombie   Gastro-intestinal nausea   Vomiting   Constipation
Diarrohea   Abnormal sensation   Other:

How disabling are the side effects: Not at all   Mild   Moderate   Severe   Most severe

S.H.
Effect of pain on quality of life: None   Mild   Moderate   Considerable
How are you coping with the pain now: No better   Better   Worse
Any changes in social circumstances which may affect pain:

EVALUATION (clinician):
Compliance: excellent   v good   good   fair   poor
What are patient's current beliefs:
Patient understanding: excellent   v good good   fair   poor

Appendix B

The answers to case studies 1–4 can be found in Tables 15–18.

TABLE 15

Answer to case study 1

---

1. Positive partnership can be increased by the PERSONAL approach
    Presentation
    Empathy
    Respect
    Support
    Organisation
    Non-judgmental
    Alliance
    Leaving taking

See the text in the chapter for further clarification

2. You can increase data gathering by using the following techniques
    Simple questions
    Open questions
    Unbiased questions
    Responsive questions
    Clarification
    Encouragement
    Summarising

See the text in the chapter for further clarification

TABLE 16

Answer to case study 2

Character of the pain
Duration/onset time
Periodicity
Severity
Site
Radiation
Provoking and relieving factors
Associated factors

See text for further details

TABLE 17

Answer to case study 3

The patient has chronic facial pain and the differential diagnosis based on the drugs suggests several diagnoses. Gabapentin and clonazepam are used for trigeminal neuralgia, amitriptyline is often used for psychogenic pain, diazepam suggests anxiety, dihydrocodeine and buprenorphine are used for acute pain of dental origin. This mixture of drugs is inappropriate as the patient is unlikely to have all these potential diagnosis. Neither the doctors nor the patient have made a careful assessment of the pain nor have they evaluated each drug in turn to see if it is effective.

TABLE 18

Case study 4

Surgery will not benefit the patient. I suggested they could both benefit from some cognitive behaviour therapy for developing coping strategies for the pain. Mrs. B declined as she said it was too difficult to travel although her husband was interested in pursuing this line of treatment. Tension is likely to rise given that they are now more isolated and Mrs. B can exert more control over her husband. Mrs. B is probably getting some secondary gain from her pain and is reluctant to let her pain go, e.g. not working, getting a new home, avoiding friends.

I also put her on antidepressants and asked her to keep a diary of her pain and stress levels.

This patient presents a very complex history and your interpretation may be very different. These are my personal views.

Appendix C. Further reading

Useful books or reports to look through.

C.1. History taking and its importance

(1) Burrows GD, Elton D, Stanley GV (eds). Handbook of Chronic Pain Management. Elsevier, Amsterdam, 1987: ISBN 0-444-80446-3. (Contains data on social aspects of pain.)

(2) Feinmann C (ed). The Mouth, the Face and the Mind. Oxford University Press, Oxford, 1999: ISBN 0-19-263062-8. (Illustrates relationship between psychiatry, psychology and dentistry. Edited by a liaison psychiatrist who works in a dental school.)

(3) Good MD, Brodwin PE, Good B, Kleinman A (eds). Pain as Human Experience: an Anthropological Perspective. University of California Press, Berkeley, CA, 1992 or 1994 for paperback: ISBN 0-520-07512-9. (This book gives an interesting perspective on pain from a non-medical view point and challenges the biomedical model.)

(4) Greenhalgh T, Hurwitz B (eds). Narrative Based Medicine. BMJ Books, London, 1989: ISBN 0-7279-1223-2. (Reminds us of the need to listen carefully to our patients and record their 'story'.)

(5) Misselbrook D. Thinking about Patients. Petroc Press, Newbury, 2001: ISBN 1-900603-49-7. (A book to challenge us and remind us of the need to practice medicine in a biopsychosocial way.)

C.2. *Communication skills*

(6) Cole SA, Bird J. The Medical Interview: the Three Function Approach, 2nd edn., Harcourt Health Sciences, St Louis, 2000: ISBN 0815119925. (Very useful book, recently updated.)

(7) Ley P. Communicating with Patients, Chapman and Hall, London, 1988: ISBN 0-412-38240-7. (Details ways of improving communication and satisfaction both by way of consultation but also using questionnaires.)

(8) Lloyd M, Bor R. Communication Skills for Medicine. Churchill Livingstone, New York, 1996: ISBN 0-443-05168-2. (Well laid out with plenty of exercises to do, very useful for teaching.)

(9) Neighbour R. The Inner Consultation. Petroc Press, Newbury, 1996: ISBN 1-900-603-950. (A more reflective book on communication skills.)

(10) Tate P. The Doctor's Communication Handbook, 3rd edn. Radcliffe Medical Press, 2001: ISBN 1-85775-550-2. (A basic easy to read book used by candidates for MRCGP examinations.)

(11) D'Ardenne P, Mathani A. Transcultural Counselling in Action. Sage, London, 1989: ISBN 0-80398-1112. (Provides details on aspects that need to be taken into account when consulting across cultures.)

(12) Phelan M, Parkman S. How to work with an interpreter. Br Med J 1995; 311(7004): 555–557.

(13) Gask L, Usherwood T. The Consultation. Br Med J 2002; 324: 1567–1569. (An excellent summary of many of the points raised in this chapter.)

(14) Report of the Royal College of Physicians of London. Improving Communication between Doctors and Patients. Report of a Working Party. Royal College of Physicians, London, 1997, pp 1–38.

(15) Report of the American Psychiatric Association. Diagnostic and Statistical Manual of Mental Disorders. IV. American Psychiatric Association, New York, 1994.

(16) Report of the World Health Organisation. The ICD 10 Classification of Mental and Behavioural Disorders. WHO, Geneva, 1992.

References

Marked as regards quality according to criteria set by author.
* Poorer quality studies but only ones in the field, old style reviews.
** Cohort studies, high quality case series with controls.
*** Randomised controlled trials, high quality original studies.

** Beckman HB, Frankel RM. The effect of physician behavior on the collection of data. Ann Intern Med 1984; 101: 692–696.
** Bird J, Cohen-Cole SA. The three-function model of the medical interview. An educational device. Adv Psychosom Med 1990; 20: 65–88.
** Bird J, Hall A, Maguire P, Heavy A. Workshops for consultants on the teaching of clinical communication skills. Med Educ 1993; 27: 181–185.

* Blau JN. How to take a history of head or facial pain. Br Med J (Clin Res Ed) 1982; 285: 1249–1251.

* Blau JN. Time to let the patient speak. Br Med J 1989; 298: 39.

* Brodwin PE, Kleinman A. The social meaning of chronic pain. In: Burrows GD, Elton D, Stanley GV (eds) Handbook of Chronic Pain Management. Elsevier, Amsterdam, 1987: 109–119.

** Carlat DJ. The psychiatric review of symptoms: a screening tool for family physicians. Am Fam Phys 1998; 58: 1617–1624.

*** Chodosh J. Diagnostic strategies acute sinusitis. ACP J Club 1999; 5: 293–302.

* Craig TKJ, Boardman AP. ABC of mental health: Common mental health problems in primary care. Br Med J 1997; 314: 1609.

* Davies T. ABC of mental health: mental health assessment. Br Med J 1997; 314: 1536.

** Davis H, Nicholaou T. A comparison of the interviewing skills of first- and final-year medical students. Med Educ 1992; 26: 441–447.

*** Drangsholt M, Truelove E. Trigeminal neuralgia mistaken as temporomandibular disorder. J Evid Base Dent Pract 2001; 1: 41–50.

** Feinmann C, Harris M. Psychogenic facial pain. Part 1: The clinical presentation. Br Dent J 1984; 156: 165–168.

* Hale AS. ABC of mental health. Anxiety. Br Med J 1997a; 314: 1886–1889.

* Hale AS. ABC of mental health. Depression. Br Med J 1997b; 315: 43–46.

** Hampton JR, Harrison MJ, Mitchell JR, Prichard JS, Seymour C. Relative contributions of history-taking, physical examination, and laboratory investigation to diagnosis and management of medical outpatients. Br Med J 1975; 2: 486–489.

** Hotopf M, Wilson-Jones C, Mayou R, Wadsworth M, Wessely S. Childhood predictors of adult medically unexplained hospitalisations. Results from a national birth cohort study. Br J Psychiatry 2000; 176: 273–280.

Kleinman A, Eisenberg L, Good B. Culture, illness, and care: clinical lessons from anthropologic and cross-cultural research. Ann Intern Med 1978; 88(2): 251–258.

* Kleinman A, Brodwin PE, Good BJ, Good MD. In: Good MD, Brodwin PE, Good B, Kleinman A (eds) Pain as Human Experience: an Anthropological Perspective. University of California Press, Berkeley, CA, 1992: 1–28.

Lazarus RA, Folkman S. Stress, Appraisal and Coping. Springer, New York, 1984.

** Maguire P. Can communication skills be taught? Br J Hosp Med 1990; 43: 215–216.

** Marvel MK, Epstein RM, Beckman HB Patients, interrupted? J Fam Pract 2000; 49: 471.

*** McAlister FA, Straus SE, Sackett DL. Why we need large, simple studies of the clinical examination: the problem and a proposed solution. CARE-COAD1 group. Clinical Assessment of the Reliability of the Examination-Chronic Obstructive Airways Disease Group. Lancet 1999; 354: 1721–1724.

** Miall LS, Davies H. An analysis of paediatric diagnostic decision-making: how should students be taught? Med Educ 1992; 26: 317–320.

** Mohamed SN, Weisz GM, Waring EM. The relationship of chronic pain to depression, marital adjustment, and family dynamics. Pain 1978; 5: 285–292.

** Novack DH, Dube C, Goldstein MG. Teaching medical interviewing. A basic course on interviewing and the physician–patient relationship. Arch Intern Med 1992; 152: 1814–1820.

* Peterson MC, Holbrook JH, Von Hales D, Smith NL, Staker LV. Contributions of the history, physical examination, and laboratory investigation in making medical diagnoses. West J Med 1992; 156: 163–165.

* Roshan M, Rao AP. A study on relative contributions of the history, physical examination and investigations in making medical diagnosis. J Assoc Phys India 2000; 48: 771–775.

* Ryle JA. The Natural History of Disease. Oxford University Press, London, 1936.

** Sandler G. The importance of the history in the medical clinic and the cost of unnecessary tests. Am Heart J 1980; 100: 928–931.

** Simpson M, Buckman R, Stewart M, Maguire P, Lipkin M, Novack D, Till J. Doctor–patient communication: the Toronto consensus statement. Br Med J 1991; 303: 1385–1387.

** Verdon ME, Siemens K. Yield of review of systems in a self-administered questionnaire. J Am Board Fam Pract 1997; 10: 20–27.

** Weissman MM, Broadhead WE, Olfson M, Sheehan DV, Hoven C, Conolly P, Fireman BH, Farber L, Blacklow RS, Higgins ES, Leon AC. A diagnostic aid for detecting (DSM-IV) mental disorders in primary care. Gen Hosp Psychiatry 1998; 20: 1–11.

*** Whooley MA, Avins AL, Miranda J, Browner WS. Case-finding instruments for depression. Two questions are as good as many. J Gen Intern Med 1997; 12: 439–445.

*** Woolf CJ, Mannion RJ. Neuropathic pain: aetiology, symptoms, mechanisms, and management. Lancet 1999; 353: 1959–1964.

Assessment and Management of Orofacial Pain
Pain Research and Clinical Management, Vol. 14
Edited by J.M. Zakrzewska and S.D. Harrison
© *2002 Elsevier Science B.V. All rights reserved*

CHAPTER 5

Examination of facial pain patients

Joanna M. Zakrzewska[*]

*Department of Clinical and Diagnostic Oral Sciences, Oral Medicine Unit, Dental Institute, Barts
and the London Queen Mary's School of Medicine and Dentistry, Turner Street, London E1 2AD, UK*

Objectives for this chapter:

This chapter will attempt to show you how to do a basic examination of the:
- Face including facial expression of pain
- Cranial nerves
- Mental state
- Mouth
- Temporomandibular joint and its muscles
- Eye

It will suggest a template for recording these findings

1. Introduction

Examination begins from the moment a patient enters the consulting room although more formal elements are performed after a full history has been elicited. The general principles of examination of the orofacial region are presented in this chapter but more detailed specific features may be found in individual chapters. It is important to repeat examinations at follow-up visits as subtle changes may occur. Patients with trigeminal neuralgia due to tumours may initially have no neurological abnormalities and only develop them later. They can be as small as the loss of the corneal reflex or a small patch of numbness and are not always noted by the patient.

The examination does not need to be done in the order in which it is presented. It may be easier to examine the mental state prior to doing a physical examination. The chapter includes some very basic features of examination as we expect the readership to come from wide clinical backgrounds, e.g. dentists, clinical psychologists, doctors. Medical students get very low exposure to teaching about the mouth and so a section on basic dental examination has been included. Equally, dentally qualified clinicians may not be using some of their neurological skills on a regular basis and may benefit from some revision.

Studies have shown that physical examination contributes 2–9% to the diagnosis but raises confidence in the diagnosis (measured on a scale of 1–10) rises from around 6 to 8 (Hampton et al., 1975; Peterson et al., 1992; Roshan and Rao, 2000). It is, therefore, more useful to invest more time in history taking than in trying to elicit clinical signs.

[*] Tel.: +44-20-7377-7053; Fax: +44-20-7377-7627;
E-mail: j.m.zakrzewska@qmul.ac.uk

2. Examination of the facies

During history taking the facies will have been examined in a general way but it is important to carry out a formal examination of the face. Examination should include the following:

- Noting of any facial swelling, salivary gland swelling, asymmetry, wasting of muscles, hypertrophy of muscles, tenderness over the sinuses
- Nose: blockage, deviation of septum, postnasal drip
- Skin colour including redness or pallor, pigmentation, texture, surface, and any lesions such as rashes, eruptions, ulcers and their distribution
- Lips: muscle tone, swelling, colour, lesions especially at the angles, competency

2.1. Facial expression and pain behaviour

Examination of the face during history taking will also give you some information of how the face is expressing pain and emotion. It is generally agreed that there are seven discrete expressions: happiness, fear, anger, sadness, disgust, surprise and contempt, but researchers consider that there are more of these including one of pain. You need to take into account not only what the face is 'doing' objectively but also how you interpret it. How you or others around react or do not react to the behaviour will further influence it as pain results in an emotional response.

Facial pain expression has been assessed as a distinct type of behaviour and there is now a considerable body of evidence to show that facial behaviour during pain shows some consistent pattern. This can be reliably identified by observers and has resulted in a facial action coding system (FACS) Ekman and Friesen (1978). The particular areas of the face that are scanned are the brow, eyes and mouth and these make up 44 action units which are then graded on a five-point scale. These measurements can be made from video recordings as well as photographs (LeResche, 1982). However training is required if observers are to be sensitive to varying

TABLE 1	
KEY FACTS: facial expressions of pain	
Vocal	Crying, screaming, sighing, moaning
Physiological	Pallor, sweating, muscle tension
Expressions	Grimacing
Postures	Rubbing area, guarding, immobility

intensities of pain in facial pain expression and this still remains mainly a research tool (Solomon et al., 1997).

Although it appears that pain expressions are universal the conditions that elicit them and the context in which they are used can be highly variable and are not correlated with pain threshold, pain tolerance or intensity (Prkachin, 1992). They will also change over time and may be different in acute and chronic pain and show more change than verbal reports of pain (LeResche et al., 1992). Facial pain expressions also appear to be the same across cultures (Ekman et al., 1987). Certain facial behaviours can be controlled but some are less amenable to voluntary control. You need to be aware that facial expression can be manipulated and you may see genuine, false, inhibited, exaggerated or mixed expressions of pain (Hadjistavropoulos et al., 1996). Healthcare professionals frequently underestimate pain because facial expression is not taken into account. This underestimation may be as high as 80% although it can be improved by training (Prkachin et al., 1994; Solomon et al., 1997). This is a source of concern as this will lead to under treatment of the pain.

Clinically, when assessing pain, we take into account facial expressions of pain, paralinguistic vocalisations, distinct movements or postures and visible physiological changes such as those listed in Table 1 key facts.

Further details on this subject can be found in Chapter 9 of Handbook of Pain Assessment (Craig et al., 2001) or in the Journal of Nonverbal Behaviour.

3. Examination of the neck and salivary glands

As well as examining the skin, as for the face, the neck should be palpated with you standing directly behind the patient.

You are especially assessing:

Lymph nodes: for size, shape, consistency, contour, edge, surface, mobility, tenderness, number

Parotid gland: palpate distal to the ascending ramus of the mandible and behind the ear (the ear lobe may be turned outward in a large swelling and intraorally between the fauces due to deep lobe extension)

Submandibular gland: must be done bimanually with two fingers in the mouth and includes examination of the ducts in the floor of the mouth

You can find further details on examination in books such as those listed at the end of the chapter.

4. General examination

This is not often necessary unless there are indications for their need in the history. Measurement of blood pressure, pulse and weight may be useful if drugs are to be prescribed which can affect the cardiovascular system.

5. Neurological examination

The following text provides a summary only. For more details we suggest you read a book such as 'Neurological examination made easy' (Fuller, 1999) which includes useful illustrations.

5.1. Cranial nerve testing

The thoroughness with which the cranial nerve functions are tested depends on the circumstances. If your patient has had a head injury or you suspect a frontal tumour then you need to test smell carefully otherwise it is sufficient to ask the patient if they have any problems with smell. The trigeminal

nerve, on the other hand, needs to be tested carefully in all patients with facial pain. Examination of the fundi may not be relevant in some lower facial pain conditions. Routine testing of the gag reflex, pharyngeal movement and sensation as well as vocal cord function is only necessary when bulbar problems are suspected and you identify some symptoms in the patient's history which suggest a dysfunction. Mirrors, good lighting and skill are required for examination of the vocal cords. Table 2 key facts is a summary of the principle functions and procedures for testing the cranial nerves.

If you are not a neurologist and do not do these tests frequently you may find the notes listed below useful when carrying out cranial nerve examinations:

- When testing *corneal reflex* you need to ensure that you are just touching the cornea and this is made easier if you ask the patient to look up and you retract the lower eyelid and touch it very lightly with a wisp of cotton wool, not touching the sclera. If you find a fifth nerve abnormality check if ophthalmoplegia is present as this could indicate lesions in the cavernous sinus.
- When assessing lesions of the *facial nerve* you need to determine whether the lesion is an upper motor neurone or lower motor neurone one. The simplest way of assessing this is to test the movement of the forehead. In supranuclear unilateral lesions (upper motor neurone) the forehead and eye closure is not as weak as in the lower face, whereas in lower motor lesions there is marked upper face weakness. This is due to bilateral representation of the forehead in the motor cortex which still remains in upper motor lesions.
- *Taste* of the anterior two-thirds of the tongue is from the VII through the chordi tympani, whereas the posterior third is from the IX. Traditionally, four tastes are used salt, sucrose, acetic acid and quinine, but these may not be discriminatory enough in patients with taste disturbance (see Chapter 16 on burning mouth for more details). Note down the location.
- When testing the *eighth nerve* remember to test each ear separately by masking the other ear with

TABLE 2

KEY FACTS: cranial nerve testing

Number	Nerve	Function and testing
I	Olfactory	Smell using several different smells
II	Optic	Visual acuity, papillary light responses, visual fields, fundoscopy
III	Oculomotor	Ocular movements, diplopia
IV	Trochlear	Light reaction, ocular movement
V	Trigeminal	Sensation of the face, muscles of mastication: corneal reflex, light touch, pin prick, strength of muscles of mastication, jaw jerk
VI	Abducens	Ocular movements, diplopia
VII	Facial	Muscles of facial expression: frown, eye closure, smile, pouting
VIII	Acoustic	Hearing whisper, watch, Rinne's and Weber's test, nystagmus
IX	Glossopharyngeal	Gag reflex applied to tonsillar fossa
X	Vagal	Palatal elevation during phonation, vocal cord function
XI	Accessory	Elevation of shoulder, neck rotation with/without resistance
XII	Hypoglossal	Deviation of tongue, fasciculation, wasting

a finger and ensure the patient cannot lip read. Conductive deafness due to disease of the middle ear as opposed to perceptive deafness (sensorineural) due to cochlea or nerve lesions can be crudely ascertained using the modified Rinne and Weber tests. These tests rely on the principle that air conduction is normally better than bone conduction. A vibrating tuning fork of 512 Hz is held in front of the ear (lateral to the external auditory meatus with the prongs aligned parallel to the meatus) and you ask the patient whether they hear this sound better in this position than when the base of the tuning fork is place on the mastoid bone behind the ear. In the Weber test, the vibrating tuning fork is placed in the middle of the patient's forehead and you ask the patient where they hear the sound best. If the sound does not localise then the test is judged normal. The sound localises to the affected ear if conductive deafness is present and to the contralateral ear in sensorineural deafness. Nystagmus is the to and fro movement of the eye which is usually due to a defect of control of the eye movement emanating from the labyrinths or to their central brain connections. It can occur in patients with multiple sclerosis which is associated with an increased risk of developing trigeminal neuralgia and patients taking drugs such as phenytoin. Nystagmus is difficult to test at the bedside as care is needed in the interpretation of the results. If any abnormality is detected then it may be useful for you to refer for formal ENT assessment.

- The *motor system* is not often examined in facial pain patients but if there is anything in the history or on gross examination that suggests some abnormality then it should be carried out.
- *Tremors* may be noticed during examination. Patients with Parkinsonism have a tremor at rest, whereas tremors caused by anxiety, drugs including alcohol and thyrotoxicosis are detected when the fingers are outstretched.
- When testing *sensation* remember to do this from the abnormal area to the normal area. When testing sensation on the face use a thin wisp of cotton wool and ask the patient to close their eyes. It is worth looking for allodynia: light touch with

wisp of cotton wool produces a sensation of pain. There may also be different areas of loss for light touch as compared to pinprick. When testing pain with a pin it is important to ask the patient to close their eyes and to ask if the pin feels sharp or blunt. Two-point discrimination requires practise as the ability to discriminate between two points is different in parts of the body e.g. sole of the foot and face. Thermal testing is not often done, but can be crudely done using a metal and rubber object. Equipment is now available to test all modalities of sensation but it tends to be used in specialised units and for research, as it is a time-consuming procedure.

6. Mental state

Not every patient needs a mental state examination but we have included it here for those occasions when it may prove to be necessary. Examination of mental state may not be achieved completely at the first interview and may need to be slowly built up. It is also liable to change and so the patient may need to be re-examined. Many of the aspects of the examination are noted while taking the history, including listening to the patients speech and observing their comprehension. Mental state needs to be considered under the following headings:

- Appearance: attire, cleanliness, posture, gait, body ornaments, hair, make up
- Behaviour: activity, facial expression, co-operation or aggression, agitation, level of arousal
- Speech and preoccupations: rate, tone, form, quality, content — is it logical, coherent and congruent with the questions being asked. Patients ability to read, write, repeat words and phrases should be tested if you suspect that dysphasia is present
- Mood: anxiety, current mood and comparison with reported mood, apathy, irritable, labile, optimistic, pessimistic, psychotic ideas, suicidal ideas, biological markers, e.g. sleep pattern, appetite, weight, tiredness
- Phobias/obsessions: avoidance of stimuli, rituals

TABLE 3
KEY FACTS: simplified hierarchy of symptoms in mental health
1. Delirium
2. Dementia
3. Schizophrenia
4. Mania and other psychosis
5. Depression and other mood disturbances
6. Anxiety, phobia, panic, neurosis
7. Personality disorder, character traits

- Thoughts/abnormal beliefs: overvalued ideas, delusions, rational, fixed, do they affect safety of patient or others
- Perceptions/abnormal experiences: illusions, hallucinations in any modality, e.g. taste, smell, touch, auditory, depersonalisation
- Intellect: cognitive and intellectual function, oriented in time, space and person, able to function at level expected from their education
- Insight/self appraisal: how does the patient explain the symptoms

The diagnostic and statistical manual DSM III or IV provides the diagnostic criteria for all psychiatric illness and enables you to make sense of the data you have collected. It will be discussed further in Chapter 8 on classification and diagnosis. The hierarchy of symptomatology of mental disorders (see Table 3 key facts) enables you to understand that personality is likely to affect all mental disorders, whereas schizophrenia which will often include anxiety and depressed mood must also include specific delusions or hallucinations.

7. Intraoral examination

If you have been dentally trained then the following section should be familiar to you. This section is primarily for the benefit of those who have not had any formal training in the examination of the mouth.

The examination of the mouth needs to be divided into two main sections: examination of the soft tissues and the hard tissues.

7.1. Soft tissue

The soft tissue examination is essential in the screening and for diagnosing of oral cancer but the examination may also reveal causes of oral pain which are not related to the teeth. There are a number of booklets and videos available on how to do this in a systematic way and most books on the subject of oral medicine will include details on how to carry out a systematic examination of the mouth. The use of two dental mirrors or wooden spatula, gloves and a good light are the basic requirements. Ask your patient to remove any removable appliances such as dentures or orthodontic plates before examining the soft tissues. Mouth piercing is becoming increasingly popular and some of the devices used can lead to dental damage, infection and pain. The examination looks to detect any colour changes such as red, white, brown, purple patches as well as lesions such as ulcers, lumps, blisters. Food substances will stain tissues and can make interpretation difficult and this is especially so in patients who use betel nut products. Interpretation of the findings can be found in textbooks of oral medicine or you can refer your patient to an oral physician or oral surgeon for further advice.

The soft tissue examination is described in Table 4 key facts.

7.2. Hard tissue examination

The hard tissues include not just the teeth and their relationship to the jaws and gingiva, but also the bony elements. The basic hard tissue examination is listed in Table 5 key facts. It is very simple and can be done in a medical environment. It is not essential to count all the teeth but just form an overall picture of the dental health of the patient. Overall oral hygiene gives you an overview of the

---

TABLE 4

KEY FACTS: intraoral soft tissue examination includes the following areas

- Lips upper and lower outer and inner to the buccal sulcus
- Right and left buccal mucosa, stretched and at rest
- Tongue, dorsum, ventral surface, lateral borders
- Floor of mouth and lingual sulci which may require retraction of the tongue
- Palate hard and soft
- Oropharynx, fauces, tonsils, uvula, posterior wall of nasopharynx
- Gingival tissues
- Salivary function: colour, quality and viscosity of saliva
- Presence of odour

---

patients' commitment to dental care. Brushing of teeth will be avoided in areas of pain and in patients with trigeminal neuralgia I have had patients who have been unable to brush one side of the mouth but have maintained good oral hygiene on the other non-painful side of the mouth. The coating of the tongue will give you an indication of the type of foods eaten, i.e. those with less fibre and more milky will result in a white coating. This type of food will be favoured in patients with intra-oral pain. Percussion of teeth (done with the tip of the mirror handle) can elicit tenderness and dullness both of which indicate inflammation. Several teeth must be tested including those presumed healthy. Dentists will carry out more detailed examinations and you can find a description of those in dental undergraduate books.

The mandible and maxilla often need to be examined using radiographs, but palpation of the jaws may elicit cystic or hard swellings and fractures. Maxillary sinus examination is dealt with in Chapter 13 on maxillary sinusitis.

TABLE 5

KEY FACTS: hard tissue examination includes the following

- Number of teeth in each arch
- Lack of teeth in each arch, unerupted, partially erupted, submerged
- Broad assessment of type of occlusion, Classes I, II or III, (primarily relationship of anterior incisors), malocclusion
- State of the teeth: caries (decayed/broken down), broken teeth, roots, wearing down of tooth substance, mobility, tilted teeth, partially erupted, response of teeth to percussion
- Restorations: present amount, e.g. little, moderate, extensive

    Type, e.g. gold, amalgam, composite (white), crowns

    State, e.g. overhangs, margins, wear, fractures, contacts
- Presence of bridges, fixed appliances, removable appliances
- Examine the appliance in and out of the mouth: type, design, age, fit, retention, occlusion, relationship to soft tissue
- Gingival tissues: colour, swelling, abscess, pocketing, recession of gingiva from teeth
- Alveolar ridges: overlying mucosal colour, texture, tenderness, degree of resorption, mobility of mucosa, retained roots
- Overall oral hygiene: presence of plaque, calculus

8. Examination of temporomandibular joint (TMJ) and muscles of mastication

The key TMJ features to be examined are sum-marised in Table 6. The TMD research diagnos-tic criteria (ROC) as proposed by Dworkin and LeResche (1992) are very comprehensive and too time-consuming for everyday practise. This can be found on the internet *www.rdc-tmdinternational.org*. When examining the muscles note any weakness, tenderness and presence of trigger points.

9. Eye

External features which should be examined include the following:

- Lids: symmetry, skin, retraction, ptosis, spasm, inflammation or swelling
- Conjunctiva: inflammation, redness, colour, dis-charge, subconjunctival haemorrhage
- Cornea: opacities, ulcers, abrasions which may need fluorescein eye drops
- Sclera: colour
- Anterior chamber: clarity
- Pupils: equal and reacting to light and accommo-dation
- Lens: opacities, arcus
- Extraocular movements
- State of lubrication
- Orbit position: exophthalmos
- Ophthalmoscopy and slit lamp examination are necessary if the history suggests eye problems
- Assess acuity

A red eye is often painful and some causes can re-sult in loss of vision (glaucoma, acute iritis, corneal ulcers). It is, therefore, important to differentiate these from more easily treated causes such as epis-cleritis, conjunctivitis and conjunctival haemorrhage. Assessment of acuity, state of the cornea and papil-lary reflexes should be sensitive enough to determine whether an urgent specialist opinion is needed. More details on examination of the eyes can be found in textbooks of ophthalmology.

TABLE 6

KEY FACTS: examination of TMJ and its muscles includes

- Measurement of maximum opening from incisive tips of incisors either in mm or fingers, lower limit 35 mm for women, 40 mm for men, lateral excursion is normally 8 mm in either direction
- Assessing the range of movements: right, left, forward
- Opening and closing of the jaw and whether it occurs in a straight line or deviates at any stage
- Listening for joint sounds: if click is heard ascertaining at which stage of opening or closing: early, middle, late
- Determining whether locking occurs and if so whether it is while opening or closing
- Palpation of joint for crepitations and tenderness
- Joint palpation of the lateral wall, posterior wall
- Palpation and testing of function of muscles at their origin and insertion on each side temporalis, masseter, medial and lateral pterygoid
- Looking for trigger spots
- Looking for evidence of bruxism intra orally

---

10. Structured notes

It is the duty of every clinician to ensure that there is a complete set of contemporaneous notes on every patient that has been seen and in Chapter 4 we provide an example of a set of structured history notes. In Appendix A, we include an example of a set of structured notes for examination purposes. Once familiar with a form it should be quick to complete and will ensure that all the basic data are collected. Such a structured examination may not be necessary at each visit but you must remember to update your clinical examination in the same way that the history is updated.

Patients with abnormal history or examination may require referral to an appropriate specialist as the abnormal findings may be incidental and not connected with the original facial pain.

11. Summary

See Table 7 for a summary of this chapter.

TABLE 7

Summary of Chapter 5

---

1. A generalised examination of the face and structures including ears, nose and eyes should be carried out

2. The trigeminal and facial cranial nerves must always be carefully examined. The others should be assessed if the history or general examination warrants it

3. A mini mental state should be done on patients in whom a psychiatric diagnosis is suspected from the history

4. Intraoral examination of hard and soft tissues should be performed

5. The functioning of the TMJ and its muscles should be performed on those with symptoms

6. Any patient with an abnormal examination may need referral to: neurologist, ENT surgeon, ophthalmologist, psychiatrist, oral and maxillofacial surgeon or dentist

---

Appendix A

Example of structured notes for recording examination of the head and neck. See also Appendix A in Chapter 4 for the structured history sheet.

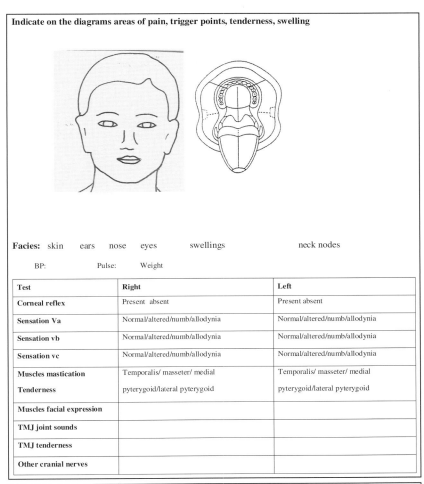

Indicate on the diagrams areas of pain, trigger points, tenderness, swelling

Facies: skin   ears   nose   eyes   swellings   neck nodes

    BP: Pulse: Weight

Test	Right	Left
Corneal reflex	Present absent	Present absent
Sensation Va	Normal/altered/numb/allodynia	Normal/altered/numb/allodynia
Sensation vb	Normal/altered/numb/allodynia	Normal/altered/numb/allodynia
Sensation vc	Normal/altered/numb/allodynia	Normal/altered/numb/allodynia
Muscles mastication **Tenderness**	Temporalis/ masseter/ medial pyterygoid/lateral pyterygoid	Temporalis/ masseter/ medial pyterygoid/lateral pyterygoid
Muscles facial expression		
TMJ joint sounds		
TMJ tenderness		
Other cranial nerves		

Mouth opening *: normal limited*   *cm opening*   *lateral excursion opening   mm*

Mouth opening : deviations - opening   closing   protrusion   to right   to left

Occlusion: Class 1   Class II div i div ii   Class III

Dentition: no teeth full dentition partially erupted teeth   roots   carious teeth

  partial dentition :most anterior teeth top R L bottom R L   most posterior teeth top R L bottom R L

  dentures: partial : top bottom   full: top bottom

Oral Hygiene: good / moderate / poor   periodontal disease: Y   N

  Conservation: *nil   little   extensive   very extensive amalgams composites bridges implants*

Soft tissue: note lesions on diagram

Appendix B. Further reading

Books which include examination of various parts of the face.

B.1. Oral and dental

(1) Birnbaum W, Dunne SM. Oral Diagnosis. The Clinician's Guide. Wright, Oxford, 2000: ISBN 0-7236-1040-1. (A very useful clearly written book on the topic.)

(2) Kidd EAM, Smith BGN. Pickard's Manual of Dentistry. Oxford University Press, Oxford, 6th edn. 1996: ISBN 0-19-262610-8. (A book on the diagnosis and management of hard tissues of the mouth.)

(3) Chestnutt IG, Gibson J (ed). Churchill's Pocketbook of Clinical Dentistry, 2nd edn. Churchill Livingstone, London, 2002: ISBN 0-443-07084-9. (A useful basic text on all aspects of dentistry.)

(4) Turk DC, Melzack R. Handbook of Pain Assessment. Guilford Press, New York, 2001: ISBN 1-57230-488-x. (Chapter 9 facial expressions of pain, chapter 25: orofacial pain.)

B.2. Ear, nose and throat

(5) Ludman H. ABC of Otolaryngology, 4th edn. BMJ Publishing, London, 1997; (Simple text and many illustrations.)

B.3. Neurology

(6) Fuller G. Neurological Examination Made Easy, 2nd edn. Churchill Livingstone, Edinburgh, 1999: ISBN 0443-06166-1 (Plenty of simple illustration to help in doing a neurological examination.)

(7) Ginsberg LD. Lecture Notes in Neurology, 5th edn. Blackwell Science, Oxford, 1999: ISBN 0632048271. (A basic neurology text.)

(8) Warlow C. Handbook of Neurology. Blackwell, Oxford, 1991: ISBN 0632011130. (A more in depth book on neurology.)

B.4. Ophthalmology

(9) Chawla HB. Ophthalmology: A Symptom-Based Approach, 3rd edn. Butterworth-Heinemann, Oxford, 1999. (A very basic approach but clearly illustrated and light-hearted text.)

B.5. General medicine

A wide variety of books are on the market and the following is just an example.

(10) Ballinger A, Patchett S. Saunders' Pocket Essentials of Clinical Medicine, 2nd edn. Saunders, Edinburgh, 2000.

(11) Report of the American Psychiatric Association. Diagnostic and Statistical Manual of Mental Disorders. APA, Washington, DC, 1987.

(12) Report of the American Psychiatric Association. Diagnostic and statistical manual of mental disorders, IV. American Psychiatric Association, New York, 1994.

References

Marked as regards quality according to criteria set by author.
* Case studies, no controls, only evidence.
** Cohort studies, high quality case series with controls.
*** Randomised controlled trials, high quality original studies.

Craig TKJ, Prkachin KM, Grunau RVE. The facial expression of pain. In: Turk DC, Melzack R, editors. Handbook of pain assessment. New York: The Guildford Press, 2001: 153–169.

Davies T. ABC of mental health: mental health assessment. Br Med J 1997; 314: 1536.

Dworkin SF, LeResche L (eds) Research diagnostic criteria for temporomandibular disorders. J Craniomandibul Disord 1992; 6: 301–355.

** Ekman P, Friesen WV. Facial Action Coding System Investigators Guide. Consulting Psychologists Press, Palo Alto, 1978.

** Ekman P, Friesen WV, O'Sullivan M, Chan A, Diacoyanni-Tarlatzis I, Heider K, Krause R, LeCompte WA, Pitcairn T, Ricci-Bitti PE. Universals and cultural differences in the judgments of facial expressions of emotion. J Pers Soc Psychol 1987; 53: 712–717.

Hadjistavropoulos HD, Craig KD, Hadjistavropoulos T, Poole

GD. Subjective judgments of deception in pain expression: accuracy and errors. Pain 1996; 65(2–3): 251–258.

** Hampton JR, Harrison MJ, Mitchell JR, Prichard JS, Seymour C. Relative contributions of history-taking, physical examination, and laboratory investigation to diagnosis and management of medical outpatients. Br Med J 1975; 2: 486–489.

* Kopelman MD. Structured psychiatric interview: psychiatric history and assessment of the mental state. Br J Hosp Med 1994; 52: 93–98.

* LeResche L. Facial expression in pain: a study of candid photographs. J Non Verbal Behav 1982; 7: 46–56

*** LeResche L, Dworkin SF, Wilson L, Ehrlich KJ. Effect of temporomandibular disorder pain duration on facial expressions and verbal report of pain. Pain 1992; 51: 289–295.

* Peterson MC, Holbrook JH, Von Hales D, Smith NL, Staker LV. Contributions of the history, physical examination, and laboratory investigation in making medical diagnoses. West J Med 1992; 156: 163–165.

*** Prkachin KM. The consistency of facial expressions of pain: a comparison across modalities. Pain 1992; 51: 297–306.

*** Prkachin KM, Berzins S, Mercer SR. Encoding and decoding of pain expressions: a judgement study. Pain 1994; 58: 253–259.

* Roshan M, Rao AP. A study on relative contributions of the history, physical examination and investigations in making medical diagnosis. J Assoc Phys India 2000; 48: 771–775.

*** Solomon PE, Prkachin KM, Farewell, V. Enhancing sensitivity to facial expression of pain. Pain 1997; 71: 279–284.

Assessment and Management of Orofacial Pain
Pain Research and Clinical Management, Vol. 14
Edited by J.M. Zakrzewska and S.D. Harrison
© *2002 Elsevier Science B.V. All rights reserved*

CHAPTER 6

Measurement of pain in adults

Toby Newton-John [*]

*Department of Clinical Psychology, Eastman Dental Hospital, Gray's Inn Road, London WC1X 8LD, and
Sub-Department of Clinical Health Psychology, University College London, Gower Street, London WC1E 6BT, UK*

Objectives for this chapter:

This chapter will attempt to show you that:
- The measurement of pain is always influenced by subjective factors, which should be taken into account when interpreting results
- The quality of an assessment tool is determined by its psychometric properties: reliability, validity and sensitivity. Other factors to take into account are whether normative data are available for different populations
- The selection of an assessment tool should be guided by its intended use: as a means of evaluating treatment outcome, to provide descriptive information about a patient group, or for analysis of individual patient presentations
- The assessment of pain is multidimensional, with measurement domains ranging from physical functioning, to psychological disturbance, to the use of coping skills and strategies

1. Introduction

There is scarcely an area of life which can remain impervious to the effects of chronic pain. Social and occupational functioning, leisure activities, domestic chores, relationships with family and friends, the provision of childcare and marital functioning are commonly reported to be adversely affected as a result of living with pain on a daily basis (Skevington, 1995). Equally, these are the domains in which positive changes are expected to be seen when the treatment of pain is successful. This raises issues about how to demonstrate these changes — when

the outcome is not as straightforward as whether the pain is present or absent.

The first aim of this chapter is to discuss the various purposes for which pain assessment is used. It will be seen that the choice of instrument or assessment tool is very much guided by the intention for its use. Secondly, the psychometric issues which should be taken into account as part of the assessment–selection process will be discussed. Finally, each of the primary domains of psychological assessment in pain will be presented, and examples of appropriate instruments within each domain will be highlighted. The emphasis of the data presented will be on the application of measures to facial pain in particular, and a case study used to illustrate the use of various measures with this population. The chapter is necessarily brief; however, if you wish to read further

[*] Tel.: +44-20-7915-2351; Fax: +44-20-7915-1194;
E-mail: toby.newton-john@uclh.org

on this topic, there are excellent texts by Turk and Melzack (2001) and Williams (1995) which offer more comprehensive coverage of the issues covered here.

2. Why measure pain?

Finding a pain clinician who is not hard pressed for time just managing his or her caseload would be a difficult task. Under such time-constrained circumstances, the measurement of pain is usually a simple inquiry of the patient as to whether the pain is better or not. The question of why one would intentionally add to the clinical demands by measuring pain in a more systematic way than just using this dichotomous outcome variable is a valid one.

There are multiple reasons for carrying out some form of standardised pain assessment (Table 1). Firstly, if we are involved in the process of delivering treatment to patients suffering from pain problems it is incumbent upon us to validate our interventions. This textbook is testimony to the importance now given to evidence-based healthcare, as 'gut feelings' or 'clinical experience' are no longer satisfactory methods of assessing treatment efficacy. Having valid and reliable measures of change in patient functioning from pre-treatment to post-treatment, and over some length of follow-up, is becoming increasingly recognised as an essential component of the treatment process.

Secondly, psychometric assessments can provide invaluable information with which to add to the routine clinical interview. Important constructs such as health locus of control and self-efficacy, which are known to influence treatment adherence and outcome, can be rapidly assessed with minimal effort. The fact that patients can complete questionnaires prior to attending the first appointment means that the clinician can amass a considerable amount of knowledge about an individual before they enter the office. Finally, standardised assessments offer a means of describing the population of patients that are seen in the particular service in a meaningful way. The reasons for assessing pain in a structured way are therefore multifactorial.

3. How is pain measured?

Notwithstanding the extent to which medical technology has advanced in the last decade, particularly with regard to body imaging and scanning techniques, pain remains an entirely subjective phenomenon. It cannot be 'shown' on any scan or investigation (although recent work examining cortical activity and pain appears promising, e.g. Derbyshire, 2000). We can therefore rely only upon the patient's report of pain to determine its existence.

The assessment of pain is most commonly conducted through self-report questionnaires. The advantages of this method are clear: patient data can be obtained rapidly from large numbers of individuals, and specific constructs can be focused upon for analysis. Questionnaires should not require complex instructions for patients to complete, and can be scored easily — although the interpretation of the score is not necessarily so straightforward, as will be discussed.

However, the assessment of pain through self-report questionnaires is by no means the only methodology available. A systematic method for observing and quantifying the frequency of pain-related behaviours, such as grimacing, groaning or holding the head or neck has been developed (Keefe and Block, 1982). The examination of health care usage in terms of number of physician visits due to pain, or the quantity of medication consumed for

---

TABLE 1

KEY FACTS: why measure pain and associated characteristics?

1. To enable you to evaluate your intervention

2. To obtain detailed information about your patient

3. To compare your patient with other patients from a similar population

4. To monitor your patient's progress over time

pain, will also provide objective data about the patient's level of function. Furthermore, including the patient's spouse or significant other in the assessment can provide important information about the impact of the pain on relationship and family functioning, which may have important treatment ramifications (Turk et al., 1985).

However, self-report questionnaires are by far and away the most common format in which to collect health outcome data, because of their convenience and expediency. The remainder of this chapter will therefore focus on this format of measurement.

4. Psychometric considerations when selecting a pain measure

The psychometric profile of a given assessment measure refers to the degree to which the instrument actually measures what it professes to, and whether it can do this reliably and sensitively. There are two points worth bearing in mind when considering assessment issues. Firstly, scores derived from self-report questionnaires are just that — numbers that are assigned a significance for the purposes of understanding a given construct. They do not directly assess that construct, they are only an attempt to represent it. Secondly, simply giving a questionnaire a certain title does not guarantee that this is what is being measured. Hence a measure labelled The Pain-Related Quality of Life Scale may not in fact be measuring quality of life at all, but assess health beliefs or anxiety symptoms or some other variable. The psychometric support for any research tool is therefore extremely important, and the following issues should be considered.

4.1. Validity

Validity broadly refers to the accuracy with which a measure assesses the construct in question. There are various forms of validity, including construct validity, content validity and predictive validity (Saw and Ng, 2001), depending upon the aspect of the assessment being considered. However, all forms rely upon a comparison of the measure in question with a 'gold standard', to determine how closely the two measures correlate. For example, the criterion validity of a new depression questionnaire might be determined by comparing questionnaire scores with the judgement of an experienced psychiatrist in diagnosing depressive illness. As there is no such external standard by which to judge the validity of pain assessment, construct validity is used. Here, the measure is evaluated against a number of theoretically related indices to determine its validity, such as mood, physical function, analgesic use, heart rate or blood pressure levels. Predictive validity is concerned with the accuracy of the assessment tool in forecasting subsequent outcomes. For example, the predictive validity of the Pain Self-Efficacy Questionnaire (see Section 7) was demonstrated by showing that patients scoring below a certain point were significantly at risk of drop out from a multidisciplinary pain management programme (Coughlan et al., 1995).

4.2. Reliability

Reliability is the extent to which you would obtain the same result if you were to administer the same measure again to the same person (or group of people) under the same circumstances. The most straightforward assessment of this is test–retest reliability: the measure is given on two separate occasions to the same cohort of subjects, and the degree to which the results are stable is computed. Certain constructs would not be expected to vary much across time, such as beliefs about the aetiology of a pain complaint (prior to the instigation of treatment), whereas pain intensity measures would not necessarily have high test–retest reliability because of expected variation from day to day. One of the indices of reliability most commonly reported in health journals is Cronbach's alpha (α). This refers to the internal consistency of the measure — the degree to which each of the individual items relate to each other. High internal consistency indicates that all items are assessing a similar construct, but offers no information about accuracy of the assessment.

TABLE 2

KEY FACTS: what to look for when considering a pain measure

1. Validity: does the test truly measure what it purports to measure

2. Reliability: are all the items within the test measuring the same construct, and will the test give the same result if repeated on different occasions

3. Sensitivity and specificity: how accurately and exclusively does the test identify the characteristic you are interested in

4.3. Sensitivity and specificity

Where the purpose of a measure is to detect the presence of a certain construct in a population, for example the prevalence of Post Traumatic Stress Disorder (PTSD) in a chronic pain patient group, it is important to know the accuracy rate with which the measure achieves this. Sensitivity refers to this accuracy — how many patients who truly have PTSD are classified as such by the measure. Specificity on the other hand refers to the probability that the measure correctly identifies those who do not have the trait in question. A measure is of little use if it has very high sensitivity but low specificity, as it will then be classifying all subjects as possessing the trait of interest. These tests offer an additional means of determining the usefulness of a given assessment tool.

Points to take into consideration when considering a pain measure are listed in Table 2

5. Contextual factors in psychosocial assessment of pain

The psychometric issues discussed above are matters which pertain to the quality of the instrument being used. However, an accurate interpretation of assessment results does not depend solely on the reliability and validity of the measure itself. Evidence has also indicated that the context in which the as-

sessment is carried out can powerfully influence the results that are obtained. For example, Levine and De Simone (1991) showed that the sex of the experimenter can influence pain intensity reports. Using an acute pain tolerance paradigm, male subjects withstood a noxious stimulus for a longer duration when the experimenter was female rather than male; the experimenter's sex made little difference for female subjects. The physical environment is also a factor, as the study of Dworkin and Chen (1982) demonstrated. They found that tooth pulp stimulation conducted in a dental clinic, with the associated anxiety-provoking cues of a dental setting, was reported to be more painful than when conducted in a research laboratory. Equally, a pain patient who feels believed and understood by his or her physician is in a better position to respond accurately during an assessment (see Chapter 9). Displays of pain behaviour during an assessment interview such as grimacing and sighing (Keefe and Block, 1982) tend to escalate as patients feel less understood.

Having covered the basic psychometric and contextual issues which need to be considered as part of the assessment process, it is now possible to outline the range of measures that are commonly used in pain research and clinical work.

6. Domains of assessment

Because pain itself is multidimensional, its assessment is equally wide-ranging. Table 3 illustrates the various domains of assessment that are typically covered. At the first level, you have the choice between a 'multiaxial' pain questionnaire which covers a range of different areas within the one questionnaire, or choosing individual measures to address specific areas.

6.1. Multiaxial questionnaires

As discussed in Chapter 4, there are a range of multiaxial instruments available each with differing degrees of detail and complexity (Table 4). The Sickness Impact Profile (Bergner et al., 1981) is a 136-

TABLE 3

Domains of psychosocial assessment in chronic pain

- Severity of pain: intensity, quality

- Emotional functioning: depression, anxiety, anger

- Coping skills: cognitive and behavioural pain management strategies

- Personality: stable traits associated with chronic pain

- Beliefs about pain: self-efficacy, catastrophising, future health status

- Physical disability: self-reported disability, objectively tested

- Family factors: spouse responses to pain behaviours, marital satisfaction

- Health care usage: medication, clinical attendances

item inventory which assesses the extent to which health problems interfere with physical and psychosocial functioning. It offers considerable detail, and may be conceptualised as a quality of life measure, but the scoring system is somewhat complex and it is time-consuming to complete and to score. By contrast, the Medical Outcome Study 36-Item Short Form Health Survey (SF-36; Ware and Sherbourne, 1992) is much briefer and also offers assessments of physical and social functioning, of mental health status, and of the limitations in roles due to physical and emotional disturbance. A particular strength of the SF-36 is its age- and sex-based normative data, which have been derived from US population surveys. However, concerns have been raised that the measure is too broad and not sufficiently sensitive to treatment effects following pain management interventions (Battie and May, 2001). The issue of questionnaire sensitivity is particularly relevant in the case of facial pain, as the SF-36 contains items such as the ability to climb stairs, walk more than a mile or problems with bathing and dressing. These kinds of mobility-related questions are unlikely to reflect the difficulties experienced by facial pain sufferers (see Section 6.4).

The measure which has dominated much of the psychological literature on chronic pain has been the West-Haven Yale Multidimensional Pain Inventory (MPI; Kerns et al., 1985). Its 56 items are arranged into three sections, which include measures of pain severity and interference and perceived life control, the response of the spouse or significant other to pain behaviours, and an activity level scale. It too has norms for a range of different ages and pain conditions (including TMD), and has been extensively psychometrically validated (Riley et al., 1999). The activity scale is especially useful — rather than documenting 'disability' or 'impairment' as in the other questionnaires, an index of how often patients engage in a range of daily activities (work in the garden, visit friends, go to a movie) is geared more towards pain treatment outcome. In support of its use with facial pain, Dahlstrom et al. (1997) showed that the subgroup classifications observed in chronic back pain patients ('adaptive coper', 'interpersonally distressed', 'dysfunctional') could be replicated in a sample of TMD patients. Rudy et al. (1994) also demonstrated the utility of the MPI as a index of treatment outcome in TMD. The MPI showed that patients receiving biofeedback made more significant longer term improvements than those receiving splint therapy.

A further option is the increasingly widely used, the Brief Pain Inventory (BPI; Cleeland, 1989), which was originally developed as a cancer pain assessment tool. The BPI uses 0–10 numerical rating scales to assess the interference of pain with mood, walking, general activity, work, relations with others, sleep and enjoyment of life. It can be administered and scored rapidly, has been translated in several languages, and has been used with chronic pain conditions such as Chronic Regional Pain Syndrome (Galer et al., 2001) and low back pain (Lin, 1998). It has not been evaluated for use with facial pain as yet. However, it has become the measure on which the Pain Audit Collection System (PACS; Weston King, 2000) database has been developed for use in pain clinics throughout the UK. This computerised database offers a user-friendly way of monitoring activity and outcome of pain clinics using standard pain relief procedures. It requires minimal computer power and familiarity, and is constantly being up-

TABLE 4

KEY FACTS: common multiaxial pain questionnaires

Name	No. of items	Comments
Sickness Impact Profile (SIP)	136	Lengthy and complex to score; broad coverage of areas; widely used in chronic pain research
Short Form Health Survey (SF36)	36	Plentiful normative data; may not be sufficiently sensitive for chronic facial pain assessment
Multidimensional Pain Inventory (MPI)	56	The 'gold standard' in many ways — strong psychometrics, norms, coping profiles available
Brief Pain Inventory (BPI)	10	Useful tool when time and resources are limited; however, the data obtained are also limited
Pain Audit Collection System (PACS)	10+	New UK developed audit and research tool; computerised data collection; nationwide database

dated and revised by the authors. The PACS package can be obtained free of charge by contacting the authors directly (*admin@westonking.com*).

Moving on from these global assessments of physical, emotional and social functioning, there are a host of individualised measures based on the domains listed in Table 4. Although presented separately for the purposes of clarity, it is important to remember that these constructs often overlap. For example, measures of pain catastrophising (see below) share common variance with general anxiety scales such as the Hospital Anxiety and Depression Scale (Zigmond and Snaith, 1983), and with specific measures of pain-related anxiety such as the Pain Anxiety Symptom Scale (McCraken et al., 1992). The choice of assessment tool in these circumstances depends upon which aspect of the construct is of most interest.

6.2. Pain intensity and quality

The simplest and most common methods for measuring the severity of pain are via Numerical Rating Scales (NRS) or Visual Analogue Scales (VRS). The NRS asks patients to record the number which best represents their pain intensity on a 0–10 or 0–100 scale, where $0 = no\ pain$, $10/100 = pain\ as\ bad\ as$ *it could be*. A VAS consists of a line, usually 10 cm long, whose end points are labelled as above. The patient is asked to indicate which point along the line best represents their pain level, with the distance from the no pain end to the patient's mark becoming the pain score.

Both of these forms of pain intensity measurement have much to commend them. They are intelligible to the majority of patients, they are simple to administer and score, and there is good evidence of their validity and sensitivity to treatment effects (Jensen and Karoly, 2001). Moreover, a NRS may be administered over the telephone, increasing its applicability.

However, despite their apparent straightforwardness, neither method has avoided criticism. Williams et al. (2000) used qualitative data analytic techniques to reveal the inconsistency that is inherent with these recording systems. Patients do not tend to use the upper end points of a NRS of VAS, making them logarithmic rather than linear scales. As noted in the paper, there is considerable idiosyncratic variation in the use of the scales to reflect internal sensations. Hence an 8/10 rating for one patient was labelled as 'average everyday pain', whereas the same rating for another patient was labelled as 'barely tolerable'. Jensen and Karoly (2001) have also questioned the ratio properties of the NRS, such that a decrease in pain from 60 to 30 does not necessarily indicate that the perceived pain intensity had halved.

A dissatisfaction with unidimensional ratings of pain such as VAS or NRS, which imply that pain can be satisfactorily measured with a single item, led to the development of the McGill Pain Questionnaire (MPQ; Melzack, 1975, 1987). The MPQ is an assessment of pain quality, as much as pain intensity, by utilising 20 sets of pain descriptors such as 'pricking', 'boring' or 'stabbing'. The later version of the MPQ contains only 15 descriptors in order to reduce administration and scoring time. There are between three and six descriptors in each set and, as each descriptor is rank ordered, the sum of the rank values becomes the overall pain rating index.

The MPQ is one of the most widely used pain assessment tools in both clinical and research settings, and has been translated into 19 different languages. It discriminates between the sensory, affective and evaluative aspects of the pain experience, and research has demonstrated the diagnostic utility of the descriptor choices. For example, Melzack et al. (1986) showed that the MPQ correctly classified 91% of trigeminal neuralgia versus 'atypical' facial pain patients. Hall et al. (1986) showed that temporomandibular joint dysfunction patients chose significantly different descriptors from patients with pain of periodontal or pulpal origin. And Turp et al. (1997) also found that the choice of descriptors distinguished chronic facial pain patients from patients suffering from other chronic pain disorders, such as cancer or chronic back pain. Facial pain patients tended to select 'radiating' and 'pressing' with a greater frequency than the other groups.

However, one of the limitations of the MPQ that I have encountered is the level of language ability that is required of patients in order to complete it accurately. For example, patients must be familiar with the terms 'lancinating', 'rasping' and 'searing', and be able to evaluate them against their own internal sensations. You can see some examples of these in Chapter 15 which were collected at a secondary care facial pain clinic. In deciding whether or not to use the MPQ you must consider whether the bulk of your patient population is capable of making these discriminations.

An interesting recent development in this assessment areas is the Leeds Assessment of Neuropathic Symptoms and Signs (LANSS; Bennett, 2001), which consists of a brief self-report pain questionnaire (five items) and a brief sensory testing examination (two items). The aim of the measure is to estimate the probability that neuropathic mechanisms are contributing to the chronic pain experienced by the patient, and it achieves this with an 83% sensitivity and an 87% specificity.

6.3. Pain affect

It has been established that there are conceptual and empirical differences between pain intensity and pain affect (Jensen and Karoly, 2001). Pain intensity refers to how much the individual hurts, whereas pain affect refers to the emotional arousal or distress that is generated by the pain. As noted above, one of the strengths of the MPQ is the ability to separate these two dimensions into Sensory and Affective subscales. However, it is possible to utilise a NRS or VAS for the same purpose by choosing appropriate wording, and thereby capture more of the multidimensional nature of the pain experience. Therefore, in addition to inquiring about pain intensity, the items detailed in Table 5 can be modified to include the question "How *distressing* is/was your pain right now/on average?"

TABLE 5

Simple pain intensity measurements

Visual analogue scale

No pain   Pain as bad as it could be

Numerical rating scale

On a scale from 0 to 100 where 0 means 'no pain', and 100 means 'pain as bad as it could be', please indicate in the space below the number that best describes your pain

(a) How intense is your pain right now/on average. . . . . . .

6.4. Physical function

The extent to which physical mobility or functioning (self-care, activities of daily living, social activities etc.) is compromised by pain is one of the most important elements of the assessment battery. It is often the domain which has the most face validity for the patients themselves, as it points to the ways in which the pain has changed their daily lives. As stated at the beginning of this chapter, one of the overriding aims of the standardised assessment is to identify areas to target in treatment. There are three broad domains of assessment regarding pain and physical functioning (Table 6), and these will be discussed in turn.

6.4.1. General disability

One might expect that the effect of facial pain on physical functioning would be qualitatively and quantitatively different from that observed in other chronically painful conditions such as musculoskeletal back pain or fibromyalgia. While limitations in sitting, standing, walking and bending are characteristic of the latter disorders (Harding et al., 1994), patients with chronic facial pain would not necessarily be expected to suffer these difficulties. Hence the appropriateness of generic disability measures that are used with heterogeneous pain patients might be open to question. Yet the evidence indicates that such measures may be reasonably used with facial pain patients. For example, the Pain Disability Index (PDI; Pollard, 1984) is a 7-item self-report questionnaire assessing the degree to which the respondent feels disabled by pain in seven life areas: recreation, family/home responsibilities, sexual activity, occupational functioning, social activity, self-care and life-supporting activities such as eating and sleeping. Bush and Harkins (1995) explored the factor structure of the PDI in a sample of 272 orofacial pain patients and found minimal differences from those observed in musculoskeletal pain patients, indicating the validity of the measure for a facial pain population. Furthermore, Auerbach et al. (2001) showed that following treatment for TMD, the PDI scores of patients demonstrated clinically significant improve-

---

TABLE 6

KEY FACTS: varieties of assessment of physical functioning

1. Self-report of general disability, e.g Pain Disability Index, MPI Activity scale

2. Self-report of facial pain-related disability, e.g. Mandibular Function Impairment Questionnaire

3. Observer assessment of disability, e.g. mouth opening

---

ments. The Multidimensional Pain Inventory (MPI; see above) has also been shown to be a valid measure for use with TMD patients.

6.4.2. Facial pain-related disability

However, specific measures of facial pain-related disability have also been developed. The Graded Chronic Pain Scale (Von Korff et al., 1992) has a facial pain modification which seeks to distinguish between pain intensity and the disability that is associated with the pain (see Chapter 9). The Mandibular Function Impairment Questionnaire (Stegenga et al., 1993) is a 17-item measure consisting of two subscales assessing masticatory and non-masticatory jaw disability. Kropmans et al. (1999) confirmed adequate test–retest reliability for the measure; however, Turner et al. (2001) found a high correlation ($r = 0.69$) between the subscales suggesting significant amounts of shared variance.

Perhaps the most intensively psychometrically investigated facial pain disability measure is the Oral Health Impact Profile (OHIP; Slade, 1997). It contains 14 items in which the respondent is asked how often in the past month have they have experienced difficulties with pronunciation, discomfort in eating, feelings of embarrassment or self-consciousness, problems with diet, and so on. Slade (1997) showed that the measure had high internal consistency and construct validity, and more recently Allen et al. (2001) confirmed the clinical sensitivity of the OHIP in detecting pretreatment to post-treatment changes. Unlike the more general measures of pain disability, the OHIP addresses the issue of social anxiety which can be a significant factor in the psychological profiles of chronic facial pain patients (Feinmann, 1999). Patients who experience difficulties in relation to eating, smiling and talking in public because of pain are at some risk of developing anxiety disorders which can require treatment in their own right.

TMD-specific self-report measures have also been developed (e.g. TMJ Scale; Levitt et al., 1994), and used to document the natural history of the disorder. Contrasting TMD patients who received treatment (splint therapy, physical therapy, counselling, and/or non-steroidal anti-inflammatory medications) with a group who declined treatment, Brown and Gaudet (1994) showed that the untreated group continued to experience pain and disability over time, rather than spontaneously improving as had been suggested. In an interesting progression in the nature of assessment, Yap et al. (2001) have also reported the development of a computerised system for assessing disability related to TMD problems.

6.4.3. Objective disability assessment

Aside from the self-report of disability, mouth opening measurement has been employed as an objective outcome measure (e.g. Turner et al., 2001). By measuring the distance in millimetres between the edges of the maxillary and mandibular central incisors, a further index of impairment can be obtained which provides additional information about function.

6.5. Emotional functioning

The fact that chronic pain can and often does interfere with most aspects of an individual's life suggests that a measure of emotional functioning will also be important component of the standardised assessment. Prevalence rates for depression in chronic pain populations are considered to be as high as 50% (Banks and Kerns, 1996), and facial pain patients suffering from elevated levels of mood disturbance do not benefit from treatment as much as those whose mood has not been compromised (Riley et al., 1999). Clearly there is a need to identify those patients in whom affective distress is a significant part of their clinical presentation.

6.5.1. Depression

However, a number of authors have commented on the inherent difficulty in the assessment of depression in chronic pain patients (e.g. Banks and Kerns, 1996; Williams, 1998) because of the somatic symptom overlap. Core depressive symptoms such as sleep disturbance, impaired concentration, and loss of energy are also frequently part of the chronic pain constellation of symptoms, and therefore do not necessarily constitute mood disturbance in a chronic pain sufferer. Korszun and Ship (1997) have also commented on this confound in chronic facial pain. Unfortunately, as the majority of self-report questionnaires assessing depression were developed and normed using non-pain patient populations, there is a risk of scores being artificially inflated due to symptom overlap.

Despite the fact that the Beck Depression Inventory (BDI; Beck et al., 1961) was normed on psychiatric patients and therefore suffers from the confounding referred to above, it remains the most widely used self-report measure of depression in the pain field and there is a vast literature upon which to draw (Beck et al., 1988). It contains 21 items rated on a 0–3 scale and includes a question about suicidal ideation which is often clinically useful. However, interpretation of the total score must be done carefully. While Beck and colleagues recommend a score of 10 as the cut-off for depression in the physically healthy population (Beck et al., 1988), a more recent predictive study of mood disorder in chronic pain suggested that 21 was the optimal cut-off score (Geisser et al., 1997).

An alternative is the Hospital Anxiety and Depression Scale (HADS; Zigmond and Snaith, 1983), which was specifically developed for use with medical and surgical patients, and does not contain items pertaining to somatic symptoms to avoid the confounding issue. Both measures are have been used to evaluate depressive symptoms in chronic facial pain (e.g. McNeil et al., 2001; Turner et al., 2001), and found to be suitably sensitive. In terms of their clinical usefulness, the HADS does not contain any cognitive items of depression which makes it less valuable in the clinic in my opinion. It may give a depression score uncontaminated by pain symptoms, but we have no idea what the patient is depressed about or why.

6.5.2. Anxiety

Aside from depression, it is anxiety that has attracted the most research interest in terms of understanding the affective dimensions of chronic pain. Perhaps stemming from the well-documented relationship between anxiety and dental treatment in general (Gatchel, 1989) anxiety has also been explored in some detail in chronic facial pain (Madland et al., 2000; McNeil et al., 2001). Measures such as the anxiety subscale from the HADS mentioned above, or the Spielberger State-Trait Anxiety Inventory (Spielberger, 1983) provide global evaluations of patient anxiety, but little in the way of specific information concerning the nature of their anxiety. Pain-specific assessment tools, such as the Pain Anxiety Symptom Scale (McCraken et al., 1992) or the Fear of Pain Questionnaire (McNeil et al., 2001) offer more information about the anxiety itself. For example, McNeil et al. (2001) showed that whilst fear of pain was a significant feature in their sample of chronic facial pain patients when compared to a group of age- and sex-matched healthy controls, there were no differences between the groups in other aspects of their psychological functioning (depression, anxiety concerning dental treatment).

6.5.3. Anger

Less well researched but equally important is the issue of anger in chronic pain (Fernandez and Turk, 1995). Pain patients may express angry feelings for a variety of reasons — the failure of the health system to provide a cure for the pain, their frustration at the effect the pain has had on their lives, and their irritation with the medical/legal/benefits systems which can appear to be undermining their efforts to cope with their situation. The clinical importance of anger was demonstrated by Burns et al. (1998), who showed that patient anger expression can significantly influence treatment outcome from multi-

disciplinary pain management, particularly amongst male chronic pain patients. Male chronic pain patients who tended to suppress their anger made fewer improvements in depression and general activities scores, whereas improvements in lifting capacity were negatively correlated with anger expression.

The most commonly used self-report anger measure is the Spielberger Anger Expression Scale (Spielberger, 1988), which has subscales of anger expression and anger suppression to discriminate between how often anger is experienced versus it being communicated or expressed. Okifuji et al. (1999) have adapted a Targets of Anger Scale for use with chronic pain patients, which assesses current anger towards nine specific targets including the person who caused the injury (if relevant), health care providers, the employer and the self. In a sample of 96 heterogeneous chronic pain patients, Okifuji et al. (1999) found that the intensity of anger overall was significantly related to pain intensity, depression levels and the extent of perceived disability, further highlighting the importance of this variable in assessment.

Common measures of emotional functioning can be seen in Table 7.

6.6. Personality assessment

The assessment of personality in relation to chronic pain has been a much discussed and highly controversial area (Gamsa, 1994; Vendrig, 2000). Psychoanalytic perspectives of pain posited that psychological disturbances could be displaced onto the body in individuals where bodily pain was seen to be less threatening than acknowledging emotional pain (Merskey and Spear, 1967). Engel (1959) suggested that a 'pain-prone personality' could be reliably detected, and would be distinguished by a number of features including conscious (or unconscious) guilt, and an unfulfilled aggressive drive state. The development of the original Minnesota Multiphasic Personality Inventory (MMPI) in the 1940s provided a means of investigating the association between chronic pain and personality structure. The so-called conversion-V profile, with elevated scores on the Hypochondriasis and Hysteria scales but a low score

TABLE 7

KEY FACTS: common measures of emotional functioning

Name	No. of items	Comments
Beck Depression Inventory	21	Most widely used depression scale; simple administration; confound with pain symptoms
Hospital Anxiety and Depression Scale	14 (7 in each scale)	Avoids confound but perhaps less clinically useful
Spielberger State-Trait Anxiety Inventory	40	Global anxiety scale; gives measure of both current and general anxiety levels
Pain Anxiety Symptom Scale	55	Lengthy; some items reverse scored; relates primarily to chronic pains
Fear of Pain Questionnaire	30	Contains scales relevant to acute dental procedures as well as chronic pains; less widely used
Spielberger Anger Expression Scale	24	Discriminates between anger experienced and anger expressed to others; little use in chronic facial pain

on Depression (indicating a denial of emotional disturbance) was originally considered to be a defining characteristic of the 'functional' as opposed to organic chronic pain patient.

A large amount of research has since been conducted using the MMPI in chronic pain (Vendrig, 2000), and the scale has also been revised (MMPI-2; Butcher et al., 1989) to remove outdated items and improve the psychometric properties. In general, the literature does not support the notion that chronic pain patients display any consistent, identifiable personality profile (Gamsa, 1994), or that the assessment of personality has much value in terms of predicting treatment outcome for chronic pain patients (Bradley and McKendree-Smith, 2001). The specific application of the MMPI to facial pain patients has not proven to be any more useful. Graff-Radford and Solberg (1993) explored the personality characteristics of atypical odontalgia patients and found all means on all subscales to be within normal limits. Steed (1998) found that treatment outcome for TMD patients was independent of their MMPI score profiles. Given that the questionnaire contains over 500 items, many of which suffer from the contamination with physical symptoms discussed above, there are many other assessment tools with stronger claims for evaluating psychological functioning in chronic pain.

As an alternative, the Symptom Checklist-90 Revised (SCL-90R; Derogatis, 1983) is a briefer measure of psychological disturbance, asking patients to rate to what extent each of the 90 psychiatric or physical symptoms has bothered them in the past week. Subscales include Interpersonal Sensitivity, Paranoid Ideation, Phobic Anxiety and Somatisation; however, there is a Global Severity Index which provides an overall measure of psychological distress. The SCL-90R is widely used in psychiatric settings but the factor structure has not been widely supported when it has been applied to chronic pain patients (Bradley and McKendree-Smith, 2001). Again, you need to consider whether a psychometric tool which has been developed and normed on an inpatient psychiatric population is the most appropriate assessment device for your purposes.

7. Pain beliefs

One of the most intriguing clinical aspects of pain management is observing differences in patient responses to pain. On being given exactly the same information about managing 'flare-ups' of pain, one individual will immediately begin to use gentle stretch and relaxation whereas another will continue to take large numbers of pain killers and lie prone for hours at a time. Cognitive behavioural theory suggests that the difference in the observed behaviour of two such patients (movement versus immobility; active versus passive coping) can be traced back to differences in their cognitive representations of the pain. In other words, differences in how each of these individuals interprets their pain and their capacity to exert influence over it. Patient beliefs or cognitions about pain are of central importance in understanding the emotional and behavioural consequences of the problem: as DeGood and Tait (2001) have stated, "Maladaptive cognitions can lie at the heart of the chronic pain problem" (p. 321).

Given the importance of pain beliefs in understanding patient adjustment, and the sheer broadness of the topic itself, many different instruments have been developed for examining pain beliefs and attitudes. The interested reader is referred to comprehensive overviews by DeGood and Tait (2001) and Skevington (1995); however, several cognitive domains will be discussed here.

Self-efficacy refers to the personal conviction that one can successfully perform certain behaviours in a specific situation. The Pain Self-Efficacy Scale (Nicholas, 1989) is a 10-item questionnaire asking about the respondent's confidence to carry out a range of different activities (socialising, household chores, coping without pain medication) despite ongoing pain. Low self-efficacy has been shown to predict drop-out from pain management for chronic low back pain (Coughlan et al., 1995); however, its value has not yet been explored in relation to chronic facial pain.

By contrast, catastrophising is a pain cognition that has been investigated in a range of chronic pain disorders including chronic facial pain. Catastrophising has been defined as "expecting or worrying about major negative consequences from a situation, even one of minor importance" (Turner et al., 2000, p. 116). The catastrophising subscale from the Coping Strategies Questionnaire (Rosensteil and Keefe, 1983) is the standard catastrophising measure, and the psychometric properties of the scale have been well established (Jensen et al., 1991; Robinson et al., 1997). It assesses the frequency of thoughts when in pain such as "It is awful and I feel that it overwhelms me" and "I worry all the time about whether it will end". Turner et al. (2001) found that catastrophising accounted for significant proportions of the variance in activity interference, jaw activity limitation and depression scores in a sample of 118 TMD patients. Madland et al. (2000) also demonstrated the importance of catastrophising in facial pain, in showing that both anxiety and depressive mood could be predicted by the frequency of catastrophic cognitions. Following successful treatment for chronic pain, patients show significant reductions in their tendency to catastrophise about their pain (Jensen et al., 2001), further highlighting the salience of this construct in the adjustment to pain.

Jensen et al. (1987) developed perhaps the most wide-ranging of the contemporary pain cognitions scales, the Survey of Pain Attitudes (SOPA). It contains seven treatment-oriented subscales which include beliefs about perceived physical disability, the degree of personal control over pain, the relationship between exercise and physical damage, and the likelihood of a medical cure for the pain. The original 57-item scale is lengthy, and with a number of items reverse scored to prevent response bias it can be cumbersome to use. However, a short form has been developed without any loss of psychometric quality (Jensen et al., 2000a,b). One of the newer areas of pain cognition assessment has been the application of the transtheoretical stages of change model to pain evaluation (Kerns et al., 1997). Originally developed to assess readiness to enter drug rehabilitation programmes, the stages of change model is being used here to determine preparedness for adopting cognitive behavioural self-management pain strategies. There has been considerable debate about whether a self-report questionnaire is capable of quantifying such a multifactorial, fluid notion (Jensen et al., 2000a,b); however, identifying patients in the initial 'precontemplation' phase has been shown to be of some value in predicting treatment outcome (e.g. Biller et al., 2000).

As a final point, it must be recognised that from a cognitive theory standpoint, an individual's beliefs about his or her pain do not exist in a cognitive vacuum. Those beliefs form a subset within a larger domain of beliefs termed the 'cognitive triad' (Beck et al., 1979) relating to the self, the world and the future. There is a reciprocal influence between these more global sets of assumptions and those specifically relating to pain, which can have important clinical ramifications. For example, if an individual holds a general (dysfunctional) assumption that "Nothing I do ever turns out properly. I can never do anything right", he or she is at an immediate disadvantage when facing the challenge of a pain management programme. Equally, a strongly held general belief that "Effort is always rewarded in life" is likely to have a positive bearing upon this form of treatment.

8. Treatment goals

Whilst all of the measures discussed to this point have their particular uses, they do not tell us anything about a fundamental aspect of clinical assessment: what does the patient hope to gain from treatment? This question is extremely important given that the obvious treatment objective — a rapid and permanent cure of the pain — is unfortunately an unlikely treatment outcome for the majority of the chronic facial pain cases that we see. By finding out what the patient would consider to be a useful outcome from treatment other than this, we can tailor our intervention to their needs more effectively. This should result in more expedient service delivery, and in greater patient satisfaction with treatment.

With this in mind, the Pain Management Goals Questionnaire (Newton-John, 2000) was developed (see Chapter 11). It contains 12 different treatment outcomes, encompassing functional activity (e.g. 'Returning to work', 'Carrying out more household chores'), social activity (e.g. 'Feeling less self-conscious in public') and emotional functioning (e.g. 'Feeling less depressed'). It also specifically addresses doctor–patient interactions, by including items regarding satisfaction with communication with the doctor, and satisfaction with knowledge about the pain complaint. Concerns about the pain being a sign of more sinister pathology are also

addressed. Respondents rate each item according to its importance to them, from 'very important' to 'doesn't apply'. The measure has yet to be psychometrically validated, but initial findings have been positive (Atkin et al., 2002). A pilot sample of 33 chronic facial pain patients rated the items concerning doctor–patient communication as highly as the ratings given to more practical issues such as remaining at work or decreasing pain medications. These results reinforce the notion that effective treatment involves much more than the type of drug prescribed or the procedure carried out.

9. Case study

The following cases in Table 8 illustrate how psychometric tests can be used to identify different characteristics in patients suffering from chronic facial pain. By identifying those differences early in the treatment process, the interventions can target the salient issues for a patient more expediently.

10. Conclusion

The plethora of methods and measures for assessing pain can be off-putting for clinicians seeking to construct their own assessment battery for use in their pain service. The sheer number of different instruments that have been developed reflects the multifaceted nature of pain itself, and also the fact that no measure is ideal. There has been and will continue to be an ongoing search to refine or improve existing assessment tools in order to overcome some of the biases and limitations that were referred to at the outset of the chapter. Nevertheless, I hope that you now have some further understanding of the principle issues involved in the psychosocial assessment of pain. There is, however, an overriding consideration to bear in mind as you begin to develop your assessment battery. Irrespective of the particular measure that you select, a score on a questionnaire has little meaning if it is interpreted independently of the context in which it was obtained. By combining psychometrically sound data with an awareness of

TABLE 8

Case study

Patient 1: Mrs. S.	Mrs. S. is a 64-year-old woman with an 18-month history of trigeminal neuralgia. She is married, has three grown up children, and retired from her secretarial job 4 years previously. She has been given an array of different medications for her pain, but has not obtained much benefit from any and experienced various side effects including constipation and drowsiness.
Patient 2: Ms. A.	Ms. A. is a 35-year-old woman with a 5-year history of TMD. She has constant pain in her jaws, neck and shoulders, and has had numerous treatments for this over the years, including mobilisations, ultrasound, a bite-raising appliance and cranial osteopathy. She now avoids chewing hard foods and yawning where possible. She works full-time as a solicitor, and is aware that her activity levels have diminished over the last 3 years.

Both patients were given the same assessment battery, and obtained the following results. How would you interpret them? Please see Table 10 at the end of the chapter for an interpretation.

Measure	Mrs. S.	Ms. A.
McGill Pain Questionnaire		
Present pain intensity	4/5	4/5
Sensory subclass	31/42	24/42
Affective subclass	6/14	12/14
Beck Depression Inventory	16/63	26/63
Oral Health Impact Profile	23/64	40/64
Pain Disability Index	18/70	27/70
Pain Management Goals Questionnaire		
Items rated very important	(b), (h), (l)	(a), (c), (d), (g),

the circumstances in which it was obtained, a careful and thorough assessment becomes an even more crucial aspect of the treatment process.

11. Summary

See Table 9 for a summary of this chapter.

TABLE 9

Summary of Chapter 6

This chapter has attempted to highlight the following:

1. The standardised measurement of pain should be considered an essential aspect of any clinical service in order to accurately assess treatment efficacy

2. There are several psychometric caveats which should be borne in mind when selecting assessment instruments. Giving a questionnaire a certain title does not guarantee that it is assessing what it purports to assess

3. Self-report questionnaires can be broadly distinguished as multiaxial (one instrument assessing a wide range of areas) or specific (questionnaire aimed at assessing a focused area)

4. Measures are available to assess pain intensity and quality, physical disability, mood and emotional state in relation to pain, beliefs and expectations about pain, as well as objective signs of facial pain-related impairment

5. Assessment is always a compromise between obtaining as much detailed information as possible, fatiguing the respondent, and fatiguing the individual responsible for administering, scoring and interpreting the material

TABLE 10

Answers to case study from Table 8

The results clearly show that despite the pain intensity levels being comparable between the two patients, the effect of pain on mood and activities of daily living is quite different. Mrs. S. describes much more vivid and intense descriptors of her pain on the McGill Pain Questionnaire, choosing words such as "lacerating", "stinging" and "shooting". However, her overall mood scores and the degree of disruption to her normal activities due to pain is considerably less than with Ms. A. The profile of Ms. A. shows a greater identification with the affective descriptors on the McGill Pain Questionnaire, such as "terrifying", "vicious" and "suffocating", rather than with the sensory subclass items. She is also reporting more severe mood disturbance and greater disability, both in relation to her facial pain and in terms of wider disruption to daily activities.

The Pain Management Goals Questionnaire then clarifies some of the issues raised by the assessment above. Mrs. S. identifies a reduction in her medication as a primary objective, a sensible choice given that she does not obtain much benefit from it. She is also keen to know that the pain is not indicative of a more sinister pathology, and would like to improve her communication with her doctor — both of these aims usually achievable by making more time in the consultation. Alternatively, the questionnaire shows that Ms. A. has somewhat different goals from treatment. She is concerned about being able to remain working with her pain problem, and identifies that her mood requires attention in treatment. She is also aware that her ability to socialise has been impaired because of self-consciousness about the pain, perhaps because of feeling that she smiles awkwardly or cannot laugh naturally due to limited mouth opening.

The differences elicited above will be due to several factors, including the type of pain problem, the difference in duration of pain (Ms. A. has had unrelenting pain and succession of failed treatments for longer which would impact directly upon mood), and their different stages of life and life interests. This profile indicates quite different areas of treatment involvement between these two patients. Yet a simple pain intensity score would not have revealed this information.

Appendix A

See Table 10 for the answers to the case study in Table 8.

Appendix B. Further reading list

The following are excellent reference texts or papers for those interested in psychosocial assessment in chronic pain.

(1) Turk DC, Melzack R. Handbook of Pain Assessment, 2nd edn. Guilford Press, New York, 2001.
(2) Skevington SM, Psychology of Pain. John Wiley and Sons, Chichester, 1995.
(3) Williams ACdeC Pain measurement in chronic pain management. Pain Rev 1995; 2: 39–63.

References

Marked as regards quality according to criteria set by author.
SR = systematic review or high quality review with methodology.
** Cohort studies, high quality case series with controls.

** Allen PF, McMillan AS, Locker D. An assessment of sensitivity to change of the Oral Health Impact Profile in a clinical trial. Commun Dent Oral Epidemiol 2001; 29: 175–182.

Atkin PA, Escudier M, Zakrzewska JM. A pilot study of patient goals in chronic facial pain. Abstract presented at the Pan European Conference of Oral Sciences, Cardiff 2002.

Auerbach SM, Laskin DM, Frantsve LM, Orr T. Depression, pain, exposure to stressful life events, and long-term outcomes in temporomandibular disorder patients. J Oral Maxillofac Surg 2001; 59: 628–633.

Banks SM, Kerns RD. Explaining high rates of depression in chronic pain: a diathesis-stress framework. Psychol Bull 1996; 119: 95–110.

Battie MC, May L. Physical and occupational therapy assessment approaches. In: DC Turk, R Melzack (eds), Handbook of Pain Assessment, 2nd Edition. The Guilford Press: New York, London 2001.

Beck AT, Ward CH, Mendelson M, Mock N, Erbaugh J. An inventory for measuring depression. Arch Gen Psychiatry 1961; 4: 561–571.

Beck AT, Rush AJ, Shaw BF, Emery G. Cognitive Therapy of Depression. Guilford Press, New York, 1979.

SR Beck AT, Steer RA, Garbin MG. Psychometric properties of the Beck Depression Inventory: twenty-five years of evaluation. Clin Psychol Rev 1988; 8: 77–100.

Bennett M. The LANSS Pain Scale: the Leeds assessment of neuropathic symptoms and signs. Pain 2001; 92: 147–157.

Bergner M Bobbitt RA, Carter WB, Gibson BS. The Sickness Impact Profile: development and final revision of a health status measure. Med Care 1981; 19: 787–805.

Biller N, Arnstein P, Caudill MA, Federman CW, Guberman C. Predicting completion of a cognitive–behavioral pain management program by initial measures of a chronic pain patient's readiness for change. Clin J Pain 2000; 16: 352–359.

Bradley LA, McKendree-Smith NL. Assessment of psychological status using interviews and self-report instruments. In: Turk DC, Melzack R (eds) Handbook of Pain Assessment, 2nd Edition. Guilford Press, New York, 2001, pp. 292–319.

** Brown DT, Gaudet EL Jr. Outcome measurement for treated and untreated TMD patients using the TMJ scale. Cranio 1994; 12: 216–222.

Burns JW, Johnson BJ, Devine J, Mahoney N, Pawl R. Anger management style and the prediction of treatment outcome among male and female chronic pain patients. Behav Res Ther 1998; 36: 1051–1062.

Bush FM, Harkins SW. Pain-related limitation in activities of daily living in patients with chronic orofacial pain: psychometric properties of a disability index. J Orofac Pain 1995; 9: 57–63.

Butcher JN, Dahlstrom WG, Graham JR. Manual for administration and scoring Minnesota Multiphasic Personality Inventory-2. Minneapolis: University of Minnesota Press, 1989.

Cleeland CS. Measurement of pain by subjective report. In CR Chapman, JD Loeser (eds), Issues in Pain Management. New York: Raven Press, 1989, pp. 391–403

Coughlan GM, Ridout KL, Williams ACdeC, Richardson PH. Attrition from a pain management programme. Br J Clin Psychol 1995; 34: 471–479.

Dahlstrom L, Widmark G, Carlsson SG. Cognitive–behavioral profiles among different categories of orofacial pain patients: diagnostic and treatment implications. Eur J Oral Sci 1997; 105: 377–383.

DeGood DE, Tait RC. Assessment of pain beliefs and pain coping. In: Turk DC, Melzack R (eds), Handbook of Pain Assessment, 2nd Editon. Guilford Press, New York, 2001, 320–345.

Derbyshire SW. Exploring the pain 'neuromatrix'. Curr Rev Pain 2000; 4: 467–477.

Derogatis L. The SCL-90R manual-II: administration, scoring and procedures. Towson MD: Clinical Psychometric Research, 1983.

Dworkin SF, Chen AC. Pain in clinical and laboratory contexts. J Dent Res 1982; 6: 772-774.

Dworkin SF, Ohrbach R. Assessment of orofacial pain. In: Turk DC, Melzack R (eds), Handbook of Pain Assessment, 2nd Edition. Guilford Press, New York, 2001, 475–498.

Engel GL. 'Psychogenic' pain and the pain-prone patient. Am J Med 1959; 26: 899–918.

Feinmann C. The Mouth, The Face, The Mind. Oxford Univ Press, 1999.

Fernandez E, Turk DC. The scope and significance of anger in the experience of chronic pain. Pain 1995; 61: 165–175.

Galer BS, Henderson J, Perander J, Jensen MP. Course of symptoms and quality of life measurement in Complex Regional Pain Syndrome: a pilot survey. J Pain Sympt Management 2001; 20: 286–292.

Gamsa A. The role of psychological factors in chronic pain. I. A half century of study. Pain 1994; 57: 5–15.

Gatchel RJ. The prevalence of dental fear and avoidance: expanded adult and recent adolescent surveys. J Am Dent Assoc 1989; 118: 591–593.

Geisser ME, Roth RS, Robinson ME. Assessing depression among persons with chronic pain using the Center for Epidemiological Studies-Depression Scale and the Beck Depression Inventory: a comparative analysis. Clin J Pain 1997; 13: 163–170.

Graff-Radford SB, Solberg WK. Is atypical odontalgia a psychological problem? Oral Surg Oral Med Oral Pathol 1993; 75: 579–582.

Hall EH, Terezhalmy GT, Pelleu GB. A set of descriptors for the diagnosis of dental pain syndromes. Oral Surg Oral Med Oral Pathol 1986; 61: 153–157.

Harding VR, Williams ACdeC, Richardson PH, Nicholas MK, Jackson JL, Richardson IH, and Pither CE. The development of a battery of measures for assessing physical functioning of chronic pain patients. Pain 1994; 58: 367–375.

SR Herrmann C. International experiences with the Hospital Anxiety and Depression Scale — a review of validation data and clinical results. J Psychosom Res 1997; 42: 17–41.

Jensen MP, Karoly P. Self-report scales and procedures. In: Turk DC, Melzack R (eds), Handbook of Pain Assessment, 2nd Edition. Guilford Press, New York, 2001, 15–34.

Jensen MP, Karoly P, Huger R. The development and preliminary validation of an instrument to assess patients' attitudes towards pain. J Psychosom Res 1987; 31: 393–400.

SR Jensen MP, Turner JA, Romano JM, Karoly P. Coping with chronic pain: a critical review of the literature. Pain 1991; 47: 249–283.

Jensen MP, Turner JA, Romano JM. Pain belief assessment: a comparison of the short and long versions of the Survey of Pain Attitudes. J Pain 2000a; 1: 138–150.

Jensen MP, Nielson WR, Romano JM, Hill ML, Turner JA. Further evaluation of the pain stages of change questionnaire: is the transtheoretical model of change useful for patients with chronic pain? Pain 2000b; 86: 255–264.

Jensen MP, Turner JA, Romano JM. Changes in beliefs, catastrophizing, and coping are associated with improvement in multidisciplinary pain treatment. J Consult Clin Psychol 2001; 69: 655–662.

Keefe FJ, Block AR. Development of an observation method of assessing pain behavior in chronic low back pain patients. Behav Ther 1982; 13: 363–375.

Kerns RD, Turk DC, Rudy TE. The West Haven-Yale Multidimensional Pain Inventory (WHYMPI). Pain 1985; 23: 345-356.

Kerns RD, Rosenberg R, Jamison RN, Caudill MA, Haythornthwaite J. Readiness to adopt a self-management approach to chronic pain: the Pain Stages of Change Questionnaire (PSOCQ). Pain 1997; 72: 227–234.

Korszun A, Ship JA. Diagnosing depression in patients with chronic facial pain. J Am Dent Assoc 1997; 128: 1680–1686.

Korszun A, Papadopoulos E, Demitrack M, Engleberg C, Crofford L. The relationship between temporomandibular disorders and stress-associated syndromes. Oral Surg Oral Med Oral Pathol Oral Radiol Endodont 1998; 86: 416–420.

Kropmans TJ, Dijkstra PU, van Veen A, Stegenga B, de Bont LG. The smallest detectable difference of mandibular function impairment in patients with a painfully restricted temporomandibular joint. J Dent Res 1999; 78: 1445–1449.

Levine FM, De Simone LL. The effects of experimenter gender on pain report in male and female subjects. Pain 1991; 44: 69–72

Levitt SR, Kundeen TF, McKinney MW. The TMJ Scale Manual. Durham, NC, Pain Resource Centre, 1994.

Lin CC. Comparison of the effects of perceived self-efficacy on coping with chronic cancer pain and coping with chronic low back pain. Clin J Pain 1998; 14: 303–310.

Madland G, Feinmann C, Newman S. Factors associated with anxiety and depression in facial arthromyalgia. Pain 2000; 84: 225–232.

McCraken LM, Zayfert C, Gross RT. The Pain Anxiety Symptoms Scale: development and validation of a scale to measure fear of pain. Pain 1992; 50: 67–73.

McNeil DW, Au AR, Zvolensky MJ, McKee DR, Klineberg IJ, Ho C. Fear of pain in orofacial pain patients. Pain 2001; 89: 245–252.

Melzack R. The McGill Pain Questionnaire: major properties and scoring methods. Pain 1975; 1: 277–299.

Melzack R. The short-form McGill Pain Questionnaire. Pain 1987; 30: 191–197.

Melzack R, Terrence C, Fromm G, Amsel R. Trigeminal neuralgia and atypical facial pain: use of the McGill Pain Questionnaire for discrimination and diagnosis. Pain 1986; 27: 297–302.

Merskey H, Spear FG. Pain: Psychological and Psychiatric Aspects. Bailliere, Tindall and Cassell, London, 1967.

Newton-John TRO. Pain Management Goals Questionnaire. Unpublished manuscript: 2000.

Nicholas MK. The Pain Self-Efficacy Questionnaire: self-efficacy in relation to chronic pain. Proceedings of the British Psychological Society Annual Conference April 1989.

Okifuji A, Turk DC, Curran SL. Anger in chronic pain: investigations of anger targets and intensity. J Psychosom Res 1999; 47: 1–12.

Pollard CA. Preliminary validity study of The Pain Disability Index. Percept Motor Skills 1984; 59: 974.

Riley JL, Robinson ME, Wise EA, Campbell LC, Kashikar-Zuck S, Gremillion HA. Predicting treatment compliance following facial pain evaluation. Cranio 1999; 17: 9–16.

Robinson ME, Riley JL, Myers CD, Sadler IJ, Kvaal SA, Geisser ME, Keefe FJ. The Coping Strategies Questionnaire: a large sample, item level factor analysis. Clin J Pain 1997; 13: 43–49.

Rosensteil AK, Keefe FJ. The use of coping strategies in low back pain patients: relationship to patient characteristics and current adjustment. Pain 1983; 17: 33–40.

Rudy TE, Turk DC, Kubinski J, Zaki H Efficacy of tailoring treatment for dysfunctional TMD patients. J Dent Res 1994; 73: 439.

Saw SM, Ng TP. The design and assessment of questionnaires in clinical research. Singapore Med J 2001; 42(3): 131–135.

Skevington SM. Beliefs, images and memories of pain. In: Skevington SM (ed) Psychology of Pain. John Wiley and Sons, Chichester, 1995: 97–130.

Slade GD. Derivation and validation of a short-form oral health impact profile. Commun Dent Oral Epidemiol 1997; 25: 284–290.

Spielberger CD. Manual for the State-Trait Anxiety Inventory (Form 1; Consulting Psychologists Press, Palo Alto, CA, 1983.

Spielberger CD. State-Trait Anger Expression Inventory Professional Manual. Psychological Assessment Resources, Odessa, FL, 1988.

Steed PA. TMD treatment outcomes: a statistical assessment of the effects of psychological variables. Cranio 1998; 16: 138–142.

Stegenga B, de Bont LG, de Leeuw R, Boering G. Assessment of mandibular function impairment associated with temporomandibular joint osteoarthrosis and internal derangement. J Orofac Pain 1993; 7: 183–195.

Turk DC, Melzack R. Handbook of Pain Assessment. Guilford Press, New York, 2001.

Turk DC, Rudy TE, Flor H. Why a family perspective for pain? Int J Fam Ther 1985; 7: 223–234.

Turner JA, Whitney C, Dworkin SF, Massoth D, Wilson L. Do changes in patient beliefs and coping strategies predict temporomandibular disorder treatment outcomes? Clin J Pain 1995; 11: 177–188.

Turner JA, Jensen MP, Romano JM. Do beliefs, coping, and catastrophizing independently predict functioning in patients with chronic pain? Pain 2000; 85: 115–125.

Turner JA, Dworkin SF, Mancl L, Huggins KH, Truelove EL. The roles of beliefs, catastrophizing and coping in the functioning of patients with temporomandibular disorders. Pain 2001; 92: 41–51.

Turp JC, Kowalski CJ, Stohler CS. Pain descriptor characteristics of persistent facial pain. J Orofac Pain 1997; 11: 285–290.

SR Vendrig AA. The Minnesota Multiphasic Personality Inventory and chronic pain: a conceptual analysis of a longstanding but complicated relationship. Clin Psych Rev 2000; 20: 533–559.

Von Korff M, Ormel J, Keefe FJ. Dworkin SF. Grading the severity of chronic pain. Pain 1992; 50: 133–149.

Ware JE, Sherbourne CD. The MOS 36-item Short Form Health Survey (SF-36). Med Care 1992; 30: 473–483.

Williams ACdeC. Pain measurement in chronic pain management. Pain Rev 1995; 2: 39–63.

SR Williams ACdeC. Depression in chronic pain: mistaken models, missed opportunities. Scand J Behav Ther 1998; 27: 61–80.

Williams ACdeC, Davies HTO, Chadhury Y. Simple pain ratings hide complex idiosyncratic meanings. Pain 2000; 85: 457–463.

Yap AU, Tan KB, Hoe JK, Yap RH, Jaffar J. On-line computerized diagnosis of pain-related disability and psychological status of TMD patients: a pilot study. J Oral Rehabil 2001; 28: 78–87.

Zigmond AS, Snaith RP. The Hospital Anxiety and Depression Scale. Acta Psychiat Scand 1983; 67: 361–370.

Assessment and Management of Orofacial Pain
Pain Research and Clinical Management, Vol. 14
Edited by J.M. Zakrzewska and S.D. Harrison

CHAPTER 7

Investigations for facial pain

Joanna M. Zakrzewska[*]

Department of Clinical and Diagnostic Oral Sciences, Oral Medicine Unit, Dental Institute, Barts and the London Queen Mary's School of Medicine and Dentistry, Turner Street, London E1 2AD, UK

Objectives for this chapter:

The chapter will attempt to:
- Show that careful clinical assessment is crucial as a guide for initiating investigations
- Show how tests merely confirm and may not give clear cut answers
- Give a brief overview of investigations commonly used in orofacial pain patients
- Give an overview of the radiological examination of the facial structures including teeth
- Demonstrate that there is a serious lack of evidence to assess the utility of different investigations

1. Introduction: reading articles on diagnostic tests

When reading this chapter you should keep in mind the following three evidenced-based questions about any of the diagnostic tests being discussed:

(1) Is the evidence about the accuracy of a diagnostic test valid?
(2) Does this (valid) evidence demonstrate an important ability of the test to accurately distinguish patients who do and do not have the specific disorder?
(3) Can I apply this test to my specific patient? (Sackett et al., 2000)

These points are further expanded in Table 1 key facts.

Consider reading the chapter on diagnosis and screening in the book 'Evidence based Medicine. How to practice and teach EBM'. There are also some useful articles in the series 'Users' of medical literature' on how to read articles on diagnostic tests and these are listed at the end of the chapter in further reading.

Many results are reported as 'normal' but it is important that you know what this can mean. Below are some definitions that are applied to tests which are then called normal:

- Gaussian: the mean ± 2 standard deviations and makes the assumption that all tests have a normal distribution, e.g. haemoglobin
- Percentile: the range is often specified as 5–95% and makes the assumption that all tests have a normal distribution
- Diagnostic: point at which the target disorder becomes a high probability

[*] Tel.: +44-20-7377-7053; Fax: +44-20-7377-7627;
E-mail: j.m.zakrzewska@qmul.ac.uk

TABLE 1

KEY FACTS: questions to ask when evaluating an article on diagnostic tests

Are the results of the study valid?

- Was there an independent blind comparison with a reference (gold) standard?

- Did the patient sample include an appropriate spectrum of patients to who the test will be applied in clinical practice?

- Did the result of the test being evaluated influence the decision to perform the reference standard?

- Were the methods of the test described in sufficient detail to permit replication?

What are the results?

- Are likelihood ratios for the test results presented or data necessary for their calculation provided?

Will the results help me in caring for my patients?

- Will the reproducibility of the test and its interpretation be satisfactory in my setting?

- Are the results applicable to my patient?

- Will the results change my management?

- Will the patients be better off as a result of the test?

When reading articles on diagnostic tests it is important to ascertain the inter operator agreement and this is done using the κ-test. κ values of 0.4 and below are considered poor, 0.4–0.6 fair, 0.6–0.8 moderate and 0.8 and above are excellent.

Unfortunately many of the tests that will be discussed in this section have not undergone rigorous evaluation as described.

There are few evaluations of the cost effectiveness of diagnostic tests and yet as medical resources become more restricted their use will become more limited to those which give the best results (Mushlin et al., 2001).

Some of the investigations are done to confirm a diagnosis, others to monitor treatment both in terms of outcome measures and monitoring of side effects or adverse reactions. Many patients are over investigated often because a careful history and examination have not been done and it is erroneously thought that the investigations will pick up everything.

2. Haematology/biochemistry tests used in orofacial pain patients

These tests are performed on many patients and often little thought is given to their relevance both in terms of diagnosis and monitoring. Sometimes unexpected results are obtained and they then need to be interpreted both in the light of the presenting complaint but also as possible unrelated factors. Hampton et al. (1975) showed in their study that the relative contribution of the laboratory investigations in the diagnosis and management of medical outpatients was 9% (7/80 new patients seen). They further showed that when physicians were asked to categorise their tests into essential, desirable and routine the highest yield of abnormal results was in those classified as essential (40%) whereas in those done routinely only 10% were abnormal. Roshan and Rao (2000) also showed that investigations were used to make a diagnosis in only 13% of patients. Attitudes towards use of investigations is extremely variable and is not necessarily linked to lack of confidence in a diagnosis-based on history and examination (Hampton et al., 1975).

There are relatively few investigations needed for facial pain patients and some of the investigations which may be of relevance to facial pain, are summarised in Table 2. Further details are to be found in textbooks of medicine.

The value of the ESR in diagnosis for temporal arteritis has been critically evaluated on the basis of reported cases in the literature and shown to be a reliable guide (Smetana and Shmerling, 2002). A negative ESR even using a high cut off point of 50 mm/h virtually rules out a positive temporal artery biopsy and hence temporal arteritis. On the other hand, a high ESR has not got such a high likelihood ratio in part due to bias in choosing only cases with raised ESR to biopsy. Anaemia was found in 44% of biopsy proven cases, but this was similar to the

TABLE 2

KEY FACTS: interpretation of results

Test	Abnormality	Possible diagnosis	Further evaluation
Haemoglobin	Lowered	Anaemia, may be related to temporal arteritis	Depends on other parameters
MCV	Raised	Vitamin B_{12}, folate deficiency, alcohol/liver disease	Serum vitamin B12, red cell folate, liver function tests, thyroid function
	Lowered	Chronic blood loss, iron deficiency anaemia, thalassaemia	Blood film, serum ferritin, reticulocyte count, electrophoresis, faecal occult bloods
MCH	Raised	Vitamin B_{12}/folate	
ESR	Raised	Elevated among others in patients with temporal arteritis	Temporal artery biopsy
	Lowered	Iron deficiency anaemia, megaloblastic anaemia, thalassaemia	
γ-Glutamyl transferase (GGT)	High	Liver disease, alcohol use, drug induced	
Alkaline phosphatase	High	Liver disease, gallstones, drug induced, bone disease	GGT, isoenzymes to determine whether due to bony abnormalities
Liver transaminases	High	Liver disease, thyroid disease, heart failure, drugs	
Autoantibody screen: anti-Ro and anti-La, thyroid		Painful trigeminal neuropathies, Sjogren's syndrome, scleroderma, thyroid disease	Labial gland biopsy for Sjogren's syndrome, thyroid hormone levels

negative biopsy number and so lack of anaemia is not helpful in ruling out disease.

Patients with depression who also have features suggestive of thyroid disease may need to be tested and antibodies assessed as this is a common disease in some parts of the world and changes may occur so subtly that patients may not complain of them. It has been suggested, but never well proven, that patients with a symptom of burning mouth may be suffering from some haematinic deficiency and these patients are therefore routinely screened for them.

Blood coagulation tests may be required in patients who have a history of bleeding problems and are due for major surgery such as a microvascular decompression for trigeminal neuralgia. Patients on warfarin need to be monitored carefully, especially if they are given carbamazepine.

Patients with a history suggestive of multiple sclerosis may need an examination of CSF to confirm the diagnosis (McDonald et al., 2001). This may be of importance in patients with trigeminal neuralgia who are being considered for surgery.

Some baseline and then monitoring tests are important for certain drugs, e.g. white cell count, urea and electrolytes, liver function and folate with carbamazepine. These will be further discussed in Chapter 9 on management, but you may wish to look at the case study in Table 3.

Renal and liver functions may need to be tested if prescribing drugs that are excreted through the kidneys or liver. Many drugs will affect liver function tests (LFT) including the γ-glutamyl transferase (GGT) especially in the first 3 months. Baseline estimates should be taken when prescribing drugs that

TABLE 3

Case studies 1 and 2

Look at these results on two patients with trigeminal neuralgia in their fifties (patient 1 has thalassaemia trait) with no relevant medical or other drug history who are taking oxcarbazepine, an anticonvulsant. What is it telling you about the drug?

Test and normal range	Patient 1a	Patient 1b	Patient 2a	Patient 2b
Daily dose OXC	1200 mg	2400 mg	300 mg	1500 mg
Daily mg/kg dose OXC	20.4 mg/kg	40.9 mg/kg	5 mg/kg	35.2 mg/kg
Hb (12–16 g/dl)	10.7	11.7	13.2	13.5
WBC (4–11 10^9 l)	4.2	5.0	5.6	5.9
MCV (80–96 fl)	67.2	70	87.6	88.9
MCHC (32–35 g/dl)	32.2	32.3	33.8	33.2
Sodium (135–146 mmol/l)	133	121	141	126
Potassium (3.5–5 mmol/l)	4.1	4.5	4.4	4.5
Urea (2.5–6.7 mmol/l)	3.9	3.7	4.1	2.8
Alkaline phosphate (25–115 U/l)	74	94	96	110
GGT (7–32 U/l)	21	27	23	31

See Table 8 at the end of the chapter for answers.

may be hepatoxic such as carbamazepine. Elevation of transaminases up to two-fold is usually acceptable, but the drug should be withdrawn if levels rise above this. Abnormal LFTs due to drugs normally resolve 3–4 weeks after withdrawal and if they do not then you need to suspect some form of liver disease or alcohol use.

3. Measurement of drug levels

Drug levels are used for assessing compliance and to forecast toxicity. We cannot use drug levels alone to guide treatment and you need to remember that plasma and tissue levels are often very different. Drug levels are not frequently used in chronic facial pain, as there is often little need to check on adherence to therapy. There are suggested dose ranges for anticonvulsants, but the ranges quoted are for use in monitoring epilepsy rather than pain. Carbamazepine serum levels do not correlate well with daily dosage, whereas oxcarbazepine serum levels do reflect daily dosage. You can measure drug levels in order to assess the development of tolerance. When measur-

ing drug levels, it is very important that the timing of the samples is correlated with the drug times. Ideally, trough levels of the drugs should be measured and these levels can then be compared over time.

4. Dental tests

4.1. Vitality tests

These are used to assess the status of the pulp, but their reliability is not high. A vital tooth retains a blood supply and there are at present no reliable ways of measuring the integrity of the pulpal blood supply in a non-destructive way so the tests currently used aim to measure this indirectly by testing the nerve supply of the pulp. Both thermal (cold and hot) and electrical testing are carried out. Temperatures of 20–25°C are normally tolerated by healthy teeth. This heat is applied through a piece of heated gutta percha. Cold is applied via a pledget of cotton wool sprayed with ethyl chloride. Electrical testing offers a more controlled graded method of testing but their efficacy rapidly diminishes when the batteries run low. Most machines have some sort of read out which can be recorded. When applying the test is essential to ensure that the teeth are dry and contact is made only with the enamel. The tests need to be applied not just on the affected or suspected teeth but other presumed normal teeth from different quadrants. Testing should begin with normal presumed healthy teeth so that patients fear is not raised leading to exaggerated responses. It is important to ensure that the test is applied to normal enamel of the tooth and not restorations or soft tissues which could act as conductors. A wide variety of effects can be expected: positive (normal result), exaggerated, i.e. brief or prolonged, negative, false positive, false negative and inconclusive when even presumed normal teeth do not give a positive result. Interpretation of the results can be found in dental books and some are discussed in Chapter 10 on dental pain. Combining results from two tests increases reliability. There appears to be little correlation between vitality testing and histological pulpal changes.

It may sometimes be necessary to drill a small cavity without local anaesthesia to assess the vitality of the pulp, but this is a destructive test and should only be used in the last resort. Grushka and Sessle (1984) have shown that a McGill pain questionnaire can yield reliable results on whether the pulpitis is reversible or irreversible and this may be more reliable than the use of these tests.

4.2. Percussion

Percussion of teeth with the tip of the handle of a dental mirror can elicit tenderness and dullness, signs of inflammation. Normal and suspected teeth need to be tested. Remember that teeth can be exquisitely tender to percussion.

4.3. Mobility

Mobility is assessed by the use of either two instruments or one instrument and a finger.

4.4. Transillumination

This method, which is useful to determine cracks in teeth and caries which are not accessible to probing, may also need to include magnification. Non-vital teeth become less translucent and this can be picked up on transillumination.

Transillumination of the maxillary sinus can be carried out in a darkened room by putting the light source on the infraorbital rim and then viewing the degree of light transmission compared through both sides of the hard palate. The techniques are operator sensitive (Williams et al., 1992) and time must be made for the operators eyes to become adjusted to the darkened room. Conflicting views are given as to the clinical value of this test (Evans et al., 1975; Spector et al., 1981). Williams et al. (1992) reported a likelihood ratio of 1.6 for unilateral opaqueness or dullness and 0.5 for bilateral normal transillumination.

4.5. Local analgesia

This can be helpful in diagnosis of both dental and non-dental pain. In some forms of pulpitis it is very difficult for the patient to localise the pain to a particular tooth, so if you give a local anaesthetic you may be able to achieve this. Patients with trigeminal neuralgia will find that an injection into their trigger point will give them complete relief for a few hours, whereas patients with atypical facial pain will not gain comparable relief.

4.6. Bacteriological viral/histological tests

The 'gold standard' for the diagnosis of sinusitis is the presence of infected secretions demonstrated by sinus puncture and lavage. For further details see the section of diagnostic strategies for common medical problems in Best Evidence (see details at end of the chapter in further reading). However, this procedure is performed infrequently.

The gold standard for diagnosis of temporal arteries is the biopsy of the temporal artery. As treatment with systemic steroids carries with it many risks, it is important to have the correct diagnosis. Biopsies are done if the history and examination is highly suggestive.

5. Radiology

Radiological investigations are commonly used in chronic facial pain, but the evidence for their usefulness has not been well validated. You should familiarise yourself with the Royal College of Radiologists and the European directives for imaging guidelines which are available both electronically and on paper. The latter incorporates all the material found in the former publication (see end of the chapter for details in further reading). Some form of guidelines for dental radiological examinations have been available since 1987 and commentary on them is to be found under an editorial entitled 'Guidelines for radiological examinations: do we have all the answers yet?' (Brooks, 1997). The American Academy of Oral and Maxillofacial Radiology have produced a position paper on imaging of the temporomandibular joint which discusses a wide range of methods but is not a systematic review (Brooks et al., 1997). It will be further discussed in Chapter 11 on temporomandibular pain. A highly specialised chapter on overall imaging of pain can be found in Melzack and Wall's 4th edition of the Textbook of Pain (see further reading at the end of the chapter).

5.1. Skull and facial plain radiographs

These are rarely useful for chronic facial pain but may pick up some bony abnormalities, e.g. skull metastases like osteolytic lesions from myeloma and osteosclerotic lesions from prostatic and breast cancers. Soft tissue shadows may also be rarely useful, e.g. an enlarged parotid gland from sarcoidosis or a stone in the salivary duct. Plain radiographs are of value in sinusitis and this is further discussed in Chapter 13. A single Water's view radiograph is probably sufficient for maxillary sinusitis, but four different views may be necessary for other sinuses

---

TABLE 4

KEY FACTS: disadvantages of CT in trigeminal nerve assessments

- Ionizing radiation in region of 1–5 mSv
- Need to use a dye to enhance image which may produce side effects
- Plaques and infections not visualized
- Bony artefacts
- Cannot differentiate between nerves and blood vessels
- Rarely able to see pre-ganglionic segments

(Hayward et al., 1990; Burke et al., 1994). Plain radiographs are also recommended for bony abnormalities of the temporomandibular joint and there is good evidence for their usefulness (see reports in further reading at the end of the chapter).

5.2. Computed tomography (CT)

Plain and enhanced brain CT enables thin cuts to be taken across the base of the skull for certain tumours like nasopharyngeal carcinomas, but is not as effective for small posterior fossa tumours where bony artifacts make interpretation difficult (Referral guidelines at the end of the chapter). CT is not as useful as MRIs in the diagnosis of multiple sclerosis (McDonald et al., 2001). Table 4 key facts lists the disadvantages of CT in the assessments of orofacial pain. CT is, however, more readily available and is much cheaper than MRI. A useful review of the use of CT in clinical practice can be found in the British Medical Journal (Garvey and Hanlon, 2002).

Although CT is highly sensitive and a normal scan virtually rules out sinus disease, the specificity of sinus CT has been questioned especially when used for paranasal sinuses (Havas et al., 1998). Patients must be carefully selected and the test interpreted using strict criteria as abnormalities are also noted in patients with common cold. Burke et al. (1994) suggest that air–fluid levels or opacification

TABLE 5

KEY FACTS: advantages of MRI scanning of the trigeminal nerve

- No ionizing radiation
- No bony artifacts
- Good soft tissue contrast
- Gadolinium contrast safe
- Visualize whole course of the nerve
- Dynamic

in sinuses is easier to pick up on CT than plain radiographs.

5.3. Magnetic resonance imaging (MRI)

A simple explanation of how MRI works can be found in the British Medical Journal (Berger, 2002). The advantages of this method for imaging the trigeminal nerve are listed in Table 5.

In order for MRI to be effective good patient co-operation is required. Any patient movement, which could be due to anxiety-related reactions, may mean that the scan images are degraded due to motion artifacts. This could then impact on the patients' perception of the quality of their care. There are several studies on anxiety-related reactions to MRI examination and Melendez and McCrank (1993) have reviewed the relevant studies. They found that 4–30% of patients might suffer a reaction, which can vary from mild apprehension to severe anxiety that results in non-appearance for the examination or curtailment of it. The anxiety is related to several factors including claustrophobia, pain, the unknown as well as apprehension about what the test will show. Further studies since have shown in 80 patients who completed questionnaires pre- and post-scan that high scores on a claustrophobia questionnaire was more sensitive than measurement of anxiety and they suggest a brief screening test with six questions which could be used to identify individuals at risk (McIsaac et al., 1998). Improved patient information and re-

laxation techniques and even cognitive behaviour therapy (Lukins et al., 1997) may be used to allay this fear.

Patients with metal parts and pacemakers may pose a problem when attempting an MRI scan as there is potential for parts to move during application of the magnetic field. MRIs are very expensive and the evidence for their utility is still lacking and is therefore important to keep up to date with current guidelines (Luxenberg, 1994).

MRI is suggested for use in smaller cerebropontine angle tumours like meningiomas and acoustic neurilemomas and in the diagnosis of multiple sclerosis, intrinsic brainstem gliomas, syringobulbia (see reports in further reading at the end of the chapter).

Depending on the criteria set and the age of the patient, the specificity and positive predictive value of MRI in the diagnosis of multiple sclerosis was shown to be acceptable (Offenbacher et al., 1993). Its sensitivity for multiple sclerosis ranges from 60 to 80% (Kent et al., 1994). MRI may, however, be negative in up to 25% of those with established multiple sclerosis (reports at the end of the chapter). The international panel for diagnosis of multiple sclerosis (McDonald et al., 2001) suggest that 3 out of 4 of the following features should be present on MRI to make a diagnosis of MS:

- One gandolinium enhancing lesion or nine T2-hyperintense lesions if there is no gadolinium enhancing lesion
- At least one infratentorial lesion
- At least one juxtacortical lesion
- At least three periventricular lesions

MRIs are also useful for extensive salivary gland masses (reports at the end of the chapter). MRIs are not as useful in sinus neoplasia due to poor resolution of bony margins (Lloyd, 1990). MRIs are also used to examine the menisci in the temporomandibular joints and are discussed further in Chapter 11.

MRIs are used in trigeminal neuralgia for assessment of vascular contact, but the quality of evidence is not high at present (Zakrzewska, 2002). Individuals who may be at risk of having a structural abnormality on MRI can be identified on the basis of history and clinical examination (Goh et al., 2001). Please also see Chapter 15 on trigeminal neuralgia for further details.

5.4. Intraarterial digital subtraction angiography

Rare cause of referred facial pain from dissected carotid or vertebral arteries may be investigated using this type of angiography. Arterial dissections are one of the commonest causes of stroke in young persons and so should always be suspected when there are no other predisposing factors. Magnetic resonance angiography is nearly as good.

5.5. Dental and temporomandibular radiology

Dental radiographs are frequently taken by general dental practitioners in general practice and guidelines for these have been published and details are given at the end of the chapter. Table 6 key facts lists some of the dental radiographs that are taken to establish pain of dental origin.

5.6. Ultrasound

The best use of ultrasound is for salivary gland masses where there is reasonable quality evidence to suggest it as the first-line investigation if local expertise is available (see report at end of chapter in further reading). Ultrasonography had shown initial promise as a non-invasive diagnostic test, but studies have not supported its use in maxillary sinus.

5.7. Arthrography

This is suggested for patients with suspected internal derangement as it is a dynamic demonstration of the joint action and the evidence for its use is of good quality (see report at end of chapter in further reading). This is a minimally invasive technique which can result in a significant radiation dose. In inexperienced hands, it can be time consuming and demanding. A small percentage of patients may be allergic to the contrast medium.

5.8. Angiography

This was the method to evaluate the presence of tumour or compressing vessels on the trigeminal nerve

---

TABLE 6

KEY FACTS: radiology used in oral diagnosis

Type of X-ray	Use and indication
Bitewings	Crowns, caries, restorations, alveolar bone
Periapicals	Root, pulp chamber, surrounding bone including lamina dura, periodontal and pulpal disease
Panoral orthopantomogram (OPG)	General view of all teeth, maxilla and mandible, TMJ
Lateral oblique	General view of all teeth, maxilla and mandible used when OPG not available
Maxillary anterior occlusal	Roots of maxillary anterior teeth
Mandibular occlusal	Calcification in floor of mouth, salivary stones, fractures
Transcranial/transmaxillary/submental–vertex and transpharyngeal open close views	One or two of these views useful for TMJ — condyles, arthritic changes, fractures, neoplasia
Occipitomental	Maxillary sinus, facial, skull bones

but has been largely superseded by MRI, which is less invasive. de Lange et al. (1986) evaluated its use using a control group and suggested that it could be used for diagnostic purposes.

5.9. Positron emission tomography (PET)

This radiological investigation provides data on the viability of tissue and/or metabolic activity of the area being examined. It relies on the ability of radionuclides to emit positively charged particles or positrons which, having travelled a short distance in tissue, interact with electrons and emit energy in the form of two high-energy γ-rays. Multiple detectors surrounding the head then detect these γ-rays. It does expose patients to relatively large radiation dosages and the short-lived nature of the radionuclide means its location needs to be near the required source. More sophisticated cameras are being developed which should increase its clinical use. Currently this technique is used to identify viable foci of tumour cells or myocardial tissue and is being developed to provide data on brain metabolism. It is in this area that it may, in the future, be of value in facial pain. Its research use has been reported in atypical facial pain patients (Derbyshire et al., 1994), trigeminal neuralgia (Jones et al., 1999) and cluster headaches (May et al., 1999). The uses of PET in determining central pain mechanisms are reviewed by Laurent et al. (2000) and they put forward some of the challenges that need to be addressed before PET becomes a clinically useful tool in the management of pain patients.

6. Thermography

This technique has been reported in patients with a variety of neurological, vascular, inflammatory and painful conditions, but few high quality reports have been produced. Although the studies had control data the studies do not fulfil all the criteria for evaluation of diagnostic tests as suggested at the start of the chapter, e.g independent observers, reproducibility, κ data, gold standard. There are no available re-

views. Thermography is non-invasive and does not involve ionising radiation. However, special equipment is required and it is a time-consuming procedure and requires a special room with a constant temperature. Its use has been evaluated in cluster headaches (Drummond and Lance, 1984; Mongini et al., 1990), headaches (Ford and Ford, 1997), temporomandibular pain (Canavan and Gratt, 1995; Pogrel et al., 1996; McBeth and Gratt, 1996), and trigeminal neuralgia (Gratt et al., 1996). It is interesting to note that Mongini et al. (1990) found that prolonged tooth clenching resulted in thermographic changes.

7. Evoked potentials

The main clinical use for these tests is in making a diagnosis of multiple sclerosis. Patients with multiple sclerosis can show delayed but well-preserved wave form on visual evoked responses and so supplement clinical data. Care is, however, needed in interpretation and clinical features play a more important role in diagnosis than this test (McDonald et al., 2001).

Somatosensory evoked potentials have been used in a wide variety of conditions and even reported in patients with trigeminal neuralgia. However, all the reports provide poor evidence as to their usefulness as there is no record of blinding the interpreters, no validation and in some cases no controls other than the other side of the patients face. The initial results claimed that these tests could be used to distinguish between a classical and atypical trigeminal neuralgia (Bennett and Jannetta, 1983; Singh et al., 1982) and that they showed which patients are likely to get good long-term effects (Bennett and Lunsford, 1984). However, there has been little in the literature on their use in trigeminal neuralgia since the early 1990s, probably because their specificity is low.

Auditory evoked potentials are used by many neurosurgeons during microvascular decompression to ensure that hearing is preserved (McLaughlin et al., 1999). This is discussed further in Chapter 15 on trigeminal neuralgia.

8. Nerve function

Quantitative sensory testing (QST) are sophisticated tests used to measure somatosensory function. They are important when measuring outcome after nerve repairs and to supplement clinical examination. The methodology is complex and often time consuming and so is not employed routinely (Greenspan, 2001). These psychophysical measures may improve our understanding of neuropathic pain and are currently being used in burning mouth patients (Svensson et al., 1993; Jaaskelainen et al., 1997), patients with atypical facial pain (Jaaskelainen et al., 1999) and trigeminal neuralgia (Nurmikko, 1991; Bowsher et al., 1997). Their use has also been reported in patients with trigeminal neuralgia to demonstrate sensory function after various surgical treatments, e.g. microvascular decompression (Miles et al., 1997), glycerol rhizotomy (Eide and Stubhaug, 1997) and after radiofrequency thermorhizotomy (Hampf et al., 1990), but evidence is not supplied on the use of blinding and independent observers.

9. Miscellaneous tests

All patients undergoing microvascular decompression (MVD) for trigeminal neuralgia are at risk of hearing loss either transient or permanent. Hearing should therefore be objectively measured using audiometric tests especially if this is a complication that could have significant quality of life implications, e.g. for a musician. Ideally, measurements should be done pre and post operatively at several time points to indicate when hearing returns to normal. Most series reporting hearing loss after MVD do not state how this was determined and yet Fritz et al. (1988) suggest that it is important to do these tests, as the pattern of hearing loss can be different and some can be avoided by appropriate technique.

10. Summary

See Table 7 for a summary of this chapter.

TABLE 7

Summary of Chapter 7

- When evaluating diagnostic tests you need to assess whether the results are valid and use what the pretest likelihood of a positive result are likely to be

- Some basic haematological and biochemical tests are likely to be important as baseline data especially if medical management is to be used

- There are a variety of dental tests that can be used including vitality, percussion, mobility, transillumination

- Bacteriological, virological and histological tests may be required in specific cases, e.g. maxillary sinusitis

- Radiographs both dental and facial are important to identify causes of facial pain and there are guidelines available of when and how they should be used

- CT and MRI are increasingly being used to evaluated causes of orofacial pain, some for presence of lesions others for relationships between vessels and nerves

- Positron emission tomography (PET) is a relatively new tool which may prove to be very useful

- Thermography, evoked potentials and nerve function tests are not being used routinely but may become increasingly important

11. Further reading

(1) Sackett DL, Straus SE, Scott Richardson W, Rosenberg W, Haynes RJ Evidence-Based Medicine. How to Practice and Teach EBM. Churchill Livingstone, Edinburgh, 2000; ISBN 0-443-06240-4. (The essential EBM book which is small enough to fit into a pocket but which is updated and expanded on the Web.)

The three following articles are essential when reading articles on diagnosis and differential diagnosis:

(2) Jaeschke R, Guyatt G, Sackett DL. Users' guides to the medical literature. III. How to use an article about a diagnostic test. A. Are the results of the study valid? Evidence-Based Medicine Working Group. J Am Med Assoc 1994; 271: 389–391.

(3) Jaeschke R, Guyatt GH, Sackett DL. Users' guides to the medical literature. III. How to use an article about a diagnostic test. B. What are the results and will they help me in caring for my patients? The Evidence-Based Medicine Working Group. J Am Med Assoc 1994; 271: 703–707.

(4) Richardson WS, Wilson MC, Guyatt GH, Cook DJ, Nishikawa J. Users' guides to the medical literature: XV. How to use an article about disease probability for differential diagnosis. Evidence-Based Medicine Working Group. J Am Med Assoc 1999; 281: 1214–1219

(5) Chodash J. Acute Sinusitis Best evidence (CD ROM). American College of Physicians American Society of Internal Medicine, Philadelphia, PA, 1999, pp 293–302. (This is part of a series in Diagnostic Strategies for Common Medical Problems and provides excellent overviews on these topics including required tests.)

(6) Ingvar M, Hsieh J. Imaging in pain. In: Wall PD, Melzack R. (eds), Textbook of Pain. Churchill Livingstone, Philadelphia, PA, 1999: 215–233. ISBN-0443-06252-8. (A very comprehensive overview of imaging and future possibilities.)

(7) Report: Referral Guidelines for Imaging. Radiation Protection 118 Published by European Communities 2001. Luxemburg, 2001: ISBN 92-828-9454-1 (Available on the web from *http://europa.eu.int* or through Royal College of Radiologist London on *http//www.rcr.ac.uk*.

(8) Report: Making the Best Use of a Department of Clinical Radiology — Guidelines for Doctors, 4th edn. Royal College of Radiologist, 1998. ISBN 1-872599-37-0. (Contains essentially similar material to the European directive and many NHS Trusts have them available for their staff on their intranet, details on how to order on the web site http://www.rcr.ac.uk

(9) Report: Selection Criteria for Radiography. Faculty of Dental Practitioners Royal College of Surgeons UK, 1998. (Due to be updated in 2001.)

(10) Guidelines: Guidelines on Radiology Standards for Primary Dental Care. National Radiological Protection Board HSMO, 1994.

(11) Kidd EAM, Smith BGN. Pickard's Manual of Dentistry, 6th edn. Oxford University Press, Oxford, 1996: ISBN 0-19-262610-8. (Useful reference for dental terminology.)

(12) Chestnutt IG, Gibson J. Churchill's Pocketbook of Clinical Dentistry, 2nd edn. Churchill Livingstone, London, 2002; ISBN 0-443-07084-9. (Provides details of investigations used in dentistry including a radiological one.)

Appendix A

See Table 8 for the answers to Table 3.

TABLE 8

Answers to case studies 1 and 2 in Table 3

These patients both show a lowering of serum sodium levels when the dose of oxcarbazepine is raised. This is a recognized side effect of oxcarbazepine and appears to be due to a re-distribution factor. As the symptoms of hyponatraemia are similar to the side effects of the drug itself it, is important to monitor the serum levels rather then rely on patients' reporting of symptoms. Despite the high doses of oxcarbazepine, there has been no change in the liver function tests. Carbamazepine in similar dosages would have resulted in a marked rise of these values as it induces liver enzymes. You would now look for evidence to evaluate the likelihood of developing hyponatraemia and whether it is a dose–response effect. You also need to determine the frequency of monitoring tests.

References

Marked as regards quality according to criteria set by author.
* Expert case studies, only studies in the field.
** Cohort studies, high quality case series with controls.
*** Randomised controlled trials, high quality original studies.

* Bennett MH, Jannetta PJ. Evoked potentials in trigeminal neuralgia. Neurosurgery 1983; 13: 242–247.
* Bennett MH, Lunsford LD. Percutaneous retrogasserian glycerol rhizotomy for tic douloureux: Part 2. Results and implications of trigeminal evoked potential studies. Neurosurgery 1984; 14: 431–435.
* Berger A. Magnetic resonance imaging. Br Med J 2002; 324: 35.
** Bowsher D, Miles JB, Haggett CE, Eldridge PR. Trigeminal neuralgia: a quantitative sensory perception threshold study in patients who had not undergone previous invasive procedures. J Neurosurg 86, 1997; 190–192.
* Brooks SL. Guidelines for radiologic examinations: do we have all the answers yet? Oral Surg Oral Med Oral Pathol Oral Radiol Endod 1997; 83: 523–524.
* Brooks SL, Brand JW, Gibbs SJ, Hollender L, Lurie AG, Omnell KA, Westesson PL, White SC. Imaging of the temporomandibular joint: a position paper of the American Academy of Oral and Maxillofacial Radiology. Oral Surg Oral Med Oral Pathol Oral Radiol Endod 1997; 83: 609–618.
** Burke TF, Guertler AT, Timmons JH. Comparison of sinus x-rays with computed tomography scans in acute sinusitis. Acad Emerg Med 1994; 1: 235–239.
* Canavan D, Gratt BM. Electronic thermography for the assessment of mild and moderate temporomandibular joint dysfunction. Oral Surg Oral Med Oral Pathol Oral Radiol Endod 1995; 79: 778–786.
* de Lange EE, Vielvoye GJ, Voormolen JH. Arterial compression of the fifth cranial nerve causing trigeminal neuralgia: angiographic findings. Radiology 1986; 158: 721–727.
* Derbyshire SW, Jones AK, Devani P, Friston KJ, Feinmann C, Harris M, Pearce S, Watson JD, Frackowiak RS. Cerebral responses to pain in patients with atypical facial pain measured by positron emission tomography. J Neurol Neurosurg Psychiatry 1994; 57: 1166–1172.
* Drummond PD, Lance JW. Thermographic changes in cluster headache. Neurology 1984; 34: 1292–1298.
* Eide PK, Stubhaug A. Sensory perception in patients with trigeminal neuralgia: effects of percutaneous retrogasserian glycerol rhizotomy. Stereotact Funct Neurosurg 1997; 68: 207–211.
** Evans FO, Syndor JB, Moore WE et al. Sinusitis of the maxillary antrum. N Engl J Med 1975; 293: 735–739.
* Ford RG, Ford KT. Thermography in the diagnosis of headache. Semin Neurol 1997; 17: 343–349.
* Fritz W, Schafer J, Klein HJ. Hearing loss after microvascular decompression for trigeminal neuralgia. J Neurosurg 1988; 69: 367–370.

** Garvey CJ, Hanlon R. Computed tomography in clinical practice. Br Med J 2002; 324: 1077–1080.
* Goh BT, Poon CY, Peck RH. The importance of routine magnetic resonance imaging in trigeminal neuralgia diagnosis. Oral Surg Oral Med Oral Pathol Oral Radiol Endod 2001; 92, 424–429.
* Gratt BM, Graff-Radford SB, Shetty V, Solberg WK, Sickles EA. A 6-year clinical assessment of electronic facial thermography. Dentomaxillofac Radiol 1996; 25: 247–255.
* Greenspan JD. Quantitative assessment of neuropathic pain. Curr Pain Headache Rep 2001; 5: 107–113.
** Grushka M, Sessle BJ. Applicability of the McGill Pain Questionnaire to the differentiation of 'toothache' pain. Pain 1984; 19: 49–57.
** Hampf G, Bowsher D, Wells C, Miles J. Sensory and autonomic measurements in idiopathic trigeminal neuralgia before and after radiofrequency thermocoagulation: differentiation from some other causes of facial pain. Pain 1990; 40: 241–248.
** Hampton JR, Harrison MJ, Mitchell JR, Prichard JS, Seymour C. Relative contributions of history-taking, physical examination, laboratory investigation to diagnosis and management of medical outpatients. Br Med J 1975; 2: 486–489.
* Hayward MW, Lyons K, Ennis WP, Rees J. Radiography of the paranasal sinuses: one or three views? Clin Radiol 1990; 41: 163–164.
* Havas TE, Motbey JA, Gullane PJ. Prevalence of incidental abnormalities on computed tomographic scans of the paranasal sinuses. Arch Otolaryngol Head Neck Surg 1998; 114: 856–859.
** Jaaskelainen SK, Forssell H, Tenovuo O. Abnormalities of the blink reflex in burning mouth syndrome. Pain 1997; 73: 455–460.
** Jaaskelainen SK, Forssell H, Tenovuo O. Electrophysiological testing of the trigeminofacial system: aid in the diagnosis of atypical facial pain. Pain 1999; 80: 191–200.
* Jones AK, Kitchen ND, Watabe H, Cunningham VJ, Jones T, Luthra SK, Thomas DG. Measurement of changes in opioid receptor binding in vivo during trigeminal neuralgic pain using [11C]diprenorphine and positron emission tomography. J Cereb Blood Flow Metab 1999; 19: 803–808.
* Kent DL, Haynor DR, Longstreth WT Jr, Larson EB. Clinical efficacy of magnetic resonance imaging in neuroimaging. Ann Intern Med 1994; 120: 856–871.
* Laurent B, Peyron R, Garcia LL, Mauguiere F. Positron emission tomography to study central pain integration. Rev Neurol (Paris), 2000; 156: 341–351.
** Lloyd GAS. CT of the paranasal sinuses: study of a control series in relation to endoscopic surgery. J Laryngol Otol 1990; 104: 477–481.
** Lukins R, Davan IG, Drummond PD. A cognitive behavioural approach to preventing anxiety during magnetic resonance imaging. J Behav Ther Exp Psychiatry 1997; 28: 97–104.
* Luxenberg J. Commentary on the clinical efficacy of magnetic resonance imaging in neuroimaging. ACP J Club 1994; 121: 49.

* May A, Buchel C, Bahra A, Goadsby PJ, Frackowiak RS. Intracranial vessels in trigeminal transmitted pain: A PET study. Neuroimage 1999; 9: 453–460.

* McBeth SB, Gratt BM. Thermographic assessment of temporomandibular disorders symptomology during orthodontic treatment. Am J Orthod Dentofac Orthop 1996; 109: 481–488.

** McDonald WI, Compston A, Edan G, Goodkin D, Hartung HP, Lublin FD, McFarland HF, Paty DW, Polman CH, Reingold SC, Sandberg-Wollheim M, Sibley W, Thompson A, van den NS, Weinshenker BY, Wolinsky JS. Recommended diagnostic criteria for multiple sclerosis: guidelines from the International Panel on the diagnosis of multiple sclerosis. Ann Neurol 2001; 50: 121–127.

** McIsaac HK, Thordarson DS, Shafran R, Rachman S, Poole G. Claustrophobia and the magnetic resonance imaging procedure. J Behav Med 1998; 21: 255–268.

* McLaughlin MR, Jannetta PJ, Clyde BL, Subach BR, Comey CH, Resnick DK. Microvascular decompression of cranial nerves: lessons learned after 4400 operations. J Neurosurg 1999; 90: 1–8.

*** Melendez JC, McCrank E. Anxiety-related reactions associated with magnetic resonance imaging examinations. J Am Med Assoc 1993; 270: 745–747.

* Miles JB, Eldridge PR, Haggett CE, Bowsher D. Sensory effects of microvascular decompression in trigeminal neuralgia. J Neurosurg 1997; 86: 193–196.

* Mongini F, Caselli C, Macri V, Tetti C. Thermographic findings in cranio-facial pain. Headache 1990; 30: 497–504.

* Mushlin AI, Ruchlin HS, Callahan MA. Costeffectiveness of diagnostic tests. Lancet 2001; 358: 1353–1355.

* Nurmikko TJ. Altered cutaneous sensation in trigeminal neuralgia. Arch Neurol 1991; 48: 523–527.

* Offenbacher H, Fazekas F, Schmidt R et al. Assessment of MRI criteria for a diagnosis of MS. Neurology, 1993; 43: 905–909.

* Pogrel MA, McNeill C, Kim JM. The assessment of trapezius muscle symptoms of patients with temporomandibular disorders by the use of liquid crystal thermography. Oral Surg Oral Med Oral Pathol Oral Radiol Endod 1996; 82: 145–151.

** Roshan M, Rao AP. A study on relative contributions of the history, physical examination and investigations in making medical diagnosis. J Assoc Phys India, 2000; 48: 771–775.

* Singh N, Sachdev KK, Brisman R. Trigeminal nerve stimulation: short latency somatosensory evoked potentials. Neurology 1982; 32: 97–101.

*** Smetana GW, Shmerling RH. Does this patient have temporal arteritis? J Am Med Assoc 2002; 287: 92–101.

** Spector SL, Lotan A, English G, Philpot I. Comparison between transillumination and the roentgenogram in diagnosing paranasal sinus disease. J Allergy Clin Immunol 1981; 67: 22–26.

** Svensson P, Bjerring P, Arendt-Nielsen L, Kaaber S. Sensory and pain thresholds to orofacial argon laser stimulation in patients with chronic burning mouth syndrome. Clin J Pain 1993; 9: 207–215.

** Williams JW, Simel DL, Roberts L, Samsa GP. Clinical evaluation for sinusitis: making the diagnosis by history and physical examination. Ann Intern Med 1992; 117: 705–710.

** Zakrzewska JM. Diagnosis and differential diagnosis of trigeminal neuralgia. J Clin Pain 2002; 18: 14–21.

Assessment and Management of Orofacial Pain
Pain Research and Clinical Management, Vol. 14
Edited by J.M. Zakrzewska and S.D. Harrison

CHAPTER 8

Classification and diagnosis of facial pain

Joanna M. Zakrzewska[*]

*Department of Clinical and Diagnostic Oral Sciences, Oral Medicine Unit, Dental Institute, Barts and
the London, Queen Mary's School of Medicine and Dentistry, Turner Street, London E1 2AD, UK*

Objectives for this chapter:

This chapter will attempt to show you:
- Why a classification system for pain is needed
- What classification systems we currently have
- How complex a task it is to devise a classification system
- How to make a diagnosis using evidence based methodologies
- How to use classification systems to make a diagnosis

---

1. Classification

1.1. Definition and current classification systems

Classification systems allow us to compare observations and carry out research knowing that they apply to the same group of individuals and the need for them is summarised in Table 1 key facts.

There are several major international classification systems for a range of diseases and conditions available as shown in Table 2 key facts, but there remains considerable difficulty in classifying orofacial pain (Woda and Pionchon, 1999) or for that matter any type of pain as any review of the literature shows (Turk and Rudy, 1992, in Handbook of Pain Assemment).

TABLE 1
KEY FACTS: classification systems for chronic pain are essential for
• Epidemiological studies
• Prescribing of treatments
• Evaluation of treatment efficacy
• Decision making and planning

1.2. Theory of classification systems

A variety of classification systems can be used but each must ensure that it is based on a series of common factors and variables, which enable one group of individuals to be consistently distinguished from another. Turk and Rudy (1992) suggest that there are two major strategies for classifications: the theoretical and the empirical. The theoretical model's approach is a deductive process which attempts to

---

[*] Tel.: +44-20-7377-7053; Fax: +44-20-7377-7627;
E-mail: j.m.zakrzewska@qmul.ac.uk

TABLE 2

KEY FACTS: classification systems for pain and psychiatric morbidity

- International Association for the Study of Pain (Merskey and Bogduk, 1994)

- International Headache Society (Anonymous, 1988)

- American Academy of Orofacial Pain Guidelines (Okeson, 1996)

- Research diagnostic criteria for temporomandibular disorders (Dworkin and Le Resche, 1992)

- The ICD 10 classification of mental and behavioural disorders (WHO, 1992)

- Diagnostic and Statistical Manual of Mental Disorders IV (American Association of Psychiatrists, 1994)

define a preconceived cluster of characteristics which is thought to be able to discriminate between different individuals. The International Classification of Diseases coding (ICD), International Society for the Study of Pain (IASP) classification and the International Headache Society (IHS) classification systems all use this approach. The empirical approach is inductive and sets out to first identify a naturally occurring set of variables which characterise each group and then by use of cluster statistics attempts to determine categories. Examples of these types of classification are the MMPI and the SCL-90 systems used in psychological assessments (see Chapter 6 for an explanation of these scales). Within both these systems there is a further division into unidimensional or multidimensional classification systems.

Some of the earliest pain classifications did little more than divide pain into those caused by physical or psychological problems and location was the primary heading. These scales then came to be extended to more categories including time, severity and location, but they remained unidimensional because of the way they were used. An example of this type of classification in the one proposed by the IHS for facial pain (Gobel, 2001). On the other

hand, the IASP classification is multidimensional as it classifies pain on 5 levels:

- body region
- system involved
- aetiology
- temporal characteristics
- intensity and duration of symptoms.

It does not however include any psychosocial or behavioural aspects.

It has long been recognised that patients with the same physical features when given the same treatment do not respond in the same way because factors such as psychosocial ones and personality also affect the outcomes. This has lead to the growing realisation that classification systems must include psychological factors within their structure if we are to make better decisions about treatments and predict outcomes. It is these factors that may be more discriminatory in chronic pain patients. Scales such as the MMPI and SCL90 (see Chapter 6) have therefore been used to categorise patients and so determine treatment choices as well as predict outcomes. Classifications have been based on cognitive factors as well as pain behaviours.

1.3. Multiaxial classification

Turk and Rudy (1992) argue that no studies using current single classification systems have shown convincingly that these systems lead to improved treatment outcomes. They have therefore proposed a multiaxial assessment of patients (MAP) classification based on three questions:

(1) What is the extent of the patient's physical pathology?
(2) What is the magnitude of the patient's disability (suffering and inability to enjoy usual activities)?
(3) Is the patient's behaviour consistent with the pathology identified or is there evidence of amplification of symptoms for any of the variety of psychological, social or economic purposes?

They have put patients into three groups: dysfunctional, interpersonally distressed and adaptive copers and suggested that this is independent of diagnosis. This system was assessed in patients with low back pain, temporomandibular disorders (Rudy et al., 1989) and head pain. It led Turk and Rudy (1992) to suggest that patients' responses to their pain are likely to be similar even if based on different medical causes. This therefore naturally suggests that treatments be based on these three categories rather than on the aetiology but the evidence is still lacking. Turk and Rudy (1992) suggest that patients should have a polydiagnostic approach which would allow them to be included in several classifications. Thus a patient can be diagnosed on the IASP classification system as having a TMJ disorder and on the MAP system as being dysfunctional. Another patient may equally be classified as having a TMJ disorder but on the MAP fits into the adaptive copers group. The treatment for these two patients could therefore be different if you manage the patients according to the MAP classification.

1.4. Other approaches

The polydiagnostic system allows for multiple classifications to be used simultaneously which would enable clinicians to think more broadly but could run into problems when only one or other classification changes (Turk, 1990). This concept has also been used to try and create a computerised pain profile for a patient, which uses pathophysiological, psychological and behavioural factors (Duncan et al., 1978).

More recently, Woolf et al. (1998) have suggested that the usual physical diagnosis should be replaced by a mechanism-based classification. Thus neuropathic pain whatever its location or cause can be potentially treated in the same way. An example of this approach can be can be seen in the trial of lamotrigine in neuropathic pains which did not attempt to differentiate between different conditions such as trigeminal neuralgia and diabetic neuropathy (McCleane, 1999).

Woda and Pionchon (1999), after a review of the literature, have suggested a set of diagnostic criteria that embraces all forms of orofacial pain including atypical facial pain, atypical odontalgia, stomatodynia and idiopathic facial arthromyalgia.

1.5. Evaluation of classification systems

The question that really must be asked when assessing any classification system is: does the assignment of an individual patient to a group facilitate treatment decisions or predict future outcomes and behaviour? It needs to be:

- reliable
- valid
- comprehensive
- generalizable

Accurate diagnostic criteria and hence classification systems will remain difficult to define in most facial pain until we have more objective means of validating the patients' history. Currently, diagnoses are reliant on patient history and this may be inaccurate either because the patient is a poor historian or because the clinician has not been able to elicit it for whatever reasons. Diagnosis can be helped by asking your patient to keep a prospective diary in which they note all the features of the pain. You need to be aware that pain diaries often only capture the sensory component of the pain and not the affective one which involves the patients emotions, fears about the pain and ability to cope (Andrasik et al., 1981).

The IHS classification provides clear criteria for each condition also including details on which ones and how many of the criteria need to be present to make a particular diagnosis. Code numbers are allocated to each condition. Many of criteria still need to be validated as has been attempted by Pfaffenrath et al. (1993) for atypical facial pain and chronic paroxysmal hemicrania (Leone et al., 1994). The system is used in clinical trials on headaches — migraine, cluster headache and tension type headaches (published in the International Headache Society's annual members handbook). The classification is currently being updated based on new evidence that has been published and collected from consensus meetings and will probably be available from 2002 in its new format.

The IASP classification describes each type of pain under the same headings of: definition, site, system main features (includes incidence, prevalence, pain quality, time pattern, intensity, usual duration), associated symptoms and signs, laboratory findings/investigations, relief, usual course, complications, social and physical disability, pathology, aetiology, summary of essential features and diagnostic criteria, differential diagnosis and a few key references. Each type of pain is then given its unique six-figure code. It does not make any attempt at suggesting which and how many features need to be present before a particular diagnosis is made.

A wide variety of other classifications are used in textbooks of facial pain but none of them are based on any sound methodology and give no evidence for their use.

2. Evidenced-based diagnosis

Classification systems become important in the making of a differential diagnosis as they enable us to compare our patients constellation of findings with other well-defined conditions. You may like to start this section with case study 1 (Table 3).

When coming to a diagnosis we should ensure that we follow five clearly defined stages as summarised in Table 4 key facts (Richardson, 1997) and elaborated on below.

TABLE 3

Case study 1: making a diagnosis

A 74-year-old woman comes to see you complaining of a recent onset of a moderately severe throbbing headache in the right temple region which is associated with neck pain. What are the steps needed to make a definitive diagnosis of giant cell arteritis? Is there some evidenced-based material that would help you? See Table 10 at the end of chapter for the answer.

TABLE 4

KEY FACTS: making a diagnosis

- Gather clinical information
- Frame clinical problem
- Select differential diagnosis
- Choose diagnostic test
- Interpret test results

The method has been elegantly illustrated in a case study attempting to differentiate between trigeminal neuralgia and temporomandibular pain by Drangsholt and Truelove (2001).

2.1. Gather information

Clinical findings can be both positive in that they show some symptom or sign or negative in that they do not show a particular symptom or sign. Once we have some idea of what the possible diagnosis could be then we can target questions more to ensure that we have gathered all the clinical findings. In the case discussed above we would enquire if the patient has any pain on eating even if she does not initially mention it as it is a key feature of temporal arteritis.

2.2. Frame the clinical problem

Once we have gathered the clinical findings from the history and examination we can then frame them into coherent groups or patterns, which are called clinical problems. These can be groupings such as pre-auricular pain, depression or clinical syndromes that include many findings e.g. trigeminal neuralgia.

2.3. Select differential diagnosis

Having identified one or several clinical problems we then proceed to make a differential diagnosis. This is when we need a list of possible causes and where classification systems can prove to be valuable. If the initial short list does not enable us to make a diagnosis then we need to turn to longer lists. This is an area for which more evidence is needed, as we want to know what is the pre-test possibility of the relevant disorder given the problems we have found.

2.4. Choose a diagnostic test

Having narrowed down the possible number of causes we now need to choose some diagnostic tests that would confirm our diagnosis or would exclude it. The tests themselves should have undergone evaluation as described in Chapter 7 on investigations.

2.5. Interpret the test results

Once we have the results from the most appropriate tests we need to be able to interpret them correctly. We then bring everything together and see how the post-test probability compares with our threshold of testing and treatment.

Is the evidence strong enough for us to:

- do no further tests and just go on to treatment
- do further tests
- abandon our initial diagnosis and go to the next one on the list
- choose new tests

3. How to make that initial differential diagnosis of facial pain

Primary care clinicians would not be expected to make accurate diagnoses on rare conditions, e.g. cluster headache. It would, however, be appropriate for them to be able to assess an orofacial pain sufficiently accurately to be able to refer it appropriately. Thus a classification system that would enable patients to be referred to a general dentist, a neurologist or pain specialist or to a specialist oral physician or oral surgeon would be a useful starting point.

Hapak et al. (1994) have proposed that a 21 self complete questionnaire, a diagram of chief pain location and digital pain scale for severity enables patients to be put into one of three broad diagnostic groups, e.g. musculoligamentous, dentoalveolar and neurological. This they suggest would categorise patients sufficiently for them to be referred to the correct secondary care specialist who would then carry out a full assessment and make the final diagnosis. The collected data was validated using trained clinicians as the gold standard. The musculoligamentous (ml) and neurological (ne) groups had specificities and sensitivities between 78 and 81% with positive predicative values of 88% (ml) and 56% (ne) and negative predicative values of 69% (ml) and 91% (ne) and κ values of 0.6% (ml) and 0.5% (ne). The data for the dentoalveolar pain were poorer with a κ value of 0.4%.

Hernandez-Gallego et al. (1993) used a craniofacial pain questionnaire of 57 questions which included location, quantity, quality, frequency, duration, family history, accompanying symptoms of craniofacial pain to differentiate migraines, tension-type headaches and other facial pains on 67 patients with facial pain. The patients were put into one of three categories by means of stepwise discriminate analysis which is not explained in sufficient detail.

Goulet (2001) proposes a three stepwise clinical decision process.

Step 1. Determining primary local origin:

intraoral
extraoral

if this can be determined then move on to:
 (a) establishing the cause or mechanism
 (b) assessing disability, behaviour and related psychosocial status
If this cannot be determined move on to step 2.

Step 2. determining whether pain is referred from:

intraoral sites
extraoral sites

if this can be determine proceed as in step 1. If this cannot be determined move to step 3.

Step 3. Consider source of pain in distant structures or organ systems:

neuropathic
vascular
cardiovascular
complex regional pain

once one of these has been chosen, establish the cause and mechanism as in step 1.

Tyrer (1992) in his book on psychology, psychiatry and chronic pain provides a scheme on assessment of psychological and psychiatric factors in chronic pain.

None of these systems take into account the epidemiology of different types of facial pain which will also affect your suspicions, e.g. trigeminal neuralgia is very rare as compared to dental pain, an older woman is more likely to have burning mouth syndrome than a young male.

4. How to make a definitive diagnosis

The next stage is to make a definitive diagnosis and this is currently difficult to do as the diagnostic criteria of all the different causes of orofacial pains have not been validated and there is considerable controversy in the literature (Woda and Pionchon, 1999). Criteria for multiple sclerosis (McDonald et al., 2001) and temporal arteritis are available (Hunder et al., 1990) and are widely discussed in the literature.

The best evidence from which to determine these diagnostic criteria are cross-sectional studies using a defined gold standard. In view of the lack of some objective diagnostic test for most facial pain the history and diagnosis become the main diagnostic test, the McGill Pain Questionnaire could be said to be a diagnostic test but it has not been validated in orofacial pain as not all the studies used control groups when evaluating it (Grushka and Sessle, 1984; Hall et al., 1986; Melzack et al., 1986). It is not consistently completed with patients wanting to use more than one descriptor per group or finding it too in-

volved (Vickers et al., 1998). These methods also exclude specific patient groups, such as migrants, children and those who cannot express themselves verbally.

Failing this, case series are needed which list all the clinical features together with their prevalence in the given population. An attempt has been made to address this shortcoming by setting up the CARE project (McAlister et al., 1999, *http://carestudy.com*). It is run by the Evidence-Based team at Oxford and could provide a way by which clinicians from round the world could contribute data on clinical features of a range of orofacial pain and then analyse it collectively. Once the diagnostic criteria have been validated and shown to be reliable and reproducible then it would be relatively simple to set up a computerised programme which would list diagnosis in order of probability. Pre-test probabilities calculate the probability of the patient having the target diagnosis based on findings in the history and examination.

5. Aids to making a diagnosis

It is useful to read the paper by Richardson et al. (2000) on how to read an article on clinical manifestations of disease as it reminds us that accurate well validated clinical manifestations of a disease will enable us to improve our ability to raise a diagnostic hypothesis, select an appropriate differential diagnosis and ultimately verify the final diagnosis. They suggest that to assess the validity of an article on clinical manifestations you need to ascertain the following:

- How the diagnosis was verified
- How the study sample relates to all patients with the disease
- How the clinical findings were sought
- How the clinical findings were characterised.

I attempted to assess this for trigeminal neuralgia and found that we do not have all the answers (Zakrzewska, 2002).

TABLE 5

KEY FACTS: major clinical classification of facial pain

Musculoligamentous/soft tissue	Dentoalveolar	Neurological/vascular
Temporomandibular (TMJ) disorders	Dentinal	Chronic tension headaches
Atypical facial pain/idiopathic orofacial pain	Periodontal	Trigeminal neuralgia
Myofascial pain	Pulpal	Migraine
Salivary gland disease	Dental abscess	Temporal arteritis
Internal derangements TMJ	Thermal sensitivities	Post-herpetic neuralgia
Nerve compression	Cracked tooth syndrome	Cluster headache
Burning mouth	Maxillary sinusitis	SUNCT
Candidiasis		Glossopharyngeal neuralgia
Cancer		Ramsay Hunt
Atypical odontalgia		Pre-trigeminal neuralgia
Oral mucosal diseases		Optic neuritis
		Acute angle glaucoma

The following tables provide some help in making an initial diagnosis which would enable a clinician to place the patient in one of three categories. The three categories are adapted from the classification of Hapak et al. (1994) and are shown in Table 5.

Benoliel et al. (1997) have put forward a suggestion that many orofacial pains can be classified as vascular orofacial pains. This is discussed in further detail at the end of Chapter 10.

All the studies suggest that location, severity and the nine features of pain (see Chapter 4 on history taking) can be sufficient to make a diagnosis or orofacial pain. Each of these will be considered in turn.

5.1. Site

Table 6 shows the predominant site for different orofacial pains.

TABLE 6

KEY FACTS: major sites of facial pain

Unilateral	Bilateral	Unilateral or bilateral
Trigeminal neuralgia	Burning mouth syndrome	TMJ
Salivary gland disease	Candidiasis	Atypical facial pain
Optic neuritis	Chronic tension headache	Myofascial
Internal derangements TMJ	Migraine	Maxillary sinusitis
Cancer		Frontal sinusitis
Most dental		Dental–anterior region
Glossopharyngeal neuralgia		Temporal arteritis
Nerve compression		
Cluster headache		
Post-herpetic neuralgia		
Ramsay Hunt		
Pre-trigeminal neuralgia		
SUNCT		

Some of these pains are very specifically located in the area of the trigeminal nerve, others radiate beyond the trigeminal area although they may still remain unilateral. Hapak et al. (1994) postulate that nine sites will provide enough discrimination.

5.1.1. Conditions in specific areas

Mostly bilateral

- Eyes, temples, forehead: chronic tension headaches, temporal arteritis
- Pre- and periauricular (lateral aspects): TMJ, parotid gland, diseases of the ear
- Middle face: maxillary sinusitis, upper dental problems
- Lower half of face: nerve compression, submandibular salivary gland disease
- Intraoral: dental, atypical odontalgia, maxillary sinusitis
- Whole face: atypical facial pain

Bilateral

- Intraoral: burning mouth syndrome, candidiasis, dental diseases
- Both eyes, temples forehead: tension headache, tension headache

Unilateral

- One eye, temple, half forehead: migraine cluster headache, SUNCT, giant cell arteritis, optic neuritis, chronic paroxysmal hemicrania, SUNCT
- One, two or three branches of trigeminal nerve: trigeminal neuralgia, atypical facial pain, post-herpetic neuralgia
- Throat, intraoral: glossopharyngeal neuralgia
- Intraoral: nerve compression, mental commonest

5.2. Character and severity

Vickers et al. (1998) have shown that the use of a visual analogue scale for intensity and the McGill pain questionnaire are sensitive enough for use in patients with orofacial pain and help to distinguish patients who may have more than one diagnosis.

Table 7 provides some characteristics of character and indication of severity of orofacial pain.

5.3. Timing of pain

In the McGill pain questionnaire, the timing of pain is put into three categories

- Brief, momentary, transient
- Rhythmic, periodic, intermittent
- Continuous, steady, constant

In the IASP classification, six categories are suggested and these have been used for orofacial pain as shown in Table 8.

5.4. Distinguishing features of orofacial pain

Some orofacial pains have specific characteristics which help in confirming the diagnosis as shown below:

- autonomic features: SUNCT, cluster headaches
- limited mouth opening and clicking joint: some TMJ pain
- drug response: opioids, local anaesthetic, indomethecin
- triggers non-nociceptic receptors and refractory pain periods are present: trigeminal neuralgia, glossopharyngeal neuralgia
- allodynia: post-herpetic neuralgia
- taste disturbance and dryness: burning mouth syndrome

TABLE 7

KEY FACTS: character and severity of orofacial pains

Most characteristic words used	Severity	In order of likely
Nagging, aching, dull, drawing	Mild to severe — atypical facial pain Mild to severe — dental pain Mild to moderate — TMJ	Dental pain especially chronic pulpal and periodontal Atypical facial pain, TMJ
Throbbing, aching and shooting	mild to severe — atypical facial pain, atypical odontalgia	Atypical facial pain, atypical odontalgia
Throbbing, pulsing, beating	Mild to moderate — pulpal Moderate to severe — temporal arteritis Severe — cluster headache	Pulpal pain Temporal arteritis, cluster headache
Sharp, shooting, stabbing	Mild to severe	Trigeminal neuralgia, glossopharyngeal neuralgia
Pressing, wrenching, tugging, tightening	Mild moderate severe	Nerve compression, chronic tension headache
Burning, tingling, tender, annoying, itching	Mild to moderate	Burning mouth syndrome, post-herpetic neuralgia
Unbearable, miserable, fearful	Moderate to severe	Trigeminal neuralgia, atypical facial pain (rare)

TABLE 8

KEY FACTS: characteristic timings of orofacial pain

Pattern	Possible diagnosis
Continuous or nearly continuous — non-fluctuating	Atypical facial pain, temporal arteritis, post-herpetic neuralgia, periodontal, bone pain
Continuous or nearly continuous — fluctuating	Atypical facial pain, post-herpetic neuralgia, burning mouth syndrome
Recurring, irregular	Dental, migraine, chronic tension, dental
Recurring, regular	Cluster headache, SUNCT
Paroxysmal	Pulpal, trigeminal neuralgia, glossopharyngeal
Sustained with superimposed paroxysms	Burning mouth syndrome

6. Summary

See Table 9 for a summary of this chapter.

TABLE 9

Summary of Chapter 8

1. Classification of orofacial pain improves management
2. Systems are available for both physical and psychological classification of pain
3. A multiaxial assessment may be more useful for management
4. Any system must be reliable, valid, comprehensive and generalizable
5. There are five key stages in the making of a diagnosis
6. Some aids to making a diagnosis are provided

Appendix A

The answers to the case study in Table 3 are given in Table 10.

Appendix B. Further reading

B.1. Books and chapters

(1) International Headache Society Members Handbook (2000) Scandinavian University Press, 1999: ISBN 82-00-37704-0. (Gives diagnostic criteria and also guidelines on clinical trials in the field of headache, updated yearly.)
(2) Tyrer S. Psychology, Psychiatry and Chronic Pain. Butterworth, Oxford, 1992: ISBN 0-7506-05731-1. (This one of the few books linking these subjects, it contains many useful models, schemata and algorithms.)
(3) Lund JP, Lavigne GJ, Dubner R, Sessle BJ (eds). Orofacial Pain, From Basic Science to Clinical Management. Quintessence Publish-

TABLE 10

Answer to case study 1 making a diagnosis in Table 3

- We looked on the CD ROM Best Evidence Issue 5 and found an article by Kantor (1999) based on a review of 32 articles and we then looked for an updates in PubMed and found Smetana and Shmerling (2002).

- Jaw claudication in persons older than 50 years is the single most specific symptom for temporal arteritis. Other highly specific features are new onset of headache and abnormal arteritis.

- This enables you to frame the clinical problem. This patient is likely to have temporal arteritis and you can ask her some supplemental questions to ascertain whether she has tenderness of the arteries, fever, anorexia or weight loss.

- You now need to select some possible differentials. These could include conditions that cause pain around the temple, e.g. cluster headache, optic neuritis, SUNCT or those that lead to weight loss such as malignancy, but these are lower down in the list.

- Now is the time to choose the appropriate test to differentiate between. The article in Best Evidence informs you that the most sensitive tests are an ESR and temporal artery biopsy. An ESR above 40 mm/h would rule in the possibility of temporal arteritis. A low ESR below 40 mm/h would rule it out but in this patient with a high pre-test probability an ESR and temporal artery biopsy will probably be needed.

- After the ESR and biopsy have been done you need to interpret the results and make a decision as to whether this patient has temporal arteritis and needs to be urgently treated with systemic steroids. When the results of the biopsy are positive the post-test probability of temporal arteritis is high. This is important as treatment with systemic steroids in elderly patients carries with it potential for severe side effects.

ing, Chicago, 2001: 167–183. (Evidence-based articles.)

(4) Richardson WS, Wilson MC, Williams JW Jr, Moyer VA, Naylor CD. Users' Guides to the Medical Literature: XXIV. How to Use an Article on the Clinical Manifestations of Disease. Evidence-Based Medicine Working Group. J Am Med Assoc 2000; 284: 869–875.

(5) Richardson WS, Wilson MC, Guyatt GH, Cook DJ, Nishikawa J. Users' Guides to the Medical Literature: XV. How to Use an Article about Disease Probability for Differential Diagnosis. Evidence-Based Medicine Working Group. J Am Med Assoc 1999; 281: 1214–1219.

(6) Richardson WS, Detsky AS. Users' Guides to the Medical Literature. VII. How to Use a Clinical Decision Analysis. A. Are the Results of the Study Valid? Evidence-Based Medicine Working Group. J Am Med Assoc 1995: 273; 1292–1295.

(7) Richardson WS, Detsky AS. Users' guides to the medical literature. VII. How to use a clinical decision analysis. B. What are the results and will they help me in caring for my patients? Evidence-Based Medicine Working Group. J Am Med Assoc 1995; 273: 1610–1613.

B.2. Major classification systems

(8) Anonymous. Classification and diagnostic criteria for headache disorders, cranial neuralgias and facial pain. Headache Classification Committee of the International Headache Society. Cephalalgia 1988; 8 (Suppl 7): 1–96.

(9) Merskey H, Bogduk N (eds), Classification of Chronic Pain. Descriptors of Chronic Pain Syndromes and Definitions of Pain Terms. IASP Press, Seattle, WA, 1994.

(10) Dworkin SF, LeResche L. Research diagnostic criteria for temporomandibular disorders: review, criteria, examinations and specifications, critique. J Craniomandib Disord 1992; 6: 301–355.

(11) Okeson JP. Orofacial pain guide: guidelines for assessment, diagnosis and management. Consensus views of American Academy of orofacial pain. Quintessence Publishing, Chicago, 1996.

(12) American Psychiatric Association. Diagnostic and Statistical Manual of Mental Disorders IV. New York, American Psychiatric Association, 1994.

(13) World Health Organisation. The ICD 10 Classification of Mental and Behavioural Disorders. WHO, Geneva, 1992.

References

Marked as regards quality according to criteria set by author.
* Poorer quality studies but only ones in the field, old style reviews.
** Cohort studies, high quality case series with controls.
*** Randomised controlled trials, high quality original studies.

* Andrasik F, Blanchard EB, Ahles T, Pallmeyer T, Barron KD. Assessing the reactive as well as the sensory component of headache pain. Headache 1981; 21, 218–221.

Benoliel R, Elishoov H, Sharav Y. Orofacial pain with vascular-type features. Oral Surg Oral Med Oral Pathol 1997; 84: 506–512.

*** Drangsholt M, Truelove E. Trigeminal neuralgia mistaken as temporomandibular disorder. J Evid Base Dent Pract 2001; 1: 41–50.

* Duncan GH, Gregg JM, Ghia JN. The pain profile: a computerized system for assessment of chronic pain. Pain 1978; 5: 275–284.

* Gobel H. Classification of headaches. Cephalalgia 2001; 21: 770–773.

Goulet JP. The path to diagnosis. In: Lund JP, Lavigne GJ, Dubner R, Sessle BJ. Orofacial Pain, From Basic Science to Clinical Management. Quintessence Publishing, Chicago, 2001: 167–183.

** Grushka M, Sessle BJ. Applicability of the McGill Pain Questionnaire to the differentiation of 'toothache' pain. Pain 1984; 19: 49–57.

** Hall EH, Terezhalmy GT, Pelleu GB Jr. A set of descriptors for the diagnosis of dental pain syndromes. Oral Surg Oral Med Oral Pathol 1986; 61: 153–157.

** Hapak L, Gordon A, Locker D, Shandling M, Mock D, Tenenbaum HC. Differentiation between musculoligamentous, dentoalveolar, and neurologically based craniofacial pain with a diagnostic questionnaire. J Orofac Pain 1994; 8: 357–368.

* Hernandez-Gallego J, Larrea J, Cubero A, Carrillo F. In: Olesen J, Schoenen J (eds), Tension-Type Headache: Classification, Mechanism and Treatment. Raven Press, New York, 1993: 33–37.

**Hunder GG, Bloch DA, Michel BA, Stevens MB, Arend WP, Calabrese LH, Edworthy SM, Fauci AS, Leavitt RY, Lie JT. The American College of Rheumatology 1990 criteria for the classification of giant cell arteritis. Arthritis Rheum 1990; 33: 1122–1128.

***Kantor SM. Temporal Arteritis. American College of Physicians-American Society of Internal Medicine, Philadelphia, PA, 1999.

*Leone M, Filippini G, D'Amico D, Farinotti M, Bussone G. Assessment of International Headache Society diagnostic criteria: a reliability study. Cephalalgia 1994; 14: 280–284.

***McAlister FA, Straus SE, Sackett DL. Why we need large, simple studies of the clinical examination: the problem and a proposed solution. CARE-COAD1 group. Clinical Assessment of the Reliability of the Examination-Chronic Obstructive Airways Disease Group. Lancet 1999; 354: 1721–1724.

*McCleane G. 200 mg daily of lamotrigine has no analgesic effect in neuropathic pain: a randomised, double-blind, placebo controlled trial. Pain 1999; 83: 105–107.

**McDonald WI, Compston A, Edan G, Goodkin D, Hartung HP, Lublin FD, McFarland HF, Paty DW, Polman CH, Reingold SC, Sandberg-Wollheim M, Sibley W, Thompson A, van den Noort NS, Weinshenker BY, Wolinsky JS. Recommended diagnostic criteria for multiple sclerosis: guidelines from the International Panel on the diagnosis of multiple sclerosis. Ann Neurol 2001; 50: 121–127.

**Melzack R, Terrence C, Fromm G, Amsel R. Trigeminal neuralgia and atypical facial pain: use of the McGill Pain Questionnaire for discrimination and diagnosis. Pain 1986; 27: 297–302.

**Pfaffenrath V, Rath M, Pollmann W, Keeser W. Atypical facial pain–application of the IHS criteria in a clinical sample. Cephalalgia 1993; 13 (Suppl 12): 84–88.

***Richardson WS. Evidence based diagnosis: more is needed. Evid-Based Med 1997; 2: 70.

**Rudy TE, Turk DC, Zaki HS, Curtin HD. An empirical taxometric alternative to traditional classification of temporomandibular disorders. Pain 1989; 36: 311–320.

***Smetana GW, Shmerling RH. Does this patient have temporal arteritis? J Am Med Assoc 2002; 287: 92–101.

*Turk DC. Strategies for classifying chronic orofacial pain patients. Anesth Prog 1990; 37: 155–160.

*Turk DC, Rudy TE. In: Turk DC, Melzack R (eds), Handbook of Pain Assessment. Guilford Press, New York, 1992: 409–428.

*Vickers ER, Cousins MJ, Woodhouse A. Pain description and severity of chronic orofacial pain conditions. Aust Dent J 1998; 43: 403–409.

*Woda A, Pionchon P. A unified concept of idiopathic orofacial pain: clinical features. J Orofac Pain 1999; 13: 172–184.

*Woolf CJ, Bennett GJ, Doherty M, Dubner R, Kidd B, Koltzenburg M, Lipton R, Loeser JD, Payne R, Torebjork E. Towards a mechanism-based classification of pain? Pain 1998; 77: 227–229.

**Zakrzewska JM. Diagnosis and differential diagnosis of trigeminal neuralgia. J Clin Pain 2002; 18: 14–21

Assessment and Management of Orofacial Pain
Pain Research and Clinical Management, Vol. 14
Edited by J.M. Zakrzewska and S.D. Harrison
© *2002 Elsevier Science B.V. All rights reserved*

CHAPTER 9

Management overview

Joanna M. Zakrzewska [*]

*Department of Clinical and Diagnostic Oral Sciences, Oral Medicine Unit, Dental Institute, Barts and
the London Queen Mary's School of Medicine and Dentistry, Turner Street, London E1 2AD, UK*

Objectives for this chapter:

This chapter will attempt to:
- Illustrate how patients can become partners in their management
- How good communication skills are needed to educate and manage patients with chronic facial pain
- Provide you with an appreciation of how patients' beliefs and expectations affect outcome
- Suggest how integrated care can provide improved outcome
- Stress the importance of a holistic approach to management that may involve a variety of different treatments
- Illustrate the importance of using data from randomised clinical trials to inform management and how this data can be improved
- Broadly evaluate the use of drugs, surgery, psychological and physiological forms of treatment for chronic facial pain patients
- Provide an overview of management of depression
- Provide information on how to find patient information and how to assess its value
- Assess factors that lead to chronicity and the need for long-term management

1. Introduction

In many respects, treatment of a chronic facial pain patient is no different from any patient with chronic pain as the psychosocial and behavioural response patterns are the same despite different medical and dental causes. However, you need to remember that the psychological and symbolic significance of the head in the development of self esteem, body image and interpersonal relationships confers special characteristics on pain in this area. The features that

* Tel.: +44-20-7377-7053; Fax: +44-20-7377-7627;
E-mail: j.m.zakrzewska@qmul.ac.uk

are common to all the forms of chronic facial pain will be discussed in this chapter. You will find more detail on specific treatments for the different types of facial pain in the individual chapters.

Although chronic pain can lead to dysfunction in some patients, you need to remember that not all patients with chronic pain are disabled and some adapt to pain and continue to function normally despite the pain.

For management to be successful it must begin with a discussion about the diagnosis or possible differential diagnosis and then move on to a review of possible treatment plans which then leads to a negotiated treatment plan to which adherence needs to be achieved. This process involves active patient participation, good communication skills and appropriate choice of treatment based on high quality evidence and increased patient information and self support. Chronic facial pain cannot always be totally abolished and so it is important to have in place long-term strategies for its management. Regular reassessment is essential and should even include a possible change in diagnosis.

We all know that clinical problems are rarely simple and we are surrounded by uncertainties and yet, traditionally, we have used linear models to break down clinical care into small divisions each of which have their precisely defined methods of management. This has led to considerable dissatisfaction and so it is important for treatment to be viewed as a highly complex science that requires a holistic approach. Chronic facial pain results from complex, dynamic and unique interactions between different components of the overall system and effective care needs to build in unpredictability and take on board not only strict guidelines but also include the intuition and experience of both the patient and the healthcare worker.

In the section on further reading two further articles are provided from the series Users Guides to the Medical Literature, one on the use of treatment recommendations and the other on the use of electronic health information resources which will help you in critically appraising the data.

2. Patients as partners in managing facial pain

2.1. Patient centred care

There is growing consensus that patients should become more involved in all aspects of their health care. Patients have become experienced consumers who understand that they have rights and have become less inclined to leave all the medical decisions to the doctors. Patient's autonomy, i.e. what the competent, informed patient wants, is more important than what the doctor thinks best for the patient. There is evidence that patient involvement in care leads to better health outcomes and this is resulting in a shift in power and in patient-centred care (Ka-

TABLE 1
KEY FACTS: level of patient involvement with treatment
• Patient wants information which includes alternatives, but delegates all decision making to the doctor
• Patient collaborates with the doctor in decision making
• Patient makes his/her own decisions after being given sufficient information

plan et al., 1989). Not only is patient-centred care extremely complex, but you also need to take into account the fact that not all patients want this approach nor do all healthcare providers wish to comply with this approach. It is, therefore, important to determine at what level patients want to be involved in their care and to review this from time to time as shown in Table 1. You may like to read more about patient-centred care in David Misselbrook's book on thinking about patients (see further reading). Price and Leaver (2002) also draw attention to the fact that all of the patient's reasons for attendance need to be elicited and that at the first consultation it is useful to be able to give patients a diagnosis, a feeling that their concerns have been addressed and some knowledge of the treatment and prognosis as this allays anxiety and improves outcomes.

Which level of involvement patients choose will depend on:

- patient's background
- clinical situation which may even vary in the same patient
- family and cultural expectations/beliefs
- the healthcarer's attitude towards patient-centred care

Patient-centred medical care emphasises the central role of the patient in deciding about their healthcare and this was one of the major recommendations made after the Bristol inquiry into the failures of performance of surgeons involved in cardiac surgery on

TABLE 2

KEY FACTS: benefits of patient centred care

- Provision of care appropriate to patients needs
- Improved patient safety: patients know what to expect from their treatment, check their own notes and results
- Reduces complaints and litigation: informed consent, improved communications
- Improves quality of care: patient-centred satisfaction surveys and increased public accountability

children. Patient-centred care can result in a number of benefits, which are shown in Table 2. Training can improve a healthcare worker's ability to deliver patient centred care as has been shown by a systematic review (Lewin et al., 2002).

In order for the patient to be more involved in their care, Hope (1996) puts forward a four-step chain:

(1) The issue needs to be of importance to patients who are making choices: patients need to be involved in identifying the issues
(2) The evidence must be of good quality: systematic reviews and randomised controlled trials are the ideals but lower quality evidence may need to be used
(3) The information should be in a form that is accessible to patients with a minimum of bias: risks and benefits need to be highlighted
(4) The information can be used by patients to enhance choice: patients need to have genuine choice free of medical bias

Empowering patients to take on more responsibility for their care means that they must be given a variety of tools:

- Recognition of their expertise, values and preferences
- Offered informed consent, not passive consent
- Be trained in shared decision-making
- Given evidence-based decision aids
- Educated in interpretation of clinical evidence

- Provided with access to their electronic health records
- Given public access to comparative data on quality and outcomes

Holman and Lorig (2000) suggest that for effective management, both the patients' individual information and the doctors' general information on the disease or condition are important. They go on to provide details of three types of programmes that have been developed to enable patients to participate more effectively in their healthcare.

(1) Self-management education: this involves patients in learning about effective use of their medication and how it influences their pain, coping with emotional reactions, adjusting their social behaviour and using other resources including learning from other patients. These programmes focus on problems experienced by patients who need to learn how to solve their own problems, set their own goals and give and receive feedback on their accomplishments. This type of programme has been evaluated in arthritis and shows that patients' confidence in their ability to cope with their disease rises substantially (Lorig et al., 1993).
(2) Group visits: patients with the same disease/condition meet on a regular basis with one doctor. The agendas are largely set by the patients and concern problems they encounter from their disease (Beck et al., 1997). One small study has been reported on the use of group therapy in 19 patients with chronic idiopathic facial pain (Harrison et al., 1997) which appeared effective but did not have a control group to improve its validity. These techniques therefore could be potentially useful in facial pain management and could prove to be cost effective.
(3) Remote medical management via the telephone or electronic communication. This is especially useful if the healthcare worker is the same and the patients live at some distance. Not only does this result in decreased costs, but also improves outcomes (Wasson et al., 1992).

2.2. Decision-making

Making decisions about treatment depends not only on the patients' understanding of the disease or condition, but also their understanding and attitude towards risk-taking. Risk-taking involves assessing the probability, severity and timing of an adverse outcome. Some patients prefer to put off bad outcomes for the future, others will accept them immediately. Patients with very severe trigeminal neuralgia will often accept any form of surgery despite the adverse effects, but if the same surgery is proposed to them during a period of remission or mild pain, they are often reluctant to take the risk and opt for medical management. Informed decision-making should increase the probability of an outcome which the patient regards as favourable while at the same time decreasing the probability of an outcome that a patient regards as being unfavourable. Patients are more likely to be involved in the decision-making process if the doctor is satisfied with his/her professional autonomy and has longer consultation times. Kaplan et al. (1996) also showed that interview skills training in primary care physicians enabled this to be achieved.

In order to help patients with decisions both on treatment and screening, a variety of decision aids have been designed and many of these are evaluated in the journal of 'Medical Decision Making'. A systematic review has been published whose objective was to determine if decision aids improved decision-making and outcomes (O'Connor et al., 1999, 2001). The review concluded that decision aids:

- Improve knowledge
- Reduce decisional conflict
- Stimulate patients to be more active in the process
- Do not increase anxiety
- Have little effect on satisfaction
- Have a variable effect on decisions
- Effect of decisions on outcome remains uncertain

Decision aids appear to be most beneficial to patients who are undecided about their treatment (O'Connor et al., 1999). Elwyn et al. (2001) provide a useful review of the current status of decision analysis in patient care which illustrates the complexity of the subject and the need for considerable research before decision analysis will have a significant impact on management of patients. Redelmeier et al. (1993) also remind us that clinicians need to understand how people reason and how emotional and cognitive factors can sometimes conflict.

3. Negotiating treatment plans

Both the patients' and the doctors' models of illness and disease (see chapter on history taking) must be taken into account when negotiating treatment plans (Kleinman et al., 1978).

In order to achieve this, your communication skills at this stage of diagnosis and treatment planning need to be as well developed as when taking a history. Good communication skills can improve physical health, psychological health, informed consent, compliance and decrease litigation. Your aim at this stage of the consultation is to share your understanding of the diagnosis of the condition, then come to a negotiated treatment plan to which the patient will adhere in order to improve outcomes. In order for this to happen successfully you need to ensure that the patient has the knowledge and relevant attitude and behaviour. At this stage, educational methodology is important and how this is done is summarised in Table 3 key facts.

Patients' feelings must be discussed and the patients need to feel that they have been understood, believed and accepted. Only then will patients begin to develop insight into their problems and find they can look at new ways of managing their pain.

Patients' pain beliefs play a vital role in management and need to be assessed at all levels. It is often the lack of attention to this detail that results in treatment failure. Skevington (1995) has shown that matching treatment to a patient's belief, unless the treatment is aimed at changing beliefs, is most successful.

Patient beliefs as to the cause of the pain can be:

- Somatic

TABLE 3

**KEY FACTS: education and management of patients
(Bird et al., 1990)**

Share understanding

Explore patients'	Knowledge/beliefs
	Attitudes and feelings
	Wishes and expectations, their illness model
Explain	Your own views, being careful not to stereotype the patient
Explore	Patient's reaction
Consolidate	Clarify common ground
	Check understanding by patient feedback and questions

Agree treatment plan

Explore	The patient's belief, feelings and expectations in the light of your explanation
Explain	Your own approach to management
Explore	Patient's reaction to your treatment plan
Consolidate	Clarify common ground
	Negotiate agreed plan
	Ask patient to repeat and consent to treatment plan

Achieve continued adherence to treatment

Explore	Adherence
	Determine reasons for adherence/non-adherence
	Determine statement on commitment
Consolidate	Negotiate solutions
	Reaffirm treatment and commitment to follow-up

- Interaction of many factors including psychological
- Caused by someone else as opposed to chance
- Symptom of more severe disease
- Benign condition of unknown cause

Fig. 1 shows how patients and doctors beliefs may overlap and the factors that influence these beliefs and need to be noted.

3.1. Treatment expectations and outcome measures

Patient treatment expectations need to be the same as delivered and yet Price and Leaver (2002) point out that there is often a mismatch, e.g.:

- Patients want to know the cause of the condition but often they are not given a clear diagnosis
- They want explanations and information that address their needs and concerns but may get a poor explanation
- They want advice and treatment and yet may not get it
- Most patients want reassurance and yet this is not always given
- They want to be taken seriously by a sympathetic doctor but often the doctor shows a lack of interest and believes the symptoms are unimportant

Treatment expectations can be varied, change with time and can include:

- Patient-led therapy with active participation
- Totally passive therapy, doctor decides
- Invasive or non-invasive therapy
- Medical rather than surgical treatment
- Somatic rather than psychological or behavioural therapy

Keefe et al. (2000) have shown that matching treatment to the individual increases participation and decreases drop out rate from treatment programmes. Treatment expectations can be assessed using a questionnaire, which the patient completes prior to the consultation. This gives the patient time to think through the issues and the questionnaire then provides you with a lead in to the topic. I find a questionnaire on treatment goals (discussed in Chapter 6) extremely useful when deciding on management as it gives me an idea of what the important issues are for the patient and in which order these need to be addressed. We have found that many of our facial pain patients are looking for improved communication about their pain with the doctor. Patients and doctors may have very different ideas of which treatments and outcomes are needed

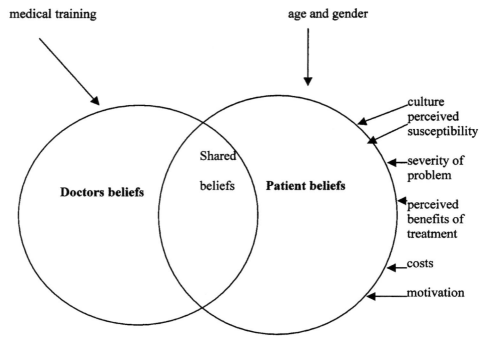

Fig. 1. Schematic representation of how patients' and doctors' health beliefs are influenced.

and this has been shown in many studies especially in the field of cancer. It is important that the patient is aware of the possible discrepancies between their model of treatment and yours and that this is discussed. Kleinman et al. (1978) suggest that the process of negotiating treatment which may include the making of compromises, e.g. take antidepressants, but also use other folk charms, can be the single most important step in gaining the patient's trust, preventing major discrepancies in evaluating outcomes, promoting adherence and reducing patient dissatisfaction.

Before continuing this section, please read the two case scenarios in the case studies box (Table 4) and then read through the answers at the back of the chapter.

We have found the following mnemonic useful when dealing with patients with idiopathic facial pain in whom no physical cause has been found.

REASON:

R   Reassurance that nothing is wrong does not help
    Relationship and understanding does

E   Emotional explanation: avoid premature explanation of an emotional cause

A   Agreement: agree that the patient is ill
    Acknowledgement of the patient's plight
    Allowing ventilation of patient's beliefs and Attribution theories

S   Stress: education about stress should be introduced gradually

O   Organic: diagnosis of positive findings will not cure the patient

N   Non-illness behaviours and communications should be reinforced

As well as determining patients' views on the types of treatment wanted, it is important to determine what outcomes are going to be important to the patient and this can be done using questions shown in Table 4 key facts box. It is important to stress that complete pain relief is often not a possibility and that patients must take some responsibility for their treatment.

Treatment needs to address not only the sensory component of the pain, such as intensity, location and quality, but also the affective ones such as patient's fears concerning issues such as ability to cope, impact on patient's social life, possibility of it becoming more serious. It is also important to search for trigger, environmental, coping and reinforcing factors that may be linked to the continuation of the pain. Management of stress factors and/or depression may be more important than dealing directly with the pain intensity. The inclusion of significant others/family members into the treatment plan as well as cultural factors will be crucially important (Kleinman et al., 1978). Dealing with the patients' illness as opposed to disease often requires primarily psychosocial interventions. As pain continues so patients tend to develop feelings of fear, confusion and frustration which lead to loss of confidence and lack of trust in the medical profession. Trust needs to be re-established. Patients with chronic facial pain may also feel stigmatised and this can further lead to ill health (Marbach et al., 1990). Healthcare workers need to be careful about contributing to this feeling by their verbal and non-verbal behaviour.

Other factors that influence treatment planning include:

- The healthcarer's relationship with the patient
- Patients' personality
- Patients' attitudes and values towards attendance
- Cost and consequences of treatment
- Patients' age
- Patients' attitude towards risk-taking
- Life-style and occupation

Having determined what outcomes the patient wishes, you then need to decide on how you will measure them. LeResche (1997) has put forward some physical and behavioural outcomes that can be used in the treatment of TMJ but which are equally applicable to other facial pain complaints. These are summarised in Table 6 and further details on their use are to be found in Chapter 6.

In order to reduce the number of scales used and to take into account both pain intensity and disability Von Korff et al. (1990) have developed a graded chronic pain scale and a modified version of it as published in Lund et al.'s book on Orofacial pain and is shown in Table 7.

3.2. Adherence to treatment

Not only do you need to ensure that the patients adhere to the treatment, but also that they persist with it until they reach the agreed target which may not need to be complete pain relief. It has been estimated that adherence to doctors' recommendations can be as low as 50% in chronic diseases and this is irrespective of age, disease or treatment. Winkler et al. (1989) showed that 44% of headache patients did not follow their physician's advice and only 40% of rheumatoid arthritis patients agreed to undergo a recommended treatment programme (Bradley et al., 1988). A higher proportion of pain clinic patients accept treatment (around 60%) (Cassisi et al., 1989), which may merely be a reflection of the chronicity of the patients attending pain clinics. Self-referred patients in the USA offered (free) treatment for back pain (following advertisements) had an 85% acceptance rate of treatment (Turner and Clancy, 1988), reflecting the difference between a physician selected and self-selected sample although it may also reflect the prohibitive cost of chronic pain programmes. It is no better when treating diseases with high mortality or morbidity (Bloom, 2001) and is a universal problem. The results of various studies to examine which patients are most likely to accept treatment for chronic pain have been equivocal. It has been suggested that between one- and two-thirds of patients enter treatment and the rest do not.

The reasons for non-acceptance of treatment are varied (Turk and Rudy, 1990). Non-compliance can be deliberate or accidental and may be caused by patients' beliefs, feelings that they can control what happens to their health, intellectual and emotional appraisal of their condition or the way the medical

TABLE 4

Case studies using treatment goals questionnaire

Read through the two case histories and look at their completed treatment goals questionnaires. How is this going to affect your management of these two patients?

Patient 1

Mr. A. was a 36-year-old male with a 2-year history of tingling in his lips which more recently had spread into his mouth and was also causing him a continuous dull aching discomfort in the throat. On the visual analogue scale his pain/discomfort was never rated as over 4/10 and he did acknowledge that on average the score was 2/10. He had had a successful repair of a hole in the heart 25 years ago, but still complained at times of pain down his arm and occasional difficulty catching his breathe. He had been told that he was cardiologically fit. A history of intermittent mild headaches and pruritus was also elicited. His family and social history revealed that his mother had died 2 years ago after bowel cancer that had been diagnosed 6 months previously. He had a very close relationship with her and still felt her loss. His wife had sarcoid and was being treated with systemic steroids and he was concerned that she had developed complications from their use. Below you see his completed treatment goals which were done prior to the consultation for his facial pain.

A.	Goal	How important is it to you?
1.	Returning to work, or remaining at work	<u>Very</u>/moderately/slightly/doesn't apply
2.	Reducing pain medication	<u>Very</u>/moderately/slightly/doesn't apply
3.	Improving mobility, e.g. walking, sitting, standing	Very/moderately/<u>slightly</u>/doesn't apply
4.	Feeling less self-conscious in public	Very/moderately/<u>slightly</u>/doesn't apply
5.	Understanding my pain problem better	<u>Very</u>/moderately/slightly/doesn't apply
6.	Decreasing my tendency to overdo activities	Very/<u>moderately</u>/slightly/doesn't apply
7.	Feeling less depressed	Very/<u>moderately</u>/slightly/doesn't apply
8.	Being reassured that my pain is not a sign of a more serious disease	<u>Very</u>/moderately/slightly/doesn't apply
9.	Carrying out more household chores	Very/<u>moderately</u>/slightly/doesn't apply
10.	Being physically intimate with partner	Very/<u>moderately</u>/slightly/doesn't apply
11.	Meeting other people with a similar pain problem	Very/<u>moderately</u>/slightly/doesn't apply
12.	Improving communication with doctors about pain	<u>Very</u>/moderately/slightly/doesn't apply
B.	The three things I would most like help with for my pain problems are:	(1) 5, (2) 8 and (3) 12

consultation is conducted. Doctors often view non-compliance as deviant behaviour and may exclude patients who do not comply. It is important that doctors reassess their methods especially in relation to communication. A non-judgmental, non-threatening approach is essential when asking patients about compliance with treatment. Patients who admit to being non-compliant are easier to manage then those who do not admit their non-adherence as in the former group it enables new strategies to be negotiated.

Chronic pain patients are often described as poorly motivated, resistant and denying. The lack of motivation is attributed to personality traits. It is suggested that they are focused upon secondary gains of financial compensation and positive reinforcement from the family. Both of these are likely to discourage patients from treatment. Treatment refusal is also related to negative patient/psychological factors, but little research has been undertaken to establish the reasons why the treatment would appear to be unacceptable or, indeed, deemed of little help to the patient.

Many patients attend with the expectation that the physical cause for their pain will be corrected so leading to pain elimination and a reduction in pain behaviours. The suggestion from the physician that

TABLE 4 *continued*

Patient 2

Mrs. P., aged 42 years, developed facial pain 1 year ago. The pain came on gradually over a period of time and was described as a dull, deep pain of mild to moderate severity. It was intermittent, lasting for a few days and then recurring again after a few days. The pain began in the right maxillary area and then spread round the whole face. No provoking factors were elicited and analgesics give some relief. It was associated with occasional tinnitus, neck pains and headaches. There was no other medical history.

Social and family history: She had come from India with her whole family when she was 6 years old. She was married with two children, 16 and 13 years old. She had worked for many years in the local school on a part-time basis supervising children, but in the last year she moved to a full time job as a welfare assistant at the school. She was very content with the job but had noticed that it had cut down the time she had available for socialising. She had altered her diet to include less hard substances so as to reduce her medication. Below you see her completed treatment goals which was done prior to the consultation for her facial pain.

A.	Goal	How important is it to you?
1.	Returning to work, or remaining at work	Very/moderately/slightly/doesn't apply
2.	Reducing pain medication	Very/moderately/slightly/doesn't apply
3.	Improving mobility, e.g. walking, sitting, standing	Very/moderately/slightly/doesn't apply
4.	Feeling less self-conscious in public	Very/moderately/slightly/doesn't apply
5.	Understanding my pain problem better	Very/moderately/slightly/doesn't apply
6.	Decreasing my tendency to overdo activities	Very/moderately/slightly/doesn't apply
7.	Feeling less depressed	Very/moderately/slightly/doesn't apply
8.	Being reassured that my pain is not a sign of a more serious disease	Very/moderately/slightly/doesn't apply
9.	Carrying out more household chores	Very/moderately/slightly/doesn't apply
10.	Being physically intimate with partner	Very/moderately/slightly/doesn't apply
11.	Meeting other people with a similar pain problem	Very/moderately/slightly/doesn't apply
12.	Improving communication with doctors about pain	Very/moderately/slightly/doesn't apply
C.	The three things I would most like help with for my pain problems are:	(1) 2, (2) 11 and (3) 12

See Table 28 at the end of the chapter for the answers.

TABLE 5

KEY FACTS: questions to ask about treatment outcomes

- What are the most important results you hope to receive from this treatment?
- Are you expecting a complete cure or just relief of pain?
- How much reduction in suffering would be acceptable if complete reduction were not possible?
- Are you looking for rapid results or are you prepared to accept slow change?
- How important is your quality of life and how much can this be compromised to achieve better pain control?
- How important is it to you to improve your physical and mental functioning?
- What help do you need to develop active coping skills?
- What do you fear most about your illness?

TABLE 6

KEY FACTS: outcome measures that can be used for facial pain patients

Pain intensity (sensory)	Physical signs, bruxism, facial expression, severity using VAS
Pain affective component	McGill pain questionnaire, multidimensional pain inventory
Emotional	Depression and anxiety using HAD, Beck depression inventory
Behavioural	Ability to socialise, sleep, taking of medication, time of work using Graded Chronic Pain Scale
Cognitive — understanding cause	Coping strategies questionnaire

VAS, visual analogue scale; HAD, hospital anxiety and depression scale.

TABLE 7

Graded chronic pain scale (Von Korff et al., 1990) and modified Von Korff scale

Question	Graded chronic pain scale (pain duration >6 months)	Modified Von Korff scale (pain duration >2 months)
1.	How would you rate your facial pain on a 0–10 scale at the present time, that is right now where 0 is 'no pain' and 10 is 'pain as bad as could be'?	As originally proposed
2.	In the past 6 months, how intense was your worst pain, rated on a 0–10 scale where 0 is 'no pain' and 10 is 'pain as bad as could be'?	In the past 2 months. . .
3.	In the past 6 months, on the average, how intense was your pain rated on a 0–10 scale where 0 is 'no pain' and 10 is 'pain as bad as could be'?	In the past 2 months. . .
1.–3.	Characteristic pain intensity = mean (pain right now, worst pain, average pain) × 10	As originally proposed
4.	About how many days in the last 6 months have you been kept from your usual activities (work, school, or housework) because of facial pain? ——— days	About how many days in the past 2 months. . .
	Disability points: 0–6 days: 0 points 7–14 days: 1 point 15–30 days: 2 points 31+ days: 3 points	*Disability points:* 0–2 days: 0 points 3–5 days: 1 point 6–10 days: 2 points 11+ days: 3 points
5.	In the past 6 months, how much has facial pain interfered with your daily activities rated on a 0–10 scale where 0 is 'no interference' and 10 is 'unable to carry on any activities'?	In the past 2 months. . .
6.	In the past 6 months, how much has facial pain changed your ability to take part in recreational, social, and family activities where 0 is 'no change' and 10 is 'extreme change'?	In the past 2 months. . .
7.	In the past 6 months, how much has facial pain changed your ability to work (including housework) where 0 is 'no change' and 10 is 'extreme change'?	In the past 2 months. . .
4.–7.	Disability score = mean (daily activities, social activities, work activities) × 10 0–29: 0 points 30–49: 1 point 50–69: 2 points 70+: 3 points Disability points: score for disability days + disability score	As originally proposed

Grade 1: characteristic pain intensity < 50, disability points < 3.
Grade 2: characteristic pain intensity > 50, disability points < 3.
Grade 3: 3–4 disability points regardless of characteristic pain intensity.
Grade 4: 5–6 disability points regardless of characteristic pain intensity.

they need to change their maladaptive and/or dysfunctional beliefs and attitudes may make patients feel threaten and uncomfortable as it is probable that these ideas are completely alien and incomprehensible to them. This hypothesis is supported by various studies including an investigation of 300 pain patients, 271 of whom felt that they did not receive adequate explanations of their symptoms and 237 thought their pain to be caused by something other than that diagnosed (Colvin et al., 1980). With such a lack of understanding of their condition, it is surprising that as many as 40% of patients can accept treatment. These patients are often labelled as unmotivated and yet it may be that they are merely confused. Most illness is described in physical terms and treated by physical means. Following one (or possibly more) consultations we are asking patients to change their lifelong conceptions and understanding of disease. It is not surprising that patients opt for treatment which appears to deal with their symptoms in a conventional way e.g. surgery or acupuncture. Patients may feel that they are already coping well with their pain and so may think that no other treatment is offered. It is therefore essential that patients understand the pain condition for which they are attending, the rationale for its treatment and come to believe that the treatment is appropriate for them. There is little data in relation to these factors in the field of facial pain.

It seems that adherence can be improved by a variety of strategies which are shown in Table 8 key facts.

Studies on adherence to medication have shown that it is related to frequency of dosage with 78% of patients complying with a once daily regime, but this is down to 40% when prescribing a four a day regimen (Bloom, 1988). You would do well to consider the use of retard formulations to reduce the number of doses needed. Reminder systems are also useful, e.g. blister packs with calendars. The other major factor affecting adherence is the incidence of unwanted side effects. The higher these are, the less likely are patients to be adherent to therapy. Relatively speaking, newer drugs are less likely to cause side effects, but they are likely to be more expen-

TABLE 8
KEY FACTS: methods of improving adherence to treatment
• Providing clear information on the origins of the pain and why it persists
• Providing the reasoning behind the proposed management
• Changing their attitude towards treatment
• Modifying schedules to suit the patients lifestyle
• Providing practical solutions to how treatment can be optimised
• Encouraging patients to take on responsibility for managing their pain
• Addressing behavioural aspects of pain management
• Involving close family members in management
• Providing clear guidelines on length of treatment and goals
• Giving patient feedback and noticing their accomplishments
• Regular follow-up appointments with user-friendly reminders if failed
• Providing treatment in the context of the patients' family and culture
• Encouraging patients to take notes during the consultation

sive. If the patient becomes pain-free, adherence to drug regimens decreases and this may explain why patients get rebound pain after stopping their medication before they have been advised to do so by their doctor.

Adherence to treatment can be measured by:

- Listening to the patient
- Counting tablets left after a treatment period
- Assessing a drug metabolite or marker in the blood, urine or faeces

However, all of these can be manipulated by patients and have proven to be unreliable (Wright, 1993).

4. Settings for treatments including integrated treatment

Care can be provided in a variety of settings both primary and secondary. The increasing availability of evidence-based guidelines means patients can be treated in the primary care sector. For example, we have developed guidelines for treatment of trigeminal neuralgia in the primary care sector in the UK under a national scheme called Prodigy (*http://guidance.prodigy.nhs. uk/trigeminal%20neuralgia*). Some patients will be treated by dentists, others by doctors, but this can be shared not only between primary care sectors, but also with the secondary care system. Increasingly, secondary care systems are providing 'fast track appointments' to patients who become unmanageable in the primary care sector. Within the secondary care system, patients may be referred to physicians, neurologists, oral surgeons, oral physicians or neurosurgeons. Patients will be referred to pain units which offer a more multidisciplinary approach.

Chronic pain patients require time and healthcare professionals need patience when working with them. Chronic pain management involves not just treatment of the pain. Most patients will have multiple complaints which will sometimes include depression, and so a single modality approach is unlikely to work. This may not only involve the use of several different methods, but also an interdisciplinary team of healthcare workers (Ashburn and Staats, 1999). Chronic pain patients need to be managed in the context of the family, ethnic/cultural group, work site and the healthcare system if treatment is to be optimised (Brodwin and Kleinman, 1987).

Interdisciplinary care ensures that each discipline contributes to the management, so making the treatment truly integrated. This approach also ensures that communication and understanding between the disciplines is established and offers an increased opportunity for learning and sharing of skills between disciplines. Most importantly, it prevents splitting where a patient will play one doctor off against another. Teams can consist of pain physi-

cian, nurse, psychologist, liaison psychiatrist, oral surgeon, anaesthetist, counsellor, pharmacist. This has also led to the development of pain management programmes to enhance these patients' physical performance and help them cope more effectively with their pain. Controlled studies show that both inpatient and outpatient programmes are effective in improving the pain, with slightly more pronounced gains after the inpatient treatment (Williams et al., 1996b). The programmes, will include progressive muscular relaxation therapy, goal-setting and pacing, group cognitive therapy and education about physiology and pharmacology of pain. Many of the programmes are aimed at patients with physical disability, such as low back pain and so include physiotherapy exercises and as such may not be appropriate for facial pain patients. You need to be aware that outcomes from such programmes are not primarily aimed at pain reduction, but look for improvements in mood, catastrophising, physical performance, overall function, and use of drug treatments. There are no reports of their efficacy in patients with facial pain and few of the evaluated programmes have included these patients and yet it would seem that with some minor modifications, they could be adapted for use in patients with facial pain.

5. Clinical trials

Decisions about treatment should all be based on the best quality evidence that can be identified and before individual treatments are considered it is useful to consider how to find and assess the available treatments. The quality of the evidence is based on a hierarchy which has been discussed in Chapter 1 (Table 7 and the appendix). Given the paucity of trials in the field of facial pain, it may be easier to use a simpler recommendation grading system as shown in Table 9 which has been used by the Royal College of Anaesthetists in producing their clinical guidelines on analgesics and uses three grades rather than four.

Although well conducted randomised control studies (RCT) are excellent sources of data, it is

TABLE 9

Grades used in recommendations for treatment

Grade	Definition
A	Based on strongest evidence available, including at least one randomised controlled trial as part of the body of literature of overall quality
B	Based on availability of well-conducted clinical studies but not randomised trials
C	Based on expert consensus of the group in the absence of studies of good quality or good quality studies but show inconclusive evidence of efficacy or high level of adverse events

TABLE 10

KEY FACTS: are the results from the study relevant to my patient?

1. Were the patients allocated to the treatment groups in a completely random way?
2. Were details of the randomisation kept concealed?
3. Were patients and clinicians blind to the treatment?
4. Were the patients analysed in the groups to which they were assigned?
5. Was the follow-up long enough and were all the patients accounted for?
6. Were the groups of patients similar at the start of the study?
7. Were all the groups treated equally except for the experimental treatment?
8. Were all the side effects and adverse events reported?
9. Were the patients similar to my patient in their characteristics?

risky to make decisions based on a single trial. Systematic reviews are, therefore, of more value as they combine all the individual trials carried out on different populations, doing a meta analysis if possible and so, it is hoped, providing a more balanced result. You should therefore start by looking for systematic reviews. These will need to be critically reviewed according to guidelines you can find in resources such as EBM toolbox as described in Chapter 1 or in a textbook on EBM (Sackett et al., 2000). If you are appraising a randomised controlled trial then you need to ask yourself several questions about the report before deciding whether the treatment they are evaluating is likely to benefit your patient. Remember that a poor RCT may not always be worth as much as a well conducted cohort study. When using a RCT for deciding on treatment you need to ask yourself the questions summarised in Table 10.

There is still a lack of well conducted, randomised controlled trials in the field of facial pain. It is essential that all new treatments, medical or surgical, are well evaluated and this may necessitate multicentre trials, especially when conditions are rare as having small samples will jeopardise the chances of a complete answer. The trials should address clinically relevant questions and to achieve this should include consumers as active members of the research team. There are a considerable number of well conducted international trials in the field

of headaches. The International Headache Society (IHS) has published not only guidelines for controlled trials in migraine, tension type headaches and cluster headaches, but also a statement on ethical issues in headache research and management which could act as a blueprint for clinicians conducting research on facial pain (IHS handbook).

It has been appreciated for many years that trials are not uniformly reported in the literature and therefore their evaluation and then subsequent comparisons are difficult. This has led to the publication of a statement on the Consolidated Standards of Reporting Trials (CONSORT) in 1996 (Begg et al., 1996). The statement was developed to help authors, peer reviewers and editors to improve the standard of published RCTs. The statement is made up of a flow diagram mapping out the progress of patients through the trial and includes a check list of 21 items that address different aspects of the RCT. It is essential that trialists report all trials soon after completion and irrespective of whether the results are positive or negative. Several journals will now publish trial protocols before completion of the trials in the hope that this will increase rapid reporting and publishing of all results, not just the positive ones.

The methodology was accepted by several journals and in 2001 a review was published which assessed the quality of reporting of trials in four major journals, three of which had accepted the CONSORT statement. It showed that those journals using the CONSORT statements had a statistically significant improvement in the reporting of trials. The CONSORT statement has been recently revised again and it is being kept updated on the web (Moher et al., 2001).

If RCTs are to affect management, their findings must be rapidly and effectively disseminated. It is important that the data are presented in a clear, short, vivid, engaging, meaningful and relevant format. Although both the Cochrane Collaboration and Clinical Evidence produce their data in a uniform way, which makes it easier to extract the required data, these may still be too complex for the busy clinician. Clinical Evidence has therefore launched a Concise version to improve usage. The Internet may also prove to be a better way of disseminating the results. Increased education among healthcare professionals, decision makers and consumers is needed if the concept of RCTs is to be understood by the end users. These groups could also put more pressure on pharmaceutical companies to conduct RCTs in rarer conditions.

Although RCTs are now the accepted way forward, this is not always possible and in some instances small poorly designed trials can be misleading. This is especially true in surgery where RCTs are difficult to conduct. McCulloch et al. (2002) have reviewed this subject in an article called 'randomised trials in surgery: the problems and possible solutions'. They suggest several reasons for the lack of RCTs in surgery. Surgeons are used to making important clinical decisions very quickly often based on little information and this, McCulloch et al. (2002) suggest, makes it difficult for them to be consciously uncertain as to which of two treatments may be best. Historically, surgeons do not have a good track record in research, do not recruit patients readily to

trials and these factors have not encouraged funding support for good quality trials. As surgery is so variable, it is often difficult to define precisely both the intervention and to establish guidelines for quality control. Surgical learning curves cause difficulty in timing and performing of RCTs of new techniques. This can clearly be seen in the technique of microvascular decompression for trigeminal neuralgia where the results have improved overall since the technique was first described. Often, the modifications are small at each stage but overall become significant in the long run. RCTs, therefore, done at stages, may not pick up this difference. Comparisons of surgical and non-surgical treatments with greatly different risks causes difficulties for patients trying to make decisions. Patients with trigeminal neuralgia find it difficult to decide between surgical and medical treatment and this is then further confounded by having to make a decision about which type of surgery to have. This could mean very slow recruitment to planned studies already made difficult by the rarity of the condition. McCulloch et al. (2002) make the following suggestions for improvements in surgical trials:

- Regular comprehensive audit of all surgical procedures
- Continuous quality control techniques to identify whether RCTs may be appropriate, improving cooperation between surgeons to improve size of trials
- Measure and control for learning curves and variations in techniques
- Incorporate non-randomised initial phases to permit these evaluations
- Determine suitable end points and allow sample size calculations

It needs to be recognised that meta-analysis of non-randomised trials may be the only way forward.

5.1. Informed consent

Any patient undergoing treatment needs to give his/her informed consent. To be valid, consent needs to ensure that the person concerned has the competence to make the decision (personal competence), that the patient gives consent correctly (procedural competence) and that the consent relates to an issue to which the patient may validly consent (material competence) (Syse, 2000). Not only do patients need to know what treatment or procedure they will be undergoing, but also the healthcare professional should outline the risks and benefits and check the patient's understanding.

For many treatments, this is done verbally, but when carrying out clinical trials, written informed consent is mandatory. What constitutes informed consent is not always easy to ascertain. In the field of cancer trials, a questionnaire called 'the Quality of Informed consent' has been designed to assess the informed consent process for cancer trials (Joffe et al., 2001; Tattersall, 2001). This has also led to a study conducted with a group of patients on what information they would like when asked to participate in clinical pain trials. This paper should be read by anyone designing trials as it highlights patients' concerns and offers advice about how these can be allayed (Casarett et al., 2001). Age, education, pain level and percentage of pain relief affect the information needs of patients. Patients were keen to know how the overall results of the study would affect their management and whether it would give them better insight into controlling their pain. Patients also thought that being part of a study would provide them with more time with a clinician, not only to discuss the study, but also their own pain. As expected, patients were keen to know what extra burdens were likely to be imposed on them when they took part in the study and whether they could continue the medication if they found it useful. There were concerns about escape medication, ability to contact personnel in an emergency and how dosage schedules would be managed to ensure rapid attainment of efficacy. Patients wanted details of side effects with particular concerns about drowsiness and addiction if the drugs were opioids. It is also important that patients are aware that clinical trials are more likely to benefit future patients than themselves.

5.2. The placebo effect

In every trial, attention needs to be paid to the possible placebo effect. Table 11 provides a definition of this phenomenon.

Placebos have been reported to provide a degree of symptomatic relief in most disorders; however, most of the available information is derived from studies where placebo administration constituted the control condition for the evaluation of another form of active treatment. The effects attributed to the placebo may, however, be the results of spontaneous fluctuations in the symptoms of the disorder (Richardson, 1995) or perhaps a result of positive reassurance. The proportion of placebo responders can vary from 0 to 100%, although the number commonly falls within the 30–50% range. In psychiatric disorders, it can be as high as 75% (Shapiro and Morris, 1978). Johnson (1994) suggests that in many drug trials, reports of placebo action lasting 3 months are common.

Placebos have been shown not only to influence clinical measures with subjectively reported symptoms, but also on objectively recorded measures and in healthy volunteers they can influence performance involving cognitive and psychomotor functions along with provoking severe adverse reactions and a small number of patients report worsening of their symptoms (Richardson, 1995). Beecher (1955) has reported that 35% of patients with severe clinical pain will respond to a placebo with a similar degree of

TABLE 11

KEY FACTS: placebos and their effects

Definition of placebo: any therapy or component of therapy that is deliberately used for its non-specific, psychological or psychophysiological effect, or is used for its presumed specific effect, but is without specific activity for the condition being treated (Shapiro and Morris, 1978).

- The effect of a placebo will depend on the condition being treated, type of treatment and the therapist

- Numerous mechanisms for its action have been suggested but remain unproven

relief that may normally be expected from 10 mg of morphine. However, Wall (1999) considers that the placebo response is directly related to the procedure being undertaken.

There does not appear to be a typical placebo responder or placebo responding personality, although many have investigated the psychological characteristics of such patients with no distinct conclusion being able to be made from the various studies (Richardson, 1995). Personality characteristics of introversion/extroversion, neuroticism, hypnotisability, suggestibility have all been investigated with contradictory results. Different individuals may respond differently on different occasions (Frank, 1968). The general consensus is that any individual may be responsive to placebo effects under the right circumstances (Skevington, 1995).

5.2.1. Type of treatment

The treatment characteristics have a significant influence upon the outcome of the placebo response. Differing physical characteristics of a tablet can influence results, some colours of pills are more effective in treatment than others (Buckalew and Ross, 1974). Treatments that appear more 'serious', e.g. surgery, appear to have a greater placebo response (Finneson 1969), larger doses appear to work better and injections have a greater therapeutic impact than tablets (Carne, 1961). The placebo effect has also been demonstrated with technically sophisticated equipment. Ultrasound has been used in an investigation to reduce post-operative swelling (following surgical removal of third molars), and was found to produce a reduction of swelling compared to those patients with no intervention; however, similar results were achieved independent of the activation of the machine (Hashish et al., 1988).

Surgery is reportedly a very powerful placebo (Beecher, 1961). Angina pectoris has been treated with ligation of the internal mammary artery with excellent results in terms of post-operative measures (exercise tolerance) and decreasing the frequency of intake of necessary medication (glycerol trinitrate); however, the results were better in the hands of those surgeons more enthusiastic about the surgery

than those who were sceptical. A blind investigation of this procedure compared with merely an operation scar in the skin, showed that up to 85% of patients improved independent of the specific procedure with improvements lasting at least 6 months. Gracely (2000) suggests that this effect is also found in patients with trigeminal neuralgia who have a microvascular decompression operation, but where no vessels are found to be compressing the nerve.

5.2.2. Effect of the therapist

Status of the therapist appears to be as important as treatment credibility and the confidence with which the placebo is administered. High status individuals administering placebos work more effectively in producing better results than those given by lower status therapists (Shapiro, 1964), this may of course reflect the confidence of a more experienced therapist. This led Shapiro (1964) to introduce the term iatroplacebogenesis (IPG) to describe the effects that a clinician can have on treatment efficacy. In the previously mentioned ultrasound study, improved results were obtained with the therapist wearing a white coat (Hashish et al., 1988). Confidence in a particular treatment, it is also suggested can improve the placebo effect from the commonly reported rate of 35% to 62% (Grevert et al., 1983). Petrie and Hazleman (1985) also found that credibility was an important factor in pain treatment in investigations of placebo transcutaneous nerve stimulation and acupuncture. Therapists beliefs, expectations or wishes may influence the patient's responses in ways which can bypass the normal constraints of a double-blind trial as shown in a trial reported by Uhlenhuth et al. (1959), where the results obtained from each of the doctor's patients was in accordance with the expectations of the doctor. Shapiro and Morris (1978) concluded that the therapist's interest in the patient, treatment and results is related to success in treatment and placebo effects, which could account for the previously mentioned increased success rate of enthusiastic surgeons undertaking internal mammary artery ligation for the treatment of angina. Further details can be found in Gracely's review article 'Charisma and the art of healing: can nonspecific factors be enough' (2000). Please also refer to Chapter 3, Section 3.9.

5.2.3. *The mechanism of the placebo response*

There are numerous theories of the mechanism involved in the placebo response, including expectancy–attribution (Ross and Olson, 1981), reporting error (Shapiro, 1964), cognitive dissonance (Totman, 1976), conditioning processes (Gleidman et al., 1957) and anxiety reduction (Evans, 1974). Many psychological processes are thought to influence pain perception and effective placebo analgesia may occur via manipulation of many of the above-mentioned processes.

Endorphins have been implicated as the chemical mediator of the placebo response, and the ability of naloxone to block opioid action has been used to investigate 'placebo responders'. Levine et al. (1978) concluded that the placebo response was mediated by endorphins. However, Wall (1999) suggests that although there is some evidence for opiate-dependent mechanisms, it does not explain how placebo responses are generated.

6. Range of treatments used for chronic facial pain

If one accepts the bio-psychosocial model for pain then treatments for chronic facial pain include not just medical or surgical therapies, but also associated behavioural, psychiatric and psychosocial therapies to change maladaptive thinking, disturbed emotions and dysfunctional behaviour. These can be grouped under the traditional categories as shown in Table 12 key facts. There is little doubt that using more than one method improves outcome.

Woolf and Mannion (1999) argue that treatment for neuropathic pain should not be managed by symptom or aetiological factors, but aimed at the mechanisms that produce the symptoms as shown in Table 13. The mechanisms are also discussed in Chapter 2. Our knowledge, however, is insufficient as yet for us to use this approach in the treatment of all neuropathic pain.

TABLE 12

KEY FACTS: treatments available for chronic facial pain

Pharmacological	Analgesics: NSAID, paracetamol up to opioids Antidepressants, anticonvulsants, other neuropathic drugs Blockage of nerve transmission: local anaesthetic, steroid, opioid
Surgical	Selective nerve destruction, decompression of nerves, arthrocentesis, arthroscopy, TMJ disc repositioning, menisectomy, TMJ reconstruction Dental treatment
Physical	Intraoral appliances
Stimulators	TENS
Acupuncture	
Behavioural	Relaxation Distraction, imagery Hypnosis Biofeedback Cognitive behaviour therapy Counselling
Self-help	Information leaflets Internet Support and self-help groups

7. Pharmacological treatment

7.1. *General principles*

Before and during treatment with drugs, it is essential that the following are observed:

- Complete medical history is taken and regularly reviewed
- Comprehensive drug history is taken and then regularly updated to include over-the-counter preparations
- Drugs are carefully selected in relation to drug history, medical history, age and patient preferences and beliefs
- Patient understands why the drug is being pre-

TABLE 13

Drugs used in neuropathic pain

Mechanism	Symptoms affected	Types of drugs used
Peripheral sensitisation	Spontaneous pain, thermal and pressure hyperalgesia	Capsaicin analogues, cytokine inhibitors, bradykinin B_1 and B_2 receptor antagonists, nerve growth factor inhibitors
Ectopic discharges	Spontaneous pain, paraesthesia, neuroma	Selective ion channel blockers: antiepileptic drugs, e.g. carbamazepine, lamotrigine
Central sensitisation	Tactile, cold and pin prick hyperalgesia	Tachykinin NK-1 and NK-2 receptor antagonists *N*-methyl-D-aspartate (NMDA) antagonists, nitric oxide synthetase inhibitors Adenosine A_1 receptor agonists
Increased transmission with reduced inhibition	Spontaneous pain, hyperalgesia	Opiates, gabapentin, clonidine, tricyclic antidepressants, SSRI

scribed and how it is supposed to work
- Route of administration and dosage schedules established and understood by the patient
- Side effects and adverse reactions discussed with the patient so they are prepared to cope with them and recognise unexpected problems
- Treatment outcomes are set, including use of diaries if relevant
- Patient consent obtained
- Regular review of treatment with adjustments
- Blood monitoring if indicated by the drug profile
- Consideration of different forms of treatment, including referral

Systematic reviews which include meta-analysis are the most useful method of selecting the best available drugs as these generally contain large numbers of patients. These reviews provide a reliable measure against which different drugs can be compared. The number needed to treat (NNT) is defined as the number of patients who need to be treated with a particular drug in order to achieve one additional good outcome. In the field of pain, a good outcome is mostly defined as >50% pain relief as it seems to be a clinically relevant effect. However, this can be changed to either 75% or 25%. The

lower the NNT, the more effective is the drug. The absolute risk increase (ARI) is the absolute arithmetical differences in rates of bad outcomes between experimental and control patients in a trial. At the same time, it is important to also look at the number needed to harm (NNH) which is defined as: the number of patients who, if they receive the experimental treatment, would lead to one additional patient being harmed, compared with patients who received the control treatment. This is sometimes subdivided into adverse reactions which preclude the use of the drug and side effects which allow for drug continuation. There has been an attempt to develop a global index of safety to assess drug safety, but at present it has only been used in one trial (Sacristan et al., 2001).

The most important consideration when choosing drugs must be the safety of the drug, then efficacy should be considered and only then should costs be taken into account.

7.2. Pain diaries for monitoring

Most patients benefit from personalised drug schedules that instruct them on the day-to-day taking of medication. This can be combined with pain diaries.

These have been used extensively in headache monitoring and are a way of ensuring that events are not forgotten and that retrospective analysis can be done. These can be either incident or calendar. With incident diaries, patients record only during times of pain. This allows for complex recording during these times but you are not always sure whether all the incidents are recorded. In a calendar diary, patients are asked to record at least once a day. Keeping such diaries up for a long time can involve considerable time involvement and so cannot be too complex. Significant others may also provide useful data. A recent study comparing paper diaries with electronic diaries has shown that with paper diaries, patients report 90% compliance, although actual compliance (measured by the use of electronic sensors) is between 11 and 20%, whereas with electronic diaries 94% compliance is achieved (Stone et al., 2002).

Peters et al. (2000) using electronic diaries over 4-week periods have shown how pain severity, duration, disability and psychological adaptation affect the daily reporting of pain. They showed that reporting of past pain experience is modified by current pain intensity. It is therefore important to capture pain episodes as they occur rather than at some future date. For clinical trials where accuracy is especially important, electronic diaries should be used (Stone et al., 2002). These will record the time patients have made entries and will also remind them when to take their medication and record their data. Studies have also shown that electronic diaries are a more reliable way of recording and transferring data to statistical programmes than pen and paper diaries, although some suffer from the lack of ability to include free text (Bolten et al., 1991; Hyland et al., 1993; Lundstrom, 1993; Carr et al., 1999). Farmer (1999) in his review of measuring and monitoring adherence, stresses the need to use more than one measure.

Fig. 2 shows an example of a diary completed by a patient with trigeminal neuralgia. It shows how pain varies on different days and how the patient has attempted to adjust her medication as a result.

These are examples of fairly rigid diaries which leave no room for patients' emotions and feelings. You may find that encouraging patients just to keep their own diary of thoughts and feelings may give you more insight into their pain than trying to measure it using formal methods.

You may find that although the overall severity of the pain has not changed, other factors may have changed, e.g. coping strategies or reduction in catastrophising which have reduced the patient's distress from the pain. As well as providing data on patient adherence to treatment, the diaries can also provide data on the temporal characteristics of different facial pains. There are no data on how the temporal aspects of facial pains are modified by other factors including stress and medication (Zakrzewska and Hamlyn, 1999).

7.3. Drugs used in pain management

A wide range of drugs is used in the management of facial pain and the major groups have been summarised in Table 14.

7.3.1. Simple analgesics for mild to moderate pain
Non-opioid analgesics for control of acute mild pain include the salicylates (aspirin and diflunisal) and para-aminophenol derivatives (paracetamol/acetaminophen). Their effectiveness has been well reviewed and Fig. 3 is the Oxford league table for analgesic efficacy. The NNT is calculated for the proportion of patients with at least 50% pain relief over 4–6 h compared with placebo in RCTs with patients with moderate to severe pain. The pain model used for many of these trials is the one of wisdom teeth. These drugs are of limited benefit in chronic facial pain and there are no RCTs to support their use in this area.

7.3.2. Non-steroidal anti-inflammatory drugs (NSAIDs)
These drugs have analgesic, anti-inflammatory and antipyretic activity to varying degrees. They are frequently prescribed and are well tolerated, being mainly indicated for musculoskeletal pain (Flower et al., 1985). The NSAIDs are a chemically diverse group of drugs which all have the ability to inhibit the enzyme cyclo-oxygenase of the prostaglandin

PAIN DIARY

Patient's name: Hospital Number:

Date of visit: 31 · 1 · 01

At the end of each day please record your pain severity and ability to do activities according to the definitions below:

a)   Pain severity.

0	**1**	**2**	**3**	**4**	**5**
No pain					Pain as bad as could be

b)   How much has the pain or side effects of the drugs interfered with your daily activities?

0	**1**	**2**	**3**	**4**	**5**
No interference					Unable to carry out activities

c)   Please enter number of tablets per day and which ones, by initial.

2 ✳ Carbamazepine (Tegretol)   100 mg (T1)   Baclofen (B)   10 mg
      Carbamazepine (Tegretol)   200 mg (T2)   Nortriptyline (N)
      Epanutin (Phenytoin)   100 mg (E) –3–   Lamotrogine (Lamactil)   25 mg (L)
      Prozac (P)   Other Gabapentin 100 mg = G 1
                                                                     300 = G·3

Date	Pain Severity	Activ-ities	No. Tabs	Side Effects	Date	Pain Severity	Activ-ities	No. Tabs	Side Effects
1·2·01	3	4	8		4·3	3	4	1	5G3	
2·2·01	4	5	8	bad back	5·3	3	4	1	5G3	
3·2	3	4	8	S gland sore back	6·3	3	3	1	5G3	
4·2	2	4	2E 3G3	" "	7·3	3	3	1	5G3	
5·2	3	4	1P3G3	" "	8·3	3	3	1	5G3	
6·2	2	4	"	still weak	9·3	3	3	1	5G3	
7·2	2	4	3G3	still A bit weak	10·3	3	3	1	5G3	
8·2	1	4	3G3	tingles h hands	11·3	3	1	5G3	
9·2	1	4	3G3	" hands/feet	12·3	4	1	6G3	
10·2	1	2	3G3	" " "	13·3	4	1	6G3	
11·2	1	2	3G3	" " "	14·3	4	1	6G3	
12·2	1	4	3G3	" " "	15·3	4·5	4	7G3	
13·2	2	3	3G3		16·3	4·5	1	7G3	
14·2	2	4	3G3		17·3	4·5	2	7G3	
15·2	1	2	3G3		18·3	5	3	7G3	
16·2	1	3	3G3		19·3				
17·2	0	1	3G3						
18·2	0	1	3G3						
19·2	0	3	3G3						
20·2	1	2	3G3						
21·2	1	2	3G3						
22·2	1	1	3G3						
23·2	1	0	3G3						
24·2	1	0	3G3						
25·2	1	0	3G3						
26·2	1	0	3G3						
27·2	2	0	3G3						
28·2	3	0	4G3						
1·3	3	0	4G3						
2·3	4	1	4G3						
3·3	4	1	5G3						

Fig. 2. Example of a pain diary completed by a patient with trigeminal neuralgia.

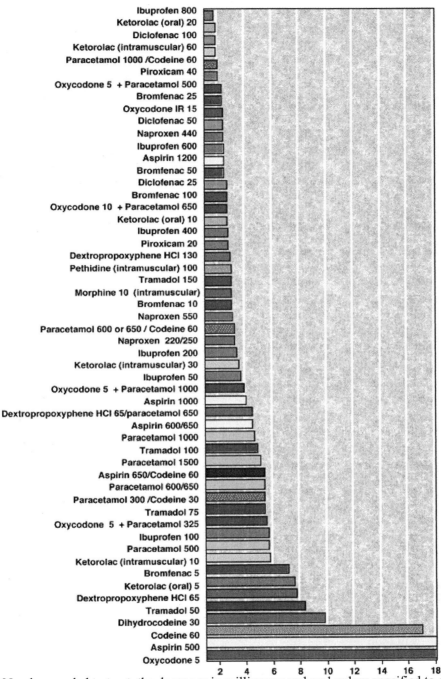

Number needed to treat, the doses are in milligrams and oral unless specified to get 50% pain relief.

Fig. 3. The Oxford leaguer table of analgesic efficacy from Bandolier *http://www.jr2.ox.ac.uk/bandolier/booth/painpag/Acutrev/Analgesics/Leagtab.html* showing number needed to treat to obtain 50% reduction in pain.

TABLE 14

KEY FACTS: drugs used for facial pain and their main indication

Group of drugs	Use
Mild to moderate analgesics	Acute dental pain, tension headaches, post operative pain
Non-steroidal anti-inflammatory (NSAID)	Musculoskeletal pain including acute TMJ pain
Opioids	Severe post operative pain
Antidepressant drugs including tricyclics (TCA), monoamine oxidase inhibitors (MAOI), selective serotonin reuptake inhibitors (SSRI)	Chronic idiopathic facial pain, TMJ pain, burning mouth syndrome, postherpetic neuralgia
Anticonvulsants	Neuropathic pain including trigeminal neuralgia, post herpetic neuralgia
Triptans	Migraine, cluster headaches

synthesis pathway. The mechanism of the irreversible cyclo-oxygenase inhibition differs for individual drugs, but results in decreased production of prostaglandins and other inflammatory mediators. NSAIDs appear to have little effect upon chronic idiopathic facial pain (Roldan et al., 1990), but are frequently used in acute exacerbations.

7.3.3. Opioids

Narcotic analgesics mimic endogenous opioids and act by causing activation of the opiate receptors. They produce analgesia, respiratory depression, sedation and euphoria. Continuous treatment with these drugs can result in tolerance and dependence and their use in chronic pain is limited and requires careful consideration (Turk and Brody, 1993), although analgesic benefit, with low risk of addiction has been shown in patients with chronic regional pain (Moulin et al., 1996). Some of the less potent opioids, e.g. codeine and dextropropoxyphene may be helpful in mild to moderate pain and frequently in combination with simple analgesics, but can still lead to dependence and are subject to abuse (Jaffe and Martin, 1985). This class of drugs is used little in chronic facial pain except with acute exacerbations and probably has no major role to play in neuropathic pain (Dickenson et al., 2002; McQuay, 2002).

7.3.4. Antidepressant drugs

Antidepressant drugs are known to act to increase the availability of the neurotransmitters, either noradrenaline (NA) or serotonin (5-HT), in the synaptic cleft of central nerve terminals, by either inhibition of reuptake into the neuronal terminal (tricyclic antidepressants and selective serotonin reuptake inhibitors) or prevention of its breakdown (monoamine oxidase inhibitors). Their action in reducing depression and possibly pain is complex involving changes in density and functional responsiveness of both adrenergic and serotoninergic receptors along with availability in the synaptic cleft, producing a cascade of events as well as changes in neuronal signal transduction beyond the receptor site (Palazidou, 1997).

Tricyclic antidepressant drugs (TCAs). These are compounds related to the dibenzazepine (imipramine) and dibenzocyclohepadiene (amitriptyline) ring structures. The potency and selectivity for inhibition of the neuronal transport varies greatly among the different agents, e.g. amitriptyline inhibits the uptake of 5-HT and NA equally well but is a less potent inhibitor of NA compared to desipramine, which is also 100–1000 times less potent as an inhibitor of 5-HT transport.

Drugs do not appear to have greater antidepressant activity than one another; however, their side effect profile is different, presumably due to their differing potencies at selected sites. The side effects are most frequently due to unwanted autonomic effects, e.g. dry mouth, blurred vision, constipation, urinary retention and hypotension (Goodman et al., 1985).

Monoamine oxidase inhibitors (MAOIs). These drugs are generally reserved for those patients who do not respond to TCAs, because of their high incidence of side effects, some of which are potentially fatal.

Second-generation antidepressants. This class of antidepressants has been developed following identification of several serotonin receptors and the production of selective agonists and antagonists. The selective serotonin reuptake inhibitors (SSRIs) are the most common class of drugs within this group; however, selective noradrenaline and monoamine inhibitors and reuptake inhibitors and serotonin-selective antagonists all appear to have useful antidepressant action. Their use in depression is now widespread, the efficacy is not greater than more traditional therapies, but there is a possible reduction of side effect profile and a lack of toxicity in overdose (Leonard, 1993).

7.3.5. Rationale for the use of antidepressants in pain and depression

It has been suggested that chronic pain and depression are different representations of a similar central neurochemical alteration. Chronic pain, it was proposed, alters brain neurotransmitter levels and that pain inhibition is dependent upon adequate circulating 5-HT and perhaps dopamine. Chronic pain depletes 5-HT, especially in the region of the dorsal raphe nucleus. This reduction of 5-HT, it is suggested, explains the apparent increase in pain with chronicity, the lack of analgesia obtained with opiates and the association with depression along with the effectiveness of tricyclics to reverse the symptoms. Acute experimental administration of TCAs (amitriptyline, imipramine or iprindole) can induce hypoalgesia as shown by prolonging the latency of the response of mice to thermal noxious stimuli, and can be blocked by naloxone. The antinociception was reduced in animals made tolerant to morphine (de Felipe et al., 1986), suggesting that TCAs ap-

pear to act in a different way to opiates and that short-chain opioids have a role in the hypoalgesic effect of TCAs (de Felipe et al., 1986). Chronic administration of TCAs has produced a selective increase in Met-enkephalin-like immunoreactivity in discrete areas of the rat brain (de Felipe et al., 1985). Amitriptyline potentiates the effects of morphine leading Botney and Fields (1983) to suggest that this increased analgesia may be by potentiation of descending antinociceptive brainstem systems and not directly at synapses. This is thought to be mediated by blocking 5-HT uptake in the CNS leading to augmented serotoninergic activity at spinal endings in the opioid-mediated intrinsic analgesia system. In addition, amitriptyline has also been shown to enhance inhibition of neurones in the trigeminal nucleus caudalis, and therefore prevent excessive firing of wide dynamic range neurones (Fromm et al., 1991), and central sensitisation in rat models is reduced by those antidepressants effective clinically (desipramine and mexiletine) against neuropathic pain and unaltered by fluoxetine (relatively ineffective clinically) (Jett et al., 1997). A wide range of chronic pains in addition to facial pain are responsive to antidepressant drugs. There is much evidence to suggest that treatment of pain with antidepressant drugs is independent of its antidepressant activity; however, some studies have found a direct correlation between depression and improvement in pain symptoms. Numerous studies have been undertaken to evaluate the effectiveness of antidepressant drugs in chronic pain, many of the patients in these trials, however, had clinical depression and the evaluation of the drugs as an analgesic is therefore complicated. Many of the trials conducted are uncontrolled and do not include the use of a placebo, only controlled studies will be discussed. A systematic review of antidepressants in neuropathic pain has provided clear evidence of an analgesic effect in several different pain syndromes (McQuay et al., 1996). Diabetic neuralgia, post-herpetic neuralgia and central pain were all reduced by TCAs, SSRIs appeared to be less effective. In studies of treatment of tension headache with antidepressants, most studies have found significant improvements, using a variety of TCAs. Okasha et al. (1973) compared amitriptyline, doxepin diazepam and placebo in 80 patients all with concomitant anxiety and/or depression. At 4 weeks, all drugs were more effective than placebo, but at 8 weeks only amitriptyline was more effective. The pain improvement correlated with the relief of symptoms of anxiety and/or depression and was produced with lower doses of drug than would usually be effective in depression. Fogelholm and Murros (1985) studied 30 patients in whom only 13 had scores indicative of depression, they found that maprotiline was more effective than placebo over 6 weeks, but patients with no or mild depressive symptoms responded better.

Lance and Curran (1964) in a study with 27 tension headache patients who had depressive symptoms, found that amitriptyline was more effective than placebo and that the presence of depression did not selectively influence the response. Pain scores were decreased whilst depressive scores did not significantly improve. Ziegler et al. (1987) in a study of 30 patients without depression found that migraine frequency decreased with amitriptyline.

Turkington (1980), in a study using an active control described 100% relief from pain and depression with imipramine and amitriptyline in 59 depressed patients with diabetic neuropathy. Max et al. (1987), using lower doses of amitriptyline than are effective in depressive illness, described pain improvement (half of the patients had depression) in patients with diabetic neuropathy. Responders had higher measured plasma concentrations of amitriptyline and its metabolites than non-responders.

Despite SSRIs, apparent ineffectiveness in neuropathic pain, fluoxetine and amitriptyline have been found to be more effective than placebo in reducing pain intensity in chronic rheumatic pain. The fluoxetine was more effective in reducing pain than amitriptyline at 4 weeks, and in addition the incidence of side effects was much reduced with fluoxetine (Rani et al., 1996).

7.3.6. Anticonvulsant drugs

The use of the word anticonvulsant or antiepileptic drugs is misleading in that these drugs not only treat epilepsy but have a wide range of activity, especially in the treatment of neuropathic pain which has both central and peripheral causes and results in hyperexcitability of the whole system. Two excellent reviews of the mode of action of anticonvulsants can be found in the European Journal of Pain (Dickenson et al., 2002; Jensen, 2002) and they are the basis for the following observations. Neuropathic pain causes a wide variety of molecular changes, but four have been identified currently which are considered to be significant and for which drugs have been developed and these are summarised in Table 15.

Although most of the anticonvulsants primarily act at the peripheral level and affect sodium channels, there are likely to be other sites of action more centrally. The majority of anticonvulsants will block sodium channels by prolonging the repolarisation phase of the voltage sensitive-sodium channels. They do it in a use-dependent manner and so reduce ectopic and other evoked peripheral activity. They have a very targeted activity which means that they do not shut down the whole of the CNS. Lamotrigine, felbamate and topiramate have a significant effect on central neurones which is larger than for the other anticonvulsants. Gabapentin may act through modulation of calcium channels found on central terminals of sensory neurones. Most of these drugs affect GABA levels but none of them have been shown to have an exclusive influence on this inhibitory amino acid. NMDA receptor antagonists have also been used in neuropathic pain,

TABLE 15

Molecular mechanisms involved in neuropathic pain on which current drug therapy is based (Jensen, 2002)

1.	Accumulation and novel expression of sodium channels in the periphery
2.	Increased activity at glutamate receptor subpopulations in particular *N*-methyl-D-aspartate receptor (NMDA)
3.	Reduction of γ-aminobutyric acid (GABA-ergic) inhibition
4.	Changes in penetration of calcium into cells

but their poor tolerability restricts their clinical use. Topiramate has been shown to have an effect on all the four major mechanisms, yet it has not clinically been shown to be effective in neuropathic pain. New therapeutic agents are also being developed that act to alter the activity in adenosine systems which play an inhibitory role in the development and maintenance of central sensitisation of spinal dorsal horn neurones. Given this range of activity, it may be important in the future to clinically measure pain more specifically, e.g. evoked pain, number and intensity of paroxysmal attacks to assess which mechanisms are most relevant and which should be targeted.

Systematic reviews of the use of anticonvulsants in neuropathic pain have been done (McQuay et al., 1995; Sindrup and Jensen, 1999) and are referred to in more detail in Chapter 15 on trigeminal neuralgia.

7.3.7. Triptans

Using triptans for treating cluster headache is the logical application of knowledge about the pathogenesis of trigeminal–autonomic pain syndromes (summarised by Goadsby and Lipton, 1997). Triptans are agonists at the 5-HT$_{1D}$ receptors and there is evidence for gene expression of this receptor on trigeminal ganglion neurones, thus predicting a role for triptans for treating these conditions. Clinically, ergotamines are known to be effective for the abortive treatment for both migraine and cluster headache. As triptans are also successful for the acute treatment of migraine attacks, it would be reasonable to employ triptans for the abortive treatment of cluster headaches. Therefore, it was no surprise that subcutaneous sumatriptan 6 mg was shown to alleviate pain completely in 74% within 15 min in patients with cluster headache as opposed to 26% of patients given placebo (Ekbom et al., 1993).

There are at least five triptans currently licensed for treating migraine. In a meta-analysis, Ferrari et al. (2001) have identified rizatriptan and almotriptan as the more potent drugs administered orally for the acute treatment of migraine attacks. For the alleviation of cluster headache, the route of administration rather than potency is more important.

An acute attack of cluster headache is extremely painful and may last no more than 20–40 min. Orally administered drugs are simply absorbed too slowly to provide meaningful relief. Of all the triptans, only sumatriptan is available for parenteral administration in the UK. The subcutaneous preparation of sumatriptan 6 mg single-dose injections is popular for treating cluster headaches. Sumatriptan nasal sprays 20 mg is has been tried. In an open labelled study directly comparing subcutaneous injection versus intranasal spray, complete alleviation of pain within 15 min was achieved in 49/52 attacks with the injections but only 7/52 with the intranasal spray (Hardebo and Dahlof, 1998). Of the orally administered triptans, only zolmitriptan has been subjected to a proper placebo controlled study (Bahra et al., 2000). Only the 10 mg doses of zolmitriptan showed statistical significance compared to placebo. This is four times the usual dose used for treating acute migraine attacks. In the absence of any other subcutaneous preparation, sumatriptan injections are the treatment of choice for cluster headaches.

8. Surgical treatments

Surgical treatments are mainly used in the management of TMJ and trigeminal neuralgia and these will be discussed in Chapters 11 and 15. Dental treatment is discussed in Chapter 10.

9. Alternative therapies

9.1. Intraoral appliances

These appliances in the form of soft or hard splints worn for a variety of time periods have been used extensively by dental professionals and yet their value has not been proven (Forssell et al., 1999). They are further discussed in the chapter on temporomandibular pain. Altering patients' parafunctional habits such as bruxism, tongue thrusting or nail biting may be helpful, but have not been formally evaluated.

9.2. Stimulators

The principle of transcutaneous electrical nerve stimulation (TENS) is based on the gate control theory of pain (discussed in Chapter 2). It is suggested that an electrical stimulus of high frequency (50–100 Hz) on the skin will stimulate low threshold touch fibres and lead to the closure of the gate and so block onward transmission of impulses signaling tissue damage and so decrease the pain. It may also stimulate the production of endorphins, the bodies own naturally occurring opioids. There are reports of its use in TMJ/myofascial pain and these are discussed in Chapter 11, but the trials are of low quality.

A TENS system basically consists of a battery powered electronic pulse generator to which two to four lead wires are connected ending in electrodes that are placed on the skin. The electrodes are fixed by the use of a gel, although some are now supplied with an adhesive tape. These can be left on and only the unit disconnected when not being used. The positioning of the electrodes is important and most patients favour placing them over the nerve innervating the painful site. Some patients, however, may prefer to have them placed further away from the painful site. The stimulation is felt as a tingling or buzzing and needs to be adjusted till the sensation is pleasant and provides relief. This is done by the use of the control box. The machine can be used as often as the patient wishes.

9.3. Acupuncture

This form of therapy has been in existence for over 5000 years in China. Ordinary acupuncture is carried out using sterile stainless steel needles, although silver and gold ones may be used. The needles can be inserted superficially or deeply and moved or left untouched for varying periods of time. There are other forms of acupuncture such as electroacupuncture, finger acupuncture (use of finger pressure only) or auricular acupuncture where the needle is applied only to the external ear.

Acupuncture may depend on a number of mechanisms for its effect which have not all been proven.

It is postulated that it works on the Aδ fibres and probably affects the opening of the gate and then also affects the descending pathways leading to a release of neurotransmitters. It is likely to have a psychological effect.

Acupuncture has been used in a wide variety of chronic pains and there is one completed systematic review on its use in idiopathic headaches (Melchart et al., 2001). A review of acupuncture in dentistry has questioned its analgesic role in dentistry, but suggests there may be some evidence for its use in treating temporomandibular joint pain (Rosted, 1998). It is also used in the management of trigeminal neuralgia as discussed in Chapter 15 (Shuhan et al., 1991).

9.4. Behavioural

A review of the effect of attention and emotion on pain processing shows these do have an effect on neuronal mechanisms and may preferentially involve pathways through the medial thalamus to the anterior cingulated cortex (Villemure and Bushnell, 2002). It may be important to start interventions early on in the development of pain to prevent establishment of poor pain behaviour. Some of the psychological basis for these treatments have been discussed in Chapter 3, Section 3.8. Table 16 lists some of the psychological therapies that are used.

Involvement of significant others can often enhance outcomes as the significant other, by understanding the goals of the treatment, can enhance its efficacy and prompt the patient to use them.

9.4.1. Relaxation techniques

Relaxation is freedom from mental and physical tension as well as stress. The rationale for relaxation therapy lies in the assumption that pain is a stressor and will increase muscle tension. Pain will also lead to the body to guard against actions that may increase the pain and this often results in more muscle tension. A vicious cycle is set up resulting in more pain. Emotions will cause arousal and activation and so can impact on pain tolerance and sensitivity. Reducing this by lowering muscle tension can be helpful. Patients may feel that this physical method

TABLE 16
KEY FACTS: types of psychological therapies

Psychological therapies may include:	Grades for recommendations
• Relaxation techniques	C
• Distraction	C
• Imagery	C
• Hypnosis	C
• Biofeedback	C
• Positive thinking	C
• Reduce catastrophising behaviour	C
• Cognitive behaviour therapy — this often involves many of the above	A

gives them control over the pain. Some patients will practice relaxation on their own, whereas others will be helped by having a therapist who will set realistic goals and give constructive positive feedback. Techniques include breathing exercises and meditation. These techniques are often included as part of cognitive behaviour therapy which has been systematically reviewed.

9.4.2. Distraction

This is a very simple procedure where patients are encouraged to focus attention on a stimulus other than pain. This is not easy to do as pain is such an attention-demanding modality that it interferes with the individual's ability to focus attention. Often another sensory modality is used e.g. touch or olfaction. This can be as simple as reading, listening to music, talking about pleasant events or breathing rhythmically. It can be used effectively while waiting for drugs to take their effect. A number of studies have shown distraction can reduce pain (Villemure and Bushnell, 2002).

9.4.3. Imagery

This differs from distraction in that it is not dependent on an external stimulus but is dependent on the mind evoking visual or other sensory images. It can be used as part of distraction. Patients can be taught the technique and they can use it for periods of 10–20 min. The patient needs to be alert and concentrating on creating a pleasant image where pain no longer exists. It can also be used incorporating the pain and suggesting images that allow the pain to flow away or transform the pain into another sensation e.g. numbness. Colour can also be used to create images and pain can be converted from the harsh red colour to more peaceful greens and yellows. If this results in a change in mood and emotional state than the perception of pain can be altered. There is no evidence for its effectiveness in chronic facial pain.

9.4.4. Metaphor

Another way both of communicating about pain and managing pain is to use metaphors. This section and the exercises are from Maguire (personal communication). Metaphors are a symbolic and profound means of communicating complex information, observations, reflections and feelings in simple ways which can implicitly connect to the listener by passing the explicit, cognitive reasoning gates. Metaphor among other things: enables people to speak of the unspeakable, is open but safe, is deeply effective, integrates the cognitive and the emotions, creates a safe place and provides a means by which patients can help themselves. You can find metaphors in phrases, poetry, images, dreams, stories and objects.

Before you try this technique with your patients it may be useful for you to explore your own process in relation to a metaphoric object to more readily understand how quickly a metaphoric object can access material that is heavily defended by cognition, tradition and conventional response. You could try this yourself with some colleagues. On a table put out a selection of pictures, postcards or objects and then ask everyone to pick one out to which they were drawn. Then go away with it individually and reflect on it:

• What has drawn you to the particular image/object, what connected you to it?
• What does it make you feel?

- What does it make you think of/feel in relation to yourself, to something you have experienced? Or perhaps you are afraid of, look forward to or wish for?
- Think of a patient you feel overwhelmed by, you feel you cannot help, you have no connection with and imagine that they gave you this image to describe their pain or something important about themselves they want you to know but could not explain it.

You will quickly become aware how quickly and deeply the patient metaphor can penetrate the emotion and pain of yourself as well as the patient.

Now you are ready to use this technique with your patients. Ask your patient to draw their pain or give it a colour or to bring a picture which could tell you something about the experience of pain. You can then work with the image to help the patient explore his/her own relationship to their own pain. The metaphor often shifts/changes over time which in itself is a metaphor of progress. If it does not change this in itself is a metaphor for the entrenchment or paralysing features of the patients' experience and you can work with it using some or all of the following:

- How would you like to change this image?
- If you could change or colour it what would it be?
- Who or what are you in the image?
- If you do not want to be here bring me an image or a picture of where you would rather be?
- So how do we get from here to there?
- What is the bridge?

9.4.5. Hypnosis

This method can be used to help patients develop positive imagery or distraction. Please see Chapter 3, Section 3.8.5 for further details.

9.4.6. Biofeedback

This is a technique whereby patients get feedback on the physiological effect that actions produce, e.g. can see their heart rate on a monitor or look at the tension in muscles on electromyography. The effect that stress and pain can have on a variety of physiological functions can be demonstrated and patients shown how they can alter them often using relaxation techniques. Please see Chapter 3, Section 3.8.4, for more details.

9.4.7. Cognitive behaviour therapy (CBT)

A meta analysis of the role of CBT in chronic pain management has shown it to be effective (Morley et al., 1999). Follow-up of between 6 months and 2 years in some of the studies has indicated that improvements may be maintained for considerable periods after treatment completion. Cognitive behavioural therapy has been introduced into pain management and can be successful in managing maladaptive behaviours associated with chronic pain and sometimes the pain itself. The CBT methods have been widely incorporated into the management of chronic pain conditions and their use in now commonplace in specialist pain clinics (Dworkin et al., 1994).

A recent innovation based on CBT principles is that referred to as minimal intervention/therapy (Glasgow et al., 1991), these emphasise the use of information and education in the form of self-help materials with brief professional guidance. This involves fewer sessions and low cost follow-up, e.g. brief telephone counselling.

A variety of components can be used in CBT which include the behavioural methods discussed above as well as goal setting, developing behavioural coping strategies, stress management and assertion skills.

Coping is a multidimensional process which is extremely complex and has been defined in many different ways. In the pain field, pain is considered to be the stressor and adjustments are made in the belief the stress will be alleviated. Jensen et al. (1991) have shown that patients who believe that they can control their pain, who avoid catastrophising about their condition and who believe they are not severely disabled appear to function better than those who do not. A systematic review of the literature on coping with chronic pain appears to show that effective coping strategies are associated with adjustments that reduce pain, but the methodology of many of the trials is poor (Jensen et al., 1991). The authors of the review suggest that coping, beliefs and adjustments must be measured individually and causal relationships between them need to be looked for. None of the studies they evaluated were related specifically to chronic facial pain patients.

The main coping strategies are summarised in Table 17.

Coping skills training includes:

- reconceptualising the pain
- developing coping strategies
- behavioural rehearsal and guiding in its effective practice
- applying the skills during pain episodes

It is not sufficient to just teach patients to cope with stress but is it is important to change pain patients attitudes and behaviour towards catastrophising, avoidance and withdrawal (Crook et al., 1988). Keefe et al. (2000) have shown how catastrophising plays a major role in pain management of patients with osteoarthritis.

Positive thinking. Patients can easily misunderstand their pain and Tyrer (1992) suggests five common errors which are shown in Table 18. It is important to identify these and ideally dispel them.

Negative thoughts about pain are important causes for maintenance of pain and pain behaviour. These can include perceived threats to ones relationships, control of emotions, role in the family, self esteem. Read through the 'thoughts' in Table 19 and identify those that are positive and those that are negative.

Therapy will depend on:

- identifying these thoughts
- questioning their accuracy
- looking for evidence to support or refute them
- challenging them to change them by taking a more objective view of the problem

9.4.8. Counselling

Some patients may benefit from less formal behavioural treatment by the use of counselling in their primary care environment. A systematic review has shown that counselling for psychological and psychosocial problems in primary care is effective and associated with high levels of satisfaction. No clear cost advantages of counselling over the usual general practice care has been shown in part due to poor methodology of the trials (Rowland et al., 2001).

Spiritual healing as therapy for chronic pain and for other health problems has been assessed but there is no reliable evidence for its efficacy (Abbot et al., 2001; Roberts et al., 2001).

10. Treatment of depression and psychiatric disorders

It is very important that patients with chronic pain and depression are treated not just for their pain but also for their depression. It is difficult to establish sometimes which came first, the pain or depression. Depression increases patients susceptibility to other somatic disorders and therefore it is important to treat it aggressively. A systematic review has shown that patients with depression and physical illness respond well to antidepressant therapy (Gill and Hatcher, 1999). Therapy will improve overall well being and so enable a patient to cope better with their pain.

TABLE 17

KEY FACTS: main coping strategies

- Increasing tolerance to pain: learning to minimise the disability
- Increasing role of patient in treatment and changing of beliefs: patients must come to feel that they are in control and they must solve their problems themselves
- Controlling mood: many pain patients feel angry, frustrated and anxious and these feelings need to be altered
- Encouraging positive thinking, reducing catastrophising

TABLE 18

KEY FACTS: typical errors in misunderstanding pain which need to be addressed (Tyrer, 1992)

Error	Example
Selective abstraction	Noticing only the times when pain is bad and forgetting the good times
Overgeneralisation	A problem which is only present occasionally being thought of as being present continuously
Dichotomous reasoning	The pain will be cured or get worse, there is no in between state
Personalisation	It is my fault that the pain is not improving and I cannot do anything to help it
Arbitrary inference	Jumping to conclusion without evidence, the pain can only get worse

10.1. Evidence-based sources

Depression can be successfully managed in primary care and medical outpatients as a variety of studies will testify. Whooley and Simon (2000) have published a review paper on managing depression in

TABLE 19

Case study: recognising positive and negative thoughts

Read through the following statements and decide which are negative and which are positive

1. I cannot be happy as I am continually in pain

2. I can manage my pain

3. As my pain is getting worse the doctors cannot have found the right cause

4. I will try anything as long as it will take away my pain

5. The doctors cannot understand how bad my pain is as they are not treating me

6. I am okay

7. To hell with this pain

8. Nobody takes me seriously

9. My doctor tells me there is nothing further he can do so I will have to suffer this pain

10. I am going to put on my favourite music when I next get a strong pain

Please see Table 29 at the end of the chapter for the answers.

medical outpatients which has several helpful figures but it must be noted that this is an old style review that does not provide details of the search strategy used to identify papers nor the criteria on which papers were selected. There are a number of systematic reviews in the Cochrane Library as well as a number of articles in Best Evidence on management of depression that you can consult. Wilson et al. (2001) in a systematic review have shown that antidepressants are better than placebo for depressed, elderly patients. There are a variety of meta analysis and randomised controlled trials to look at the effectiveness of different types of antidepressants especially tricyclic antidepressants as compared to selective serotonin-re-uptake inhibitors which are to be found in the ACP journal (Mulrow et al., 2000) or Clinical Evidence. A summary of management of depression in relation to pain is provided in Table 20.

10.2. Drug therapy

The main criteria used when selecting appropriate antidepressant drugs are its possible side effects, interactions, overdose and current medical history. Antidepressants divide broadly into:

- tricyclic antidepressants (TCAs)
- monoamine oxidase inhibitors (MAOIs)
- newer selective serotonin reuptake inhibitors (SSRIs)

TABLE 20

KEY FACTS: management of depression in relation to pain

Treatment	Recommendation grade
• Use of drugs including:	
tricyclic antidepressants (TCAs)	A
monoamine oxidase inhibitors (MAOIs)	A
selective serotonin reuptake inhibitors (SSRIs)	A
	A
St. John's wort	A
• Providing pain relief	C
• Cognitive behaviour therapy	A
• Changing attitude and behaviour	C
• Educating, providing information, support groups	C
• Regular review and encouragement	C
• Referral to specialists if outcome remains poor	C

TCAs should not be used in patients with cardiac conditions (especially recent myocardial infarctions), narrow angle glaucoma, prostatic obstruction and care should be exercised in the elderly as they may cause postural hypotension. MAOIs interact with certain drugs and foods. SSRIs can increase the chances of upper gastrointestinal bleeding in the elderly and interfere with drugs such as warfarin.

Hale (1997) and Whooley and Simon (2000) provide some useful data on the available antidepressants including their side effects. New drugs are likely to have fewer side effects and the SSRIs are likely to be safer in the elderly as they have fewer cardiovascular side effects. It has also been noted that the correct dose of SSRIs are more likely to be prescribed, not only because the lowest dosage are more effective, but also because the fewer side effects mean that higher, more effective dosages can be achieved faster without the need for a slow escalation (Donoghue and Tylee, 1996). If your patients do not want to take these types of drugs, then they may be persuaded to use St. John's wort. A meta-analysis has shown that more patients with depression respond to extracts of St. John's wort than respond to either placebo or antidepressant medications. The number of side effects in patients who take St. John's wort is similar to that of patients who take placebo but less than that of patients who take active medication (Linde and Mulrow, 2000).

To help primary care physicians prescribe more effectively, various toolkits have been devised and their evaluation has shown them to be effective in providing evidence-based care for depression (Rubenstein et al., 1999; Brody et al., 2000).

10.3. Alternative forms of treatment

There is evidence that treatment other than antidepressants can be effective in the management of depression. Gloaguen et al. (1998) in a meta analysis have shown that in patients with mild-to-moderate depression, cognitive therapy has a beneficial effect equivalent to that of behaviour therapy and that of antidepressants and a group of other miscellaneous therapies. Katon (1996), in a small study of adult patients with minor and major depression in primary care, showed that patients who had multifaceted interventions showed improved adherence and satisfaction with care and a reduction in depressive symptoms when compared with usual care. Interventions included printed and videotaped information on depression, antidepressant medication, brief solution-focused cognitive behavioural therapy, and counselling to improve adherence (four to six visits).

10.4. Ensuring improved outcomes

Brody et al. (1994) have suggested the following simple strategies that primary care physicians may use to help patients with depression:

- Encouraging relaxation techniques
- Participating in enjoyable activities daily

TABLE 21

KEY FACTS: strategies to improve adherence to antidepressants

- Start with a low dose

- Increase to target dose in 5–10 days

- Reduce dosages in the elderly and those with hepatic and renal impairment

- Use for 3–4 weeks and increase dose if no improvement noted at that time

- If intolerable side effects occur or no improvement noted after another 3–4 weeks consider changing to another antidepressant

- Full therapeutic effects will not be seen for 4–6 weeks

- Most side effects wear off after 1–4 weeks

- Regular review to encourage continuation with medication — monthly initially

- Treatment may need to continue for 6–24 months

- Gradual withdrawal of therapy with regular review

- Education

- Identifying exaggerated negative or self-critical thoughts
- Developing more realistic self perceptions
- Breaking current life problems into smaller manageable components
- Helping deal with problems

Patient education is crucial and includes removing the stigma of depression and highlighting that depression causes physical symptoms which can be reduced. There are a variety of patient support groups and internet resources which are provided at the end of the chapter to which you can direct your patients.

In Table 21, some hints on the use of antidepressants are provided which may help to improve adherence which tends to be very low, may be as low as 50% (Hale, 1997).

Patients with more severe depression, persistence of symptoms and prior depressive episodes are more likely to have a recurrence of their depression and they must be encouraged to report a return of their symptoms. These patients may need treating for several years (Hale, 1997).

Monitoring by telephone may be useful if this includes feedback to the doctor and adjustment to treatment and it may be cost effective as it reduces visits to the clinic (Simon et al., 2000).

10.5. When to refer patients with depression for specialist help

Although a high percentage of patients will improve on the above treatments, some will not respond and will need referral to a psychiatrist (Craig and Boardman, 1997; Hale, 1997). The following features may suggest a need for referral:

- History of mania or psychosis
- Poor response to two medications
- Patients who will need combination therapy
- Drug or alcohol abuse
- Suicidal risk: severe anhedonia or hopelessness
- Severe life events, social problems
- Severe physical illness or personality disorder
- Patients at increased risk: male, young

Patients with post-traumatic stress may require specialised help.

10.6. Somatisation

Patients who somatise their psychological problems need to be managed with care. It is important for them to feel that they are not being blamed for the symptoms and to explain the problem in tangible terms linking the physical symptoms with the emotional problems. (Salmon et al., 1999). A RCT of cognitive behaviour therapy in patients with medically unexplained physical symptoms has been shown to be effective for at least 1 year (Speckens et al., 1995). Goldberg et al. (1992) have put forward some practical suggestion for how these patients can be managed in primary care and they stress the need for good communication skills and an understanding of how to manage depression and anxiety.

11. Patient information

11.1. How to prepare patient information

One way of improving patient-led care is to ensure the availability of good quality information which is free of medical jargon and is available either in the printed form or on the internet. This has led to the formation of a range of organisations which aim to both help in supplying high quality information to consumers and in preparing it. Some are country specific and so address the particular needs of its citizens. One such organisation in the UK is 'The Help for Health Trust', *http://www.hfht.org/index.htm*. The Trust is an independent, not-for-profit charitable organisation which aims to provide a range of quality information services and database products. It includes the Centre for Health Information Quality which was established in 1997 as part of the Patient Partnership Strategy, a UK NHS initiative acknowledging, accepting and understanding the need to 'put patients first'.

The Trust also includes a section on research and one on consumers in NHS research. From organisations such as these, guidelines on how to prepare patient information can be accessed. The Centre for Health information at *www.hfht.org/chiq/guidelines.htm* has drawn up a check list on producing and maintaining patient information as shown in Table 22 key facts. It also provides further information on how this can be achieved and where to find the resources for this. A bulletin on readability provides details on the most commonly used readability tests such as Flesch and Gobbledygook and quality tools for assessment of the material.

NHS Direct *www.nhsdirect.nhs.uk* carries a number of patient information leaflets which have fulfilled all the criteria shown in Table 22 key facts.

At the end of the chapter in the appendix some useful organisations that provide information are listed, but for a more comprehensive review of internet pain resources take a look at Martelli et al. (2000) article on chronic pain resources on the internet or the book, 'The Patients Internet Handbook'

TABLE 22

KEY FACTS: check list for producing and maintaining patient information on conditions and treatments from the Centre of Health Information Quality

Theme	Objective
Accessibility	The information is in an appropriate format for the target audience
Accuracy	The information is based on the best available evidence
Appropriateness	The information communicates relevant messages and low cost follow-up, e.g. brief telephone counselling.
Availability	The information is available to the widest possible audience
Continuity	The information is presented in context with other resources
Currency	The information is up-to-date
Legibility	Written information is clearly presented
Originality	Information has not already been produced for the same audience and in the same format
Patient involvement	The information is specifically designed to meet the needs of the patient
Readability	Words and sentences are kept short where possible. Jargon is minimised
Reliability	The information addresses all essential topic areas

both listed at the end of the chapter. I also use a computer-based explanation of facial pain prepared in powerpoint which gradually builds up the 'story' of how the gate control therapy of pain can be used to explain facial pain. I print out the final page for patients to take home and a preliminary version is shown in Fig. 4. Patients can be encouraged to fill/add to the boxes or can even try to make up the picture themselves. They could also add in the emotions that the pain experience evokes in them, e.g. fear, anxiety, anger, and guilt. It would also benefit from the use of colour and this could be used to chart the patient's progress over time. Professor Patrick Wall's book on 'Pain the science of suffering' is a short readable book for lay people which can be used to prepare material in jargon-free terms.

11.2. How to assess resources for patients

Once the information has been found it then has to be assessed from a variety of quality aspects. This is a particular problem with material on the internet which is not subject to any verification. As Rigby et al. (2001) point out "products in health information are unregulated with regard to safety and efficacy". Gagliardi and Jadad (2002) have identified 98 instruments used to assess quality of websites, but only a handful had any evidence that they had been validated and so there continues to be a need for looking at other ways to assess quality.

Risk (2002), director of Health Research and Development, has suggested the following generic criteria for all sites:

- Quick and easy to find and remember
- Well defined purpose
- Clean, clear and pleasing design
- No gimmicks, audio, pop-up boxes etc.
- No uninvited intrusion
- Adherence to Health Code of ethics

  (1) Candour
  (2) Honesty
  (3) Quality: accurate, current disclaimers, referenced, cautions
  (4) Respect for the need to obtain informed consent of the reader
  (5) Respect for readers' privacy
  (6) Professionalism
  (7) Responsible partnering
  (8) Accountability

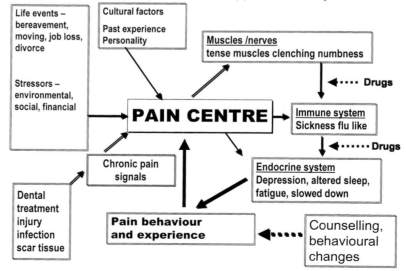

Fig. 4. An example of a patient diagram to explain chronic pain and the factors that affect this. This is a computer diagram that is gradually built up in front of the patient.

Wilson (2002) has attempted to classify the various tools available and this is summarised in Table 23.

Many of these produce their special logos and these can be seen on the web pages. Fig. 5 shows those at the bottom of the US TNA website. Fig. 6 shows a page from a leaflet.

Delamothe (2000) has argued that all these kitemarks are not required as the consumer will cope with the internet just as they have with other media. Table 24 shows an example of one of these user guides.

Attempts have also been made to produce instruments that would reliably check those information sources that provide information on treatment choices. An example of one of these is shown below. The DISCERN instrument has been devised to help judge the quality of written consumer health information on treatment choices (Charnock et al., 1999). Its handbook can be accessed through its website *www.discern.org.uk* which includes the evaluation forms on which the information is graded. They provide the following list of items that should be included on a good quality publication:

(1) Have explicit aims
(2) Achieve its aims
(3) Be relevant to consumers

TABLE 23

KEY FACTS: classification of tools rating quality of web sites from Wilson (2002)

Tool	Example	Address	Comment
Code of conduct	Internet health coalition	www.ihealthcoalition.org/ethics/ethics.html	
	American medical association	www.ama-assn.org/about/guidelines	
	Health summit working group	www.mitretek.com	American organisation
	Europe	http://europa.eu.int/ISPO/iap/	Trying to develop a trustmark
Quality label	Health on the Net Foundation (HON)	www.hon.ch	Used by the trigeminal neuralgia groups
	Hi ethics	www.hiethics.com/Principles/index.asp	Mainly used by commercial sites
User guide	DISCERN	www.discern.org.uk	See below for details
	Netscoring	www.chu-rouen.fr/dsii/publi/critqualv2.html	
	QUICK	www.quick.org.uk	Developed for children, see example below
Filter	OMNI	www.biome.ac.uk/guidelines/eval/factors	Provides a gateway to quality health and medicine resources
Third party certification	Medcertain	www.medcertain.org	European pilot scheme to award trust marks
	TNO QMIC	www.health.tno.nl/en/news/qmic-uk.pdf	European pilot scheme
	URAC	www.urac.org/	US scheme

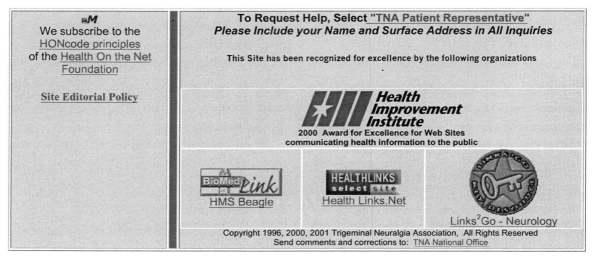

Fig. 5. Web page of the US trigeminal neuralgia association showing various kitemarks to verify that a code of ethics has been adhered to in the preparation of the site.

Other causes of chronic facial pain

These conditions are considered together because they have many common features. Many sufferers will have pain not only in the face but also in other parts of the body, e.g. the neck, back or stomach. They may also have itchy skin or ringing in the ears.

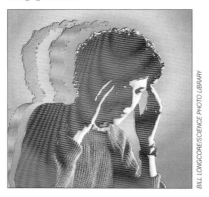

Temporo mandibular joint dysfunction

This condition is sometimes called *facial arthromyalgia* or *Costen's Syndrome*. It also has a number of other names.

The pain is in the form of a dull ache that affects the jaw and muscles in the side of the face. It may also cause clicking of the jaw and difficulty in opening the mouth because of **spasm** in the jaw muscles. The pain may extend over the side of the head and down into the neck. Often pain may be felt in the ear, where there may also be a sense of fullness or buzzing. It may sometimes be accompanied by dizziness.

The cause of this pain is unknown, although for some the problem is a product of disease in the jaw joint. It can also occur when the teeth do not align

properly. This can happen when teeth have been lost or if dentures do not fit well. Treatment will therefore begin with a careful assessment by a dental specialist.

Atypical face pain

This term is used to describe facial pain for which no cause can be found and which does not respond to painkillers. The pain can be intermittent and of varying intensity. It may affect a small area, commonly the cheek and nose, but it can also spread across the whole of the face and mouth. This is the commonest form of facial pain and occurs most frequently in young women. There are no tests to aid in the diagnosis of this condition, and any investigations that are performed will produce negative results, so doctors are very reliant on an accurate description of the symptoms. Tiredness and stress often make the pain worse.

Atypical odontalgia

Odontalgia is a medical word for toothache. Atypical odontalgia is a severe and continuous discomfort in the teeth or a tooth socket that is not caused by any apparent dental problems. Oddly the pain may be made worse if dental treatment is pursued, though it is very common for teeth to have been removed by the time the diagnosis becomes clear. The pain often begins after a tooth has been taken out or following a root filling.

Oral dysaesthesia – burning mouth syndrome

This is a group of problems that include a burning or altered sensation in the tongue and gums. It may be associated with a nasty taste. Some people have a sense that they produce too much or too little saliva. Dentures, crowns and bridges may become uncomfortable to such a degree that it is impossible to wear them despite all attempts to modify the shape. A severe burning sensation in the lips and cheeks may also be experienced, especially in the case of older women with the condition. Some people may develop a "phantom bite" whereby they feel the teeth do not meet properly.

Fig. 6. A page from the Brain and Spine Foundation leaflet on facial pain.

TABLE 24

KEY FACTS: quality information check list from *www.quick.org.uk* **Oct 2001**

1.	Is it clear who has written the information?	Who is the author? Is it an organisation or an individual person? Is there a way to contact them?
2.	Are the aims of the site clear?	What are the aims of the site? What is it for? Who is it for?
3.	Does the site achieve its aims?	Does the site do what it says it will?
4.	Is the site relevant to me?	List five things to find out from the site.
5.	Can the information be checked?	Is the author qualified to write the site? Has anyone else said the same things anywhere else? Is there any way of checking this out? If the information is new, is there any proof?
6.	When was the site produced?	Is it up to date? Can you check to see if the information is up to date and not just the site?
7.	Is the information biased in any way?	Has the site got a particular reason for wanting you to think in a particular way? Is it a balanced view or does it only give one opinion?
8.	Does the site tell you about choices open to you?	Does the site give you advice? Does it tell you about other ideas?

(4) Make sources of information explicit

(5) Make date of information explicit

(6) Be balanced and unbiased

(7) List additional sources of information

(8) Refer to areas of uncertainty

(9) Describe how treatment works

(10) Describe the benefits of treatment

(11) Describe the risks of treatment

(12) Describe what would happen without treatment

(13) Describe the effects of treatment choices on overall quality of life

(14) Make it clear there may be more than one possible treatment choice

(15) Provide support for shared decision-making

At the end of the day, consumers need to learn to search and assess information in a critical way as most already do with printed material where details of authors, publisher etc. are used to assess quality. Everyone has different needs and so the same standards may not be used by all consumers.

12. Self-help groups/support groups

Self-help groups began in the 1970s and aimed to provide their members with mutual aid and support. An essential ingredient of a self-help group is for members to do things together in the context of shared experience and understanding in order to give members a new meaning to life and their place in it. Groups explicitly focus on certain specific, but simple, technical problems, while implicitly addressing a whole range of everyday problems of living. Technically, professionals are not involved, although their indirect support is often required. Rootes and Aanes (1992) have put forward the following criteria for such groups:

- Members learn from each other
- Decisions are made by the whole group
- Professionals must not exercise authority over the group
- Members must accept responsibility for change

within themselves and this then encourages others in the group to help each other

- It has a single purpose which has been agreed on by all
- Membership is voluntary
- Members must be committed to personal change
- Anonymity and confidentiality must be maintained by the members

Patients need a forum in which they can discuss their feelings and emotions, but professionals are often concerned that groups such as these may result in wrong information being passed to other patients and also that disclosure of psychological problems could lead to problems when there is nobody in the group able to help (Kelleher, 1991). On the other hand, these groups may give patients increased confidence to ask questions and for them to compare their management with others being treated by a different doctor or hospital.

Support groups, on the other hand, do not attempt to change individuals, but provide information, not only to sufferers but also to the community at large and healthcare professionals in order to gain more awareness of the condition as shown in Table 25. Many of them help to reduce an individual's isolation by providing contact with others through a variety of means e.g. meetings, telephone or electronic and showing that there are others who care. It is important that access to them is easy, e.g. through national databases, cost-free or low cost and that they are not time limited. A very comprehensive survey of self-help groups was carried out in Kansas involving a sample of 253 self-help groups (Wituk et al., 2000). They showed that these groups have shared leadership, actively recruit members, receive support from professionals and are linked to national or local organisations which provide guidance and information. They suggest that these groups have a significant role to play and that awareness of them should be raised, especially among social workers. The setting up and evaluation of a headache support group has been described by Klapper et al. (1992) and there are support groups for patients with temporomandibular joint pain patients (Garro et al.,

---

TABLE 25

KEY FACTS: aims of self-help vs support groups

Self-help groups aim to:

- Decrease patients' sense of isolation
- Show that there are others who care
- Provide new ways of coping
- Provide a forum for sharing feelings
- Increase confidence in asking questions from healthcare providers

Support groups aim to:

- Provide information about the disease
- Increase public and professional awareness of the condition
- Put patients in touch with each other
- Look for available resources for treatment

1994). However, I could not find any evidence for the value of these groups in the management of facial pain.

Before referring patients to these groups it is important to check that they are still in existence.

Support groups coupled with the increasing amounts of patient information have enabled patients with chronic conditions to possess a wealth of knowledge and experience about their particular condition. These so-called expert patients could be used to take a lead in managing their condition rather than just being the recipients of care as this has been shown to increase health outcomes. This has led the UK Chief Medical Officer to launch the Experts Patients Programme which will "help to create a new generation of patients who are empowered to take action with the healthcare professional caring for them, for example, reduce pain, improve the use of medication and enhance their overall quality of life. Patients will receive the support to help them take more control of their own health and treatment, to make more appropriate use of health and social services and be more empowered" (*www.ohn.gov.uk*,

2001). These initiatives are very applicable to facial pain patients, e.g. patients with trigeminal neuralgia and much can be done to help chronic facial pain patients become expert patients.

13. Chronicity and long-term management

We know that the same nociceptive stimulus may result in no pain in some individuals, whereas in others it can result in excruciating pain. We have also come to appreciate that chronic pain is often out of proportion to the initial injury (if it occurred), it is unrelenting and often persists after treatment has finished. Chronic pain is often defined in terms of time to distinguish it from acute pain, but the basic distinction lies in the body's inability to restore itself to normal function. We have seen that the way the brain processes pain producing information and responds to it is influenced by numerous afferent inputs such as pathogenic and somatosensory inputs, cultural factors, personality variables and attention. Learned experiences, expectations and stress will also affect the interaction between the neuromatrix and the periphery and lead to altered responses.

In some cases, response pathways that developed due to acute pain may persist and so lead to chronic pain. We also know that the longer the pain persists the more inevitable it is that other factors will become superimposed on it and so both increase the intensity of the pain and result in its persistence. Once pain is perceived it results not only in an expression of pain (behaviour) but also a subjective experience of suffering. Chapman and Gavrin (1999) remind us that pain and suffering are not synonymous as suffering is a much broader state which encompasses pain as well as other factors. Suffering is defined as perceived damage to the integrity of the self which is a psychological construct that represents a subjective sense of identity. Unrelieved pain causes suffering in that it changes the individual and results in loss of self esteem. Persistent pain results in impaired performance at work, home and in the community. A disparity, therefore, results between self expectations and actual performance so resulting in damage to self. As the disparity between what the patient believed themselves to be before the illness and what they are now increases so an extra stressor is added and results in even more disability. It is this increase that leads to chronicity, greater difficulty in controlling pain and increasing feeling of hopelessness and fear. A reassuring, understanding physician can do much to reduce pain; offers hope and hence reduce suffering.

Keefe et al. (2000) has suggested that you can use the concept of the wheel of change to help patients deal with their pain. All pain management involves a change and so it may be appropriate to consider patients views on whether they are changing their attitudes and behaviour towards their pain. Some patients may already be changing their behaviour, others may have changed and need encouragement to maintain this change, but there may be others who are still pre-contemplators and so will need considerable input to convince them to change. It is these latter that are at greatest risk of continued pain and suffering and it may be essential to get professional help for them so they realize that they must change in order to relieve their pain.

13.1. Why may there be patients with special needs who do not respond to treatment?

Not all patients will respond to treatment and it can be due to a wide variety of reasons. Below are listed some that you may want to consider:

- Limited verbal communication
- Lack an advocate or translator
- Have different culture and beliefs from healthcare worker treating them
- Feel stigmatised
- React to drug therapy
- Develop emotional or physical dependence

13.2. When should patients with facial pain be referred to a specialist?

Stohler (2001) suggests using the modified Von Korff scale to determine which patients can be treated in

TABLE 26

KEY FACTS: indicating a need for a referral to a specialist clinic

- Disability far exceeds that expected from the physical disability
- Patients make excessive demands for investigations and treatments
- Show evidence of psychological disturbance
- Poor adherence to treatment, excessive self-treatment, lack of response, development of tolerance
- Dentists may not be able to prescribe the range of drugs needed; primary care physicians may not have provision for psychosocial support

primary care and which should be referred to a specialist clinic. Some indications for referral to a specialist are shown in Table 26.

How we ultimately manage each individual patient depends on sound research information based on the best available evidence but which takes into consideration the values and preferences of all involved and which takes into account the circumstances prevailing at the time that the decision is made. Collaborative decision-making will yield the best results.

14. Summary

See Table 27 for a summary of this chapter.

Appendix A

The answers to case studies are shown in Tables 28 and 29.

TABLE 27

Summary of Chapter 9

- Patients who become equal partners and negotiate their management of pain are more likely to have improved outcomes
- Effective communication based on understanding and agreeing a treatment plan will result in improved adherence to treatment
- Identifying the reasons why patients do not adhere to treatment plans enables strategies to be put in place for dealing with them
- Treatments for the majority of chronic facial pain patients needs to be integrated and requires more than one modality
- Treatments should be based on evidence from systematic reviews and randomised controlled trials
- Pharmacological treatments can include any of the following groups of drugs: analgesics, anticonvulsants, antidepressants, triptans
- Alternative therapies include TENS and acupuncture
- Psychological therapies include cognitive behaviour therapy, relaxation, biofeedback, coping strategies and reduction of catastrophising
- Depression, if found, must be treated using evidence from systematic reviews
- Patients should be directed to relevant support groups for further information and patient contact

TABLE 28

Answer to case study in Table 4

It could be that Mr. A. was concerned that he could also have cancer that nobody was recognising this, but you would need to question him more about this anxiety, e.g. does he often perform checks on himself. He also wanted reassurance as shown by his request for better communication with the doctor and this could have included not just his pain but also about possibilities of cancer. He was reluctant to take drugs because of his wife's experience and he was very relieved that he did not need any drug therapy. Explicit reassurance was sufficient.

Mrs. P. was aware that her pain was not due to some serious condition, but socialising with her friends was something very important to her and we note that her pain coincided with the start of a full-time post. Her treatment goals also relate to her need to be able to socialise.

TABLE 29

Answers to the case study in Table 19

Negative thoughts are numbers 1, 3, 4, 5, 8, 9

Positive thoughts are numbers 2, 6, 7, 10

Appendix B. Resources

In addition to some of these national organisations, there are often many local groups that can help put patients in contact with each other. These were all accessed between October 2001 and March 2002.

Google is a good search engine to use to find internet resources.

B.1. General pain organisations

B.1.1. American Pain Foundation

Founded in 1997, the American Pain Foundation is an independent non-profit organisation serving people with pain through information, education and advocacy. Their aim is to improve the quality of life for people with pain by raising public awareness, providing practical information, promoting research, and advocating to remove barriers and increase access to effective pain management.

Website: *http://www.painfoundation.org/*

B.1.2. Brain and Spine Foundation

Information and support for people with neurological disorders. They have published many booklets including: Face Pain, Back and Neck Pain, Brain Tumor, CT Scan, Head Injury and Concussion, Headache, MRI Scan, Multiple Sclerosis, Stroke.

Address: 7 Winchester House, Kennington Gardens, Cranmer Road, London SW9 6EJ, UK. Tel.: +44-20-7793-5900; Fax: +44-20-7793-5939; Helpline: 0808-808-1000 (free call) weekdays from 09.00 to 13.00 h, except Wednesday from 10.00 to 18.00 h; E-mail: *info@brainandspine.org.uk*; website: *www.brainandspine.org.uk*

B.1.3. Carolina Oral and Facial Pain Centre

The purpose of this site is to provide useful information about facial pain disorders to patients and healthcare professionals. Information on a wide variety of topics is available, but the current focus is on TMJ disorders.

Address: 6340 Quadrangle Drive, Chapel Hill, NC 27514, USA. Website: *www.ncpain.com*

B.1.4. Pain Concern

A registered charity offering information, and support to pain sufferers and their cares

Address: PO Box 13256, Haddington EH 41 4YD, UK. Tel. +44-1620-822572.

E-mail: *painconcern@btinternet.com*;

Website: *http://www. painconcern.org.uk*

B.1.5. Pain Relief Foundation

Charity funding research and education on chronic pain in the UK. They also publish leaflets and tapes for patients, including trigeminal neuralgia, facial pain migraines, dental pain, shingles.

The Pain Relief Handbook (Self-Help Methods for Managing Pain) by Dr. Chris Wells and Graham Nown. Vermilion, London, 1996. Available from the Pain Relief Foundation at £9.99 + £1.00 postage and packing or from all good book shops.

Pain helpline: 'Healthwise' freephone: 0800-66-55-44.

Address: Pain Relief Foundation, Clinical Sciences Centre, University Hospital Aintree, Lower Lane, Liverpool L9 7AL, UK. Tel.: +44-151-523-1486; Fax: +44-151-521-6155;

E-mail: *pri@liv.ac.uk*;

Website: *http://www.painrelieffoundation.org*.

B.1.6. Pain.com

Web-based US organisation providing information on all types of pain.

Website: *http://www.pain.com/*

B.1.7. SHIP Self-Help In Pain

Run by Rosalie Everatt, this is a self-help pain management program.

Address: 33 Kingsdown Park, Tankerton, Kent CT5 2DT, UK. Tel.: +44-227-264677.

B.2. Specific pain type

B.2.1. The Neuropathy Trust

This is a UK registered charity providing support and information for people affected by peripheral neuropathy and neuropathic pain.

Address: PO Box 26, Nantwich, Cheshire CW5 5FP, UK. Tel.: +44-1270-611828;

E-mail: *info@neuropathy-trust.org*;

Website: *http//www.neuropathy-trust.org*

B.2.2. TMJ Association

The TMJ Association is a patient-based advocacy organisation whose mission is to provide information to patients, health professionals and the public on temporomandibular (jaw) joint diseases, commonly known as TMJ. The Association's goal is to establish safe and effective means of diagnosis, treatment and prevention of these diseases — ultimately to 'change the face of TMJ'.

Address: The TMJ Association, PO Box 26770, Milwaukee, WI 53226, USA. Fax: +1-414-259-8112; E-mail: *info@tmj.org*;

Website: *http://www.tmj.org/*

B.2.3. Trigeminal Neuralgia Association (USA)

This large American support group aims to address this problem in the following ways:

- To provide information, mutual aid, support and encouragement to patients and families
- To reduce the isolation of those affected by the disorder
- To increase public awareness and understanding of the problem
- To serve as a resource and information centre for current TN data
- To facilitate and promote research on trigeminal neuralgia
- To advocate for public policy which is supportive of the needs of those with rare disorders

Address: TNA, 2801 S.W. Archer Road, Suite C, Gainesville, FL 32608, USA. Tel.: +1-352-376-9955; Fax: +1-352-376-8688;

Website: *http://www.tna-support.org*

They have produced a book for patients 'Striking back' the trigeminal neuralgia handbook. Cost £15.

They provide chat rooms and E-mail contact as well as a wide range of publications.

There are numerous local support groups throughout the US which meet on a regular basis and the Association run a national meeting every two years that is attended by consumers and healthcare professionals.

B.2.4. Trigeminal Neuralgia Association UK

This charity organisation runs on the same lines as the American one and was started in 1999. The two organisation are in close contact with each other.

Address: TNA UK, PO Box 413, Bromley, Kent BR2 9EP, UK. Tel.: +44-20-8462-9122; Website: *www.tna-uk.org.uk*

A help line, E-mail service and leaflets are available to members. Meetings of patients and healthcare professionals are also held.

B.2.5. Cluster headaches resources

Website: *http://www.chhelp.org*. A relatively new patient support group site with numerous links. Good information on understanding the disease but also advice on choosing a new doctor and choosing treatment. A lot of information is specific to the United States, like help on insurance and legal rights. Also some links to well known physicians with special interest in cluster headaches and good links to allow patients to communicate with doctors.

Website: *http://www.clusterheadaches.org.uk*. This is the website for the United Kingdom cluster headache support group OUCH UK with registered office in Leicester. A good site for communicating with other cluster headache sufferers and much more relevant to UK residents.

Website: *http://www.clusterheadaches.com*. This is another large cluster headache support group website based in the United States. Provides a description of the 'Kip scale' described by Bob Kipple which is a patient's perspective of the severity of their cluster headache attacks. There is a 'ask Doc Greg' section where questions can be posed to a doctor who is a CH sufferer himself. Some interesting answers in this section, like Doc Greg's interpretation of the gate theory of pain and explanation for the efficacy of oxygen for treating acute CH attacks. Good information about medicotherapy and general information for CH. Over 3000 persons listed by country on this site. Curiously, the Isle of Wight is listed as separate country on its own!

Website: *http://www.clusterheadaches.org/*. Incorporating US, UK, Italian and German OUCH. Provides a link to the support groups of these countries.

B.2.6. The Shingles Support Society

This is a sub-group of the Herpes Viruses Association a UK-based organisation, formed to give help to people with pain following shingles: post-herpetic neuralgia. Provides written material and a helpline.

Address: Herpes Association, 41 North Road, London N 9DP, UK, Tel.: +44-20-7609-9061; Website: *http://www.herpes.org.uk/shingles.htm*

B.3. Psychiatric support groups

MIND Mental Health Charity of England and Wales. Lealfets on a very wide range of topics are available including depression, anxiety, suicide, self esteem, stress. Help lines and email

Address: Mind Publications, Granta House, 15-19 Broadway, London E15 4BQ.
E-mail publications@mind.org.uk
Website: http://www.mind.org.uk

B.3.1. MIND-National Association for Mental Health
Tel.: +44-181-519-2122.

B.3.2. Samaritans
Twenty-four hour emergency line: +44-170-874-0000.

B.4. General organisations

B.4.1. NHS Direct
Medical advice and information on NHS Services. Tel.: +44-0845-4647;
Website: *www.nhsdirect.nhs.uk*
Leaflets From NHS Executive, Mental Illness, PO Box 643, Bristol BS99 1UU, UK

B.4.2. The Expert Patient Programme
Contact: Jo Harding, Room 534, Wellington House, 133–155 Waterloo Road, London SE1 8UG, UK. Tel.: +44-20-7972-4467; Website: *www.ohn.gov.uk*

B.4.3. National Institute of Dental and Craniofacial Research (NICDR)
This organisation, based in the USA, serves to liase with international agencies involved in global oral health and it has an organisation called the friends of NIDCR.

Address: 1555 Connecticut Ave. NW, Suite 200, Washington, DC 20036-1126, USA. Website: *www.nidcr.nih.gov*

Appendix C. Further reading

C.1. Guide to reading the literature critically

(1) Guyatt GH, Sinclair J, Cook DJ, Glasziou P. Users' guides to the medical literature:

XVI. How to use a treatment recommendation. Evidence-Based Medicine Working Group and the Cochrane Applicability Methods Working Group. J Am Med Assoc 1999; 281: 1836–1843.

C.2. Classic books/articles to read on pain management

(2) Keefe FJ, Lefebvre JC. Behavioural therapy. In: Wall PD, Melzack R (eds) Textbook of Pain, ISBN-0443-06252-8. Churchill Livingstone, Philadelpia, PA, 1999: 1445–1462.

(3) Turk DC, Okifuji A. A cognitive behaviour approach to pain management. In: Wall PD, Melzack R (eds) Textbook of Pain. ISBN-0443-06252-8, Churchill Livingstone, Philadelphia, PA, 1999: 1431–1445.

(4) Feinmann C. The Mouth, the Face and the Mind, Oxford University Press, Oxford, 1999, ISBN 0-1926630628.

(5) Lund JP, Lavigne GJ, Dubner R, Sessle BJ. Orofacial Pain, from Basic Science to Clinical Management, Quintessence Publishing, Chicago, 2001: ISBN 0-867-15-381-4.

(6) Skevington SM. Psychology of Pain, Wiley, Chichester, 1995: ISBN 0-471-95771-9.

(7) Tyrer S. Psychology, Psychiatry and Chronic Pain. Butterworth, Oxford, 1992: ISBN 0-7506-05731-1.

C.3. Books/papers on communication

Please also see selection in Chapters 4 and 5.

(8) Levy P. Communicating with Patients. Chapman and Hall, London, 1993: ISBN-0-412-38240-7.

(9) Misselbrook D. Thinking about Patients. Newbury Petroc Press, 2001: ISBN 1-900603. (Challenges our role as doctors.)

(10) Gask L, Usherwood T. The consultation. Br Med J 2002; 324: 1567-1569 and Price J, Leaver L. Beginning treatment. Br Med J 2002; 325: 33–35. (Excellent articles which form part of a series on ABC of psychological medicine

and due to be published as a book winter 2002.)

(11) Cole SA, Bird J. The Medical Interview: the Three Function Approach, 2nd edn., Harcourt Health Sciences, St. Louis, 2000: ISBN 0815119925.

C.4. Books or articles on use of the internet

(12) Hunt DL, Jaeschke R, McKibbon KA. Users' guides to the medical literature: XXI. using electronic health information resources in evidence-based practice. Evidence-Based Medicine Working Group. J Am Med Assoc 2000; 283: 1875–1879.

(13) Kiley R, Graham E. The Patient's Internet Handbook. RSM Press, London, 2001: ISBN 1-85315-498-9.

(14) Br Med J issue 9 March 2002 'Trust me. I'm a web site' this contains many articles and commentaries on internet material.

C.5. Books for patients to read, also see Chapter 15

(15) Wall PD. Pain. The Science of Suffering. Weidenfeld and Nicolson, London, 1999: ISBN 0-297-84255-2.

(16) Sternbach R. Mastering pain. Arlington Books, London, 1987: ISBN 0-85140-716-1. (A 12-step guide to how chronic pain can be managed.)

References

Marked as regards quality according to criteria set by author.

SR = systematic review or high quality review with methodology

* Poorer quality studies but only ones in the field, old style reviews.

** Cohort studies, high quality case series with controls.

*** Randomised controlled trials, high quality original studies.

*** Abbot NC, Harkness EF, Stevinson C, Marshall FP, Conn DA, Ernst E. Spiritual healing as a therapy for chronic pain: a randomized, clinical trial. Pain 2001; 91: 79–89.

* Ashburn MA, Staats PS. Management of chronic pain. Lancet 1999; 353: 1865–1869.

** Bahra A, Gawel MJ, Hardebo JE, Millson D, Breen SA,

Goadsby PJ. Oral zolmitriptan is effective in the acute treatment of cluster headache. Neurology 2000; 54: 1832–1839.

*** Beck A, Scott J, Williams P, Robertson B, Jackson D, Gade G, Cowan P. A randomized trial of group outpatient visits for chronically ill older HMO members: the Cooperative Health Care Clinic. J Am Geriatr Soc 1997; 45: 543–549.

* Beecher HK. Powerful placebo. J Am Med Assoc 1955; 159: 1602–1606.

* Beecher HK. Surgery as placebo. J Am Med Assoc 1961; 176: 1102–1107.

*** Begg C, Cho M, Eastwood S, Horton R, Moher D, Olkin I, Pitkin R, Rennie D, Schulz KF, Simel D, Stroup DF. Improving the quality of reporting of randomized controlled trials. The CONSORT statement. J Am Med Assoc 1996; 276: 637–639.

Bird J, Cohen-Cole SA. The three-function model of the medical interview. An educational device. Adv Psychosom Med 1990; 20: 65–88.

** Bloom BS. Direct medical costs of disease and gastrointestinal side effects during treatment for arthritis. Am J Med 1988; 84: 20–24.

* Bloom BS. Daily regimen and compliance with treatment. Fewer daily doses and drugs with fewer side effects improve compliance. Br Med J 2001; 323: 647.

* Bolten W, Emmerich M, Weber E, Fassmeyer N. Validation of electronic by conventional pain diaries. Z Rheumatol 1991; 50 (Suppl 1): 55–64.

* Bradley LA, Young LD, Anderson KO, Turner RA, Agudelo CA, McDaniel LK, Semble EL. Effects of cognitive–behavioral therapy on rheumatoid arthritis pain behavior: one-year follow-up. In: Dubner R, Gebbart GF, Bond MR (eds) Proceedings of the Vth World Congress on Pain, Elsevier, Amsterdam, 1988: 310–314.

* Botney M, Fields HL. Amitriptyline potentiates morphine analgesia by a direct action on the central nervous system. Ann Neurol 1983; 13: 160–164.

* Brodwin PE, Kleinman A. In: Burrows GD, Elton D, Stanley GV (eds) Handbook of Chronic Pain Management. Elsevier, Amsterdam, 1987: 109–119.

* Brody DS, Thompson TL, Larson DB, Ford DE, Katon WJ, Magruder KM. Strategies for counselling depressed patients by primary care physicians. J Gen Intern Med 1994; 9: 569–575.

* Brody DS, Dietrich AJ, deGruy F III, Kroenke K. The depression in primary care tool kit. Int J Psychiatry Med 2000; 30: 99–110.

* Buckalew LW, Ross S. Relationship of perceptual characteristics to efficacy of placebos. Psychol Reports 1974; 48: 3–8.

* Carne S. The action of chorionic gonadotrophin in the obese. Lancet, 1961; ii: 1282–1284.

Carr AJ, Green D, Kidd B. Electronic measurement of pain: a comparative study of an electronic pain diary and existing pain measures. Abstract at Br Rheumtol conference, 1999.

** Casarett D, Karlawish J, Sankar P, Hirschman KB, Asch DA. Obtaining informed consent for clinical pain research:

patients' concerns and information needs. Pain 2001; 92: 71–79.

** Cassisi JE, Sypert GW, Salamon A, Kapel L. Independent evaluation of a multidisciplinary rehabilitation program for chronic low back pain. Neurosurgery 1989; 25: 877–883.

* Chapman CR, Gavrin J. Suffering: the contributions of persistent pain. Lancet 1999; 353: 2233–2237.

* Charnock D, Shepperd S, Needham G, Gann R. DISCERN: an instrument for judging the quality of written consumer health information on treatment choices. J Epidemiol Community Health 1999; 53: 105–111.

* Colvin DF, Bettinger R, Knapp R, Pawlicki R, Zimmerman J. Characteristics of patients with chronic pain. South Med J 1980; 73: 1020–1023.

* Craig TKJ, Boardman AP. ABC of mental health: Common mental health problems in primary care. Br Med J 1997; 314: 1609.

* Crook J, Tunks E, Kalaher S, Roberts J. Coping with persistent pain: a comparison of persistent pain sufferers in a specialty pain clinic and in a family practice clinic. Pain 1988; 34: 175–184.

de Felipe MC, de Ceballos ML, Gil C, Fuentes JA. Chronic antidepressant treatment increases enkephalin levels in n. accumbens and striatum of the rat. Eur J Pharmacol 1985; 112: 119–122.

* de Felipe MC, de Ceballos ML, Fuentes JA. Hypoalgesia induced by antidepressants in mice: a case for opioids and serotonin. Eur J Pharmacol 1986; 125: 193–199.

* DeGood DE, Shutty MS. Assessment of pain beliefs, coping and self efficacy. In: Turk DC, Melzack R (eds) Handbook of Pain Assessment. Guilford Press, New York, 1992: 221.

* Delamothe T. Quality of websites: kitemarking the west wind. Br Med J 2000; 321: 843–844.

* Dickenson AH, Matthews EA, Suzuki R. Neurobiology of neuropathic pain: mode of action of anticonvulsants. Eur J Pain 2002; 6: 51–60.

* Donoghue JM, Tylee A. The treatment of depression: prescribing patterns of antidepressants in primary care in the UK. Br J Psychiatry 1996; 168: 164–168.

** Dworkin SF, Turner JA, Wilson L, Massoth D, Whitney C, Huggins KH, Burgess J, Sommers E, Truelove E. Brief group cognitive–behavioral intervention for temporomandibular disorders. Pain 1994; 59: 175–187.

** Ekbom K, Monstad I, Prusinski A, Cole JA, Pilgrim AJ, Noronha D. Subcutaneous sumatriptan in the acute treatment of cluster headache: a dose comparison study. The Sumatriptan Cluster Headache Study Group. Acta Neurol Scand 1993; 88: 63–69.

* Elwyn G, Edwards A, Eccles M, Rovner D. Decision analysis in patient care. Lancet 2001; 358: 571–574.

* Evans FJ. The placebo response in pain reduction. In: Bonica JJ (ed) Advances in Neurology, Vol. 4. Raven Press, New York, 1974: 289–296.

* Farmer KC. Methods for measuring and monitoring medication regimen adherence in clinical trials and clinical practice. Clin Ther 1999; 21: 1074–1090.

SR Ferrari MD, Roon KI, Lipton RB, Goadsby PJ. Oral triptans (serotonin 5-HT(1B/1D) agonists) in acute migraine treatment: a meta-analysis of 53 trials. Lancet 2001; 358: 1668–1675.

*Flower RJ, Manceda S, Vane JR. Analgesic–antipyretics and anti-inflammatory agents. In: Goodman AG, Goodman LS, Rall TW, Murad F (eds) Goodman and Gilman's The Pharmacological Basis of Therapeutics, 7th edn. MacMillan Publishing Company, New York: 1985: 674–715.

Finneson BE. Diagnosis and management of pain syndromes. Philadelphia: W.B. Saunders, 1969.

**Fogelholm R, Murros K. Maprotiline in chronic tension headache: a double-blind cross-over study. Headache 1985; 25: 273–275.

SR Forssell H, Kalso E, Koskela P, Vehmanen R, Puukka P, Alanen P. Occlusal treatments in temporomandibular disorders: a qualitative systematic review of randomized controlled trials. Pain 1999; 83: 549–560.

*Frank JD. The role of hope in psychotherapy. Int J Psychiatry 1968; 5: 383–395.

*Fromm GH, Nakata M, Kondo T. Differential action of amitriptyline on neurons in the trigeminal nucleus. Neurology 1991; 41: 1932–1936.

SR Gagliardi A, Jadad AR. Examination of instruments used to rate quality of health information on the internet: chronicle of a voyage with an unclear destination. Br Med J 2002; 324: 569–573.

*Garro LC, Stephenson KA, Good BJ. Chronic illness of the temporomandibular joints as experienced by support-group members. J Gen Intern Med 1994; 9: 372–378.

SR Gill D, Hatcher S. A systematic review of the treatment of depression with antidepressant drugs in patients who also have a physical illness. J Psychosom Res 1999; 47: 131–143.

*Glasgow RE, Hollis JF, McRae SG, Lando HA, LaChance P. Providing an integrated program of low intensity tobacco cessation services in a health maintenance organisation. Health Educ Res 1991; 6: 87–99.

Gleidman LH, Gantt WH, Teitelbaum HA. Some implications of conditional reflex studies for placebo research. Am J Psychiatry 1957; 113: 1103–1107.

SR Gloaguen V, Cottraux J, Cucherat M, Blackburn IM. A meta-analysis of the effects of cognitive therapy in depressed patients. J Affect Disord 1998; 49: 59–72.

SR Goadsby PJ. The clinical profile of sumatriptan: cluster headache. Eur Neurol 1994; 34 (Suppl 2): 35–39.

Goadsby PJ, Lipton RB. A review of paroxysmal hemicranias, SUNCT syndrome and other short-lasting headaches with autonomic feature, including new cases. Brain 1997; 120: 193–209.

*Goldberg RJ, Novack DH, Gask L. The recognition and management of somatization. What is needed in primary care training. Psychosomatics 1992; 33: 55–61.

Goodman WK, Charney DS. Therapeutic applications and mechanisms of action of monoamine oxidase inhibitor and heterocyclic antidepressant drugs. J Clin Psychiatry 1985; 46(10 Pt 2): 6–24.

*Gracely RH. In: Devor M, Rowbotham MC, Wiesenfeld-Hallin

Z (eds) Proceedings of the 9th World Congress on Pain. IASP Press, Seattle, WA, 2000; 16: 1045–1067.

*Grevert P, Albert LH, Goldstein A. Partial antagonism of placebo analgesia by naloxone. Pain 1983; 16(2): 129–143.

*Hale AS. ABC of mental health. Depression. Br Med J 1997; 315: 43–46.

*Hardebo JE, Dahlof C. Sumatriptan nasal spray (20 mg/dose) in the acute treatment of cluster headache. Cephalalgia 1998; 18: 487–489.

**Harrison S, Watson M, Feinmann C. Does short-term group therapy affect unexplained medical symptoms? J Psychosom Res 1997; 43: 399–404.

**Hashish I, Hai HK, Harvey W, Feinmann C, Harris M. Reduction of postoperative pain and swelling by ultrasound treatment: a placebo effect. Pain 1988; 33: 303–311.

*Holman H, Lorig K. Patients as partners in managing chronic disease. Partnership is a prerequisite for effective and efficient health care. Br Med J 2000; 320: 526–527.

SR Hope T. Evidence-Based Patient Choice. Kings Fund Publishing, London, 1996.

*Hyland ME, Kenyon CA, Allen R, Howarth P. Diary keeping in asthma: comparison of written and electronic methods. Br Med J 1993; 306: 487–489.

*Jaffe JH, Martin JR. Opioid analgesics and antagonists. In: Goodman AG, Goodman LS, Rall TW, Murad F (eds) Goodman and Gilman's The Pharmacological Basis of Therapeutics, 7th edn. MacMillan Publishing Company, New York, 1985: 491–532.

SR Jensen MP, Turner JA, Romano JM, Karoly P. Coping with chronic pain: a critical review of the literature. Pain 1991; 47: 249–283.

SR Jensen TS. Anticonvulsants in neuropathic pain: rationale and clinical evidence. Eur J Pain 2002; Suppl 6: 61–68.

**Jett MF, McGuirk J, Waligora D, Hunter JC. The effects of mexiletine, desipramine and fluoxetine in rat models involving central sensitization. Pain 1997; 69: 161–169.

SR Joffe S, Cook EF, Cleary PD, Clark JW, Weeks JC. Quality of informed consent in cancer clinical trials: a cross-sectional survey. Lancet 2001; 358: 1772–1777.

*Johnson AG. Surgery as a placebo. Lancet, 1994; 344: 1140–1142.

*Kaplan SH, Greenfield S, Ware JE Jr. Assessing the effects of physician-patient interactions on the outcomes of chronic disease. Med Care 1989; 27: S110–S127.

*Kaplan SH, Greenfield S, Gandek B, Rogers WH, Ware JE Jr. Characteristics of physicians with participatory decision-making styles. Ann Intern Med 1996; 124: 497–504.

*Katon W. The impact of major depression on chronic medical illness. Gen Hosp Psychiatry 1996; 18: 215–219.

**Keefe FJ, Lefebvre JC, Kerns RD, Rosenberg R, Beaupre P, Prochaska J, Prochaska JO, Caldwell DS. Understanding the adoption of arthritis self-management: stages of change profiles among arthritis patients. Pain 2000; 87: 303–313.

*Kelleher DJA. Patients learning from each other: self-help groups for people with diabetes. J R Soc Med 1991; 84: 595–597.

*Klapper J, Stanton J, Seawell M. The development of a support group organization for headache sufferers. Headache 1992; 32: 193–196.

Kleinman A, Eisenberg L, Good B. Culture, illness, care: clinical lessons from anthropologic and cross-cultural research. Ann Intern Med 1978; 88: 251–258.

** Lance JW, Curran DA. Treatment of chronic tension headache. Lancet 1964; 1: 1236–1239.

* Leonard BE. The comparative pharmacology of new antidepressants. J Clin Psychiatry 1993; 54 (Suppl) 3–15.

* LeResche L. Assessment of physical and behavioral outcomes of treatment. Oral Surg Oral Med Oral Pathol Oral Radiol Endod 1997; 83: 82–86.

* Levine JD, Gordon NC, Fields HL. The mechanism of placebo analgesia. Lancet 1978; 2: 654–657.

SR SR Lewin SA, Skea ZC, Entwistle V, Zwarenstein M, Dick J. Interventions for providers to promote a patient-centred approach in clinical consultations. Cochrane Database Syst Rev 2002; 3: CD003267

SR Linde K, Mulrow CD. St John's wort for depression. Cochrane Database Syst Rev 2000; CD000448.

** Lorig KR, Mazonson PD, Holman HR. Evidence suggesting that health education for self-management in patients with chronic arthritis has sustained health benefits while reducing health care costs. Arthritis Rheum. 1993; 36: 439–446.

* Lundstrom S. Electronic patient diaries. Technol Update 1993; 2: 35–38.

* Marbach JJ, Lennon MC, Link BG, Dohrenwend BP. Losing face: sources of stigma as perceived by chronic facial pain patients. J Behav Med 1990; 13: 583–604.

* Martelli MF, Liljedahl EL, Nicholson K, Zasler ND. A brief introductory guide to chronic pain resources on the Internet. NeuroRehabilitation 2000; 14: 105–121.

** Max MB, Culnane M, Schafer SC, Gracely RH, Walther DJ, Smoller B, Dubner R. Amitriptyline relieves diabetic neuropathy pain in patients with normal or depressed mood. Neurology 1987; 37: 589–596.

McCulloch P, Taylor I, Sasako M, Lovett B, Griffin D. Randomised trials in surgery:problems and possible solutions. Br Med J 2002; 324: 1448–1451.

SR McQuay H. Neuropathic pain: evidence matters. Eur J Pain 2002; 6: 11–18.

SR McQuay H, Carroll D, Jadad AR, Wiffen P, Moore A. Anticonvulsant drugs for management of pain: a systematic review. Br Med J 1995; 311: 1047–1052.

SR McQuay HJ, Tramer M, Nye BA, Carroll D, Wiffen PJ, Moore RA. A systematic review of antidepressants in neuropathic pain. Pain 1996; 68: 217–227.

SR Melchart D, Linde K, Fischer P, Berman B, White A, Vickers A, Allais G. Acupuncture for idiopathic headache. Cochrane Database Syst Rev 2001; CD001218.

* Moher D, Schulz KF, Altman D. The CONSORT statement: revised recommendations for improving the quality of reports of parallel-group randomized trials. J Am Med Assoc 2001; 285: 1987–1991.

Morley S, Eccleston C, Williams A. Systematic review and meta-analysis of randomized controlled trials of cognitive behaviour therapy and behaviour therapy for chronic pain in adults, excluding headache. Pain 1999; 80(1–2): 1–13.

*** Moulin DE, Iezzi A, Amireh R, Sharpe WK, Boyd D, Merskey H. Randomised trial of oral morphine for chronic non-cancer pain. Lancet 1996; 347: 143–147.

SR Mulrow CD, Williams JW Jr, Chiquette E, Aguilar C, Hitchcock-Noel P, Lee S, Cornell J, Stamm K. Efficacy of newer medications for treating depression in primary care patients. Am J Med 2000; 108; 54–64.

* O'Connor AM. A call to standardize measures for judging the efficacy of interventions to aid patients' decision making. Med Decis Making 1999; 19: 504–505.

* O'Connor AM, Drake ER, Fiset V, Graham ID, Laupacis A, Tugwell P. The Ottawa patient decision aids. Eff Clin Pract 1999; 2: 163–170.

SR O'Connor AM, Stacey D, Rovner D, Holmes-Rovner M, Tetroe J, Llewellyn-Thomas H, Entwistle V, Rostom A, Fiset V, Barry M, Jones J. Decision aids for people facing health treatment or screening decisions (Cochrane Review). Cochrane Database Syst Rev 2001; 3: CD001431.

** Okasha A, Ghaleb HA, Sadek A. A double blind trial for the clinical management of psychogenic headache. Br J Psychiatry 1973; 122: 181–183.

* Palazidou E. Development of new antidepressants. Adv Psychiatric Treat 1997; 3: 46–51.

* Peters ML, Sorbi MJ, Kruise DA, Kerssens JJ, Verhaak PF, Bensing JM. Electronic diary assessment of pain, disability and psychological adaptation in patients differing in duration of pain. Pain 2000; 84: 181–192.

** Petrie J, Hazleman B. Credibility of placebo transcutaneous nerve stimulation and acupuncture. Clin Exp Rheumatol 1985; 3: 151–153.

Price J, Leaver L. Beginning treatment. Br Med J 2002; 325: 33–35.

** Rani PU, Naidu MU, Prasad VB, Rao TR, Shobha JC. An evaluation of antidepressants in rheumatic pain conditions. Anesth Analg 1996; 83: 371–375.

* Redelmeier DA, Rozin P, Kahneman D. Understanding patients' decisions. Cognitive and emotional perspectives. J Am Med Assoc 1993; 270: 72–76.

* Richardson P. Placebos: their effectiveness and modes of action. In: Broome AK (ed) Health Psychology Processes and Application. Chapman and Hall, London, 1995.

* Rigby M, Forsstrom J, Roberts R, Wyatt J. Verifying quality and safety in health informatics services. Br Med J 2001; 323: 552–556.

* Risk A. Commentary: on the way to quality. Br Med J 2002; 324: 601–602.

SR Roberts L, Ahmed I, Hall S. Intercessory prayer for the alleviation of ill health. Cochrane Database Syst Rev 2000; CD000368.

* Roldan OV, Maglione H, Carriers R, Mainieri S. Piroxicam, diazepam and placebo in the treatment of temporomandibular joint dysfunction. Double blind study. Rev Asoc Odontol Argentina 1990; 78: 83–85.

* Rootes LE, Aanes DL. A conceptual framework for under-

standing self-help groups. Hosp Commun Psychiatry 1992; 43: 379–381.

* Ross M, Olson JM. An expectancy–attribution model of the effects of placebos. Psychol Rev 1981; 88: 408–437.

SR Rosted P. The use of acupuncture in dentistry: a review of the scientific validity of published papers. Oral Dis 1998; 4: 100–104.

SR Rowland N, Bower P, Mellor C, Heywood P, Godfrey C. Effectiveness and cost effectivenss of counselling in primary care (Cochrane Review; Cochrane Database Syst Rev 2001; 3: CD001025.

SR Rubenstein LV, Jackson-Triche M, Unutzer J, Miranda J, Minnium K, Pearson ML, Wells KB. Evidence-based care for depression in managed primary care practices. Health Aff (Millwood) 1999; 18: 89–105.

SR Sackett DL, Straus SE, Scott Richardson W, Rosenberg W, Haynes RJ. Evidence-Based Medicine. How to Practice and Teach EBM. Churchill Livingstone, Edinburgh, 2000.

* Sacristan JA, Gomez JC, Badia X, Kind P. Global index of safety (GIS): a new instrument to assess drug safety. J Clin Epidemiol 2001; 54: 1120–1125.

* Salmon P, Peters S, Stanley I. Patients' perceptions of medical explanations for somatisation disorders: qualitative analysis. Br Med J 1999; 318: 372–376.

* Shapiro AK. Etiological factors in the placebo effect. J Am Med Assoc 1964; 187: 712–714.

* Shapiro AK, Morris LA. The placebo effect in medical and psychological therapies. In: Bergin AE, Garfield S (eds) Handbook of Psychotherapy and Behavioral Change, 2nd edn. John Wiley and Sons, New York, 1978: 369–410.

* Shuhan G, Benren X, Yuhuan Z. Treatment of primary trigeminal neuralgia with acupuncture in 1500 cases. J Tradit Chin Med 1991; 11: 3–6.

*** Simon GE, Von Korff M, Rutter C, Wagner E. Randomised trial of monitoring, feedback, management of care by telephone to improve treatment of depression in primary care. Br Med J 2000; 320: 550–554.

SR Sindrup SH, Jensen TS. Efficacy of pharmacological treatments of neuropathic pain: an update and effect related to mechanism of drug action. Pain 1999; 83: 389–400.

* Singer EJ, Sharav Y, Schmidt E, Dionne RA, Dubner R. The efficacy of diazepam and ibuprofen in the treatment of chronic myofascial pain. Pain 1987; 31: 183–185.

*** Speckens AE, van Hemert AM, Spinhoven P, Hawton KE, Bolk JH, Rooijmans HG. Cognitive behavioural therapy for medically unexplained physical symptoms: a randomised controlled trial. Br Med J 1995; 311: 1328–1332.

** Stone AA, Shiffman S, Schwartz JE, Broderick JE, Hufford MR. Patient non-compliance with paper diaries. Br Med J 2002; 324, 1193–1194.

Stohler CS. Management of persistent orofacial pain. In: Lund JP, Lavigne GJ, Dubner R, Sessle BJ Orofacial Pain, From Basic Science to Clinical Management. Quintessence Publishing Chicago, 2001: 193–210.

* Syse A. Norway: valid (as opposed to informed) consent. Lancet 2000; 356: 1347–1348.

* Tattersall MH. Examining informed consent to cancer clinical trials. Lancet 2001; 358: 1742–1743.

* Totman R. Cognitive dissonance in the placebo treatment of insomnia — a pilot experiment. Br J Med Psychol 1976; 49: 393–400.

* Turk DC, Brody MC. Chronic opioid therapy for persistent noncancer pain: panacea or oxymoron? Am Pain Soc Bull 1993; 1: 4–7.

* Turk DC, Rudy TE. Neglected factors in chronic pain treatment outcome studies — referral patterns, failure to enter treatment, attrition. Pain 1990; 43: 7–25.

* Turkington RW. Depression masquerading as diabetic neuropathy. J Am Med Assoc 1980; 243: 1147–1150.

Turner JA, Clancy S. Comparison of operant behavioral and cognitive-behavioral group treatment for chronic low back pain. J Consult Clin Psychol 1988; 56(2): 261–266.

SR Turner JA, Clancy S, McQuade KJ, Cardenas DD. Effectiveness of behavioral therapy for chronic low back pain: a component analysis. J Consult Clin Psychol 1990; 58: 573–579.

** Uhlenhuth EH, Canter A, Neustadt JO, Payson HE. The symptomatic relief of anxiety with meprobamate, phenobarbital and placebo. Am J Psychiatry 1959; 115: 905–910.

* Villemure C, Bushnell MC. Cognitive modulation of pain: how do attention and emotion influence pain processing? Pain 2002; 95: 195–199.

* Von Korff M, Dworkin SF, Le Resche L. Graded chronic pain status: an epidemiologic evaluation. Pain 1990; 40: 279–291.

* Wall PD. Placebo and placebo response. In: Wall PD, Melzack R (eds) Textbook of Pain. Churchill Livingstone, Philadelphia, PA, 1999: 1419–1430.

* Wasson J, Gaudette C, Whaley F, Sauvigne A, Baribeau P, Welch HG. Telephone care as a substitute for routine clinic follow-up. J Am Med Assoc 1992; 267: 1788–1793.

SR Whooley MA, Simon GE. Managing depression in medical outpatients. N Engl J Med 2000; 343; 1942–1950.

SR Williams AC, Pither CE, Richardson PH, Nicholas MK, Justins DM, Morley S, Diamond A, Linton S, Vlaeyen J, Nilges P, Eccleston C. The effects of cognitive–behavioural therapy in chronic pain. Pain 1996a; 65: 282–284.

*** Williams AC, Richardson PH, Nicholas MK, Pither CE, Harding VR, Ridout KL, Ralphs JA, Richardson IH, Justins DM, Chamberlain JH. Inpatient vs. outpatient pain management: results of a randomised controlled trial. Pain 1996b; 66: 13–22.

SR Wilson K, Mottram P, Sivanranthan A, Nightingale A. Antidepressant versus placebo for depressed elderly (Cochrane Review). Cochrane Database Syst Rev 2001; 2: CD000561.

* Wilson P. How to find the good and avoid the bad or ugly: a short guide to tools for rating quality of health information on the internet. Br Med J 2002; 324: 598–602.

** Winkler R, Underwood P, Fatovich B, James R, Gray D. A clinical trial of a self-care approach to the management of chronic headache in general practice. Soc Sci Med 1989; 29: 213–219.

* Wituk S, Shepherd MD, Slavich S, Warren ML, Meissen G. A

topography of self-help groups: an empirical analysis. Soc Work 2000; 45: 157–165.

Woolf CJ, Mannion RJ. Neuropathic pain: aetiology, symptoms, mechanisms, and management. Lancet 1999; 353(9168): 1959–1964.

*Woolf CJ, Bennett GJ, Doherty M, Dubner R, Kidd B, Koltzenburg M, Lipton R, Loeser JD, Payne R, Torebjork E. Towards a mechanism-based classification of pain? Pain 1998; 77: 227–229.

*Wright EC. Non-compliance — or how many aunts has Matilda? Lancet 1993; 342: 909–913.

SR Zakrzewska JM, Hamlyn PJ. In: Crombie IKCPR, Linton SJ, LeResche L, Von Korff M (eds) Epidemiology of Pain. IASP, Seattle, WA, 1999: 171–202.

**Ziegler DK, Hurwitz A, Hassanein RS, Kodanaz HA, Preskorn SH, Mason J. Migraine prophylaxis. A comparison of propranolol and amitriptyline. Arch Neurol 1987; 44: 486–489.

Assessment and Management of Orofacial Pain
Pain Research and Clinical Management, Vol. 14
Edited by J.M. Zakrzewska and S.D. Harrison
© *2002 Elsevier Science B.V. All rights reserved*

CHAPTER 10

Dental pain

Behnam Aghabeigi [*]

Department of Oral and Maxillofacial Surgery, Eastman Dental Institute, 256 Gray's Inn Road, London WC1X 8LD, UK

Objectives for this chapter:

This chapter will attempt to:
- Describe some dental causes of pain that can mimic non-dental pain including:
  - Tooth hypersensitivity
  - Reversible pulpitis
  - Irreversible pulpitis
  - Cracked tooth syndrome
  - Acute periapical periodontitis
  - Lateral periodontal abscess
  - Pericoronitis
  - Dry socket (alveolar osteitis)
- List the key features of dental pain
- Provide an outline of treatment strategies

1. Introduction

The most common cause of pain from the mouth is inflammatory disease of the dental pulp or periodontal tissues. However, inflammation of the dental pulp and the periapical tissues is not always painful. In fact, severe pain sufficient to warrant presentation to the dentist may occur in only a small proportion of cases. Many inflammatory periapical lesions are detected by chance with no history of previous pain. Pain of non-dental origin can present as toothache and pain originating from the teeth can be referred to or spread to other structures. Inability to identify the

cause of the pain, can lead to unnecessary restorations, root canal treatment, apicectomies and extractions. The accurate diagnosis of orofacial pain may necessitate input from several clinical disciplines. Conditions mimicking dental pain are described in other chapters. However, a brief description of the recently proposed diagnostic category of vascular orofacial pain (VOP) which could mimic dental pulpitis will be presented at the end of this chapter. Investigation of dental pain has been discussed in Chapter 7. An overview of the innervation of dentine and theories of dentinal sensitivity have been discussed in Chapter 2. The key clinical features of dentally related pains are summarised in Table 1.

[*] Tel.: +44-20-7915-1275; Fax: +44-20-7915-1259;
E-mail: b.aghabeigi@eastman.ucl.ac.uk

TABLE 1
Differential diagnosis of dental pains

Aetiology	Pain character and timing	Pain intensity	Provoking factors	Relieving factors	Associated features
Tooth hypersensitivity	sharp, stabbing, stimulation evoked	mild to moderate	thermal, tactile chemical, osmotic	removal of the stimulus	attrition, erosion
Reversible pulpitis	sharp, stimulation evoked	mild to moderate	hot, cold, sweet	removal of the stimulus	caries, restorations
Irreversible pulpitis	sharp, throbbing, intermittent/continuous	severe	hot, chewing, lying flat	cold in late stages	deep caries
Cracked tooth syndrome	sharp, intermittent	moderate to severe	biting, 'rebound pain'	—	trauma, parafunction
Periapical periodontitis	deep, continuous, boring	moderate to severe	biting	removal of trauma	periapical redness, swelling, mobility
Lateral periodontal abscess	deep continuous aching	moderate to severe	biting	—	deep pockets redness and swelling
Pericoronitis	continuous	moderate to severe	biting	removal of trauma	fever, malaise imprint of upper tooth
Dry socket (acute alveolar osteitis)	continuous 4–5 days post extraction	moderate to severe	—	irrigation	loss of clot, exposed bone

2. Tooth hypersensitivity

2.1. Definition and mechanism

Tooth hypersensitivity, or more precisely dentinal sensitivity or hypersensitivity, is described clinically as pain arising from exposed dentine, typically in response to chemical, thermal, tactile or osmotic stimuli that cannot be explained as arising from any other form of dental defect or pathology (Addy, 1990). Curro (1990) considers the condition as allodynia, i.e. pain resulting from a non-noxious stimulus and proposes the term 'allodontia' to describe dentinal hypersensitivity. The mechanism responsible for dentine sensitivity is the movement of fluid along dentinal tubules (see Chapter 2 for more details), activating nociceptors in the inner dentine or outer pulp.

2.2. Clinical features

The pain is described as a sharp 'nerve' type pain which occurs immediately following application of the stimulus and is reasonably well localised (the patient can point to the area and often the tooth involved). Loss of enamel occurs by attrition associated with occlusal function and may be exaggerated by habits or parafunctional activity such as bruxism; by abrasion from dietary components or habits such as toothbrushing. Loss of enamel can also occur by the process of chemical erosion secondary to a high acid diet or gastric reflux. Exposed dentine is often but not always sensitive.

2.3. Management

Effective treatment includes covering the open dentinal tubules and perhaps applying agents that inactivate pulpal nociceptors. It is unclear to what extent inflammatory changes in the underlying pulp contribute to the sensitivity, although the finding that replacement of apparently sound restorations in patients complaining of sensitive dentine substantially reduces the sensitivity suggesting that the latter is due to microleakage. Fluoride salts can be applied to dentinal tubules using dental office procedures. Fluoridated toothpastes and mouthwashes complement this effect (Gaffar, 1990). Potassium salts reduce the excitability of pulpal axons (Orchardson and Gillam, 2000) and the inclusion of potassium salts in desensitising toothpastes may induce this effect if the ions diffuse into the pulp. Adhesive restorative materials, such as glass ionomer cements that cover exposed dentine are also effective.

2.4. Prognosis

These various treatments often provide a substantial relief of sensitivity but may not eliminate it completely. Patient education in relation to dietary habits and brushing techniques may prevent the recurrence of exposed dentine.

3. Reversible pulpitis

3.1. Definition and mechanism

Inflammation of the dental pulp is usually caused by dental caries and the early phases might be reversible. This condition may be difficult to distinguish from hypersensitive dentine. A toothache occurs in approximately 0.26% of high altitude fliers (Kollmann, 1993). This aerodontalgia or barodontalgia is thought to be a result of reduced atmospheric pressure causing pressure changes within the pulp chamber that stimulates an inflamed pulp. Early sinusitis can produce similar symptoms.

3.2. Clinical features

The pain is described as sharp, which is provoked by thermal or osmotic stimuli and is relieved when the stimulus is taken away. The absence of any exposed dentine together with the presence of some aetiologic factor such as caries or a leaking restoration aids the clinician in suspecting an inflammatory change in the underlying pulp. From a clinical point, unfortunately the relation between the signs and symptoms and the histological condition of the pulp is weak. For a time, the term pulpalgia was used to describe pain from pulpal causes, as this did not assume a relationship with any particular pathologic condition. The pain is poorly localised and the patient may be unable to distinguish whether the pain originates from the lower or the upper jaw. As a diagnostic aid, pain can usually be duplicated by controlled application of cold or hot stimuli to various teeth in the suspected area.

3.3. Management

Treatment of reversible pulpitis is by removal of the carious lesion, protection of the pulp by a dressing and a permanent restoration after a few weeks if the tooth remains asymptomatic. If removal of all the caries is likely to lead to a pulp exposure, one option is to remove most of the caries and place a dressing to seal off the remainder from the oral environment. This has a modest positive prognosis but may be worth attempting if the alternatives of root canal therapy or extraction are unattractive.

4. Irreversible pulpitis

4.1. Definition and mechanism

This condition implies irreversible pulpal changes and usually leads to pulpal necrosis and suppurative pulpitis. As the pulpal inflammation spreads, compression of pulpal blood vessels by the inflammatory oedema leads to necrosis. Although pain is the most common symptom of a diseased pulp, no correlation exists between specific pain characteristics and the histopathological status of the pulp. Many pulps die quietly and only present for treatments a result of periradicular symptoms or a radiolucency extending from a non-vital tooth. The concept of 'silent pulpitis' has thus been developed, implying that many of the pain afferents in the pulp are, in some circumstances, inactive. This suggests that there may be local antinociceptive mechanisms that block the transmission of stimuli in some circumstances.

4.2. Clinical features

Pain is spontaneous, strong and often throbbing. A history of prolonged intense pain ending suddenly is not unusual. It has been a commonly held belief that, if the evoked pain outlasts the stimulus (unlike stimulus induced pain of reversible pulpitis), the pulp is irreversibly damaged. Objective evidence for this is not strong. The pain is poorly localised and the localisation becomes even more difficult when the pain intensity increases. Pain tends to radiate or refer to the ear, temple and cheek, but does not cross the midline. Pain may be described by patients in different ways and a continuous dull ache can be periodically exacerbated (by stimulation or spontaneously) for short (minutes) or long (hours) periods. Pain may increase and throb when the patient lies down and in many instances wakes the patient from sleep (Sharav et al., 1984). The pain of pulpitis is frequently not continuous and ends spontaneously. This interrupted, sharp, paroxysmal, non-localised pain may lead to the misdiagnosis of other conditions that may mimic pain of pulpal origin (e.g. trigeminal neuralgia).

4.3. Management

The definitive treatment for irreversible pulpitis that is painful is root canal therapy or extraction. If dental treatment is not immediately available, the pain will require analgesic therapy. A combination of peripherally acting and centrally acting analgesics may be required to produce maximal effect.

5. Cracked tooth syndrome

5.1. Definition and mechanism

Pain associated with single or multiple cracks involving enamel, dentine and pulp either in isolation or in combination may prove a puzzling and frustrating condition for both patient and dentist. The crack may involve the crown alone or extend into the root of the tooth. Cracks involving only enamel are usually symptomless. Cracks usually result from an unexpected encounter with a hard object during mastication, or a blow to the chin.

5.2. Clinical features

Diagnosis of a cracked tooth is difficult as the affected tooth is poorly localised and radiographs are unhelpful (Homewood, 1998). Patients usually complain of a sharp pain, elicited by biting that ceases when pressure is removed from the teeth. This suggests a periodontal origin, whereas the true cause may be pulpal trauma caused by the shearing forces applied to the tooth. Occasionally, the pain may be worse on relief of a biting force than on application of the force. This is known as 'rebound pain' and is thought to be due to dentine surfaces rubbing together causing tubular fluid movement. The patient may also complain of pain and discomfort associated with cold and hot stimuli in the area, due to stimulation of the pulp via the fracture line. The following measures may help in diagnosis:

(1) Fibreoptic transillumination and magnification to visualise the crack
(2) Painting the tooth with a dye such as methylene blue or washable ink may allow entry of the dye into the opened crack. The dye will remain in the crack when the tooth is cleaned
(3) Percussing the cusps of the suspected teeth at different angles
(4) Asking the patient to bite on individual cusps using a fine wooden stick or a rubber dam may allow the crack to open, cause pain and thus allow the affected tooth to be identified
(5) Probing firmly around margins of fillings and in suspected fissures

5.3. Management

Vertically fractured teeth usually require extraction. Placement of adhesive restorations may be effective in preventing propagation of the fracture line and placement of a full veneer crown to splint the remaining tooth structure have been suggested.

5.4. Prognosis

The success rate of the variety of the restorative procedures described above is usually low. Occasionally hemisection (removal of one root of a molar tooth) may be indicated.

6. Periodontal pain

6.1. Periapical periodontitis

6.1.1. Definition and mechanism
Although inflammation extending from the coronal aspect of the periodontal tissue is rarely painful, inflammation of the supporting tissues around the apex of the tooth often is. Acute periradicular periodontitis can arise from trauma but more commonly as an extension of pulpal inflammation and necrosis.

6.1.2. Clinical features
Pain associated with acute periapical inflammation is spontaneous and moderate to severe in intensity for long periods of time. Pain is exacerbated by biting on the tooth and, in more advanced cases, even by closing the mouth and bringing the affected tooth into contact with the opposing teeth. The affected tooth feels extruded and is sensitive to touch. The periodontal pain is less intense than the paroxysmal and excruciating pulpal pain. In contrast to the poorly localised pain of pulpal origin, the patient is usually able to locate the periodontally affected tooth precisely. This has been attributed to the proprioceptive and mechanoreceptive sensibility of the periodontium which is lacking in the pulp. Although localisation of the affected tooth is usually precise, in approximately half the cases the pain is diffuse and spreads into the jaw on the affected side of the face (Sharav et al., 1984).

On clinical examination, the affected tooth is tender to percussion and is non-vital, i.e. does not respond to thermal stimuli or electric pulp stimulation. However, pulpal as well as periapical involvement could occur at the same time. In these cases, although the periapical area has been invaded by pain mediators spreading from the pulp, the pulp has not yet completely degenerated and can still react to stimuli such as temperature changes. As the infection spreads beyond the periapical area, rupturing the periosteum of the bone around the affected tooth, the pain diminishes in the intensity and the inflammation spreads to orofacial soft tissue spaces.

In the early stages, there are no radiographic changes detectable. Few radiographically detectable lesions are painful unless there is a reactivation of a chronic periapical lesion.

6.1.3. Management

Treatment consists of elimination of the source of irritation by root canal treatment. Grinding the tooth to prevent traumatic contact from the opposing teeth also relieves the symptoms. If cellulites, fever and malaise are present, systemic administration of antibiotics is recommended. If pus is present, incision and drainage should be instituted.

6.2. Lateral periodontal abscess

6.2.1. Definition and mechanism

Lateral periodontal abscess is usually the result of acute periodontitis of gingival origin (as compared to the apical periodontitis). Periodontal disease is usually painless. As the disease progresses, and once periodontal pockets are formed, there is an increasing possibility of an acute exacerbation of pain associated with abscess formation. This usually results from a blockage of drainage from a periodontal pocket and is frequently associated with a deep infrabony pocket and teeth with root furcation involvement.

6.2.2. Clinical features

The pain is continuous, moderate to severe in intensity and is exacerbated by biting on the affected tooth. The pain is well localised. Although pain characteristics, ability to localise and pain provoking factors are similar to those in acute periapical periodontitis, these lateral periodontal abscesses need to be differentiated as treatment is very different.

On clinical examination, the tooth pulp is usually vital, i.e. it reacts normally to temperature changes

and electrical stimulation. Occasionally retrograde spread of infection may lead to pulpitis and pulpal pain may develop. Swelling and redness of gingiva may be noticed, usually located more coronally than in the case of the acute periapical lesion. In more severe cases, cellulitis, fever and malaise may occur. A deep periodontal pocket is usually located around the tooth; once probed, there is pus exudation and subsequent relief.

6.2.3. Management

Treatment consists of irrigation and curettage of the pocket. The tooth is ground in order to avoid contact with the opposing teeth. In the presence of systemic symptoms, systemic antibiotic administration is required. If the abscess cannot be approached through the pocket, direct incision and drainage are recommended.

7. Periocoronitis

7.1. Definition and mechanism

This is defined as inflammation associated with a partially erupted tooth. Mandibular third molar (wisdom tooth) is most commonly involved. The accumulation of food debris and plaque on and around the crowns of partially erupted teeth leads to inflammation of soft tissues in the area.

7.2. Clinical features

The pain may be severe and is occasionally referred to other teeth. On clinical examination, the flap of gingiva covering the tooth is acutely inflamed, red and oedematous. Frequently, an indentation of the opposing tooth can be seen imprinted on the gingival flap. Fever, malaise and lymphadenopathy may be associated with the infection.

7.3. Management

Treatment includes irrigation of debris between the flap and the affected tooth, eliminating trauma by the opposing tooth (by grinding or extraction). Systemic antibiotic administration is commonly recommended. Once the infection has settled, the extraction of the tooth needs to be considered.

8. Dry socket (acute alveolar osteitis)

8.1. Definition and mechanism

Local infections sometimes occur after dental extractions. This is more common in association with difficult lower third molar extractions.

8.2. Clinical features

This complication usually occurs 2 or 3 days after tooth extraction. The extraction socket is usually empty or filled with debris. Granulation tissue is absent and the surface of the bone is visible. The pain intensity is described as moderate to severe.

8.3. Management

The treatment consists of gentle irrigation and an antiseptic dressing.

9. Vascular orofacial pain

9.1. Definition and mechanism

This condition is a vascular pain which predominantly affects intraoral structures. Neurogenic inflammation similar to the process occurring in migraine and other vascular type headaches is proposed as an underlying cause.

9.2. Clinical features

This condition has been introduced by Sharav et al. (1999) as a distinct diagnostic entity characterised by strong throbbing episodic, unilateral, intraoral pain. Pain may last from minutes to hours or can go on for days. Pain can be accompanied by various local autonomic signs such as tearing or nasal congestion or by other phenomenon such as photo- or phonophobia and nausea (Benoliel et al., 1997). The onset of VOP is around 40–50 years of age and females are affected more commonly than males. Differential diagnosis includes dental pain, trigeminal neuralgia and primary vascular type headaches.

9.3. Management

Successful treatment has been achieved with non-steroidal anti-inflammatory drugs and sodium naproxen has proved effective. Prophylactic treatment using tricyclic antidepressants and the use of β-adrenergic blocking agents are effective (Sharav et al., 1999). Management of dental pain is summarised in Table 2.

Now you have read through this section, please read through the case study in Table 3.

TABLE 2 KEY FACTS: management of dental pains	
Tooth hypersensitivity	Coverage of exposed dentine, fluoride, potassium salts
Reversible pulpitis	Removal of the cause (e.g. caries), sedative dental dressing and review
Irreversible pulpitis	Removal of the cause, root canal therapy, dental extraction
Cracked tooth syndrome	Adhesive restorations, splinting the tooth by a crown or onlay, root canal therapy, hemisection or extraction
Periapical periodontitis	drainage and root canal treatment, antibiotic treatment
Lateral periodontal abscess	drainage and periodontal treatment, antibiotic treatment
Pericoronitis	Irrigation under operculum, extract the upper wisdom tooth, antibiotic treatment
Dry socket	Irrigation of the socket. Eugenol based (e.g. Alvogyl) dressing

TABLE 3

Case study 1

A 45-year-old female patient complains of an intermittent sharp, shooting pain of the lower left mandible. The pain sometimes lasts for hours and keeps her awake at night. She cannot localize the pain. The pain is provoked by biting, drinking cold water and emotional stress and she admits to clenching her teeth when under stress. The pain began more than a year ago. Eighteen months ago she sustained a bilateral mandibular fracture after a collapse. This was treated by intraoral plating of the bony injuries. She feels that her pain started a few months after the injury. She has consulted her general dental practitioner who could not find any obvious clinical or radiographic dental pathology that could explain her symptoms. The dentist provided her with a soft splint in relation to her clenching habit. Her general medical practitioner, prescribed her anti-migraine medication as in her past medical history she suffers from occasional migraine attacks. She has been taking non-steroidal anti-inflammatory drugs and anti-migraine medication which provide some relief, but her symptoms continue to persist. In her social history, her sister died of a long illness 18 months ago.

Based on the above history, what is your differential diagnosis? What is the key clinical and investigative information needed to arrive at a diagnosis?

Please see Table 5 at the end of the chapter for the answer.

10. Summary

A summary of this chapter is given in Table 4.

TABLE 4

Summary of Chapter 10

1. Attention to detail in history taking will enable a differential diagnosis to be made with greater ease

2. Dental examination requires a good light and special equipment generally found only at a dentist

3. Treatment for dental problems can range from extractions, removal of pulp, use of topical medications or systemic drugs

Appendix A

The answer to the case study is given in Table 5.

TABLE 5

Answer to case study in Table 3

Based on the pain history the following pain conditions should be considered:

- Pain of dental or periodontal origin
- Post-traumatic neuropathic pain
- Vascular pain
- Atypical odontalgia
- TMJ and masticatory muscle pain

Clinical examination should involve examination of cranial nerves, temporomandibular joints and masticatory muscles. This should be supplemented with a thorough intraoral examination. Tooth vitality testing and a provocation test, biting on a cotton roll or hard plastic between single pairs of teeth, percussing the cusps of the suspected teeth at different angles and probing firmly around margins of fillings and in suspected fissures. Radiographic examination including orthopantomogram and periapical dental X-rays did not show any abnormality.

In this case, biting on a fine wooden stick produced a sharp pain in relation to the lower right first molar and there was evidence of a very fine crack in the mesiodistal direction.

Comment: Diagnosis of a cracked tooth can be difficult as there are minimal detectable clinical and radiographic findings. However, a history of acute or chronic trauma (in this case fall and bruxism) in addition to the nature of pain should alert the clinician to the diagnosis. In this patient, the situation is further complicated by the clear presence of other co-existing types of pain which may lead the clinician to overlook subtle dental pathology. The dental pain is initially caused by mechanical stimulation of tooth pulp nociceptors. In the absence of effective treatment, continuous stimulation of nociceptors could lead to peripheral and/or central sensitisation resulting in a continuous pain.

Appendix B. Further reading

(1) Birnbaum W, Dunne SM. Oral Diagnosis, The Clinician's Guide. Oxford. 2000: ISBN 0723610401. (A very useful, clearly written book on the topic.)

(2) Lund JP, Lavigne GJ, Dubner R, Sessle BJ (eds) Orofacial Pain, from Basic Science to Clinical Management. Quintessence Publishing, Chicago, 2001: ISBN 0-86715-381-4. (This book from some of the leading basic science research workers brings together basic science, research and their clinical applications.)

(3) Cohen S, Burns RC (eds) Pathways of the Pulp, 8th edn. Mosby, London, 2001: ISBN 0323011624. (This is a classic endodontic textbook which includes chapters on basic science as well as diagnostic procedures in relation to dental pain.)

References

Marked as regards quality according to criteria set by author.
* Case studies, no controls, only evidence.
** Cohort studies, high quality case series with controls.

* Addy M. Etiology and clinical implications of dentine hypersensitivity. Dent Clin North Am 1990; 34: 503–514.
** Beese A, Morley S. Memory of acute pain experience is specifically inaccurate but generally reliable. Pain 1993; 53: 183–189.
* Benoliel R, Elishoov H, Sharav Y. Orofacial pain with vascular-type features. Oral Surg Oral Med Oral Pathol Oral Radiol Endodont 1997; 84: 506–512.
* Curro FA. Tooth hypersensitivity in the spectrum of pain. Dent Clin North Am 1990; 34: 429–437.
* Dionne RA, Snyder J, Hargreaves KM. Analgesic efficacy of flurbipfofen in comparison with acetaminophen, acetaminophen plus codeine, and placebo after impacted third molar removal. J Oral Maxillofac Surg 1994; 52: 919–924.
* Eliav E, Gracely RH. Sensory changes in the territory of the lingual and inferior alveolar nerves following third molar extraction. Pain 1998; 77: 191–199.
* Gaffar, A. Treating hypersensitivity with fluoride varnish. Compend Contin Educ Dent 1990; 20: 27–33.
* Hall EH, Terezehalmy GT, Pelleu GB. A set of descriptors for the diagnosis of dental pain syndromes. Oral Surg Oral Med Oral Path 1986; 61: 153–157.
* Homewood CI. Cracked tooth syndrome – incidence, clinical findings and treatment. Aust Dent J 1998; 43: 217–222.
* Kollmann W. Incidence and possible causes of dental pain during simulated high altitude flights. J Endod 1993; 19: 154–159.
* Orchardson R, Gillam DG. The efficacy of potassium salts as agents for treating dentine hypersensitivity. J Orofac Pain 2000; 14: 9–19.
* Seymour RA. The use of pain scales in assessing the efficacy of analgesics in post operative dental pain. Eur J Clin Pharmacol 1982; 23: 441–444.
* Sharav Y, Sleviner E, Tzukert A, McGrath PA. The spatial distribution, intensity and unpleasantness of acute dental pain. Pain 1984; 20: 363.
* Sharav Y. Orofacial pain. In: Wall P, Melzack R (eds) Textbook of Pain, ISBN 0-443-06252-8. Churchill Livingstone, London, 1999; 711–737.

Assessment and Management of Orofacial Pain
Pain Research and Clinical Management, Vol. 14
Edited by J.M. Zakrzewska and S.D. Harrison
© *2002 Elsevier Science B.V. All rights reserved*

CHAPTER 11

Temporomandibular joint pain

Sheelah D. Harrison [*]

Department of Oral and Maxillofacial Surgery, Eastman Dental Hospital, 256 Gray's Inn Road, London WC1X 8LD, UK

Objectives for this chapter:

This chapter will aim to:
- Demonstrate that definitions for TMJ pain are not universally used
- Demonstrate that TMJ pain can be associated with a number of signs and symptoms and is frequently described as part of many syndromes
- Show how little good quality research has been undertaken in this area and that much of the evidence therefore is anecdotal
- Discuss numerous treatment modalities that appear to be effective in this condition
- Explain that the treatment can be perhaps tailored to the individuals needs and perceptions

1. Introduction

There is a host of varying terminology associated with chronic temporomandibular joint (TMJ) pain in the literature, with the differing descriptions having numerous names and definitions associated with each, some associate dysfunction of the mandible and others associate internal derangement of the joint itself. No consensus has been reached as to which specific signs and symptoms are important in this disorder. Three currently (commonly used) accepted conditions and their associated definitions of chronic TMJ pain are:

(1) Temporomandibular pain and dysfunction syndrome (International Association for the Study of Pain; Merskey and Bogduk, 1994)

Aching in the muscles of mastication, sometimes with an occasional brief severe pain on chewing, often associated with restricted jaw movement and clicking or popping sounds.

(2) Oromandibular dysfunction (International Headache Society; Olesen, 1988)

Three or more of the following should be present:
- temporomandibular joint noise on jaw movements
- limited or jerky jaw movements
- pain on jaw function
- locking of jaw on opening
- clenching of teeth
- gnashing of teeth (bruxism)
- other oral parafunction (tongue, lips or cheek biting or pressing)

(3) Facial arthromyalgia (FAM) (Harris, 1987)

* Tel.: +44-20-7915-1021; Fax: +44-20-7915-1259;
E-mail: sharrison@eastman.ucl.ac.uk

TABLE 1

Common terms for pain associated with the TMJ

1.	Temporomandibular pain and dysfunction syndrome (TMD)
2.	Oromandibular dysfunction
3.	Facial arthromyalgia

A chronic or intermittent pain of the temporomandibular joint and/or of its associated musculature.

The first two are by definition associated with some form of TMJ dysfunction whereas the third is a chronic pain condition not necessarily associated with dysfunction of the joint (Table 1).

It should also be noted that TMJ pain may be acute, little mention of this is made in the literature. In this chapter the aim is to include all of these similar but different named conditions using the broadest of definitions:

- pain of the temporomandibular joint and/or of its associated musculature

It would be ideal if a more precise definition could be used encompassing elements of the aetiology of the disorder and specific diagnostic criteria; however, the following chapter will hopefully show that despite so much having been written on the subject, the evidence is mostly of poor quality and hence little is actually known about this pain.

2. Epidemiology

There is a paucity of data regarding the incidence of chronic facial pain as a whole and that of the TMJ is no exception, to date there are no controlled studies. Most of the so called 'epidemiological data' available focus upon nonrepresentative groups of the population or upon patients seeking treatment. A number of studies exist reporting prevalence of facial pain in specific populations, mainly clinic samples. These are obviously biased populations (Cohen and Cohen, 1984) and have consequently not been reviewed here. There have been a number of attempts to assess the incidence of orofacial pain in the general population, but an adequate estimate of the incidence and prevalence is still not available. Most of the surveys that have been undertaken use self-report questionnaires and therefore are not able to give a diagnosis but merely the location of pain and they tend to lack measurement of the duration of the symptoms and, consequently, acute and chronic pain symptoms are reported without discrimination in the same study. Some of the more relevant studies are briefly described.

Brattberg et al. (1989) investigated pain by postal questionnaire in a randomly selected population aged 18–84 in a county of Sweden. The duration of pain was assessed and 8.9% of respondents reported having had pain in the head, face or mouth for more than 6 months. The total prevalence was reported to be 14.6% for those with pain for over 1 month. Unfortunately the all too common headache was not distinguishable from other possible causes of pain.

Chronic pain of greater than 3 months duration has been assessed by postal questionnaire in two Swedish health care districts (Andersson et al., 1993). The survey of 1806 residents aged 25–74 found that head and face pain was present in 6.2% of men and 7.7% of women in the previous 3 months. This appears to give the most information upon the presence of chronic pain; however, headache is again combined with facial pain and it is uncertain why a lower age limit of 25 years was used, as other surveys indicate that significant numbers of the population between 15 and 24 years report symptoms of orofacial pain (Helkimo, 1974; Solberg et al., 1979; Schiffman et al., 1992).

Agerberg and Carlsson (1972) investigated 1106 randomly selected residents of a Swedish city, by postal questionnaire. Facial pain and headache was reported by 24% of respondents, 12% reported pain on wide opening of the mouth, 7% limitation of mouth opening, 39% noise when moving the mandible and 2% with joint pain and stiffness. Nineteen percent of those who returned questionnaires

(91%) took analgesics for their head or facial pain. The frequency of men and women reporting symptoms was found to be similar. No questions were asked however concerning symptom duration.

Three hundred and twenty one Lapps in the north of Finland, being investigated as part of a WHO biological programme (concerning the adaptation of human beings to the arctic environment), were interviewed and examined clinically to investigate masticatory system function. It was reported that overall 14% of women and 10% of men experienced facial and jaw pain, again duration and frequency of the symptoms or actual diagnosis were not reported. The highest frequency of facial and jaw pain was found within the 35–44 year age group, with 23% reporting such pain (Helkimo, 1974).

Six hundred Hungarian individuals aged 12–85 years were investigated by self-report questionnaires for recent pain in the face, neck or around the ears in a population-based study. The prevalence reported in the study was 8.3% in women and 3.2% in men (Szentpetery et al., 1986). The study combines the acute and chronic pain sufferer.

A representative sample of the City of Toronto population completed postal questionnaires (Locker and Grushka, 1987). Of the 628 respondents 9.1% reported pain in the jaw joints, 7.6% with pain in the jaw joint when opening and chewing and 4.5% with prolonged burning sensation in the tongue or other parts of the mouth. A measure of severity, but not duration was made.

In the USA the National Centre for Health Statistics used data from a large-scale general health survey to estimate prevalence of facial pain (Lipton et al., 1993). The survey involved interviews of 42,370 individuals from non-institutionalised, nonmilitary populations in their own homes. The individuals were asked "During the past six months, did you have more than once. . . " followed by a list of symptoms. The results were as follows:

pain in the jaw joint or in front of the ear (7% in women and 3.5% in men)	5.3%
a dull aching pain across your face or cheek (excluding sinus pain)	1.4%

The highest rates of pain in the jaw or in front of the ear were in individuals 18–34 years of age and the rates decreased with decreasing age. Clearly this is not a survey of chronic pain, just repeated pain, but perhaps represents a sample of those patients likely to seek treatment.

Some selected populations have been investigated, the results from three large non-clinic populations are given briefly. A study of members of a health care organisation (whose population demographics were similar to the geographic region) were investigated using a postal questionnaire (Von Korff et al., 1988). Eight percent of male and 15% of female respondents reported pain in the TMJ or facial muscles in the previous 6 months. In a study of 739 US college students 26% were described as having symptoms of mandibular dysfunction and 76% had signs associated with dysfunction (Solberg et al., 1979), only half of them with symptoms found that they were troublesome. In a further study of trainee nurses, 57% had symptoms related to the temporomandibular joint, of these only 6.7% had sought treatment while 46% stated that the symptoms did not bother them (Schiffman et al., 1992). No statement of pain presence or chronicity are made. These selected populations appear to have a greater frequency of symptoms than the random samples described earlier, and may give an indication of the prevalence.

A lower prevalence exists in children. Again only a few reports of population-based studies exist, most report pain in only adolescents. Nilner and Lassing (1981) and Nilner (1981) report on two groups of children attending dental clinics in Sweden. A prevalence of TMJ pain was reported in 3% of 7–14 year olds and 4% in 15–18 year olds respectively.

It has been estimated that 24% of the population experience this condition (Agerberg and Carlsson, 1972) at some point in their lives.

2.1. Natural history of TMJ pain

Although the natural history of TMJ pain has not been documented it could be extrapolated from the low incidence in children that possible biological and

TABLE 2

Risk factors for TMJ pain

Psychosocial	Biological
Stress	Reproductive hormones
Somatic distress	Menstrual cycle
Depression	Hormonal Oral contraceptive pill

TABLE 3

Aetiology of TMJ pain — theories [a]

1.	Psychogenic
2.	Occlusal
3.	Traumatic (meniscal displacement)

[a] The clinical evidence to support these theories is lacking.

psychosocial risk factors are either not in evidence until after puberty or require significant exposure in healthy individuals. It has also been suggested that children's tissues may offer a greater potential for healing and adaptation compared to adults (LeResche et al., 1997). The risk of orofacial pain in adult women appears to decrease with age (Macfarlane et al., 2002).

A whole host of risk factors have been suggested, based upon experts' views of the patients seen in their respective clinics. But these views are more likely to reflect concurrent psychosocial interactions and biological conditions (LeResche et al., 1997). The presently available epidemiological data only suggest that women are more likely to suffer from TMJ pain than men and most frequently between the age of 18 years and middle age, and those who report orofacial pain are more likely to report symptoms associated with menstruation (Macfarlane et al., 2002). The potential risk factors cited are shown in Table 2.

3. Aetiology

Much controversy surrounds the aetiology of this condition and little controlled work has been undertaken to establish pathogenesis.

A syndrome of TMJ pain and dysfunction was originally ascribed to Costen (1934), but there are many earlier references. He hypothesised that his patients had missing teeth or inadequate dentures which led to 'overclosing of the mandible' and found

that restoration of the bite proved helpful. The theory of overclosure was disproved 14 years later by an anatomist named Sicher (1948). Since that time many theories of aetiology have been suggested, but none has good supporting evidence. The main theories are shown in Table 3 and will be discussed below.

3.1. Psychogenic

There is some anecdotal evidence to suggest that stress, adverse life events and vulnerable personality types predispose to TMJ pain (Feinmann and Harris, 1984). The same study also suggested that TMJ pain may manifest itself as a single clinical entity or as part of a 'chronic pain syndrome', where many body systems are affected by pain.

In 1959 a psychophysiological model was described by Schwartz where emotional tension was considered as a predisposing factor, where pain and masticatory muscle spasm developed into a self-perpetuating feedback loop accounting for most of the patients symptoms (Schwartz, 1959). This was later modified by Laskin (1980), who proposed that limited joint movement and joint sounds developed as a consequence of a psychophysiological disorder.

An aetiological role was suggested for the following psychological factors: sleep disturbance, muscle hyperactivity, parafunctional habits, anxiety and stress, patients perception and tolerance of pain, secondary gain and personality characteristics. The evidence for these factors' involvement in the aetiology is poor.

Chronic pain patients who show sleep disturbance are more likely to show more psychopathology and to respond less readily to treatment (Harness and Peltier, 1992). Although this would appear to be a common symptom of all chronic pain patients (Pilowsky et al., 1985) and it is suggested that sleep disturbance is a likely predictor of psychopathology in chronic facial pain patients, good evidence does not appear to exist to suggest such an aetiological relationship.

Stress induction experiments have yet to confirm any direct relationship between stress and muscle activity. Yemm (1969a,b, 1971) found that patients with FAM responded to stress with a greater degree of masseter muscle contraction than controls, and muscle fatigue was suggested as a cause of pain. These results were not supported by nonsignificant findings of Moss and Adams (1984). Although it has been proposed that excess stress or emotional states can lead to or accompany masticatory muscle hyperactivity expressed as parafunctional habits with high force activities leading to muscle and joint pain, limited movement and joint sounds (Haber et al., 1983). Under experimental stress pain patients showed an increased heart rate and systolic blood pressure than control patients; at rest they reported more anxiety and greater feelings of muscle tension (Carlsson et al., 1993).

The prevalence of bruxism has been reported in a random population sample, i.e. 20% were aware of jaw clenching and 10% of grinding their teeth (Agerberg and Carlsson, 1972), where only 12% of the population had pain and 7% had restricted mouth opening. Bruxism has been linked to emotional stress and periods of difficult life change (Rugh and Solberg, 1976). Most nocturnal bruxism appears to occur during rapid eye movement (REM) and stage 2 sleep irrespective of occlusal status (Dahlstrom, 1989). Investigation of patient with the Minnesota multiphasic personality inventory has not shown any association with bruxism and psychopathology (Harness and Peltier, 1992).

An higher prevalence of certain chronic pains or illnesses, such as neck, back and shoulder pain, migraine, pruritus, colitis and asthma has been found in TMJ pain patients compared to the general population (Berry, 1969). But again these studies were not of good quality.

An increased incidence of psychiatric symptoms, mostly of anxiety or depression has been described (Fine, 1971) in these patients. Personality analysis as investigated using the Minnesota multiphasic personality inventory, showed that patients with FAM had increased evidence of neurotic disorders, were somatically concerned, had increased scores of anxiety and depression and showed increased anger. The scores were greater for those patients whose pain was associated with muscle tenderness than those with internal derangement alone. The increase in scores has been noted by many investigators (Harness et al., 1990), and their profile has been described as similar to other groups of chronic pain patients (Harkins et al., 1991; Parker et al., 1993). It has been suggested that concurrent depression alters treatment outcome and concurrent treatment for depression will increase successful outcome (Tversky et al., 1991).

Speculand et al. (1984) has found a higher incidence of major life events in the 6 months preceding pain onset compared to controls. It would appear that a wide range of psychological characteristics may play an aetiological role by increasing emotional problems and difficulties in coping with life events along with pain experience being a major psychological stressor. It is of course debatable whether these psychological/psychiatric states have a causal relationship or are merely a result of chronic pain. Needless to say, the research necessary to give evidence to either of these viewpoints has not been undertaken and given the long-term nature of the appropriate study, is unlikely to be carried out in the very near future.

3.2. Occlusal

This theory was first suggested by Costen in 1934. He suggested that occlusal factors play a major aetiological role in patients pain. Since that time a number of investigators (with poor quality research) have supported this theory. Ramjford (1961) found that occlusal equilibration provided good relief and removal of occlusal interferences. Magnusson and Carlsson (1983) provided further support for this theory. However, these reports were uncontrolled and in a controlled trial Dao et al. (1994) found that occlusal splints were as effective in treating TMJ pain as placebo splints, suggesting that the role of occlusion is limited. Thomson (1971) had found no difference in malocclusion incidence between controls and patients with TMJ pain, which has also been confirmed by other workers (e.g. Dworkin et al., 1990). It has been suggested that malocclusion is in fact the 'normal' state as some studies have found that over 95% of the population had some form of malocclusion (Greider, 1972). Mock equilibration of the occlusion has proved to be as successful as actual treatment (Goodman et al., 1976), suggesting that the effect of treatment upon these patients may merely reflect the placebo effect.

3.3. Meniscus displacement theory

Juniper (1993) has suggested that as EMG studies of patients with TMJ pain have concluded that the lateral pterygoid muscle is responsible for the positioning of the meniscus within the joint, that stress and muscle hyperactivity of this muscle would result in the meniscus being placed in an anteriomedial position, the retrodiscal tissue become overstretched and attachment of the lateral pole of the condyle lost. It was thought that the joint may then become unstable and pain occur along with the occlusion being disturbed, the continued stress and muscle hyperactivity leading to progressive damage and degenerative joint disease becoming established. The relationship is however not one of cause and effect. Magnetic resonance imaging of the TMJ has revealed a prevalence of 32% of anterior displacement of the meniscus in asymptomatic patients (Kircos et al., 1987), and a randomly selected sample of a Swedish population reported clicking or noises when moving the mandible in 39% of subjects; only 12% however reported pain and 7% limitation of mouth opening (Agerberg and Carlsson, 1972).

4. Clinical features

The following clinical cases show a variety of features frequently found, read through these and decide how you would manage them (Table 4). The follow up of these patients and management is discussed at the end of the chapter.

4.1. History

Data from population-based studies to support the symptoms required for each specific diagnosis (associated with TMJ pain) based on fulfilment of diagnostic criteria is currently lacking. Hence most reports of clinical features are probably biased and dependent upon the clinical source of the patients (anecdotal reports or respected authorities), control data are not available. It should be noted that a diagnosis of either TMD or oromandibular dysfunction can be made without the presence of pain (Table 5).

This pain is often described as a dull ache or throbbing pain which can have elements of a sharp pain associated with movement of the joint located over the TMJ and/or associated muscles. It can be persistent or intermittent and may be associated with limited movement of the mandible and meniscal displacement or internal derangement of the TMJ. The latter being described as mandibular dysfunction, which may give rise to noises described as grating or clicking. The level of mandibular dysfunction is not related to the presence or absence of TMJ internal derangement (Schiffman et al., 1992). Internal derangement is usually attributed to anterior displacement of the meniscus producing auscultative joint sounds during translatory movements of the mandible.

4.2. Examination

Examination of the patient with TMJ pain is as for all patients. It includes a comprehensive medical history, physical examination and imaging; to ascertain the specific diagnosis it may be necessary to undertake additional specific tests and imaging. For the purposes of this chapter only an affirmative answer to the question "Do you have pain in or around your

TABLE 4

Case studies

Read through these cases and decide how you would manage them. You will find the answers within the chapter in Section 6 on management.

Case 1

Name	AB
Age	37
Gender	Female
Development of pain	Following removal of wisdom teeth 2 years ago. No real change in symptoms since that time. Has had numerous drugs prescribed none of which really helped, used jaw exercises and wears a bite guard at night
Character	Throbbing, sharp, aching, heavy
Site/radiation	Both jaw joints, face and temples, radiating to the neck
Severity	VAS 7.7/10 cm
Duration, periodicity	Continuous, tends to be worse first thing in the morning and later in the day
Provoking factors	Opening mouth, eating, chewing and tiredness
Relieving factors	Nil
Associated factors	Clicking of both jaw joints
Medical history	Fit and well
	Previous hysterectomy
Current medication	Nurofen and solpadeine
Social factors	Divorced 3 years. Two children aged 7 and 9 years (eldest has severe Rheumatoid arthritis). Works full time as a care assistant. Does not smoke. Drinks alcohol socially (less than 14 units per week).
Examination	Tender over both TMJs and masseter and temporalis muscles. Clicking evident upon mouth opening (both right and left). Mouth opening 35 mm (normal range 30–60 mm). Well restored dentition. Linea alba (white line on buccal mucosa in relation to the occlusal surfaces of the teeth thought to be evidence of cheek biting) present bilaterally.
Investigation	Orthopantomogram – unremarkable

Case 2

Name	BC
Age	58
Gender	Female
Development of pain	Spontaneous 6 months ago, no real change since that time, has taken over-the-counter medication which did not really help
Character	Throbbing, aching, heavy, grinding
Site/radiation	Right jaw joint, radiating to the head
Severity	VAS 5.7/10 cm
Duration, periodicity	Intermittent, tends to be worse in the cold weather and upon waking
Provoking factors	Opening mouth, eating, chewing
Relieving factors	Nil
Associated factors	Noises/creaking of right jaw joint
Medical history	Hypertension
Current medication	Bendrofluazide
Social factors	Single. Has not returned to work following a back injury. Does not smoke or drink alcohol.
Examination	Tender over right TMJ. Mouth opening 45 mm. Well restored dentition.
Investigation	Orthopantomogram – evidence of erosion of the mandibular condyle

TABLE 4 *continued*

Case 3	
Name	CD
Age	47
Gender	Female
Development of pain	Intermittent over many years, no real change, has not taken any medication for it as it was not that bad
Character	Aching
Site/radiation	Right jaw joint
Severity	VAS 2.3/10 cm
Duration, periodicity	Intermittent, tends to be worse in the cold weather
Provoking factors	Opening mouth, eating, chewing
Relieving factors	Nil
Associated factors	Nil
Medical history	Rheumatoid arthritis
Current medication	Naprosyn and ranitidine
Social factors	Married with 2 grown-up children. Works as a architect part time. Does not smoke, drinks 2–3 glasses of wine per day.
Examination	Mouth opening 48 mm, well restored dentition
Investigation	Orthopantomogram – evidence of almost complete destruction of the condyle (reported as typical of Rheumatoid arthritis)

TABLE 5

Features of TMJ pain

Duration	Days to many years [a]
Periodicity	Muscle tenderness upon waking, 8% (Locker and Slade, 1988)
	Stiffness/fatigue of muscles upon waking, 21% (Locker and Slade, 1988)
Character	Dull, throbbing, aching and occasionally sharp [a]
Site	TMJ, in front of the ears and masticatory muscles [a]
Radiation	Head, neck, shoulders and across face [a]
Severity	Mild to severe [a]
Provoking factors	Difficulty with wide opening, 7% (Locker and Slade, 1988), 6% (Locker and Grushka, 1987)
	Worse with chewing, 8% (Locker and Grushka, 1987)
Relieving factors	Resting the joint, soft diet, local heat [a]
	Antidepressants drugs (Feinmann and Harris, 1984; Sharav et al., 1987; Harrison et al., 1997)
	Diazepam (Jagger, 1973)
Associated factors	Crepitus, 26% (Agerberg and Carlsson, 1972), 3% (Mohlin, 1983), 21% males and 37% females (Szentpetery et al., 1986)
	Clicking, up to 60% in adolescents (Riolo et al., 1987), 70% (Agerberg and Carlsson, 1972), 27% (Mohlin, 1983)
	Luxation, 6% of men (Helkimo, 1974)
	Locking, 6.4% (Locker and Slade, 1988)
	Joint sounds, 39% (Agerberg and Carlsson, 1972), 25% (Locker and Slade, 1988)
	Grinding of the teeth, 10% (Agerberg and Carlsson, 1972)
	Clenching of the teeth, 20% (Agerberg and Carlsson, 1972)
	Frequent headaches, 17% (Locker and Slade, 1988)

[a] Anecdotal/expert evidence + Harrison (1999).

jaw joint or the muscles of your face or just in front of the ear?" is necessary for a diagnosis of TMJ pain. If a more specific diagnosis is required then an examination to ascertain presence or absence of a number of clinical signs is needed. There is unfortunately no specific diagnostic test which is both reliable and accurate, and indeed the commonly undertaken examination for clinical signs lacks objectivity and has not been tested for reliability in TMJ pain patients. The examination must exclude dental causes of pain. In early stages of acute dental pain the pain is poorly localised and may be difficult to differentiate from TMJ pain.

Common clinical signs detected along with TMJ pain include:

- pain upon palpation of the TMJ and
- pain upon palpation of the muscles of mastication
- decreased mouth opening
- altered lateral jaw movements
- clicking of the TMJ
- crepitus of the TMJ

Epidemiological studies have not assessed the frequency with which these signs are found. They have been used in a number of different classification systems to give 'accurate' diagnoses along with measurements of pain scores and psychological status. Few of these classification systems have been tested for reliability, utility and validity despite being widely used by numerous authors. The research diagnostic criteria for TMD (Dworkin and LeResche, 1992) employs a standardised examination and self-report questions to assign a specific diagnosis to a patient, it has been tested for reliability and clinical utility. Table 6 lists clinical findings commonly associated with TMJ pain.

It should be noted that it is unknown how many of these findings cause or relates to the TMJ pain. The evidence of association is low, and on the whole is that of anecdotal reports.

5. Investigations

Numerous devices have been used to aid in assessment of TMJ pain patients. None have been proven to meet reliability and validity standards.

TABLE 6

KEY FACTS: possible findings with TMJ pain

Finding	Likely diagnosis	Possible causes
Bulging facial muscles	Muscle hypertrophy	Biological variant
		Parafunction
Limited mouth opening		Biological variant
		TMJ ankylosis
		Meniscal displacement
		Muscular pain
		Joint pain
Noise in TMJ	Crepitus (creaking)	Osteoarthritis
		Rheumatoid arthritis
	Clicking	TMJ internal derangement, or meniscal displacement
Jerky mandibular movements	Deviation upon opening	TMJ internal derangement, or meniscal displacement
White line on buccal mucosa	Linea alba	Parafunction
Scalloped tongue edge	Tongue plication	Parafunction
Excessive tooth wear	Attrition	Parafunction
		Teeth grinding

TABLE 7

Investigations to be considered in patients with TMJ pain

Radiograph	Dental Orthopantomogram Tomograms TMJ views – transcranial, transpharyngeal	Exclude dental disease, destructive arthritis
CT scan		Exclude ankylosis
MRI scan		Inform of meniscal position
Blood tests	ESR, Rheumatoid factor etc., C reactive protein	Indicate possible disease process, e.g. temporal arteritis, arthritis

Radiographs, MRI and CT scans are now commonly used in TMJ assessment. The use of radiographs is limited by its 2-dimensional image (unless tomographic techniques are employed) and other methods are less readily available.

A small retrospective study investigating the usefulness of radiographic tomograms found that although diagnoses were changed in 24% of cases following the radiographic report, this only minimally affected the management of this group of patients. Radiographs may detect routine dental pathology missed by examination and may therefore provide a useful screening tool (Table 7).

The evidence for any of these tests is low, except for ESR to rule out temporal arteritis (low ESR would exclude temporal arteritis).

The use of MRI scans is debated, although interobserver agreement in MRI interpretation images is reasonable amongst all categories of TMJ meniscal position. The relationship of imaging findings to pain and dysfunction is unknown, 32% of asymptomatic patients were reported to have anterior displacement of the TMJ meniscus (Kircos et al., 1987).

6. Management of TMJ pain (not associated with arthritis)

The prevailing recommendation of the American Dental Association is that only conservative, reversible forms of treatment should be undertaken (Griffiths, 1983), despite many treatment modalities being available. This has been supported by a more recent National Institute of Health Technology Assessment Conference Statement (1996).

It has however been suggested that the condition may be self-limiting, and that there would be spontaneous improvement of three quarter of cases within 3 months (Toller, 1976). Epidemiological evidence would appear to support this in that there is little evidence of TMJ pain in the elderly population members. Investigation of a group of patients seeking treatment compared to controls suggested that in this condition, that is typically episodic, most change seen in clinical practice may be due to regression to the mean (due to homeostatic processes, random within-subject variation, or measurement error), rather than due to specific and nonspecific effects of treatment (Whitney and Von Korff, 1992).

In this section an attempt has been made to only mention management modalities with good evidence to support it; however, if this is not available expert opinion will be quoted. The principles of some of these techniques are discussed in Chapter 9.

6.1. Conservative treatments

6.1.1. Reassurance

Little work has been undertaken upon the use and effectiveness of positive reassurance; however, it has been suggested that the advice upon rest of the joint, appropriate adjustment of diet and use of self-prescribed analgesics along with an explanation of the symptoms can produce improvement in 80%

of patients (Toller, 1976). The National Institute of Health suggests supportive patient education (1996).

6.1.2. Exercises

Exercises are recommended following an acute phase of TMJ pain when there may be some stiffness of the muscles of mastication or a tendency to deviate the mandible upon opening. There is some controversy as to whether these exercises should be carried out when the patient is pain free (Bradley, 1987); however, many authors recommend them in order to increase range of movement and increase muscle strength (Clark et al., 1990; Carlsson et al., 1991) in order to stabilise the joint.

6.1.3. Physical therapy

This can include heat, shortwave diathermy (Clark, 1987), transcutaneous electrical nerve stimulation (TENS) and ultrasound (Hargreves and Wardle, 1983). Reports of the efficacy of these treatment modalities are uncontrolled, studies of ultrasound reported it to be effective in 82% of patients (Esposito et al., 1984); however, more recently Tsang (1988) found no improvement.

There are many types of physical therapy that can be used in the management of chronic facial pain; however, most of the treatments appear to be recommended "because these therapies had been shown to be effective for other pain conditions", but no direct evidence of effectiveness exists (Clark et al., 1990). Many studies have been undertaken, but few have fulfilled criteria for well conducted clinical trials (Feine et al., 1997), and post-treatment and follow up data are almost uniformly lacking. No one treatment appears to be more effective than another; however, large numbers of patients appear to have been effectively treated by thermal therapy, acupuncture, low intensity laser, TENS, manipulation and exercise (Dahlstrom, 1992) in the short term. Following a meta-analysis of nonmedical treatments for chronic pain, Malone and Strube (1988) suggested that there was "a uniform efficacy of treatments", probably "attributable. . . to the features they share in common" which included identification of the psychological factors that exacerbate pain, contact

with an empathetic professional and provision of hope for relief of symptoms.

As these treatments are irreversible, noninvasive, relatively cheap and provide patients with useful relief and reassurance, they may be helpful in the short term.

6.1.4. Relaxation

Voluntary relaxation has been used to treat many 'stress related' conditions (Dohrmann and Laskin, 1978), either alone or in conjunction with biofeedback. Learning muscle relaxation techniques may take many weeks to enable a therapeutic result, it can be used in patients with TMJ pain to produce a better rate of improvement than controls. However, both methods appear to be equally effective (Funch and Gale, 1984).

6.1.5. Biofeedback

This involves teaching patients with a myofascial element to their pain to relax their masseter muscle with visual or auditory electromyographic (EMG) feedback. Budzynski and Stoyva (1973) found that both feedback methods resulted in lower masseter muscle activity than under controlled conditions. Further controlled studies found that TMJ pain patients were able to reduce their masseter EMG levels and consequently pain and mouth opening (Dohrmann and Laskin, 1978). The mechanisms behind this therapy are explained in Chapter 3.

6.1.6. Occlusal splints

The aim of these removable appliances is that of correcting parafunctional habits and relaxation of the masticatory musculature (Beard and Clyton, 1980; Sheikholeslam et al., 1986) along with correcting for any premature contacts (Bradley, 1987). There are numerous reports with various types of splints with favourable results producing a decrease in pain and an increase in function (Greene and Laskin, 1972; Dahlstrom et al., 1982; Sheikholeslam et al., 1986).

Few of these studies incorporate controls or estimate the effect of a placebo response or have long-term follow up. A systematic review has shown that, although the overall quality of the trials analysed was fairly low, there was some evidence to suggest that an occlusal splint (hard) may be of some benefit in the treatment of TMD (Forssell et al., 1999). Placebo appliances appear to be equally effective to splints (Greene and Laskin, 1972; Dao et al., 1994). No sustained improvement in pain measures has been shown in any controlled study (Eversole et al., 1985; Dao et al., 1994).

6.1.7. Drugs

Non-steroidal anti-inflammatory drugs. Despite these drugs being frequently used there is little evidence to support their efficacy. Only one controlled study investigating the use of NSAIDs in TMJ pain was found, the researchers reported no difference in pain levels following treatment between piroxicam and a placebo (Roldan et al., 1990).

Sedatives (muscle relaxants). This group of drugs, which have anxiolytic and muscle relaxant properties are frequently used for patients with TMJ pain. The effect of diazepam was shown to be superior to that of placebo by Jagger (1973), but not by Roldan et al. (1990).

Antidepressants. This group of drugs are now very commonly used in chronic pain management and numerous excellent studies report effectiveness using many different individual drugs (McQuay et al., 1996). Antidepressants have been the subject of many meta-analyses which confirm their effectiveness in reduction of pain. They have been used for the treatment of AFP (atypical facial pain) since 1966 (Lascelles, 1966) in the form of monoamine oxidase inhibitors; more recently, however, they were tried for the treatment of TMJ pain, in the form of the tricyclic antidepressants. The first indication that they may be an effective treatment was shown by Gessel (1975) where amitriptyline was given in an uncontrolled fashion to eight patients of whom five benefited. In a randomised controlled trial (RCT), dothiepin, when compared to an occlusal splint, and a placebo produced a pain-free state after 9 weeks treatment in 71% of patients (46% of those taking the placebo were pain free) (Feinmann and Harris, 1984). These same groups of patients were followed up for 4 years and 80% of patients were pain free

either with or without medication (Feinmann, 1993). Sharav et al. (1987) also produced an improvement of patients pain with amitriptyline and found that low doses were as effective as larger doses and confirmed that the analgesic activity is independent of any antidepressant effect. Harrison et al. (1997) found that fluoxetine was effective in reducing pain in a randomised controlled trial of 178 chronic facial pain patients (who were not depressed). The patient group was mixed TMJ pain ($n = 133$) and atypical facial pain ($n = 30$, and mixed diagnoses $n = 15$); the results however were similar when the pain groups were subdivided into the two specific diagnostic categories.

6.1.8. Psychological interventions

The placebo effect. A placebo has been defined as "any therapy or component of therapy that is deliberately used for its nonspecific, psychological or psycho-physiological effect, or that is used for its presumed specific effect, but is without specific activity for the condition being treated" (Shapiro and Morris, 1977). Chapter 9 deals with the issue of placebo response and its use in treatment of patients.

Placebos have been reported to provide a degree of symptomatic relief in most disorders; however, most of the available information is derived from studies where placebo administration constituted the control condition for the evaluation of another form of active treatment. For interest Table 8 shows the placebo response in the RCTs of antidepressant drugs for TMJ pain.

Cognitive behavioural (CB) therapy (CBT). This treatment modality is discussed in detail in Chapters 3 and 9.

A recent innovation based on CB principles is that referred to as minimal intervention/therapy (Glasgow et al., 1991), these emphasise the use of information and education in the form of self-help materials with brief professional guidance. This involves fewer sessions and low cost follow up, e.g. brief telephone counselling. The use of this has been investigated in patients with TMJ pain prior to the usual treatment. It was found that the improved results found compared to routine treatment were de-

TABLE 8

Treatment and placebo response in TMJ patients

Treatment	Placebo response	Treatment response
Dothiepin (Feinmann and Harris, 1984)	45% pain free	70% pain free
Amitriptyline (Sharav et al., 1987)	VAS[a] reduced by 60/100	VAS reduced by 30/100
Fluoxetine (Harrison et al., 1997)	Median pain severity score reduced by 33%	Median pain severity score reduced by 45%

[a] VAS, visual analogue scale; see Chapter 6 on assessment for details on its use.

layed, at 3 months both groups had similar results for pain but during the 3–12 month review the minimal intervention group continued to improve as with routine CBT. There was no effect seen in patient mood or somatisation.

Routine CBT has been undertaken in a set of TMJ dysfunction patients who had failed to respond to routine treatment (Oakley et al., 1994). The study was poorly controlled, but showed possibly useful mood changes and improvements in perception of pain. A RCT of mixed facial pain patients combined management with antidepressants and CBT, although pain score reduction was not achieved with CBT, the patients who had undergone CBT as part of their management showed less interference with and more control over their lives than those patients who had either placebo or drug treatment (Harrison et al., 1997).

6.2. Invasive therapy

6.2.1. Occlusal rehabilitation

This is undertaken to restore the lost occlusal surfaces of teeth and provide a balanced occlusion which is without interferences. It may involve replacement restorations, crowns, bridges and selective grinding of tooth surfaces (Clark and Adler, 1985). There is no controlled study which supports the use of this type of therapy. Forssell et al. (1999) suggested that evidence for use of occlusal adjustment was lacking in their systematic review.

6.2.2. Intra-articular injections

Numerous substances have been injected into the TMJ aimed at either reducing the inflammatory re-

sponse or washing out the joint (arthrocentesis). Corticosteroid injections have been shown to be effective in eliminating pain in 46% of patients whilst producing useful reduction in another 22% of patients with TMJ pain (uncontrolled study) (Toller, 1977). It has been suggested that no more than two of these injections be given so as to prevent bony erosion of the condyle (Poswillo, 1970). Irrigation of the TMJ has been performed with lactated Ringer's solution in patients with restricted mouth opening as a feature of their TMJ pain and was found to be effective in re-establishing normal mouth opening and relieving pain for a follow up of up to 14 months (Nitzan et al., 1991). Local anaesthetics are able to give short-term relief of pain (Danzig et al., 1992).

6.2.3. Arthroscopy

This provides endoscopic access to the TMJ and is useful as both a diagnostic and therapeutic tool. It was first introduced for use in the TMJ in 1970 by Ohnishi (1980) being initially used in the knee joint in 1918. Initially its use was in diagnosis of pathological conditions; however, it became apparent that it was useful therapeutically in patients with limited mouth opening (Murakami et al., 1996). Accuracy of diagnosis has been confirmed by using cadaveric specimens and also the use of arthroscopy prior to open joint surgery (McCain, 1988). Much arthroscopic surgery is now being performed, the success of this treatment modality for closed lock is established (Sanders, 1986), and other techniques are still being investigated. Long-term outcome and controlled studies are however lacking as with most surgical techniques.

6.2.4. Surgery

A host of surgical procedures have been reported as successful treatment for TMJ pain and internal derangement; none have, however, been controlled prospective studies. Surgery is presently only recommended by some when all other conservative methods have failed and there is intractable pain (Juniper, 1993). The estimates of the need for surgery have, however, ranged from 1 to 17% of patients (Dunn et al., 1981). Surgery was first described for internal derangement of the TMJ in 1887 by Annadale performed to secure the TMJ meniscus (meisectomy). Ninety percent of Costens patients underwent condylectomy and since that time a variety of similar operations were described, the main function of which appeared to be to increase the amount of space within the joint and relieve irritation upon the nerve bearing tissues (Henry and Baldridge, 1957). Other procedures included eminectomy, menisectomy with a variety of interpositional grafts, discoplasty, condyloplasty, condylotomy and reconstructive arthroplasty. Numerous reports of success rates of condylotomies have been published (e.g. Ward, 1961). Banks and MacKenzie (1975) reported a 91% cure or improvement with surgery; follow up of patients, however, showed a high prevalence of persistent pain and dysfunction (Poker and Hopper, 1990). Menisectomy has been reported favourably by many authors (Dingman and Moorman, 1951; Husted, 1966; Agerberg and Lundberg, 1971); however, subsequent development of complications such as crepitation, headache and extensive joint remodelling had led to a decline in the popularity of this procedure. More recently a variety of alloplastic and autogenous interpositional grafts and implants have been used for meniscal replacement with varying success (Poker and Hopper, 1990), and the use of surgery at all has been questioned when there is little or no evidence of its success or of its rationale (Juniper, 1993; Harris, 1996).

7. Prognosis

Again there is no epidemiological study to advise us of the likely prognosis with a given set of present-ing features. The cohort study of Whitney and Von Korff (1992) suggests that patients improve irrespective of treatment received and perhaps suggests that the condition is self-limiting. All of the epidemiological studies quoted previously have a decreased prevalence in the elderly population, supporting the theory that TMJ pain is self-limiting. Expert opinion has suggested that three quarters of individuals will have their symptoms resolve in three months (Toller, 1976).

8. Summary

Table 9 summarises the whole chapter.

TABLE 9

Summary for Chapter 11

- Experts cannot agree upon terms to be used in this group of patients
- TMJ pain is not uncommonly seen in clinical practice It is often associated with   limited mouth opening
                                                                                        joint noises
- Little good quality evidence concerning any aspect of TMJ pain is available in the literature
- – Anecdotal evidence suggests that:
  – the onset may be acute or gradual
  – may present intermittently throughout the day or be worse a.m. or p.m.
  – may be constant with exacerbations associated with joint movement/chewing
  – often described as a dull ache, but may be a sharp or shooting pain
  – can radiate to muscles of mastication, towards head or neck
  – can be relieved by analgesics, rest, soft diet and local heat
- Investigations to exclude pathology — radiological or haematological
- Assess nature and severity of pain along with psycholog- ical aspects (anxiety and depression, coping skills)
- Manage in conjunction with and according to patients perceptions:
  – Reassurance
  – Exercises
  – Physical therapy (if available)
  – Bite guard
  – Psychological therapy (cognitive behaviour therapy, stress management etc)
  – Antidepressants (analgesics)

TABLE 10

Answers to case studies in Table 4

Case 1: AB

This patient had TMJ pain following surgery, which had not resolved despite her original surgeon assuring her it would. The patient was not keen to take (sedative) antidepressants because of her work and children. She appeared depressed. Extensive discussion with the patient revealed a number of concurrent life events with which she was not coping well. Following a consultation with our liaison psychiatrist, she was started on Fluoxetine 20 mg and enrolled in a CBT programme. CBT enlightened the patient to a number of pain-provoking factors and numerous ways in which she might be able to deal with these to reduce exacerbations of the pain and daily "life stresses". The patient was not keen to continue on the Fluoxetine and stopped the tablets some time before advising us that it was affecting her libido. Nortriptyline was started initially in a dose of 30 mg nocte. This was increased to 100 mg; this dose had good effect upon the pain, but once the drug dose was reduced, the pain returned. It was necessary to maintain the patient on 100 mg Nortriptyline nocte. The patient was keen to undergo surgery for the pain throughout treatment. It was felt that because of her psychological state this was not indicated in spite of her obvious internal derangement. She continues under review of our liaison psychiatrist.

Case 2: BC

This patient appeared to have osteoarthritis of the TMJ. She also had back pain which was debilitating and had received little help for this. We prescribed Ibuprofen for the TMJ pain, which was very effective. A consultation with our liaison psychiatrist revealed depression and significant problems relating to the back pain. Suggestions were made to the patient's GMP to address the back pain issues.

Case 3: CD

This patient had obvious rheumatoid arthritis affecting the TMJ, but little pain associated with it (she was already taking naprosyn for her rheumatoid arthritis). She was happy managing the pain by limiting mouth movements when the pain was as its worst. Her main concern was the "disappearing" jaw. She wondered if she would require joint replacement or similar in the future. She had little functional impairment and was therefore kept under review. The condition remains unchanged and no active treatment is planned at present.

Appendix A

See Table 10 for a discussion of the case studies in Table 4.

Appendix B. Further reading

(1) Drangsholt, LeResche L. Temporomandibular disorder pain. In: Crombie IK, Croft PR, Linton SJ, LeResche L (eds) Epidemiology of Pain, 1st edn. IASP, Seattle, WA, 1999, pp 203–233. (This is an excellent systematic review of the epidemiology of TMJ and includes details on clinical features.)

(2) Dworkin SF, LeResche L. Research diagnostic criteria for temporomandibular disorders: review, criteria, examinations and specifications, critique. J Craniomandib Disord 1992; 6: 301–355. (These criteria can also be accessed through the web on *http://www.rdc-tmdinternational.org/* They include a very comprehensive history and examination form.)

References

Marked as regards quality according to criteria set by author.
SR = systematic review or high quality review with methodology
*** Randomised controlled trials, high quality original studies.

*** Agerberg G, Carlsson GE. Functional disorders of the masticatory system. Acta Odont Scand 1972; 32: 597–613.
Agerberg G, Lundberg M. Changes in the temporomandibular joint after surgical management. A radiological follow-up

study. Oral Surg 1971; 32: 865–875.

*** Andersson HI, Ejlertsson G, Leden I, Rosenberg C. Chronic pain in a geographically defined general population: studies of differences in age, gender, social class and pain localisation. Clin J Pain 1993; 9: 174–182.

Banks P, MacKenzie I. Condylectomy. A clinical and experimental appraisal of a surgical technique. J Maxillofac Surg 1975; 3: 171–181.

Beard CC, Clyton JA. Effects of occlusal splint therapy on TMJ dysfunction. J Pros Dent 1980; 44: 324–335.

Berry DC. Mandibular dysfunction pain and chronic minor illness. Br Dent J 1969; 127: 170–175.

*** Brattberg G, Thorsland M, Wilkman A. The prevalence of pain in a general population. The results of a postal survey in a county of Sweden. Pain 1989; 37: 215–222.

Bradley PF. Conservative treatment for temporomandibular joint pain dysfunction. Br J Oral Maxfac Surg 1987; 25: 125–137.

Budzynski T, Stoyva J. An electromyographic feedback technique for teaching voluntary relaxation of the masseter muscle. J Dent Res 1973; 52: 116–119.

Carlsson CR, Okeson JP, Falace DA, Nitz AJ, Anderson D. Stretch-based relaxation and the reduction of EMG activity among masticatory muscle patients. J Craniomandib disord 1991; 5: 202–212.

Carlsson CR, Okeson JP, Falace DA, Curran SL, Anderson D. Comparison of psychologic and physiologic functioning between patients with masticatory muscle pain and matched controls. J Orofac Pain 1993; 7: 15–22.

Clark G. Diagnosis and treatment of painful temporomandibular disorders. Dent Clin N Am 1987; 31: 645–674.

Clark GT, Adachi NY, Dornan AR. Physical medicine procedures affect temporomandibular disorders: A review. JADA 1990; 121: 151–161.

Clark GT, Adler RC. A critical evaluation of occlusal therapy: occlusal adjustment procedures, JADA 1985; 110: 743–750.

Cohen P, Cohen J. The clinician's illusion. Arch Gen Psych 1984; 41: 1178–1182.

Costen JB. A syndrome of ear and sinus symptoms dependant upon disturbed function of the temporomandibular joint. Ann Rhinol Laryngol 1934; 43: 1–15.

Dahlstrom L. Electromyographic studies of craniomandibular disorders: A review of the literature. J Oral Rehab 1989; 16: 1–20.

Dahlstrom L. Conservative treatment methods in craniomandibular disorder. Swed Dent J 1992; 16: 217–130.

Dahlstrom L, Carlsson GE, Carlsson SG. Comparison of effects of electromyographic biofeedback and occlusal splint therapy on mandibular dysfunction. J Scand Dent Res 1982; 90: 151–156.

Danzig W, May S, McNeill C, Miller A. Effect of an anesthetic into the temporomandibular joint space in patients with TMD. J Craniomandib Disord 1992; 6: 288–295.

*** Dao TTT, Lavigne GJ, Charbonneau A, Feine JS, Lund JP. The efficacy of oral splints in the treatment of myofascial

pain of the jaw muscles: a controlled clinical trial. Pain 1994; 56: 85–94.

Dingman RO, Moorman WC. Meniscectomy in the treatment of lesions of the temporomandibular joint. J Oral Surg 1951; 9: 214–224.

Dohrmann RJ, Laskin DM. An evaluation of electromyographic biofeedback in the treatment of myofascial pain dysfunction syndrome. JADA 1978; 96: 656–652.

Dunn MJ, Benz R, Moan D. Temporomandibular joint condylectomy: a technique and post-operative follow up. Oral Surg 1981; 51: 363–374.

Dworkin SF, Huggins KH, LeResche L, Von Korff M, Howard J, Truelove E, Sommers E. Epidemiology of signs and symptoms in temporomandibular disorders: clinical signs in cases and controls. JADA 1990; 120: 273–281.

*** Dworkin SF, Turner JA, Wilson L, Massoth D, Whitney C, Huggins KH, Burgess J, Sommers E, Truelove E. Brief group cognitive–behavioral intervention for temporomandibular disorders. Pain 1994; 59: 175–187.

Esposito CJ, Veal SJ, Farman AG. Alleviation of myofascial pain with ultrasonic therapy. J Pros Dent 1984; 51: 106–108.

Eversole LR, Stone CE, Matheson D, Kaplan H. Psychometric profiles and facial pain. Oral Surg Oral Med Oral Pathol 1985; 60: 269–274.

Feine JS, Widmer CG, Lund JP. Physical therapy: A critique. Oral Surg, Oral Med, Oral Pathol, Oral Radiol Endod 1997; 83: 123–127.

*** Feinmann C. The long-term outcome of facial pain treatment. J Psychosom Res 1993; 37: 381–387.

*** Feinmann C, Harris M. The diagnosis and management of psychogenic facial pain disorders. Clin. Otolaryngol 1984; 9: 199–201.

Feinmann C, Harris M, Cawley R. Psychogenic facial pain, presentation and treatment. Br Med J 1996; 288: 436–438.

Fine E. Psychological factors associated with non-organic temporomandibular joint dysfunction syndrome. Br Dent J 1971; 131: 402–404.

SR Forssell H, Kalso E, Koskela P, Vehmanen R, Puukka P, Alanen P. Occlusal treatments in temporomandibular disorders: a qualitative systematic review of randomized controlled trials. Pain 1999; 83: 549–560.

Funch DP, Gale EN. Biofeedback and relaxation therapy for chronic temporomandibular joint pain: predicting successful outcomes. J Consult Clin Psychol 1984; 52: 928–35.

Funch DP, Gale EN. Predicting treatment completion in a behavioral therapy program for chronic temporomandibular pain. J Psychosom Res 1986; 30: 57–62.

Gessel AH. Electromyographic feedback and tricyclic antidepressants in myofascial pain syndrome. JADA 1975; 91: 1048–1052.

Glasgow RE, Hollis JF, McRae SG, Lando HA, LaChance P. Providing an integrated program of low intensity tobacco cessation services in a health maintenance organisation. Health Educ Res 1991; 6: 87–99.

Goodman P, Green CS, Laskin DM. Response of patients with

myofascial pain dysfunction syndrome to mock equilibration. J Am Dent Assoc 1976; 92: 755–758.

Greene CS, Laskin DM. Splint therapy for the myofascial pain–dysfunction syndrome: a comparative study. JADA 1972; 84: 624–628.

Greider A. An applied psychology in dentistry. In: Cinoti WR, Greider A, Springbob HK (eds) The Mosby Company, St Louis, MO, 2nd ed, 1972.

Griffiths RH. Report of the president's conference on the examination, diagnosis and management of temporomandibular disorders. JADA 1983; 106: 75–78.

Haber JD, Moss RA, Kuczmierczk AR, Garrett JC. Assessment and treatment of stress in myofascial pain–dysfunction syndrome; a model for analysis. J Oral Rehab 1983; 10: 187.

Hargreves AS, Wardle JJM. The use of physiotherapy in the treatment of temporomandibular disorders. Br Dent J 1983; 155: 121–124.

Harkins SW, Bush FM, Price DD, Hamer RM. Symptom reporting orofacial pain patients; relation to chronic pain, experimental pain, illness behavior, and personality. Clin J Pain 1991; 7: 102–113.

Harness DM, Donlon WC, Eversole LR. Comparison of clinical characteristics in myogenic, TMJ internal derangement and atypical facial pain patients. Clin J Pain 1990; 6: 4–17.

Harness DM, Peltier B. Comparison of MMPI scores with self-report of sleep disturbance and bruxism in the facial pain population. Cranio 1992; 10: 70–74.

Harris M. The surgical management of idiopathic facial pain produces intractable iatrogenic pain. Br J Oral Maxfac Surg 1996; 34: 1–3.

Harris M. Medical versus surgical management of temporomandibular joint pain and dysfunction. Br J Oral Maxillofac Surg 1987; 25: 113–120.

Harrison SD. The Management of Chronic Idiopathic Facial Pain. PhD thesis, University of London, 1999.

*** Harrison SD, Glover L, Feinmann C, Pearce SA, Harris M. A comparison of antidepressant medication alone and in conjunction with cognitive behavioural therapy for chronic idiopathic facial pain. In: Jensen TS, Turner JA, Wiesenfeld-Hallin Z (eds) Proceedings of the 8th World Congress on Pain, Progress in Pain Research and Management. IASP Press, Seattle, WA, 1997; pp 663–672.

*** Helkimo M. Studies on function and dysfunction of the masticatory system. Age, sex distribution of symptoms of dysfunction of the masticatory system in Lapps in the north of Finland. Acta Odont Scand 1974; 32: 255–267.

Henry FA, Baldridge OL. Condylectomy for the persistently painful temporomandibular joint. J Oral Surg 1957; 15: 24–31.

Husted E. Surgical management of temporomandibular joint disorders. Dent Clin N Am 1966; 10: 607–610.

*** Jagger RG. Diazepam in the treatment of temporomandibular joint dysfunction syndrome: a double blind study. J Dent 1973; 2: 37–40.

Juniper R. Whither the treatment for the TMJ? Br J Oral Maxillofac Surg 1993; 31: 137–138.

Kircos LT, Ortendahl DA, Mark AS, Arakawa M. Magnetic resonance imaging of the TMJ disc in asymptomatic volunteers. J Oral Maxillofac Surg 1987; 45: 852–854.

*** Lascelles RG. Atypical facial pain and depression. Br J Psych 1966; 112: 651–659.

Laskin, DM. Myofascial pain dysfunction syndrome: Etiology. In: Sarnat BG, Laskin DM (eds) The Temporomandibular Joint. A Biological Basis for Clinical Practice. Charles C. Thomas, Springfield, IL, 1980.

LeResche L, Saunders K, Von Korff MR, Barlow W, Dworkin SF. Use of exogenous hormones and risk of temporomandibular disorder pain. Pain 1997; 69: 153–160.

*** Lipton JA, Ship JA, Larach-Robinson D. Estimated prevalence and distribution of reported orofacial pain in the United States. JADA 1993; 124: 115–121.

Locker D, Grushka M. Prevalence of oral and facial pain and discomfort: preliminary results of a mail survey. Comm Dent Oral Epidemiol 1987; 15: 169–172.

*** Locker D, Slade G. Prevalence of symptoms associated with temporomandibular disorders in a Canadian population. Comm Dent Oral Epidemiol 1988; 16: 310–131.

*** Macfarlane TV, Blinkhorn AS, Davies RM, Kincey J, Worthington HV. Association between female hormonal factors and oro-facial pain: study in the community. Pain 2002; 97: 5–10.

Magnusson T, Carlsson GE. Occlusal adjustment in patients with residual or recurrent signs of mandibular dysfunction. J Pros Dent 1983; 49: 706–710.

SR Malone MD, Strube MJ. Meta-analysis of non medical treatments for chronic pain. Pain 1988; 34: 231–244.

McCain JP. Arthroscopy of the human temporomandibular joint. J Oral Maxillofac Surg 1988; 46: 648–655.

SR McQuay HJ, Tramer M, Nye BA, Carroll D, Wiffen PJ, Moore RA. A systematic review of antidepressants in neuropathic pain. Pain 1996; 68: 217–227.

Merskey H, Bogduk N. Classification of Chronic Pain. Descriptions of Chronic Pain Syndromes and Definitions of Pain Terms. IASP Press, Seattle, WA, 1994.

Mohlin B. Prevalence of mandibular dysfunction and relation between malocclusion and mandibular dysfunction in a group of women in Sweden. Eur J Orthodont 1983; 5: 115–123.

Moss RA, Adams HE. Physiological reactions to stress in subjects with and without myofascial pain dysfunction symptoms. J Oral Rehab 1984; 11: 219–232.

Murakami K, Moriya Y, Goto K, Segami N. Four-year follow-up study of temporomandibular joint arthroscopic surgery for advanced stage internal derangements. J Oral Maxillofac Surg 1996; 54: 285–290.

National Institutes of Health Technology Assessment Conference Statement. Management of temporomandibular disorders. JADA 1996; 127: 1595–1603.

Nilner M. Prevalence of functional disturbances and diseases of the stomatognathic system in 15–18 year olds. Swed Dent J 1981; 5: 189–197.

Nilner M, Lassing SA. Prevalence of functional disturbances and diseases of the stomatognathic system in 7–14 year olds. Swed Dent J 1981; 5: 173–187.

Nitzan DW, Dolwick MF, Martinez GA. Temporomandibular joint arthrocentesis: a simplified treatment for severe, limited mouth opening. J Oral and Maxillofac Surg 1991; 49: 163–1167.

Oakley ME, McCreary CP, Clark GT, Holston S, Glover D, Kashima K. A Cognitive–Behavioural approach to temporomandibular dysfunction treatment failures: a controlled comparison. J Orofac Pain 1994; 8: 397–401.

Ohnishi M. Clinical application of arthroscopy in the temporomandibular joint diseases. Bull Tokyo Med Dent Univ 1980; 27: 141–150.

Olesen J. Classification and diagnostic criteria for headache disorders, cranial neuralgias and facial pain. Cephalalgia 1988; 8: suppl 7.

Parker MW, Holmes EK, Terezhalmy GT. Personality characteristics of patients with temporomandibular disorders: diagnostic and therapeutic implications. J Orofac Pain 1993; 7: 337–344.

Pilowsky I, Crettenden I, Townley M. Sleep disturbance in pain clinic patients. Pain 1985; 23: 27–33.

Poker ID, Hopper C. Surgery for temporomandibular joint pain. Dent Update 1990; 17: 291–297.

Poswillo DE. Experimental investigation of the effects of intraarticular hydrocortisone and high condylectomy in the mandibular condyle. Oral Surg, Oral Med Oral Path 1970; 30: 161.

Ramjford SP. Dysfunctional temporomandibular joint and muscle pain. J Pros Dent 1961: 11: 354–374.

Riolo ML, Brandt D, TenHave TR. Associations between occlusal characteristics and signs and symptoms of TMJ dysfunction in children and young adults. Am J Orthod Dentofacial Orthop 1987; 92: 467–477.

*** Roldan OV, Maglione H, Carriers R, Mainieri S. Piroxicam, diazepam and placebo in the treatment of temporomandibular joint dysfunction. Double blind study. Rev Assoc Odont Argent 1990; 78: 83–85.

Rugh JD, Solberg WK. Psychological implications in temporomandibular pain and dysfunction. Oral Sci Rev 1976; 7: 3–30.

Sanders B. Arthroscopic surgery of the temporomandibular joint: treatment of internal derangement with persistent closed lock. Oral Surg, Oral Med, Oral Path 1986; 62: 361–372.

Schiffman EL, Anderson GC, Fricton JR, Lindgren BR. The relationship between level of mandibular pain and dysfunction and stage of temporomandibular joint internal derangement. J Dent Res 1992; 71: 1812–1815.

Shapiro AK, Morris LA. Placebos in psychiatric therapy. Curr Psychiatr Ther 1977; 17: 157–163.

*** Sharav Y, Singer E, Schmidt E, Dionne RA, Dubner R. The analgesic effect of amitriptyline on chronic facial pain. Pain 1987; 31: 199–209.

Sheikholeslam M, Holmgren K, Riise C. A clinical and electromyographic study of the long term effects of an occlusal splint of the temporal and masseter muscles in patients with functional disorders and nocturnal bruxism. J Oral Rehab 1986; 13: 137–145.

Schwartz L. Disorders of the Temporomandibular Joint. W.B. Saunders, Philadelphia, PA, 1959.

Sicher H. Temporomandibular articulation in mandibular overclosure. JADA 1948; 36: 131–139.

Solberg WK, Woo MW, Houston JB. Prevalence of mandibular dysfunction in young adults. JADA 1979; 98: 25–34.

Speculand B, Hughes AO, Gross AN. The role of stressful life experience in the onset of temporomandibular joint pain dysfunction. Comm Dent Oral Epidemiol 1984; 12: 197.

*** Szentpetery A, Huhn E, Fazekas A. Prevalence of mandibular dysfunction in an urban population in Hungary. Comm Dent Oral Epidemiol 1986; 14: 177–180.

Thomson H. Mandibular dysfunction syndrome. Br Dent J 1971; 130: 187–193.

Toller PA. Non-surgical treatment of dysfunctions of the temporomandibular joint. Oral Science Rev 1976; 7: 70–85.

Toller PA. Use and misuse of intra-articular corticosteroids in treatment of temporomandibular joint pain. Proc R Coll Med 1977; 70: 461–463.

Tsang CCA. Ultrasound Treatment for Facial Arthromyalgia. M.Sc. Thesis, University of London, 1988.

Ward TG. Surgery for the Temporomandibular Joint. Ann R Coll Surg 1961; 18: 139–152.

Tversky J, Reade PC, Gerschman JA, Holwill BJ, Wright J. Role of depressive illness in the outcome of treatment of temporomandibular joint pain–dysfunction syndrome. Oral Surg Oral Med Oral Pathol 1991; 71: 696–699.

Whitney CW, Von Korff M. Regression to the mean in treated versus untreated chronic pain. Pain 1992; 50: 281–285.

Von Korff M, Dworkin SF, Le Resche L, Kruger A. An epidemiologic comparison of pain complaints. Pain 1988; 32: 173–183.

Yemm R. Masseter muscle activity is stress — adaptation of response to a repeated stimulus in man. Arch Oral Biol 1969a; 14: 1437.

Yemm R. Temporomandibular dysfunction and masseter muscle response to experimental stress. Br Dent J 1969b; 127: 508.

Yemm R. Comparison of the electrical activity of the masseter and temporal muscles of human subjects during experimental stress. Arch Oral Biol 1971; 28: 45–46.

Assessment and Management of Orofacial Pain
Pain Research and Clinical Management, Vol. 14
Edited by J.M. Zakrzewska and S.D. Harrison

CHAPTER 12

Headache syndromes presenting with facial pain and autonomic features

M.S. Chong[*]

The Medway Hospital NHS Trust, Gillingham, Kent, and King's College Hospital NHS Trust, London, Mapother House, London SE5 9AZ, UK

Objectives for this chapter:

This chapter will attempt to show you that:
- There are a number of headache syndromes with autonomic features
- A very careful history needs to be taken when making a diagnosis and differentiating between these conditions
- Making a correct diagnosis is important because these conditions respond to specific treatment
- Effective treatments are available for patients with cluster headaches

1. Introduction

This chapter will concentrate on the predominantly primary headache syndromes with associated autonomic features during attacks. These include cluster headache (which can be further subdivided into episodic, chronic and secondary forms) paroxysmal hemicrania and SUNCT (*S*hort-lasting *U*nilateral *N*euralgiform headaches with *C*onjunctival injection and *T*earing). Making a link between headache and the associate autonomic symptoms is relatively easy. However, differentiating between these syndromes even with a good description of the attacks can be difficult. Important differentiating features include the duration and periodicity of pain as well as the degree of autonomic dysfunction with each attack.

Making an accurate diagnosis is important both to provide optimal treatment as well as counselling the patients about the prognosis of their condition. This is only possible by taking a careful history from the patient or witnesses to an attack. Physical examinations and investigations in these patients are usually less helpful except in secondary headache syndromes.

2. Cluster headaches (CH)

2.1. Definition

Cluster headache (CH) is a distinct pain syndrome with associated features which are helpful in making the diagnosis. The International Association for the Study of Pain (IASP) defined this condition as "Unilateral, excruciatingly severe attacks of pain

* E-mail: mschong@doctors.org.uk

principally in the ocular frontal and temporal region. . . " Part of the definition also stated that this condition occurs "*usually* with ipsilateral lacrimation, conjunctival injection, photophobia and nasal stuffiness and/or rhinorrhea". CH is given the code of 004.X8a. This is less precise than the International Headache Society (IHS) classification. The IASP classification also separated CH from chronic CH where it is defined as attacks " *usually* occurring more frequently than twice a week and for more than 1 year". Chronic CH is given the code of 004.X8b.

The IHS classification of cluster headaches that is summarised below is more commonly used and by demanding certain signs, gives a more exact definition. A lot of other general symptoms associated with CH like nausea, photophobia and phonophobia (see below) are not included in the IHS definition. It would be interesting to see if these symptoms are recognised in the updated IHS definitions which are due to be released soon. The present IHS criteria also recognise that episodic and chronic CH are closely related to the extent that one form may develop into the other (see below). CH is also known by numerous names including Horton's or more confusingly 'migrainous' neuralgia. Now that CH is recognised as a primary headache syndrome separate from migraine (even though they may co-exist), it is possible to make a more precise diagnosis. This has helped to improve our understanding of the susceptibility, treatment and prognosis of this condition (Tables 1 and 2).

2.2. Epidemiology

In a large survey carried out in San Marino, the prevalence was 69/100,000 (D'Alessandro et al., 1986) and incidence of CH was 2.5/100,000 per year of the population (Tonon et al., 2002). Extrapolating data from a study of army recruits in Sweden, CH was estimated to affect 0.4% of patients seen in headache clinics (Kudrow, 1980). CH predominantly affects men with first attacks occurring in the second to third decade of life. Previous large case series have reported that the ratio of men to women affected varies from 5 : 1 (Kudrow, 1980) to 6.7 : 1 (Horton, 1956). More recent studies have reported a reduction in the ratio down to 2.1 : 1 (Manzoni, 1997). Whether this reflects the recognition of different manifestations of CH in women as opposed to men (see below) or the changing role of women in society which predisposes them to CH is unclear. Women who developed CH, however, usually do so much later in life compared to men. In their retrospective analysis of 168 patients, Mosek et al. (2001) reported an incidence of 15% women (26 patients) and the mean age of onset was 61 years.

Many studies have highlighted a relationship between certain lifestyle and behavioural characteristics amongst patients with CH (Levi et al., 1992; Manzoni, 1999). One of the latest and largest series by Manzoni (1999) examined this relationship in 374 patients. A large number of his patients also reported head injuries either with (13.4% cases) or without (23.5%) loss of consciousness preceding the onset of CH. As in other reports (Reik, 1987; Turkewitz et al., 1992), these studies are prone to recall bias and any causative link between head injury and CH remains unproven. The link between heavy alcohol, cigarette, coffee consumption and CH, however, is more robust. As much as 80% of his patients are smokers with 13% of episodic CH and 20% of chronic CH patients smoking over 30 cigarettes a day. In addition, 16% of his patients with episodic CH and 27% of chronic CH patients admit to abusing alcohol (Manzoni, 1999).

The genetic link in CH is also well studied. It is estimated that first-degree relatives of a person with CH has a 14-fold increased risk of developing CH and the risk is 2-fold in second-degree relatives. In a large study of 220 Italian families, 20% of patients have a family history. The calculated risk was 39-fold increased risk in first-degree relatives (Leone et al., 2001). This strong genetic link was further emphasised by the monozygotic twin studies that have reported 100% concordance rate for CH (Sjaastad et al., 1993).

In an effort to identify the gene(s) involved, researchers have initially investigated possible links between CH and mutations of other genes known to be associated with other neurovascular headaches. A missense mutation of the P/Q type calcium chan-

TABLE 1

KEY FACTS: definitions of cluster headache

International Association for the Study of Pain
Unilateral excruciatingly severe attacks of pain, principally in the ocular frontal, and temporal areas, recurring in separate bouts with daily or almost daily, attacks for weeks to months, usually with ipsilateral lacrimation, conjunctival injection, photophobia, and nasal stuffiness and/or rhinorrhoea.

International Headache Society Classification
Diagnostic criteria:
At least 5 attacks fulfilling B through to D
A.　Severe unilateral orbital, supraorbital and/or temporal pain lasting 15 to 180 min untreated.
B.　Headaches associated with at least one of the following signs which have to be present on the side of pain:
　　1.　Conjunctival injection
　　2.　Lacrimation
　　3.　Nasal congestion
　　4.　Rhinorrhoea
　　5.　Forehead and facial sweating
　　6.　Miosis
　　7.　Ptosis
　　8.　Eyelid oedema
C.　Frequency of attacks: from one every other day to eight a day
D.　At least one of the following:
　　1.　History, physical examination and neurologic examination do not suggest another disorder.
　　2.　History and/or physical and/or neurologic examinations do suggest such disorders but it is ruled out by appropriate investigations.
　　3.　Such disorder is present, but cluster headache does not occur for the first time in close temporal relation to the disorder.

Episodic cluster headache
Occurs in period lasting 7 days to 1 year separated by pain-free periods lasting 14 days or more.
Diagnostic criteria:
A.　All the lettters heading 3.1.
B.　At least 2 periods of headaches (cluster periods) lasting (untreated patients) from 7 days to 1 year separated by remissions of at least 14 days.

Chronic cluster headache
Attacks occur for more than 1 year without remission or with remissions lasting less than 14 days.
Diagnostic criteria:
A.　All the letters heading 3.1.
B.　Absence of remission phases for 1 year or more with remissions lasting less than 14 days.

nel alpha-1 subunit (CACNA1A), for example, is known to be responsible for certain types of familial hemiplegic migraine. In a study of 75 patients with sporadic CH and 108 controls, Sjostrand and colleagues failed to find an association between the CH and the CACNA1A gene (Sjostrand et al., 2001). Another study in a family with CH has reported similar results.

2.3. Aetiology and pathophysiology

The primary mechanism for CH attacks was thought to be an inflammatory vascular process in the cavernous sinus (Moskowitz, 1988; Hardebo, 1994). This inflammation then causes disruption of venous drainage which affects the sympathetic nerves around the carotid artery and its branches. This was

TABLE 2

Terminology for description of cluster headaches [a]

Cluster headache or cluster attack	Individual attack of cluster headache usually lasting 60–90 min.
Cluster period	Time where there is occurrence of recurrent cluster attacks. May last weeks, months, even years.
Episodic cluster headache	Cluster periods lasting for 1 week to 1 year with pain-free remission of at least 14 days.
Chronic cluster headache	Cluster periods lasting for over 1 year without any remission or remission lasts for less than 14 days.

[a] After Dodick and Campbell (2001) and IHS Classification of Headaches (1988).

thought to give rise to the autonomic signs and symptoms associated with CH attacks. This theory is supported by the discovery of dilatation of the ophthalmic artery and increased intraocular pressure during CH attacks. In addition, the potent vasodilator nitroglycerin is a potent trigger of CH attacks.

The evidence against this 'vasculitis' theory is the absence of any definite structural changes on MRI scans in patients with CH. Furthermore, SPECT scans which outlined increased activity around the cavernous sinus during acute CH attacks are nonspecific and similar changes are seen in many primary and secondary headache syndromes including migraine and tension headaches. It is likely that these vascular changes are an epiphenomenon.

Instead, a neural mechanism as the primary trigger for acute CH attacks is now gaining support. The hypothesis behind this neural theory is that CH attacks are generated by activity in the circadian regions of the central nervous. This then leads to excitation of sensory afferents in the ophthalmic division of the trigeminal nerve causing pain while the autonomic signs and symptoms (see below) are due to the cranial parasympathetics that run via the facial nerve. The pathogenesis of CH attacks resulting from such a 'generator' would explain the circadian rhythmicity of these attacks. Evidence for the anatomical correlate for such a structure comes from positron emission tomographic (PET) scanning. May et al. (1998) reported activation of the ipsilateral hypothalamic grey matter in patients who had attacks of CH provoked by nitroglycerin. Indirect evidence that the

hypothalamus plays a role in the pathogenesis of CH includes the reports of reduced testosterone levels in men (Kudrow, 1976) and the reduced and blunted nocturnal peaks of melatonin secretion during a CH period (Leone et al., 1995). More direct evidence has also emerged with morphometric studies of the hypothalamus of patients with CH, once again reported by May et al. (1999). An increase in volume of the inferior posterior hypothalamus was found in 25 CH patients compared to matched controls. This area also coincides with the site of SPECT activation during acute CH attacks that was previously reported.

The hypothalamus undoubtedly plays an important role in the pathogenesis of CH and also SUNCT (see below). The complete circuitry underlying CH attacks however remains to be determined. In a recent case report, apparent complete section of the ipsilateral trigeminal nerve failed to prevent CH attacks (Matharu and Goadsby, 2002) [1]. One possible explanation for this is that the innervation of structures where pain is felt is either bilateral or there are more diffused pathways rather than via the trigeminal nerve trunk itself. Persistence of autonomic symptoms in this patient also suggested that

---

[1] Interesting case studies that pose more questions than provide answers. In a patient with apparent complete sectioning of the trigeminal nerve root, pain and autonomic symptoms are still experienced with cluster attacks and more intriguingly, the attacks respond to sumatriptan.

rather than a simple trigeminovascular and cranial parasympathetic reflex, the afferent arm is not necessary to trigger the autonomic signs and symptoms of an acute CH attack. It is also obvious that the sympathetic nervous system is in some way affected as well during acute CH attacks as up to half of the patients describe an associated Horner's syndrome. Whether this is secondary to the 'vascular congestion' as previously postulated or a primary phenomenon arising from altered activity in the hypothalamus is unclear.

2.4. Clinical features

The key clinical features of CH are summarised in Table 3 below.

2.4.1. Character
Many patients with CH use descriptors like 'tearing', 'penetrating', 'deep boring', 'sharp burning' when asked about their pain (like a hot red poker pushed and twisted into the eye). Using the McGill Pain

Questionnaire (MMPQ), Jerome et al. (1988) found that patients with CH employ different pain descriptors to describe their attack compared to patients with migraine and mixed headaches (for details of MMPQ see Chapter 6). In their study of 388 patients, the pain qualities, thermal (hot-searing), punctate (pricking – drilling-lancinating) and the absence of dull (dull-heavy) descriptors are effective in identifying 73% of patients with cluster headache.

2.4.2. Periodicity, timing, duration, onset
Most patients with episodic CH report between 1 and 4 daily cluster attacks during a period of exacerbation. A mean maximum number of between 4 and 5 attacks were reported in a 24 h period during a cluster bout (Bahra et al., 2002). Attacks build up within 5–10 min to reach a peak that lasts for up to 2 h. The mean duration of CH attacks is 45 min although the range varies greatly (Sjostrand et al., 2000). A recent study has reported mean maximum duration of 2.5 h and a mean minimum duration of

TABLE 3

KEY FACTS: clinical features of cluster headaches

Character	Thermal (hot-searing), punctate (pricking – drilling)
Site and radiation	Retro-orbital, temple, upper teeth, forehead, jaw, cheek, lower teeth, neck and nose
Periodicity, onset, duration	1–5 daily attacks during a period of exacerbation. Attacks build up within 5–10 min to reach a peak that lasts for up to 2 h. The mean duration of CH attacks is 45–70 min.
Severity	More intense than migraine or mixed headaches. Comparable to the pain of trigeminal neuralgia.
Provoking factors	REM sleep, longest and shortest days of the year, high altitude, alcohol and vasodilating drugs
Relieving factors	Acute attacks: oxygen inhalation. Drugs: subcutaneous and intranasal sumatriptan, oral zolmitriptan; intravenous and rectal ergotamine; intranasal lignocaine. Prophylaxis: verapramil, lithium, corticosteroids, methylsergide, gabapentin, topiramate
Associated factors	Lacrimation, conjunctival injection, nasal congestion, rhinorrhoea, ptosis/eyelid oedema, forehead and facial sweating, miosis, Horner's syndrome
Clinical examination	Normal in between attacks, residual Horner's syndrome very rarely found
Prognosis	Episodic cluster headaches: average cluster period 6–12 weeks with pain-free remission of 12 months Chronic cluster headache: cluster period of over 1 year with less than 14 days of remission. This may continue for years but 50% may evolve into episodic form.

72 min for cluster attacks (Bahra et al., 2002). Riess et al. reported that one half of their sample of 52 cluster headache sufferers had attacks lasting 15 min to 1 h while the other half experienced attacks of 1–3 h in duration (Riess et al., 1998).

2.4.3. Site and radiation

The pain is strictly unilateral and usually affects the same side of the head although it has been known to affect the other side during subsequent bouts. The most frequent sites for pain are the orbital, retro-orbital or deep fronto-temporal areas. In a prospective study of 230 patients with cluster headache reported by Bahra et al. (2002), the pain of an acute attack was strictly unilateral in all patients. Sixty percent of sufferers had pain on the right and 32% on the left side. The pain changed sites in between or within a bout in nearly 20%. It is rare for pain to change sides during an attack and only two sufferers reported such an experience. Pain in the retro-orbital site occurred in 92% of their group of sufferers during a cluster attack. Other common sites of pain were the ipsilateral temporal region (70%), upper teeth (50%), forehead (46%), jaw (45%), cheek (45%), lower teeth (32%) and neck (30%). Pain in the nose (20%), ear (17%), shoulder (13%), vertex (7%), occiput (6%) and parietal area (1%) was also reported. Ekbom in his comparison of cluster headaches and migraine described the upper and lower subtypes of CH. In the upper syndrome, patients describe pain radiating from the eye to the forehead, temple and parietal regions. In the lower syndrome, pain radiates from the eye to the upper teeth, jaw and even ipsilateral parts of the neck (Ekbom, 1970).

2.4.4. Severity

The pain of CH is notoriously severe, sometimes described as the 'worse pain' known to men. In the study of Jerome et al. (1988) where authors employed the McGill Pain Questionnaire as mentioned above, it was found that patients with CH report pain that is more intense than that for patients with other headaches. On a simple 0–100 visual analogue scale, the mean pain intensity reported by patients with cluster headache was 79.2. In the same study,

patients with migraine and mixed headache reported pain intensity scores of 62.3 and 57.5 respectively. Women with cluster headaches have reported that the pain of cluster headache is worse than that of childbirth.

2.4.5. Provoking and relieving factors

Spontaneous attacks usually happen in the early hours of the morning within 90 min of the patient going to sleep which coincides with the onset of Rapid Eye Movement (REM) sleep (Kudrow et al., 1984). Other vulnerable times include periods of rest when the patient is relaxing, particularly at the end of the day. Each bout may occur at roughly the same time of the day, to the extent that CH is also termed 'clockwork headache'. This cyclical pattern is also seen with 'clusters' of attacks coming on at certain times of the year, most commonly in January and July. In a prospective study reported by Kudrow (1987) in 400 patients who underwent nearly 900 cluster bouts, the peak incidence of cluster period was within 2–3 weeks of the longest and shortest days of the year in temperate countries. Nearly half of the patient sufferers reported a seasonal propensity for their cluster bouts in a recent study (Bahra et al., 2002). It would be interesting to study whether such a cyclical pattern exists in patients living outside temperate climates. Other factors which may provoke CH attacks include high altitude, alcohol and vasodilating drugs like nitroglycerin (Ekbom, 1968). A recent reported study found that 90% of those who drank alcohol reported that this triggers a cluster attack during an active bout (Bahra et al., 2002). The glare of bright light and stress are also reported triggers for cluster attacks (Riess et al., 1998).

2.4.6. Associated factors

The associated autonomic symptoms are very useful in making the diagnosis although each bout may have varying degrees of these symptoms. In a prospective study, tearing was the most common autonomic accompaniment to an acute cluster attack and was reported by 91% of patients. Seventy seven percent of sufferers also noticed conjunctival injection while nasal congestion (75%), ptosis/eyelid swelling (74%) and rhinorrhoea (72%) were also commonly reported symptoms (Bahra et al., 2002). A Horner's syndrome may be present in up to half of cluster attacks and rarely may even be seen between attacks. Some patients described feeling hot and flushed all over with each attack. It is estimated however that 3% of patients may have CH without the overt autonomic manifestations (Nappi et al., 1992).

This severe pain renders the patient very agitated causing the sufferer to rock, pace around or even strike their head against an object. They do not appear to find any comfort in any particular position they adopt (Blau, 1993). Most sufferers would admit to being apprehensive to any discomfort around the eye for the fear that this may be the harbinger of an attack. Migrainous symptoms like nausea and vomiting, photophobia and phonophobia were thought to be uncommon during CH attacks. In the study by Jerome and colleagues, the incidence of nausea was 24% in patients with cluster headaches and 43% in those with migraine (Jerome et al., 1988). This view has been challenged in a recent study by Rozen (2001) and his colleagues that compared manifestations of CH attacks in 69 male and 32 female patients (Rozen et al., 2001). They also found that nasal congestion and lacrimation was equally common in both men and women. Miosis and ptosis were more commonly reported by men while nausea affects over 60% of women. Nearly half of the women reported vomiting during CH attacks. Similarly, over three quarters of their patients report photophobia during an attack and in half, also phonophobia. This is supported by the larger prospective study reported by Bahra et al. (2002). In their series of 230 sufferers, half reported nausea associated with their cluster attack while 56% experienced photophobia in at least one attack. Phonophobia (43%) and osmophobia (26%) were less commonly encountered.

2.4.7. Psychological associations and quality of life
Patients with cluster headaches are described as having hard driving, ambitious, energetic personalities. However, at least three formal studies using the Minnesota Multiphasic Personality Inventory (MMPI) have failed to report any significant psychopathology amongst these patients (Kudrow and Sutkus, 1979; Andrasik et al., 1981; Cuypers et al., 1981).

The impact of cluster headaches on a patient's quality of life has not been extensively studied. Most investigators compared the quality of life between patients with other headache types versus cluster headache. In a study by Solomon and colleagues, for example, they used the Short Form Health Survey (SF-20) to compare the effects of migraine, mixed headache, tension type against cluster headache (Solomon et al., 1994). This study was carried out by recruiting patients from a headache clinic and is not strictly community-based. Their findings were that patients with cluster headache have a relatively higher pain score and greater limitations on their social functioning. In spite of this, patients with cluster headache demonstrated a better preservation of their physical functioning and have better health perception. This perception is supported by the study reported by Riess et al. (1998) who found that over 90% of patients with cluster headache described their condition as having no major impact on their occupation and none have lost a job because of their condition.

2.4.8. Findings on examination
During an attack the autonomic features (as described above) may be apparent. A reversible Horner's syndrome together with conjunctival injection may be seen. Facial flushing and periorbital swelling is commonly described by the patient and is only sometimes seen during an attack. A residual Horner's syndrome may rarely persist even after an attack (Lance and Anthony, 1971) and if present, often leads to extensive investigations to exclude any structural abnormalities along the sympathetic pathway (Table 3) (see Section 2.6).

2.5. Natural history

The sub-classification of cluster headache depends on the pattern of the clusters (see below). Episodic CH can remit and there are pain-free periods without either spontaneous or provoked attacks. The majority of patients (over 80%) with episodic CH experience cluster periods lasting 20–30 days. During this period, nearly half will experience at least one attack a day with a further 10% with two attacks. A substantial number of patients (nearly 50%) will experience remission periods lasting a year and up to 5 years has been reported (Kudrow, 1980). The study by Bahra and colleagues has reported a frequency of one bout a year in 182 sufferers of episodic cluster headache (Bahra et al., 2002).

Chronic CH by definition are daily bouts lasting longer than 1 year with less than 14 attack-free days. Chronic CH may evolve from episodic CH or may start as chronic CH from onset. Factors which increase the risk of transformation from episodic to chronic CH include late onset of CH, presence of sporadic attacks, high frequency of cluster periods and short duration of remissions (Torelli and Manzoni, 2002). Manzoni and colleagues in their follow-up study of nearly 200 patients over 10 years reported that up to 50% of patients with chronic CH may evolve into episodic CH but this tends to happen after many years (Manzoni et al., 1991). Chronic CH is usually extensively investigated to differentiate it from secondary CH. Structural abnormalities of the middle cranial fossa near the midline, particularly the cavernous sinus, have been reported to cause secondary cluster headaches. Vascular malformations, carotid and anterior communicating artery aneurysms as well as primary (parasellar meningioma, pituitary adenoma) and secondary (pharyngeal carcinoma) neoplasms have been reported to cause a syndrome similar to CH. However, in these secondary forms of CH the duration, frequency and pattern of attacks are usually atypical and/or these patients may have fixed neurological deficits.

You may now like to see if you can diagnose the patient described in case study 1 in Table 4.

2.6. Differential diagnosis

Apart from paroxysmal hemicrania and SUNCT (see below) there are a number of primary and secondary syndromes that can be confused with CH and these are summarised in Table 5 below. Atypical trigemi-

---

TABLE 4

Case study 1

Please read through the case. What is the diagnosis and would you do any investigations?

Mr. RM is a 21-year-old security guard who was referred from the local Ophthalmology A + E department with left-sided facial pain. This started 10 days ago while at work. He experienced a gradual onset of pain over the left side of his face that took 2 h to reach maximum severity. The maximum pain was felt over the left eye but this radiates to above his eye and also to the back of his head. He took some analgesics which alleviated the pain. The next day, he woke up with a similar pain and took himself to see his general practitioner. It was noted by his friends and his GP that his left eyelid was a little droopy. A diagnosis of ear infection was made and he was treated with analgesics and antibiotics. This made little difference to his pain which persisted and he attended the ophthalmic hospital. When he was seen there, his main complaint was a constant background discomfort around his left eye. Two to three times a day, the pain becomes more severe with watering of the left eye and conjunctival injection. He says his nose is always blocked during winter and there has not been any change in this symptom. The pain is 6–7 on a visual analogue scale and the drooping of his left eyelid remains the same in between attacks. He has no past medical history but on direct questioning, can remember having had 2 days of neck pain 1 month ago. He thought he had slept awkwardly. On examination, he had a left Horner's syndrome with ptosis and miosis of the left eye. There was no papilloedema.

Please read the answer at the end of the chapter in Table 15.

---

nal neuralgia with autonomic symptoms can also be confused with CH. The presence of provoking factors like talking, eating or touching the face which trigger these attacks are useful to refine the diagnosis. This syndrome appears to be distinct from SUNCT (see below) although response to treatment with appropriate drugs may be the same. Temporal arteritis may also be misdiagnosed as CH especially when the headache is intermittent. The later age of onset of this condition as well as specified symptoms like jaw claudication (see Chapter 17) as well as physical signs like the presence of a tender thickened temporal artery on examination

TABLE 5

KEY FACTS: differential diagnosis for cluster headache

Paroxysmal hemicrania

SUNCT

Temporal arteritis

Atypical trigeminal neuralgia

Secondary causes: 'Raeder's Paratrigeminal Syndrome'

Ophthalmological: acute glaucoma and orbital cellulitis/myositis

are useful differentiating features. Unilateral orbital myositis has also been reported to cause pain, tearing, nasal congestion and respond to treatment similar to CH (Lee and Lessell, 2002). Prolonged pain in between bouts which is atypical for CH helps to refine the diagnosis. Raeder's paratrigeminal syndrome is commonly cited as a differential diagnosis of cluster headaches. This syndrome merely described the site of pathology around the middle cranial fossa and many pathological processes can cause a constellation of pain, ptosis and miosis with variable associated trigeminal sensory loss and intact forehead sweating. In Raeder's original paper, trauma and a parasellar tumour was the reported pathology (Raeder, 1924). Once again, the character and pattern of pain in these secondary headache syndromes are usually different from that of CH and may also change with time (see Chapter 17).

There are a number of patients that appear to suffer from 'forme-fruste' of two different types of primary headache syndromes. Some patients with typical CH bouts also experience prolonged headache afterwards with nausea and vomiting reminiscent of migraine without aura. In women especially, it can be difficult to differentiate between chronic CH and episodic CH with migrainous symptoms. These patients may respond to medications usually used as migraine prophylaxis. Where the diagnoses are not sufficiently well delineated, these cases give

rise to the erroneous conclusion that medications effective for preventing migraine like tricyclics antidepressants may be useful for treating CH. Alternatively, there are some patients where there is a true co-existence of migraine and cluster headaches (D'Amico et al., 1996).

The co-existence of typical trigeminal neuralgia attacks associated with CH is also reported (Monzillo et al., 2000). This so-called cluster-tic syndrome consists of attacks longer than SUNCT and are different from atypical trigeminal neuralgias with autonomic symptoms. The importance of recognising this is to employ a combination of therapies in an attempt to alleviate pain.

Acute close angle glaucoma can sometimes masquerade as the first cluster of CH. It is important to rule out this potentially treatable condition that if not quickly treated, can lead to permanent visual loss. Dental causes may also need to be looked at (Penarrocha et al., 2001) (Table 5).

2.7. Investigations

There is little evidence to base any recommendation regarding investigation of patients with CH. As part of a general medical assessment, routine blood tests for full blood count, ESR, urea and electrolytes and liver function tests would be useful. Many of these patients are heavy smokers and a chest X-ray to look for underlying abnormalities particularly a Pancoast tumour would be appropriate. Electrocardiography would also be useful to exclude atrial fibrillation or heart block. This has been reported during an acute attack of CH (Russell and Storstein, 1984). In their study, there was an increase in heart rate before onset of a cluster attack to be followed by a relative reduction during the attack. Cardiac dysrhythmias were seen in 5/27 patients and these include frequent premature ventricular beats (2), transient runs of atrial fibrillation (1), first-degree atrio-ventricular block (1) and sino-atrial block (1). The practical importance of an interictal ECG is because many of the medications used for acute as well as prophylactic treatment of CH can cause cardiac dysrhythmias as well and this coupled with changes seen during a cluster attack as mentioned above may just precipitate a more serious cardiac disorder.

Manzoni et al. (1983) carried out routine plain skull X-rays in all their 180 patients with cluster headaches. Up to 40% had abnormalities, the most common is either opacification or polyposis of the paranasal sinuses. Whether this is a cause or consequence of cluster headaches is not clear. In their conclusion, the authors did not believe that a skull X-ray contributed anything to the clinical care of these patients and did not think this investigation to be justified.

Frishberg (1997) reviewed the extensive literature on the utility of neuroimaging in patients with common types of headaches. His conclusion was that in patients with typical episodic CH, imaging is not necessary. This is supported by the report of Sjaastad and Rinck (1990). In this study, MRI scans were performed in 14 patients, with 13 having the episodic and 1 the chronic cluster headaches. No abnormalities were found which could explain their symptoms. In spite of this, the author recommended more sophisticated methods of magnetic resonance imaging like 3-dimensional and angiographic scans. There is simply little evidence to recommend the use of any neuroimaging for investigating patients with cluster headaches.

However, any headaches with a progressive course or where there is a change in pattern of CH would need a brain scan. Any patients with neurological abnormalities apart from a Horner's syndrome between cluster attacks would also need to be investigated. Similarly, because it is thought to be relatively rare in women, those with CH are more likely to be investigated as are those with a known risk factor of secondary pathology like patients with a history of neoplasm or known to be HIV-positive. In spite of the insufficient data to base any firm recommendations, the practice of defensive medicine would dictate that most patients with CH will have a brain scan at some time in the course of their illness. This is also supported by the rare case where treatment of an underlying cause like a vascular malformation can cure secondary cluster headaches (Gawel et al., 1989). The neuroimaging of choice would still be an

---

TABLE 6

Case study 2

Please read through the case and suggest how you would manage this patient.

A 46-year-old man who is the husband of a member of staff requests to see you urgently just before Christmas. He was diagnosed as having cluster headaches in the past. For the past week, he has been woken up in the early hours of the morning with severe pain around the right eye which lasted for half an hour. During these attacks, he cries with the pain. His general practitioner has prescribed tramadol without any benefit. He is desperate for help and his wife had made a personal plea to you.

Please see Table 16 at the end of the chapter for the answer.

MRI scan because it gives a better definition of the course of the sympathetic pathway especially around the cavernous sinus. Very infrequently, intra-arterial digital subtraction angiography may need to be performed to look at the carotid vessels and also exclude aneurysms especially around the circle of Willis.

2.8. Management

Before reading through the next section please read through case 2 in Table 6 and see if you could manage this patient.

2.8.1. Non-pharmacological

Treatment of underlying cause(s) for secondary clusters and the avoidance of trigger factors would be the first logical step in helping patients to deal with their cluster headaches. During a cluster bout, patients are advised to abstain from drinking alcohol as this is a common trigger. The inhalation of volatile substances like solvents, petrol, oil-based paints can also trigger cluster attacks and are best avoided. Patients should also be informed that having a nap in the afternoon may trigger an attack and those who indulge in this should consider changing their sleep pattern. Relative hypoxaemia at high attitudes may also trigger cluster attacks and patients should avoid travel in aeroplanes in the middle of a cluster bout. There is little evidence that stopping smoking helps but counselling patients to give up tobacco would be beneficial, if only on general health grounds.

Pharmacotherapy: abortive treatment. The pain of CH is so severe that many patients are desperate for treatment that can abort an attack. The triptans is the drug of choice for alleviating cluster attacks. The route of administration is crucial.

Subcutaneous sumatriptan. Subcutaneous sumatriptan 6 mg is very effective and acts rapidly. In a placebo controlled study, 74% of patients had complete relief of their cluster attack with subcutaneous sumatriptan compared with 26% of patients on placebo (Ekbom et al., 1981). The recommended dosing regime is no more than two doses in every 24 h. It is however common for patients to greatly exceed this dose. Unlike treatment for migraine where persistent use of triptans has been shown to cause tachyphylaxis and rebound headaches, this was not seen in the majority of patients with CH. In long-term open-labelled studies, the efficacy of subcutaneous sumatriptan remained the same (Ekbom et al., 1995; Gobel et al., 1998). Patients with chronic CH, however, appear to have a lower and slower response rate to subcutaneous sumatriptan compared with those with episodic CH (Gobel et al., 1998). Subcutaneous sumatriptan should be used with caution in patients with cardiovascular disease particularly patients with CH who are also heavy tobacco consumers.

Nasal sumatriptan. Intranasal sumatriptan 20 mg has also been shown to be more effective than placebo (Van Vliet et al., 2001) but less than subcutaneous sumatriptan. In an open-labelled randomised study comparing these two routes of administration, 49/52 injections result in complete pain relief within 15 min compared with only 7/52 nasal administration (Hardebo and Dahlof, 1998). In another study of 10 patients who experienced 154 attacks, only 58% of attacks were alleviated within 30 minutes after 20 mg of inhaled sumatriptan. In spite of this relatively poor result, when interviewed 6 months later, 4/7 patients continue to use inhaled sumatriptan and only 2/7 elected to use the subcutaneous preparation (Schuh-Hofer et al., 2002).

Oral triptans. Oral triptans are generally less effective probably because absorption is too slow. Oral zolmitriptan at 10 mg which is four times the normal dose used for treating migraine attacks has been shown to be effective for alleviating cluster attacks in patients with episodic cluster headaches (Bahra et al., 2000). The effect is however modest and less than that seen with oxygen inhalation (see below). It is obvious that patient choice is an important factor in choosing abortive treatment for CH and although the subcutaneous route of administration is most effective, many patients prefer not to have an injection.

Ergots. The ergots can also be effective for alleviating cluster attacks but once again, the route of administration is important. The ergotamine aerosol is treatment of choice because drug bioavailability is highest when administered via this route. In the study reported by Ekbom et al. (1983), serum ergotamine levels peaked at 5 min when given as an inhalation as opposed to 60 min when the drug was administered as a suppository. Levels were virtually undetectable when ingested as an effervescent tablet. This confirmed an earlier study where the bioavailability of ergotamine at a dose of 2–4 mg/day administered orally was less than 1% (Ekbom et al., 1981). Three puffs of the Ergotamine Medihaler at the beginning of an attack is the treatment of choice as intravenous ergots are not available in the United Kingdom. In the United States, a 1 mg dose of dihydroergotamine administered intravenously has been reported to abort most cluster attack within 5 min (Raskin, 1988). This is unfortunately impractical in most circumstances, as patients are unable to self-administer via this route. The side-effects of ergots are also considerably more than those for triptans, so that apart from cost, subcutaneous sumatriptan is the treatment of choice for the treatment of cluster attacks. There is however a role for regular ergotamine as a short-term prophylaxis (Mather et al., 1991). As regular intravenous injections are not practical, one or two milligrams of ergotamine taken either orally or as a suppository before bedtime can be used instead and has been reported to be an effective prophylaxis for night time cluster attacks (Horton, 1956). However, there are no randomised controlled studies to support this. Furthermore, prolonged use of ergots is not recommended because of the risk of developing side-effects. For example, rectal ergotamine has been reported to cause anal strictures (Safar, 2002).

Intranasal lignocaine. The early report of five patients by Kittrelle et al. (1985) has demonstrated that intranasal lignocaine can be effective for treating cluster headache as well. When administered ipsilaterally as a 4% spray or a viscous liquid, 40–60 mg of lignocaine intranasally has been shown to be effective in reducing the pain of cluster attacks. Complete relief is rare (Robbins, 1995) and intranasal lignocaine is only useful as an adjunctive treatment (see below).

Inhaled oxygen. Inhalation of oxygen for the relieve of cluster attacks was introduced in 1956 by Horton. Pure oxygen inhaled at a rate of 7–12 l/min using a tight fitting non-rebreathing mask for 15–20 min has been shown to be effective. A small placebo controlled study has also confirmed the efficacy of inhaling oxygen for relief of cluster attacks (Fogan, 1985). Another placebo controlled study of 14 patients also reported that hyperbaric oxygen at 2 atm pressure is effective (Di Sabato et al., 1993). The practical problem with this method of treatment is the supply of oxygen and the availability of high flow oxygen regulators which would need to be purchased separately. Generally, oxygen inhalation tends to be more effective in younger patients with episodic CH.

Olanzapine. Another medication reported to be effective in the abortive treatment of CH is the atypical anti-psychotic drug olanzapine. In a study of five patients, Rozen (2001) has reported that 5–10 mg olanzapine administered orally reduced cluster pain by 80% within 20 min of taking the drug and 2/5 patients were pain free. Drowsiness was the main side-effect and this drug deserves further study.

Analgesics. A variety of opioid and non-steroidal analgesics are often prescribed in an attempt to alleviate cluster attacks. There is no evidence that any of these medications work and there is always a risk that prolonged use may induce analgesia overuse headaches. It can however be difficult to resist such demands. In an interesting report by Gallagher et al. (1996), patients when given the choice seem to prefer analgesics even though they report that it is ineffective. Similarly, only one third of their 60 patients continue to use oxygen even though it alleviated their cluster attacks.

Pharmacotherapy prophylaxis. The abortive treatment of cluster attacks are rarely completely effective and as attacks can be so frequent, prophylactic treatments which aim to suppress or shorten the cluster bout should be initiated early on. Prophylaxis for CH can be divided into short-term and long-term prevention.

Steroids. Short-term prevention of choice is the use of corticosteroids (Couch and Ziegler, 1978), although once again, this has not been subjected to vigorous testing with placebo controlled studies. A starting dose of between 40 and 60 mg prednisolone for 5 days is then followed by a tapering course where the drug is reduced by 10 mg every 3 days. Usual courses are for up to 3 weeks. Higher doses up to 80 mg a day can be tried in some patients who do not respond after 4–5 days of conventional treatment. The disadvantages of this treatment are the side-effects of steroids with prolonged use and the high incidence of relapse usually when the dose is reduced below 20 mg a day. To avoid using steroids for long periods of time, it would be sensible to start steroids in conjunction with one of the longer-term prophylactic medications at the start of a cluster bout (see below).

Methylsergide. Methylsergide is another effective prophylaxis for CH. Up to 70% of patients respond to treatment with methylsergide (Watson and Evans, 1987). The starting dose of 1 mg a day is increased by 1 mg every 3 days until a dose of 2 mg three times a day. In doses above 6 mg, the dose escalation is slowed down to 1 mg a day every week. Some patients can tolerate a dose of up to 12 mg a day. Side-effects of methylsergide include nausea, abdominal pain, muscle cramps, ankle swelling. Prolonged use of methysergide is associated with the development of retroperitoneal, pericardial and pleural fibrosis. A 1-month drug holiday every 6 months is recommended to reduce the risk of this. Methysergide is also a pro-drug of methylergometrine and can theoretically accentuate the effects of other vasoconstrictive agents like ergots and even triptans. There is also some evidence that this drug becomes less effective with repeated use (Kudrow, 1980). Methylsergide is therefore most suitable for young patients with episodic CH early on the course of their illness.

Verapramil. Long-term prophylactic agents are drugs that can be prescribed for the whole duration of the anticipated cluster bout. As mentioned above, they should be initiated at the same time as corticosteroids. The drug of choice for this purpose is verapramil. One of the earliest studies was an open-labelled trial where 33/48 patients treated with verapramil reported improvement by more than 75% (Gabai and Spierings, 1989). In a placebo controlled study, verapramil at 360 mg a day reached statistical significance in reducing headache frequency and analgesic consumption (Leone et al., 2000a,b). There appears to be a dose–response relationship and controlled release preparation of verapramil may be prescribed up to 720 mg a day. This medication is generally well tolerated although at high doses, there is a risk of bradycardia and heart block. Baseline electrocardiographic followed by regular monitoring is necessary when more than 240 mg of verapramil a day is to be prescribed.

Lithium. Lithium is also an effective prophylactic agent, particularly for chronic CH. In an earlier analysis of the literature, Ekbom (1981) collected 28 clinical trials involving over 460 patients. Three hundred patients had chronic CH and the response rate to lithium was 78% and lithium was effective even after 4 years of treatment (Manzoni et al., 1983). In the other 164 patients with episodic CH, the response rate was 63% with lithium. Equal efficacy was reported in a double-blind placebo controlled study comparing verapramil 360 mg a day and lithium 900 mg a day (Bussone et al., 1990).

Before initiating treatment with lithium, it is important to check thyroid and renal function. The starting dose is usually 300 mg twice a day with titration to 900–1200 mg a day. Regular monitoring of drug level is necessary, with the aim of keeping serum levels between 0.4 and 0.8 meq/l. Lithium can be a dangerous drug to use as a fatal overdose can happen particularly if there is inadvertent co-prescription of diuretics, carbamazepine or any drugs that may cause hyponatraemia. Patients taking lithium are advised to remain well hydrated and to seek medical help if they develop diarrhoea, polyuria or tremor.

Others. There are case reports and small studies of numerous other medications, especially the anticonvulsants as prophylaxis of CH. Sodium valproate, gabapentin and topiramate has been reported to be effective in some patients where other medications have failed. Melatonin levels has been reported to be low in patients with CH and has led to trials where its supplementation has been reported to be effective in preventing CH (Leone et al., 1996; Peres and Rozen, 2001). These reports are difficult to interpret as CH is mainly an episodic disorder and apparent success in preventing the attacks may simply be part of the natural cycle of remission. Large placebo controlled studies are the only reliable way to assess the drugs properly. For example, a recent placebo controlled study has concluded that sodium valproate is ineffective as a prophylaxis for cluster headache (El Amrani et. al., 2002) in spite of the previous case series that suggest a possible therapeutic effect.

Where a single prophylactic agent has failed, it is reasonable to combine two drugs together. Verapramil together with methylsergide or lithium are possible drug combinations. Where more than two drugs are used however (for example the addition of ergotamine to one of the combinations mentioned above) the risks of side-effects increase dramatically and is not a long-term option. A trial of the newer anticonvulsants either alone or in combination with another more established treatment would then be necessary.

2.8.2. Surgery

Surgical treatment of CH has not been evaluated as thoroughly as medical therapies. Surgery should only be contemplated in patients where medical treatment even in combinations have failed and where the cluster attacks are strictly unilateral. In patients where cluster attacks alternate between both sides, surgery may simply cause contralateral recurrence of attacks. Most surgical procedures are directed towards interruption of the trigeminal sensory pathways, similar to that employed for treating trigeminal neuralgia (see Chapter 15). Percutaneous radiofrequency thermocoagulation of the trigeminal ganglion has been reported to give good to excellent result in up to 75% of patients (Mathew and Hurt, 1988). The recurrence rate after this procedure has been reported to be 20% (Taha and Tew, 1995). Radiofrequency lesions to the sphenopalatine ganglion has also been reported to be effective for both episodic and chronic CH (Sanders and Zuurmond, 1997). Microvascular decompression of the trigeminal root and sometimes combined with decompression or sectioning of the nervus intermedius has been reported to be effective in 22/30 procedures performed (Lovely et al., 1998). Long-term follow-up, however, showed a marked decline of efficacy with time. A more destructive procedure is the complete rhizotomy at the trigeminal sensory root entry zone. One study reported 12/14 patients achieved complete pain relief (Kirkpatrick et al., 1993). All these surgical procedures are reported case series with varying length of follow-up. Transient and even long-term side-effects are considerable. In particular, destruction of the ophthalmic division of trigeminal nerve abolishes the blink reflex and can cause severe corneal damage. Iatrogenic damage to sensory nerves can also cause neuropathic facial pain.

One study that tried to answer some of these worries and included long-term data was that reported by Pieper et al. (2000). In their cohort of 18 patients with chronic CH who underwent glycerol rhizotomy, 9/18 patients had over 50% pain relief after first injection. Repeated injections had to be carried out in another 4 patients. Of all the 15 patients who reported pain relief, the Kaplan–Meier curve over 7 years showed over 65% success. The loss of pain relieve appears to occur in the first 2 years after surgery and then appears to remain stable. Sensory loss was reported in eleven patients for which in eight, this was permanent but anaesthesia dolorosa was not reported.

A recent case study by Leone et al. (2002) has suggested that stereotactic stimulation of the hypothalamus may be effective in alleviating CH. In their report, a 39 year old patient with predominant right-sided attacks underwent rhizotomy of the right trigeminal nerve. This resulted in identical CH attacks on the contralateral side. An implantable electrode was then placed in the left posterior inferior hypothalamic grey matter. Stimulation at this side gave relief from CH attacks even after 13 months. This is clearly a technique that deserves further study. Overall, the efficacy of surgical treatment for CH is uncertain and this method of therapy should only be undertaken in patients with stable personalities who can properly understand and evaluate the risks.

2.8.3. Summary on treatment

The present evidence supports the use of subcutaneous sumatriptan 6 mg injections for treating acute cluster attacks. As prophylaxis, verapramil up to 360 mg a day appears to be effective for both episodic and chronic cluster headaches. Both these treatment options have class A evidence. A lot of other treatment options are also employed for which oxygen inhalation at 7 1/min, oral zolmitriptan 10 mg and intravenous intranasal lignocaine 4% are preferred simply because of the low potential for side-effects and there is class B evidence. For the prophylaxis of cluster attacks, lithium 900–1200 mg a day (depending on blood levels) and corticosteroids have some class B evidence. Many other prophylactic agents like methylsergide, nimodipine, transdermal clonidine, baclofen, intranasal capsaicin, gabapentin and topiramate have class C evidence. All these treatment options need to be explored because there are inevitably patients who fail to respond to the first-line treatments. Combination pharmacotherapy can then be tried although the evidence for this is even more sparse. Many surgical procedures are described for the treatment of cluster headaches. Present evidence would suggest that glycerol rhizolysis is the best option when long-term efficacy is balanced against side-effects (Pieper et al., 2000). You will find a summary of the RCTs that have been conducted in CH patients in Table 7.

You will find a summary of studies which have reported on acute treatment for CH in Table 8 and of prophylactic treatment for CH in Table 9.

2.9. Prognosis

Cluster bouts are unpleasant and disruptive so that patients are interested to know what to expect. In a long-term study of over 20 years, Kudrow (1982) found that one third of patients with episodic CH went into remission. In another third, attacks were attenuated to the extent that they no longer need medications while in the last third, the pattern of attacks remained the same. In a Japanese study of 68 patients over 18 years, the frequency, duration and associated symptoms of headache attacks changed with time. The remission periods were increased from a mean of 1.1 to 3.3 years (Igarashi and Sakai, 1996).

Another report by Manzoni et al. (1991) studied 189 consecutive patients with CH over a 10 year period. About 13% of their patients with episodic CH developed into the chronic form while another 6% evolved into an intermediate form. The remaining 80% remained with episodic CH. Of their patients with chronic CH from onset, half of the patients developed episodic or intermediate CH with time. In a subsequent study they also reported that high frequency of cluster bouts, cluster attacks and short remission between bouts as predictive factors for the evolvement of episodic to chronic CH (Torelli et al., 2000).

A slightly more optimistic scenario was reported by Sjostrand et al. (2000) in their cohort of 60 patients with a single cluster bout. Of the 49 patients they managed to follow-up, 26% did not have a recurrence of their cluster attack even after 9 years. According to the IHS classification, this group of patients cannot strictly be diagnosed as having CH. In the remaining patients with episodic CH, only 17% had another cluster bout within 3 years.

The evidence so far seems to indicate that here are some patients with a single cluster bout with a low risk of recurrence. In those with a second bout and diagnosed as having episodic CH, a small number develop chronic CH while the majority continue to experience relapses but the frequency of these bouts reduces with time. For those patients with chronic CH from onset more than half will go on to develop episodic CH.

2.10. Complications

A number of patients with CH appear to have a permanent Horner's syndrome between attacks. It is unclear whether this can be explained by permanent damage to the sympathetic nervous system after repeated episodes of CH. The study by Havelius (2001)[2] appears to contradict this. In his series of 57 patients, 7 had a permanent Horner's syndrome and 5 of these patients had attacks confined to one side. Ipsilateral Horner's syndrome was apparent in photographs taken many years before the onset of CH. This seems to indicate that in these patients, there was damage to the sympathetic nervous system a long time before the development of CH.

Attacks of CH have also been associated with obstructive sleep apnoea (Chervin et al., 2000). In their report, the authors suggest that obstructive sleep apnoea may trigger CH. There are two relevant points about this association. Firstly, treatment of sleep apnoea reduces night time hypoxaemia and day time drowsiness and may alleviate CH. Secondly, in the group of patients susceptible to CH, i.e. middle aged heavy smoking men, sleep apnoea is an important risk factor for developing strokes and heart attacks. Dealing with sleep apnoea may greatly reduce morbidity and mortality in these patients.

Before reading the next section go through case study 3 in Table 10 and see if you can come to a diagnosis.

3. Paroxysmal hemicrania

The syndrome of chronic paroxysmal hemicrania (CPH) was first described by Sjaastad and Dale (1974). CPH was subsequently incorporated into the IHS classification of headaches in 1988. There are however also episodic types of paroxysmal hemicrania (PH). The relationship between these two

---

[2] Interesting study that seems to indicate that damage to the sympathetic nervous system manifesting as a Horner's syndrome predisposes to cluster headaches rather than the other way round.

TABLE 7

High quality randomised, double-blind, placebo controlled trials of drugs used in spontaneous cluster headaches

Type of trial (No. treated)	Active drug, daily dosage	Other arm(s)	Trial duration	Efficacy evaluation	Number improved (NNT)	Side-effects/withdrawals no. of side-effects in reports (NNH)	Comments/level of recommendation	Reference
Randomised placebo controlled cross-over (49 patients)	Sumatriptan 6 mg S/C	Isotonic saline	2 attacks	Mild or no pain within 15 min of injection	Sumatriptan 29/39, Placebo 10/39, NNT 2.1	17/49 dizziness on active treatment	Level A evidence for the efficacy of S/C sumatriptan for cluster headaches	Sumatriptan Cluster Headache Study Group, 1991
2-period, 3-arm cross-over study (134 patients)	Sumatriptan 6 mg or 12 mg, subcutaneous	Placebo	268 acute cluster attacks	Headache improvement 15 min after injection.	6 mg dose 69/92 attacks (2.25); 12 mg dose 70/88 attacks (2.2); Placebo 30/88	No withdrawals. 6 mg 31/92 (5.6); 12 mg 40/88 (3.4); Placebo 14/88	Level A evidence. Largest placebo controlled trial for abortive treatment of CH.	Ekbom et al., 1993
Placebo controlled 2-period cross-over study (118 patients)	Sumatriptan 20 mg, intranasal	Placebo	2 acute attacks	Headache response at 30 min	Combined data on first and second attack: 47/86 on sumatriptan and 26/82 placebo achieved end point (4.2)	No serious side-effects reported	Modest effect of intranasal sumatriptan	Van Vliet et al., 2001
Randomised placebo controlled 3 arms (124 patients) 91 ECH 33 CCH	Zolmitriptan 5 mg and 10 mg, oral	Placebo	At least 1 cluster attack treated with study medication	Improvement in headache intensity of at least 2/5 points at 30 min	ECH 10 mg 50/79, 5 mg 45/83, Plac. 36/83; CCH 10 mg 15/32, CCH 12/31, Plac. 16/32	10 mg dose 1 withdrawal; 43/111 mild S/E; 5 mg 32/114; Plac. 17/115	Zolmitriptan statistically effective at 30 min for ECH only at 10 mg oral dose	Bahra et al., 2000
Placebo controlled ECH (22 patients)	Dihydroergotamine 1 mg nasal spray	Placebo	3–8 treated attacks	Complete or greatly reduced pain	DHE 51/137 attacks; Placebo 19/133; NNT 4.4	No dropouts or reported S/E	Intranasal DHE appears to be effective	Andersson and Jespersen, 1986
Placebo controlled cross-over (19 patients)	Breathing oxygen at 6 l/min for 15 min	Air	137 attacks treated (74 on oxygen, 63 with air)	50% patient's evaluation of pain relief on 4-point scale in at least half of attacks	9/16 on oxygen; 1/14 on air	None reported	Not properly randomised but one of the studies that tried to perform placebo controlled trial of oxygen for acute CH	Fogan, 1985
Randomised placebo controlled (28 patients)	Intranasal civamide 50 mcg/day	Placebo	1 week then F/U for 20 days post-treatment	Cluster attacks during treatment and post-treatment week		Nasal burning 14/18 and lacrimation 9/18 on civamide, 1/18 on placebo	Short duration trial only modest benefit	Saper et al., 2002

TABLE 7 *continued*

Type of trial (No. treated)	Active drug, daily dosage	Other arm(s)	Trial duration	Efficacy evaluation	Number improved (NNT)	Side-effects/with-drawals no. of side-effects in reports (NNH)	Comments/level of recommendation	Reference
Randomised, placebo controlled prophylaxis for reduction in daily CH attacks (30 patients)	Verapramil 360 mg/day	Placebo	2 weeks	50% reduction in daily CH attacks	12/15 on verapramil (1.25); 0/15 on placebo	No withdrawals. 13/15 on verapramil (1.9), 5/15 on placebo	Short duration trial, small numbers but level 1 evidence	Leone et al., 2000a,b
Randomised, placebo controlled prophylaxis study (169 patients)	Sumatriptan 100 mg tds orally	Placebo	1 week	50% reduction in number of cluster attacks	20/89 on sumatriptan and 17/79 on placebo achieved end point	Sumatriptan: 2 withdrew from S/E. 21/89 S/E reported. Placebo 8/79 had S/E.	Oral sumatriptan ineffective as 'pre-emptive' agent for CH	Monstad et al., 1995
Placebo controlled trial for prophylaxis of CH (27 patients)	Lithium 800 mg/day	Placebo	3 weeks	Number of patients whose CH attacks cease after 1 week	No statistical difference in primary end point or improvement in their cluster attacks	No withdrawals. Minor NNH 7/13 on lithium 2/14 placebo.	Not fully randomised. Study stopped early because lack of efficacy. Dose of lithium (blood levels) too low and end point too strict	Steiner et al., 1997
Randomised, placebo controlled trial for 73 ECH and 17 CCH 5 unspecified (96 patients)	Sodium valproate 1–2 g/day	Placebo	2 weeks	50% reduction in cluster attacks	25/50 on valproate and 29/46 on placebo achieved end point	Valproate 2/50, Placebo 1/46 withdrew. S/E Val 20/50, Plac. 13/46.	Valproate ineffective as prophylaxis for CH	El Amrani et al., 2002

TABLE 8

Studies of acute treatment of cluster attacks

Study method and number of patients	Drug and dosage	Outcome reported in each study	Side-effects/withdrawals	Comments	Reference
Open labelled study 63 CCH 75 ECH (138 patients) total 9130 attacks. All patients had at least 1 treated attack, 57 continued for over 3 months.	S/C sumatriptan 6 mg	Median 96% of patients rated their attacks as none or mild pain 15 min after injection. No difference in efficacy with long term use.	1 patient withdrew due to S/E. 94/138 reported other S/E.	S/C sumatriptan is a safe and effective treatment for CH even with long term use	Ekbom et al., 1995
Open labelled 57 patients 2031 cluster attacks over 1 year	S/C sumatriptan 6 mg	88% of attacks improved, 57% pain-free 15 min after injection	91 non-serious side-effects in 32/52 patients. 4/52 patients withdrew due to S/E. 7/52 reported increased incidence of cluster attacks.	Long-term efficacy of subcutaneous sumatriptan established. A small but worrying number of patients noticed increased number of attacks when on sumatriptan injections.	Gobel et al., 1998
26 patients, 4 cluster attacks each. Random sequential treatment.	S/C sumatriptan 6 mg injection vs. inhaled sumatriptan 20 mg	S/C drug, all attacks alleviated within 15 min. Intranasal drug only 25/52 achieved this.	8/52 attacks bitter taste with intranasal drug. No withdrawals or serious side-effects.	Clear superiority of S/C over intranasal route of administration for alleviating acute cluster attacks	Hardebo and Dahlof, 1998
10 patients, 154 cluster attacks. Open labelled study over 6 months.	Intranasal sumatriptan 20 mg	Headache response 42/152 attacks at 15 min. And 76/152 attacks or 8/10 patients had over 50% response at 30 min.	Side-effect experienced in 6/154 attacks. Bitter taste most common.	Intranasal sumatriptan effective when measured as response 30 min after drug administration	Schuh-Hofer et al., 2002
Placebo controlled study ECH (13 patients)	Hyperbaric oxygen up to 2.5 atm vs. air	6/7 on treatment responded. None on air.	None reported	Good evidence for efficacy of hyperbaric oxygen. Randomisation not stated.	Di Sabato et al., 1993
Open labelled study 4 CCH 1 ECH (5 patients)	Oral olanzapine 2.5–10 mg. At least 2 treated attacks.	4/5 had >80% reduction pain within 20 min	Drowsiness reported	This needs to be tested in larger placebo controlled studies	Rozen, 2001
Open labelled study 2 CCH 20 ECH	10% Intravenous magnesium sulphate 1–2 g over 5 min	38 infusions given 9/22 reported improvement	Flushed feeling during all infusions	Correlation found between symptom improvement and blood magnesium levels	Mauskop et al., 1995
Open labelled study of nitroglycerin induced cluster attacks then spontaneous attacks (11 patients)	Cocaine flakes 50 mg to the sphenopalatine foramen for induced attacks, 5–10% cocaine solution for 3–7 days for spontaneous attacks	10/11 patients reported. 50% relief with cocaine for their induced attacks. 'Most patients' also reported relief from their spontaneous attacks when used at home.	No serious side-effects. 1 patient used above-recommended dose and reported CNS excitation.	Interesting but impractical treatment at present	Barre, 1982
Spontaneous and nitroglycerin induced cluster attacks in 5 patients	1 ml intranasal lignocaine 4% ± decongestant. Repeat application if pain persistent.	4/5 patients reported at least 75% pain alleviation with intranasal lignocaine	No side-effects reported	Intranasal lignocaine alleviated cluster attacks and authors recommended early treatment with repeat application with or without decongestant	Kittrelle et al., 1985

TABLE 8 *continued*

Study method and number of patients	Drug and dosage	Outcome reported in each study	Side-effects/withdrawals	Comments	Reference
Open labelled ECH (30 patients)	4–6 sprays of 4% lignocaine intranasally over 2 attacks	Only 8/30 reported moderate pain relief. The rest had mild or no relief.	2/30 reported being dizzy or weak after lignocaine	Results not as good as that of Kittrelle et al. The nasal dropper may be a better method of drug delivery?	Robbins, 1995
3-arm double-blind placebo controlled in 9 patients with nitroglycerin-induced cluster attacks	1 ml of intranasal cocaine 10%, lignocaine 10% or placebo	All attacks treated with cocaine or lignocaine pain-free at 35 min while pain still present in patients treated with saline	No side-effects reported	Intranasal lignocaine beneficial but not as fast acting as 10% cocaine in aborting induced cluster attacks	Costa et al., 2000
Placebo cross-over study (19 patients)	Prednisolone 30 mg for acute attacks and 20 mg/day for prophylaxis	17/19 on active treatment improved	Not stated	Outcome not properly defined and data lacking on many aspects in this report	Anonymous, 1988
Placebo and active controlled cross-over study of 3 arms (8 patients)	Somatostatin i.v. 25 μg/min for 20 min; Placebo or ergotamine 250 μg i.m.	Pain intensity reduced by 18% with somatostatin, 14% by ergotamine. Pain duration reduced 40% ergot, 29% somatostatin.	Nausea reported for both ergotamine and somatostatin	Treatment with somatostatin impractical as can only be administered i.v. Beneficial effects also modest.	Sicuteri et al., 1984

TABLE 9

Studies of prophylactic treatment for cluster headaches

Study method and number of patients	Drug and dosage	Outcome reported in each study	Side-effects/withdrawals	Comments	Reference
Single-blind placebo controlled cross-over (28 patients)	Pizotifen 1–4 mg/day	16/28 on pizotifen at least 50% improvement	2 withdrew. Sedation in 10 and weight gain 8 on active treatment.	Some evidence for pizotifen but side-effects also considerable	Ekbom, 1969
Case series of 60 patients reported. 49 treated with methylsergide. Case studies (6)	Methylsergide mean 6 mg/day. Methylsergide 2–6 mg.	18/49 immediate improvement sustained. >1 month in 16/49. 'satisfactory improvement' 5/6.	7 patients discontinued therapy from S/E	This was a reported case series without control or randomisation. Duration of satisfactory improvement unknown.	Watson and Evans, 1987; Pearce, 1980
Open labelled ECH (33) CCH (15)	Verapramil 120–1200 mg/day (mean 354)	24/33 ECH and 9/15 CCH had >75% improvement. 9/33 did not respond or dropout.	3 patients drop out from adverse effects. 12/45 reported milder side-effects.	Good evidence for the use of verapramil for the prophylaxis of ECH and CCH.	Gabai and Spierings, 1989
Randomised cross-over study. Prophylaxis for CCH (30 patients).	Verapramil 360 mg/day vs. lithium carbonate 900 mg/day. 23 weeks (2 week washout in between).	Verapramil arm: improvement in 12/24 of patients within 1 week. Lithium: only 9/24.	3/24 on verapramil and 7/24 on lithium reported side-effects. None dropped out because of side-effects.	Verapramil is at least as good as lithium for CCH	Bussone et al., 1990
Open labelled (ECH 13 patients)	Nimodipine 30 mg qds 10–30 days	7/13 patients, cluster attacks ceased within 10 days (mean 5)	No side-effects reported	Spontaneous resolution of cluster in some of these patients? Some early data to suggest a possible efficacy of nimodipine.	De Carolis et al., 1988
Double-blind cross-over and open labelled (8 patients)	Nimodipine 60 vs 120 mg/day then Nifedipine 30–180 mg/day or verapramil 160–720 mg/day	Reduction in mean no. attacks with all 3 agents. Nifedipine and nimodipine appear better than verapramil.	S/E reported in all groups: 40% on nimodipine; 60% nifedipine; 50% verapramil.	Calcium channel blockers are effective prophylaxis for cluster headache	Meyer and Hardenberg, 1983
Open labelled ECH (9), CCH (10)	Prednisone 10–80 mg/day for 10–30 days	Complete relief 11/19 patients. At least 50% better in another 3/19.	Weight gain reported	Prednisone is effective prophylaxis for both ECH and CCH	Couch and Ziegler, 1978
Case study 1 patient	Intravenous methylprednisolone 0.5 g weekly followed by 1 g i.v. every 2–3 weeks	Substantial alleviation of cluster attacks	No serious side-effects reported	Very large doses of steroids administered and impractical because in-patient treatment necessary	Cianchetti et al., 1998
Open labelled ECH (8), CCH (12), 1 first cluster (21 patients)	Lithium 300–1500 mg/day	Absolute improvement 11/21, partial 5/21. No improvement 5/21.	2 patients withdrew from S/E. 3 others transient S/E reported.	Lithium equally effective in CCH and ECH	Damasio and Lyon, 1980
Open labelled ECH (11), CCH (8)	Lithium sulphate. F/U CCH 1–36 (mean 13) months ECH 2 weeks–2 years.	Remission (75% reduction attacks) in CCH patients. ECH patients average 15% improvement at week 1. 3 did not respond at all.	Tremor, polydipsia, diarrhoea reported. 2 patients with ECH withdrew because of tremor.	CCH early results were good. Long term only 3/8 continued for over 1 year: reduced efficacy and change to ECH. ECH results variable, effective in some, none or little in 7/11.	Ekbom, 1981

Study	Treatment	Results	Side-effects	Comments	Reference
Open labelled CCH (32 patients)	Lithium carbonate 600–900 mg. 4 week titration. Up to 32 weeks follow-up.	27/28 patients who completed study had reduction in number of cluster attacks	4 dropouts. 8/28 patients who continued experienced side-effects.	Strong evidence for a beneficial effect of lithium for prophylaxis of CCH especially first week of treatment	Kudrow, 1977
Open labelled CCH (17), ECH (14) (31 patients)	Lithium carbonate 600–1200 mg/day. 2 weeks to 4 months.	20/31 patients reported over 60% benefit. 4/31 no response.	1 patient reported lethargy	Reduced duration, frequency and severity of attacks in over half of treated patients	Mathew, 1978
Open labelled ECH (68), CCH (22) (90 patients)	Lithium carbonate 600–1200 mg/day. Most patients 900 mg/day. CCH patients follow-up 3–48 months (22). ECH treated until 1 week after cessation of cluster bout.	CCH patients 18/22 better by 90% within 1 week. Long-term F/U 4/22 relapsed. 11/22 continued benefit, 7/11 changed to ECH. ECH patients 3/4 patients improved by more than 60%. No significant change in cluster period.	2 patients developed goitre. 35/90 patients experienced side-effects. No dropouts from side-effects.	Long-term benefit of lithium in CCH and efficacy of lithium for ECH even with repeated bouts. Side-effects preclude long-term treatment?	Savoldi et al., 1983
Open labelled study (9 patients)	Baclofen 5–10 mg tds	6/9 patients responded by having reduced cluster attacks by end of week 1. 1 other by end of week 2.	No serious side-effects and no dropouts.	Interesting observation that need to be tested in placebo controlled trials	Hering-Hanit and Gadoth, 2001
Open labelled CCH (1), ECH (12) patients	Chlorpromazine 75–700 mg/day. F/U 1 month to 3 years.	12/13 had complete relief, 9 of these withdrew from treatment within 2–3 weeks	'unpleasant oppressive feeling' reported. 1 patient had sedation.	Small study, some early evidence for chlorpromazine as CH prophylaxis but considerable potential side-effects. Safer drugs now available for the same indication.	Caviness and O'Brien, 1980
Placebo controlled ECH (18), CCH (2)	Melatonin 10 mg/day vs. placebo for 2 weeks	5/8 ECH and 0/2 CCH on melatonin improved. None on placebo did.	None reported	Randomisation not stated. Some evidence for efficacy of melatonin.	Leone et al., 1996
Case reports CCH (2 patients)	Melatonin 9 mg/day	Both patients improved	None reported	Melatonin may also work on patients with CCH	Peres and Rozen, 2001
Open labelled (20 patients)	Methylergonovine 0.2 mg 3–4 times a day as add on to other prophylaxis agent	19/20 patients reported. 50% improvement of their cluster attacks within 1 week.	2/20 reported side-effects	This is an ergot derivative and provides some evidence for the use of ergot prophylaxis in intractable cluster headache	Mueller et al., 1997
Case series CCH 4 patients	Hyperbaric Oxygen, 10 sessions of 70 min each over 2 weeks	2/4 reduced duration and frequency of attacks. 1 only frequency and 1 no response.	Not reported	All patients also on lithium during treatment. Some evidence for prophylactic effect of HBO.	Pascual et al., 1995
Case series ECH (23), CCH (31) (54 patients)	Dihydroergotamine 0.5–1 mg i.v. tds. Up to 5 days.	62 admissions, all patients were headache free. 58/64 treatments headache free within 3 d.	8/54 reported nausea, 2/54 had chest tightness	Regular doses of ergots can be an effective prophylaxis in this case series	Mather et al., 1991

TABLE 9 continued

Study method and number of patients	Drug and dosage	Outcome reported in each study	Side-effects/withdrawals	Comments	Reference
Open labelled study ECH (13), CCH (2) (15 patients)	Sodium valproate 600–1200 mg/day	11/15 reported headache improvement	Mild nausea 3/15	This study now superseded by placebo controlled study where valproate was no better than placebo	Hering and Kuritzky, 1989
Single case study	Gabapentin 300 mg b.d.	Substantial improvement and resolution of cluster attacks	No serious side-effects reported	Small dose of gabapentin for reported effect	Tay et al., 2001
Open labelled study CCH and ECH (12 patients)	Gabapentin up to 900 mg a day. ECH for 60 days, CCH for 6 months.	Shortening of cluster bout and alleviation of CCH reported	2/12 patients reported drowsiness	Preliminary indication to suggest that gabapentin may be effective as a CH prophylaxis	Leandri et al., 2001
Open labelled study 2 CCH 7 ECH, Cluster-tic 1 (10 patients)	Topiramate 50–125 mg/day	Cluster remission within 1–3 weeks in 9/10 patients	Mild S/E reported by 3/10. None had to discontinue treatment from S/E.	Early suggestion for possible use of topiramate as CH prophylaxis	Wheeler and Carrazana, 1999
Open labelled 3 CCH and 2 ECH (5 patients)	Topiramate 75–200 mg	Cluster remission in 3/5 patients	2 withdrew from S/E.	Relatively rapid escalation in dosage of topiramate caused S/E	Forderreuther et al., 2002
Open labelled study ECH (8) CCH (5)	Transdermal clonidine patches delivering 0.2–0.3 mg/d for 1 week	Mean halving of the intensity and frequency of attacks. 2/13 patients did not respond.	Tiredness in 6/13 patients	Transdermal clonidine may be useful as prophylaxis for CH	D'Andrea et al., 1995
Open labelled study ECH (16 patients)	5 mg clonidine patches releasing 0.2 mg/day for 7 days or 7.5 mg patches	5/15 patients who completed study became attack free	1 patient drop out because of increased no. attacks. Mild to moderate tiredness 14/16 patients.	Modest benefit only from transdermal clonidine	Leone et al., 1997
Single blind study of ipsilateral and contralateral application (70 patients)	0.1 ml of 10 mMol capsaicin applied intranasally every day. Follow-up period for 60 days.	Contralateral application had no effect. Ipsilateral application: 21/26 ECH and 15/19 CCH had at least 50% reduction in attacks.	Burning pain from capsaicin lasting up to 20 min. This decreased after 5–8 applications.	Interesting but potentially very uncomfortable application of capsaicin. Vallinoid analogues that do not cause such burning may be more promising.	Fusco et al., 1994
Double-blind placebo controlled 8 CCH 5 ECH (13 patients)	Intranasal 0.025% Capsaicin cream + Camphor 3% vs. Camphor 3% in vehicle.	Statistical reduction in headache severity in those given capsaicin. Individual patients not reported.	None reported	Difficult to compare as all ECH patients were randomised to active group.	Marks et al., 1993
Case report 1 patient	Naratriptan 2.5 mg b.d.	Complete remission	None reported	First evidence for the efficacy of oral naratriptan as cluster prophylaxis	Eekers et al., 2001
Case report 1 patient	Naratriptan 2.5 mg b.d.	Complete remission	None reported	Very preliminary evidence and surprising because larger trials have found oral sumatriptan taken regularly to be ineffective	Loder, 2002

TABLE 10

Case study 3

Please read the following. What is the differential diagnosis and how should he be treated?

You are requested to give a second opinion on a 51-year-old man admitted for further investigations. For the past 11 months, he experienced daily, severe unilateral pain over the right temple 5–6 times a day lasting between 20 and 30 min. The pain radiates to his upper molar teeth and is associated with tearing and erythema of his eye as well as a blockage of his right nostril. He has consulted and undergone dental and ophthalmologic treatment without any relieve for his pain. He smokes 20–30 cigarettes a day but avoids drinking alcohol as this may precipitate an attack of his headache. Physical examination was normal. MRI scan of his head revealed two high signal lesions in the cerebral hemispheres. These were reported to be nonspecific changes. Full blood count, ESR, Vit. B_{12}, folate, urea and electrolytes, liver and thyroid function tests and autoantibody screen were all normal or negative. Lumbar puncture revealed normal opening pressure and CSF constituents.

Please see Table 17 at the end of the chapter for the answer.

patterns is still unclear as episodic PH can evolve into CPH.

Over 100 cases has been described in the literature and the diagnosis may not be as uncommon as initially thought. The considerable overlap of some of the symptoms of episodic PH with CH means that there is always a chance of misdiagnosis. Whether these two conditions are separate entities or two extremes of a spectrum of headache is unclear. There are many reports where the distinction between PH and CH is blurred (Hochman, 1981; Rapoport et al., 1981) and response to treatment is used as the final arbitrator in deciding diagnosis.

3.1. Definition

The first cases described by Sjaastad and Dale (1974) were patients who experienced repeated episodes of short-lasting unilateral head and face pain. These attacks occurred many times a day and persisted for years. It was later found that there is another variation to these headaches where some patients may experience periods of pain-free remission. The original syndrome was termed chronic paroxysmal hemicrania (CPH) and episodic paroxysmal hemicrania (EPH) is used to describe the latter patterns of attacks.

3.2. Epidemiology

Unlike CH, CPH appears to be more common in women with a reported gender ratio of 2 : 1 and even 3 : 1. EPH however has been reported to show no gender preference. The age of onset of PH varies greatly, and cases from childhood to the ninth decade have been reported. In general, this is a condition affecting young adults with onset most common in the third decade. Unlike CH, there does not appear to be a genetic link and only one familial series has been diagnosed (by Manzoni and mentioned in Antonaci and Sjaastad, 1989).

3.3. Aetiology and pathophysiology

The pathogenesis of this condition is unknown. Goadsby and Lipton (1997) have summarised the investigation findings in patients with paroxysmal hemicrania. They concluded that these attacks are associated with parasympathetic activation mediated through the facial nerve with second-order neurones from the greater superficial petrosal efferents. They did not find any convincing difference in the pathophysiology between cluster headaches and CPH. They have pointed out however that the shorter duration and higher frequency of attacks together with less profound autonomic signs and symptoms seen in patients with CPH may imply a different central nervous system mechanism for CPH compared to that for cluster headaches.

3.4. Clinical features

All the clinical information about the paroxysmal hemicranias come from case series collected over

TABLE 11

KEY FACTS: clinical features of paroxysmal hemicrania

Character	Clawing, throbbing, pulsatile and pressure
Site and radiation	Orbits, temporal, cheek, forehead, neck/shoulder, occiput
Periodicity, onset, duration	8–15 attacks daily. Mean of 10 attacks a day. Pain builds up to a peak and lasts between 15 and 30 min (mean 20 min)
Severity	Excruciating in majority. Less than 5% moderately severe.
Provoking factors	Neck flexion, rotation, pressure over C2 root, drinking alcohol
Relieving factors	Menstruation, stress, joy
Associated factors	Lacrimation, nasal congestion, rhinorrhoea, conjunctival injection
Clinical examination	Ipsilateral ptosis, conjunctival injection during an attack. Interictal facial erythema and eyelid oedema.
Prognosis	Mostly chronic, may be episodic attacks. Virtually all respond to treatment usually with indomethacin.

many years. The key features are summarised in Table 11 below. No systemic investigation has been performed to validate the clinical features in these patients simply because no investigator has collected a large enough series of patient. It is hoped that as more clinicians recognise this condition, many more patients would be diagnosed and better in-depth studies can be done.

3.4.1. Character and severity

In their summary of 84 cases, Antonaci and Sjaastad (1989) have reported that 'clawing' pain was the most common descriptor and experienced by nearly half of the patients. The next commonest descriptors were throbbing, dental pain, boring and pressing. There were no reports of large numbers of patients being assessed using common tools for studying pain like the McGill Questionnaire. However, even with the relatively small numbers of patients reported so far, there appears to be a difference in the quality of pain between PH and CH patients (see Tables 3 and 14).

3.4.2. Periodicity, timing, duration, onset

It is the frequency of the attacks that helps to differentiate paroxysmal hemicrania from cluster

headaches. Patients with CPH may experience at least 5 and up to 40 attacks a day. For EPH, patients have been reported to suffer up to 30 attacks a day (Antonaci and Sjaastad, 1989). On average, patients report 15 attacks a day where each attack lasts between 2 and 30 min. Attacks can occur anytime during the day and it is not uncommon for patients to be woken up from sleep with an attack.

The daily frequency of attacks may change from day to day. In CPH, patients may experience at least 1 attack a day for years without remission. In EPH, patients may experience daily attacks in bouts that last from 2 weeks to 4 months. They may then go through a pain-free remission from 1 month to 3 years.

3.4.3. Site and radiation

Like CH, the pain of paroxysmal hemicrania is strictly unilateral. This may change with pain affecting the contralateral side during subsequent attacks. There is one report of bilateral pain which has similar characteristics and response to treatment as CPH (Pollmann and Pfaffenrath, 1986). The orbit, periorbital region and the temples are usual sites of pain. Pain is most commonly felt within the area innervated by the ophthalmic division of the trigeminal nerve. Pain outside this site, namely in the cheek and back of the head, has also been reported. The pain may also radiate to the ipsilateral shoulder and arm.

3.4.4. Severity
The pain severity was reported to be excruciating at the peak of an attack by the majority of patients. Less than 5% of patients describe their pain as moderately severe (Antonaci and Sjaastad, 1989). During an attack, pain may build up quickly. Pain severity is reported to vary from one attack to another even throughout the day.

3.4.5. Provoking–relieving factors
In 20% of patients, neck movement has been reported to provoke an attack. Similarly, pressure over the transverse processes of the most rostral cervical vertebrae or the occipital nerve may trigger an attack. In some patients, drinking alcohol has also been reported to provoke an attack of paroxysmal hemicrania (Antonaci and Sjaastad, 1989). During an attack, the pain has been reported to be accentuated by coughing and performing the Valsalva manoeuvre. The attacks are said to improve with menstruation in women. Both stress as well as joy and expectation of good news can also improve PH attacks (Antonaci and Sjaastad, 1989).

3.4.6. Associated features
Acute attacks of paroxysmal hemicrania are invariably associated with autonomic symptoms. In the IHS classification of CPH, one of the main diagnostic criteria is the association of pain with at least one of the following six autonomic symptoms: conjunctival injection, lacrimation, nasal congestion, rhinorrhoea, ptosis or eyelid oedema. It is estimated that during acute attacks, 60% of patients experience ipsilateral lacrimation. The next most common associated symptoms are nasal congestion (42%) and rhinorrhoea (36%) (Newman, 2001). Increased forehead sweating ipsilateral to the pain and a generalised increase in sweating has also been reported. There are also some patients with typical attacks of paroxysmal hemicrania and response to treatment that do not experience the usual autonomic symptoms nor signs

(Bogucki et al., 1984; Pareja et al., 1995).

3.4.7. Findings on examination
Ipsilateral ptosis and conjunctival injection has been reported in one third of patients during an attack of paroxysmal hemicrania (Newman, 2001). Otherwise, the interictal physical examination is usually normal except in patients with secondary paroxysmal hemicrania.

3.5. Differential diagnosis

Other conditions can mimic attacks similar to PH. Vascular malformations, aneurysms as well as structural lesions around the cavernous sinus have been reported to cause secondary PH. There are also single case reports of raised intracranial pressure (Hannerz, 1993) and a Pancoast tumour (Delreux et al., 1989) giving rise to attacks typical for CPH. CPH has been reported to be associated with trigeminal neuralgia (Caminero et al., 1998; Centonze et al., 2000; Zukerman et al., 2000), migraine (Pareja and Pareja, 1992) and trauma (Matharu and Goadsby, 2001, 2002).

3.6. Investigations

Although paroxysmal hemicrania is thought to be a relatively rare condition, the true incidence is unknown. Similarly, the proportion of patients with intracranial structural abnormalities that may mimic CPH and EPH is also not known. A number of secondary causes have already been reported (see above). For these reasons, it would be reasonable to perform neuroimaging, preferably an MRI scan as routine investigation for patients who experience headaches suggestive of paroxysmal hemicrania. For most patients with paroxysmal hemicrania, cranial MRI scans have been reported to be normal. Narrowing of the ophthalmic veins has been reported as an associated feature in some patients (Antonaci, 1994) but this is not a consistent finding and the relevance is unclear.

Blood tests recommended for investigating patients with suspected paroxysmal hemicrania include a full blood count to exclude thrombocythaemia and erythrocyte sedimentation rate to exclude vasculitis (Goadsby and Lipton, 1997). In patients who experience pain on both sides, a lumbar puncture to exclude raised intracranial pressure may also be useful. A chest X-ray should also be performed to exclude a Pancoast tumour. Electrocardiographic monitoring is useful in some patients to exclude a bundle branch block or cardiac dysrhythmias which are reported abnormalities associated with paroxysmal hemicrania.

3.7. Management

One of the most important characteristic and according to the IHS classification, a diagnostic criterion for PH is its response to indomethacin. The usual starting dose is 25 mg tds orally and the dose can be doubled if there is none or incomplete response after 2 weeks. Changes may be necessary to find the minimum effective dose. The side-effects of indomethacin include fluid retention and renal impairment although gastric irritation is the most troublesome. Patients should be prescribed a H2 antagonist or misoprostol prophylactically. The rectal preparation of indomethacin is not free from this adverse effect either. For patients with night time PH, long acting indomethacin can be an effective treatment. Patients with episodic PH usually need a high dose of indomethacin that is then reduced very gradually. Patients with chronic PH may need long-term treatment although prolonged remission of CPH after discontinuation of indomethacin has been reported (Sjaastad and Antonaci, 1987).

Where patients did not respond to indomethacin, the diagnosis should be reviewed. If patients do respond but are unable to tolerate indomethacin, other medications can be considered. Acetylsalicylic acid, verapramil, steroids, naproxen and acetazolamide have been reported to be effective in one case series (Evers and Husstedt, 1996). There is also a case report of a patient with CPH who responded to treatment with the COX-2 inhibitor celecoxib (Mathew et al., 2000). This class of drugs are reported to have a reduced tendency to cause stomach

irritation and may be an alternative to using other non-steroidals. The utility of the triptans for treating paroxysmal hemicranias remain unclear. There is a case report of a patient with CPH who responded to subcutaneous sumatriptan. Yet a more detailed study of seven patients with CPH found that 6 mg subcutaneous sumatriptan was ineffective (Antonaci et al., 1998). Until more patients with this condition are identified and a large placebo controlled study is performed, it would be reasonable to use other non-steroidals drugs in patients who are allergic or unable to tolerate indomethacin.

Please read through case study 4 in Table 12 before continuing reading.

4. SUNCT

4.1. Definition

This syndrome is the acronym for *S*hort-lasting *U*nilateral *N*euralgiform headaches with *C*onjunctival injection and *T*earing (Pareja et al., 1997). This name provides a description of the symptoms experienced by patients with this condition. This disorder was first described in 1978 and remains one of the rarer primary headache syndromes.

4.2. Epidemiology

The age of onset has been reported to be from 22 to 73 with a mean around 51. In one of the largest series of patients described, there is a male preponderance with mean age of onset of 51 years (Pareja and Sjaastad, 1997).

4.3. Aetiology and pathophysiology

The pathogenesis of SUNCT is unclear but in at least one patient, SPECT scans have revealed activation of the same area in the hypothalamus similar to that seen in patients with CH (May et al., 1999). It is possible that all the primary neurovascular syndromes cluster headache, paroxysmal hemicra-

TABLE 12

Case study 4

Has this patient got migraine and how may you be able to help him?

A 52-year-old right-handed commercial property investor consulted you in the outpatient clinic. He was involved in a road traffic accident 25 years ago where he was said to sustain a whiplash injury to his neck. Since then, he has developed episodes of 'migraine'. The frequency and character of attacks have remained the same except that in the last 2–3 years, they appear to be triggered by drinking alcohol. On average, he gets 6 attacks a month although he may experience 2–3 attacks 1 week and then none for the next 2–3 weeks. A typical attack starts around at between 3 and 4 a.m. with discomfort around his left shoulder followed quickly by severe pain around the left eye. The pain is confined to one side only and he states that 97 out of 100 attacks would be on the left. The attack is described as a sharp poking pain in the eye associated with a sensation of blockage of the ipsilateral ear and sometimes the nose. He does not tear and he has not noticed erythema of his eye or drooping of the lid. He normally paces around with the pain, putting pressure on the eye. Each episode may last up to 3 h and normally terminated when he either vomits, loses awareness with the pain or both. Apart from alcohol, pressure over his neck or a flare up of his neck pain for whatever reason would also precipitate an attack. Taking naproxen can sometimes abort an attack. His headache has never responded to oral triptans. He was treated with amitriptyline as headache prophylaxis without any discernible benefit. He also smokes 5 cigarettes and 1 cigar a day and still drinks a bottle of wine a day. He has consulted numerous specialists and tried many treatments for his migraine without any benefit and came in with a large package of MRI scans of his head and spine, all which were normal. He has seen a physiotherapist privately who informed him that there are 'scars' in his neck that are causing these headaches.

Please see Table 18 at the end of the chapter for some solutions.

sopharyngeal nerve rather than first division of the trigeminal nerve appears to be activated. This case report also illustrates the close connections between the trigeminal and glossopharyngeal nerves as well as the special visceral or autonomic nuclei within the brain stem. There may only be a difference in the pattern of activation of the 'generator' giving rise to all these related but not the same types of headaches.

4.4. Clinical features

The characteristic features of SUNCT are repeated short lasting attacks of unilateral pain centred around one eye with autonomic signs and symptoms. The number of attacks varies greatly from one a day to 30 an hour (Pareja and Sjaastad, 1997). Each attack lasts between 10 and 60 s although some attacks may be up to 5 min in duration. The attacks are accompanied by ipsilateral tearing, nasal discharge, nasal obstruction and conjunctival erythema. Pain intensity during attacks is moderate to severe and pain descriptors during attacks include burning, sharp, electric shock-like. A small number of patients also experience a status-like pattern of attacks where repeated bouts of up to 60 attacks lasting hours (Leone et al., 2000a,b) or even up to 3 days (Pareja et al., 1996) may occur. Most patients are pain free in between these bouts although some described persistent dull discomfort. Attacks can occur throughout the day but a bimodal pattern with more attacks during the morning and late afternoon/evening may also be evident. Some patients have attacks during the night. These symptomatic periods may last days to months. The frequency of symptomatic periods also varies greatly and may be as infrequent as only twice a year. Pain-free remission can be as short as a few weeks or as long as 7 years in duration (Pareja and Sjaastad, 1997). It averages a few months a year.

Numerous provoking factors have been identified (Pareja and Sjaastad, 1997). Touching, stroking the face and hair in the ipsilateral trigeminal distribution of these attacks are the most common triggers. The majority of cases were primary syndromes although

nia and SUNCT share the same anatomical correlates. This is supported by the case reported by Wingerchuk et al. (2000). In their case study, a 41 year old woman had pain in the throat rather than around the eye yet experienced autonomic symptoms typical for CPH. In this patient, the glos-

TABLE 13

KEY FACTS: clinical features of SUNCT

Character	Burning, stabbing, piercing electric-like
Site and radiation	Ocular, periorbital spreading to forehead or temple
Periodicity, onset, duration	Abrupt onset, maximal severity within 3–5 s. Attacks last less than 2 min. Between 1 and 30 attacks a day. Pain free in between attack.
Severity	Moderate to severe
Provoking factors	Neck movement, touching trigger area: forehead, hair, chewing, blowing nose, brushing teeth
Relieving factors	None consistently reported
Associated factors	Lacrimation, conjunctival injection, rhinorrhoea, nasal obstruction, eyelid oedema
Clinical examination	Hypoaesthesia over ophthalmic division of trigeminal nerve with reduced corneal reflex reported in a small number of patients between attacks
Prognosis	Remissions usually observed but some bouts may last many months and even years

structural abnormalities around the cerebellopontine angle, especially vascular malformations, can cause symptoms similar to SUNCT (De Benedittis, 1996; Pareja and Sjaastad, 1997).

The key features of SUNCT are summarised in Table 13.

4.5. Differential diagnosis

There are numerous similarities between SUNCT and ophthalmic division trigeminal neuralgia. Both conditions are characterised by episodic unilateral short attacks triggered by innocuous mechanical stimuli. Anticonvulsants are effective for treating both conditions (see below). There is a hypothesis that SUNCT may just be a type of transformed first division trigeminal neuralgia with autonomic symptoms (Sjaastad et al., 1993; Bouhassira et al., 1994; Benoliel and Sharav, 1998). In his series of 22 patients with trigeminal neuralgia, Sharav reported six patients with ipsilateral lacrimation. Sjaastad et al. (1997) attempted to clarify this by carefully studying the character of attacks in patients with first division trigeminal neuralgia and comparing them with SUNCT. Half of the 16 patients with first division TG had lacrimation but only 2 had conjunctival in-

jection and rhinorrhoea. In general, the attacks of SUNCT last longer than TG and autonomic features, when present, tend to be less pronounced. The anatomical sites where pain radiates to and the trigger areas are different for SUNCT and trigeminal neuralgia. They concluded that SUNCT and TG are essentially separate conditions (Sjaastad et al., 1997).

4.6. Management

SUNCT was thought to be resistant to treatment and until recently only carbamezepine and steroids has been reported to have some effect (Pareja et al., 1995; Pareja and Sjaastad, 1997). Recent case studies however have reported that lamotrigine (Leone et al., 2000a,b; D'Andrea et al., 2001) as well as gabapentin (Graff-Radford, 2000) were effective in alleviating SUNCT attacks. Hannerz and Linderoth (2002) also reported surgical treatment for SUNCT. In their three patients, retrogasserian glycerol rhizotomy provided complete pain relieve for between 2 and 4 years. In all of these patients, a repeat procedure was necessary. Two had repeat glycerol rhizotomy and a third underwent a compressive rhizotomy by balloon inflation.

TABLE 14

KEY FACTS: differences and similarities between CH, PH, SUNCT and TG

Features	Cluster headache	Paroxysmal hemicrania	SUNCT	Trigeminal neuralgia
Prevalence	40–100,000	Rare	Very rare	Point 0.1%
Sex F : M ratio	1 : 6	2 : 1	1 : 10	1.5 : 1
Age of onset	20–40	6–81	30–68	60–80
Site of maximal pain	Orbit/temple	Orbit/temple	Periorbital	V1 and V2 territory
Radiation	Upper teeth/jaw	Cheek, forehead, neck, shoulder, occiput	Forehead, temple, nose, cheek	Not outside trigeminal area
Number of daily attacks	0–8	0–40	0–80	0 to hundreds
Duration of attacks	15–180 min, average 20–45 min	2–120 min, average 2–30 min	15–250 s, average 10–60 s	seconds
Autonomic features	Most profound	Yes but less than CH	Yes but short lasting like the attacks	none
Precipitating factors	Alcohol, volatile gases, low atmospheric pressure, nitroglycerin	Neck movement, sometimes alcohol	Trigger areas outside trigeminal territory, neck movement. NOT alcohol.	Light touch
Successful acute treatment(s)	Subcutaneous sumatriptan, oxygen inhalation	Indomethacin, naproxen, diclofenac		Carbamazepine
Successful prophylaxis	Verapramil, lithium, corticosteroids	?Prednisone	Carbamezepine, steroids, lamotrigine, gabapentin	None

5. Overview

There are numerous clinical similarities between all three headache syndromes described above and these are summarised in Table 14. They can also co-exist, as in the two patients with CPH and CH described by Tehindrazanarivelo et al. (1992). As pointed out by Goadsby and colleagues, the mechanism and pathogenesis of these conditions may also be similar (Goadsby and Edvinsson, 1994; Goadsby and Lipton, 1997). As previously described, functional imaging has shown that the same area of the ipsilateral hypothalamic grey matter appears to be activated during an attack of SUNCT as in patients with cluster headache (May et al., 1999). Learning to differentiate between these conditions is useful in optimising treatment but may sometimes be difficult and in some patients a therapeutic challenge is necessary to clarify the diagnosis. The important thing about these conditions is to recognise and appreciate how easy it is to attribute them to another cause. For example, both CPH and CH have been reported to be misdiagnosed as dental disorders (Delcanho and Graff-Radford, 1993; Penarrocha et al., 2001). These conditions, although rare, must be considered in any differential diagnosis of facial pain. An overview of their management is provided in Fig. 1. For answers to case studies see Tables 15–18.

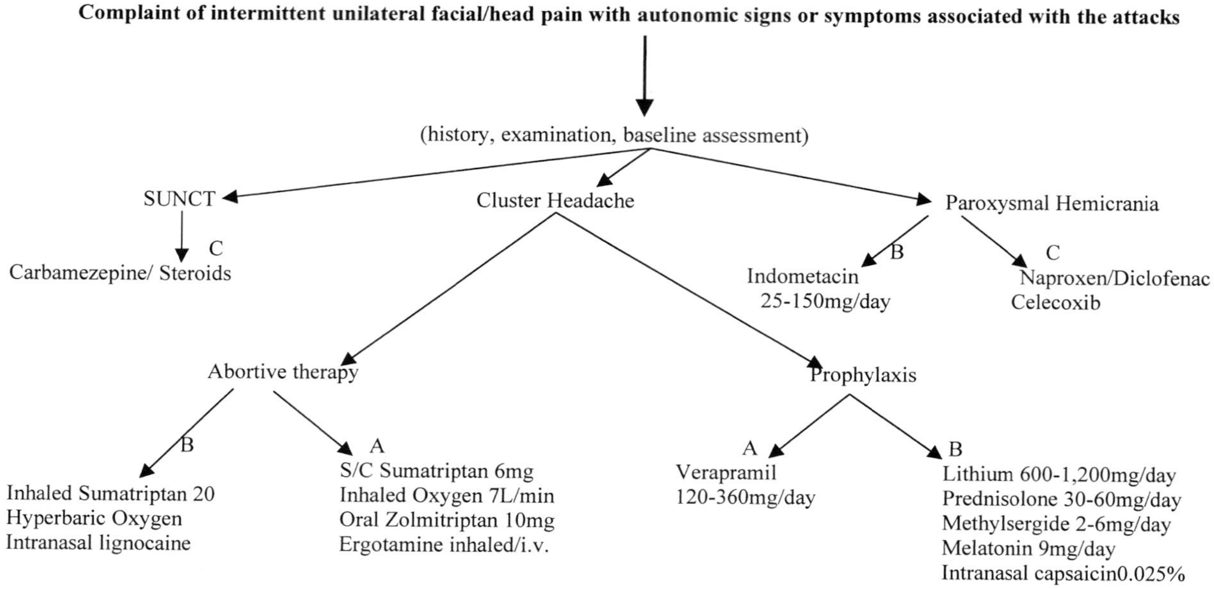

Complaint of intermittent unilateral facial/head pain with autonomic signs or symptoms associated with the attacks

(history, examination, baseline assessment)

SUNCT ← Cluster Headache → Paroxysmal Hemicrania

SUNCT:
C
Carbamezepine/ Steroids

Paroxysmal Hemicrania:
B
Indometacin
25-150mg/day

C
Naproxen/Diclofenac
Celecoxib

Cluster Headache:
Abortive therapy — Prophylaxis

Abortive therapy:
B
Inhaled Sumatriptan 20
Hyperbaric Oxygen
Intranasal lignocaine

A
S/C Sumatriptan 6mg
Inhaled Oxygen 7L/min
Oral Zolmitriptan 10mg
Ergotamine inhaled/i.v.

Prophylaxis:
A
Verapramil
120-360mg/day

B
Lithium 600-1,200mg/day
Prednisolone 30-60mg/day
Methylsergide 2-6mg/day
Melatonin 9mg/day
Intranasal capsaicin0.025%

Fig. 1. Algorithm on management of cluster headaches, paroxysmal hemicrania and SUNCT including level of evidence.Footnote. As you have seen there is good quality evidence and most is based on case reports and expert opinions. It is therefore difficult to call the schemata presented above as anything more than a suggestion based on my reading of the current literature and my own clinical practise.Grade of evidence:A, based on strongest evidence available, including at least one randomised controlled trial as part of the body of literature of overall quality.B, based on availability of well conducted clinical studies but not randomised trials.C, based on expert consensus of the group in the absence of studies of good quality *or* good quality studies but show inconclusive evidence of efficacy of high level of adverse events.

TABLE 15

Answer to case study 1 in Table 4

This man had a recent onset of painful Horner's syndrome and episodes of pain suggestive of cluster headaches. Investigations are necessary to exclude potential causes of this painful Horner's syndrome. He underwent an MRI scan of his head which was reported not to show any abnormality of the brain. An MR angiogram showed evidence of left carotid artery dissection. He was heparinised then started on warfarin. In addition, he was treated with verapramil to try and control his cluster headaches.

Learning points from this case study:

- Recent onset Horner's syndrome, especially painful needs to be investigated.

- Although attacks are typical for CH, the presence of neurological deficit between attacks means that the threshold for investigation is lower.

- The treatment for symptomatic cluster headache is the same as for idiopathic CH as long as the underlying condition is also addressed.

- Response to treatment does not mean that it is simply idiopathic CH. There is at least 1 case report of carotid artery dissection where pain was improved by administration of a triptan (Leira et al., 2001).

TABLE 16

Answer to case study 2 in Table 6

Cluster headache is such a debilitating condition that I do try to see patients urgently when they appear to experience a bout. The first step is to confirm the diagnosis and exclude any other cause of episodic periorbital pain. He was seen by another neurologist in the past and even had a normal MRI scan of his head. His last bout was 3 years ago and he is no longer on medications. Attacks occurring around the longest and shortest day of the year are common and it was interesting to note that his last bout was in the early summer. He had ascribed the nasal blockage and tearing to crying during these attacks. Physical examination was normal and he was sent to have an ECG before being started on verapramil, a course of corticosteroids for 3 weeks and given a supply of subcutaneous sumatriptan injections. Oxygen therapy would be considered if these attacks are not adequately controlled in spite of large doses of sumatriptan.

TABLE 17

Answer to case study 3 in Table 10

This patient was initially diagnosed as having cluster headache. The large number of attacks during a bout together with the relatively short duration and less prominent autonomic symptoms make episodic paroxysmal hemicrania a possible diagnosis. This man was given a trial of indomethacin 75 mg a day. At 2 months follow up, he reported that the duration of his headache was much reduced by the medication. For the first 4 weeks, he experienced a single attack of pain a day that lasted less than a minute. Later, duration of pain gradually became longer but he would still only have one attack a day lasting for about 10 min with the medication. He was advised to double the dose of indomethacin. A therapeutic response like this, even though incomplete alleviation of pain, still supports the diagnosis of paroxysmal hemicrania.

6. Summary

The chapter is summarised in Table 19.

TABLE 18

Answer to case study 4 Table 12

Stereotypic episodes like these which are strictly unilateral associated with marked agitation are unlikely to be migraine. This is partially supported by the lack of benefit from taking medications usually used to treat migraine. Cluster headaches are possible. These attacks may be precipitated by alcohol, they are centred around the eye and the character of pain and behaviour during an attack is typical. These attacks are however not associated with very profound autonomic symptoms. Another possible diagnosis is a forme fruste of paroxysmal hemicrania with migrainous features. Paroxysmal hemicrania has been reported to be triggered off after trauma and the character as well as response to naproxen would support this diagnosis. His attacks are also triggered by pressure and movements of his neck.

Neurological examination was normal with no evidence of a Horner's syndrome. The investigations were reviewed and it was confirmed that no structural abnormalities were found. This man was carefully counselled. The nature of his work means that avoiding alcohol is likely to be impractical. It was explained to him that he may have either cluster headaches or paroxysmal hemicrania. This man refuses to take any further medications regularly but would be willing to try indomethacin first during an attack. If this fails, he will be reviewed and can then be persuaded to carry a small supply of subcutaneous sumatriptan with him.

It can be difficult with some headache syndromes to give a precise diagnosis, especially when the patient no longer takes note of his symptoms. He has accepted the diagnosis of migraine and his aim in coming to clinic was to look for other treatments for his migraine. He did not expect any doubts to be raised regarding this diagnosis.

Appendix A. Internet resources

http://www.chhelp.org A relatively new patient support group site with numerous links. Good information on understanding the disease but also advice on choosing a new doctor and choosing treatment. A lot of information is specific to the United States, like help on insurance and legal rights. Also some links to well known physicians with special interest

TABLE 19

Summary for Chapter 12

- Cluster headache, paroxysmal hemicrania and SUNCT are uncommon causes of facial pain and headache

- Making a correct diagnosis is important to guide treatment and predict prognosis

- Most of these syndromes are of unknown cause but structural abnormalities around the cavernous sinus and brainstem can also cause similar symptoms

- There is insufficient evidence to recommend investigations for patients with these symptoms

- There is good evidence to recommend subcutaneous sumatriptan as treatment of choice for acute cluster attacks. Inhalation of oxygen is also effective.

- Verapramil is the first line and while lithium is an alternative for the prevention of cluster headache

- Treatment of choice for the paroxysmal hemicranias is indomethacin

- Numerous surgical procedure are described for treating these conditions. Few have long-term follow-up and most of the reported series did not report important data.

- More research is needed to elucidate the pathogenesis and of primary syndromes

in cluster headaches and good links to allow patients to communicate with doctors.

http://www.clusterheadaches.org.uk This is the website for the United Kingdom cluster headache support group OUCH UK with registered office in Leicester. A good site for communicating with other cluster headache sufferers and much more relevant to UK residents.

http://www.clusterheadaches.com This is another large cluster headache support group website based in the United States. Provides a description of the 'Kip scale' described by Bob Kipple which is a patient's perspective of the severity of their cluster headache attacks. There is an 'ask Doc Greg' section

where questions can be posed to a doctor who is a CH sufferer himself. Some interesting answers in this section, like Doc Greg's interpretation of the Gate Theory of Pain and explanation for the efficacy of oxygen for treating acute CH attacks. Good information about medicotherapy and general information for CH. Over 3000 persons listed by country on this site. Isle of Wight listed as separate country on its own!

http://www.clusterheadaches.org/ Incorporating US, UK, Italian and German OUCH. And provides a link to the support groups of these countries.

Appendix B. Further reading

(1) International Headache Society Handbook, published yearly. Scandinavian University Press Oslo ISBN 82-00-37704-0. (Contains a wealth of information on headaches.)

(2) Merskey H, Bogduk N (eds) Classification of chronic pain. Descriptors of chronic pain syndromes and definitions of pain terms. IASP Press, Seattle, WA, 1994, ISBN 0-931092-05-01.

(3) Anonymous. Classification and diagnostic criteria for headache disorders, cranial neuralgias and facial pain. Headache Classification Committee of the International Headache Society. Cephalalgia 1988; 8(Suppl 7): 1–96.

(4) Lipton RB, Micieli G, Russell D, Solomon S, Tfelt-Hansen P, Waldenlind E. Guidelines for controlled trials of drugs in cluster headache. Cephalalgia 1995; 15: 452–462. (Excellent text to understand the design of trials in the field.)

(5) Ekbom K. Treatment of cluster headache: clinical trials, design and results. Cephalalgia 1995; 15(Suppl 15): 33–36.

(6) Pareja JA, Sjaastad O. SUNCT syndrome. A clinical review. Headache 1997; 37: 195–202. (An overview of the condition.)

(7) Sjaastad O. Cluster Headache. In series Major Problems in Neurology, Saunders, London, 1992. (A book written by an expert.)

References

Marked as regards quality according to criteria set by author.
*Poorer quality studies but only ones in the field, old style reviews.
**Cohort studies, high quality case series with controls.
***Randomised controlled trials, high quality original studies.

**Andersson PG, Jespersen LT. Dihydroergotamine nasal spray in the treatment of attacks of cluster headache. A double-blind trial versus placebo. Cephalalgia 1986; 6: 51–54.

Andrasik F, Blanchard EB, Ahles T, Pallmeyer T, Barron KD. Assessing the reactive as well as the sensory component of headache pain. Headache 1981; 21: 218–221.

Antonaci F. Chronic paroxysmal hemicrania and hemicrania continua: orbital phlebography and MRI studies. Headache 1994; 34: 32–34.

Antonaci F, Sjaastad O. Chronic paroxysmal hemicrania (CPH): a review of the clinical manifestations. Headache 1989; 29: 648–656.

*Antonaci F, Pareja JA, Caminero AB, Sjaastad O. Chronic paroxysmal hemicrania and hemicrania continua: lack of efficacy of sumatriptan. Headache 1998; 38: 197–200.

***Bahra A, Gawel MJ, Hardebo JE, Millson D, Breen SA, Goadsby PJ. Oral zolmitriptan is effective in the acute treatment of cluster headache. Neurology 2000; 54: 1832–1839.

Bahra A, May A, Goadsby PJ. Cluster headache: a prospective clinical study with diagnostic implications. Neurology 2002; 58(3): 354–361.

*Barre F. Cocaine as an abortive agent in cluster headache. Headache 1982; 22: 69–73.

Benoliel R, Sharav Y. Trigeminal neuralgia with lacrimation or SUNCT syndrome? Cephalalgia 1998; 18: 85–90.

Blau JN. Behaviour during a cluster headache. Lancet 1993; 342: 723–725.

Bogucki A, Szymanska R, Braciak W. Chronic paroxysmal hemicrania: lack of pre-chronic stage. Cephalalgia 1984; 4: 187–189.

Bouhassira D, Attal N, Esteve M, Chauvin M. 'SUNCT' syndrome. A case of transformation from trigeminal neuralgia? Cephalalgia 1994; 14: 168–170.

***Bussone G, Leone M, Peccarisi C, Micieli G, Granella F, Magri M, Manzoni GC, Nappi G. Double blind comparison of lithium and verapamil in cluster headache prophylaxis. Headache 1990; 30: 411–417.

Caminero AB, Pareja JA, Dobato JL. Chronic paroxysmal hemicrania-tic syndrome. Cephalalgia 1998; 18: 159–161.

Caviness VS Jr, O'Brien P. Cluster headache: response to chlorpromazine. Headache 1980; 20(3): 128–131.

Centonze V, Bassi A, Causarano V, Dalfino L, Centonze A, Albano O. Simultaneous occurrence of ipsilateral cluster headache and chronic paroxysmal hemicrania: a case report. Headache 2000; 40: 54–56.

*Cianchetti C, Zuddas A, Marchei F. High dose intravenous methylprednisolone in cluster headache. J Neurol Neurosurg Psychiatry 1998; 64: 418.

Chervin RD, Zallek SN, Lin X, Hall JM, Sharma N, Hedger KM. Timing patterns of cluster headaches and association with symptoms of obstructive sleep apnea. Sleep Res Online 2000; 3: 107–12.

**Costa A, Pucci E, Antonaci F, Sances G, Granella F, Broich G, Nappi G. The effect of intranasal cocaine and lidocaine on nitroglycerin-induced attacks in cluster headache. Cephalalgia 2000; 20: 85–91.

*Couch JR Jr, Ziegler DK. Prednisone therapy for cluster headache. Headache 1978; 18: 219–221.

Cuypers J, Altenkirch H, Bunge S. Personality profiles in cluster headache and migraine. Headache 1981; 21: 21–24.

D'Alessandro R, Gamberini G, Benassi G, Morganti G, Cortelli P, Lugaresi E. Cluster headache in the Republic of San Marino. Cephalalgia 1986; 6: 159–162.

*Damasio H, Lyon L. Lithium carbonate in the treatment of cluster headaches. J Neurol 1980; 224: 1–8.

*D'Amico D, Leone M, Moschiano F, Bussone G. Familial cluster headache: report of three families. Headache 1996; 36: 41–43.

*D'Andrea G, Perini F, Granella F, Cananzi A, Sergi A. Efficacy of transdermal clonidine in short-term treatment of cluster headache: a pilot study. Cephalalgia 1995; 15: 430–433.

*D'Andrea G, Granella F, Ghiotto N, Nappi G. Lamotrigine in the treatment of SUNCT syndrome. Neurology 2001; 57: 1723–1725.

De Benedittis G. SUNCT syndrome associated with cavernous angioma of the brain stem. Cephalalgia 1996; 16(7): 503–506.

*De Carolis P, de Capoa D, Agati R, Baldrati A, Sacquegna T. Episodic cluster headache: short and long term results of prophylactic treatment. Headache 1988; 28: 475–476.

Delcanho RE, Graff-Radford SB. Chronic paroxysmal hemicrania presenting as toothache. J Orofac Pain 1993; 7(3): 300–306.

Delreux V, Kevers L, Callewaert A. Paroxysmal hemicrania preceding Pancoast's syndrome. Rev Neurol (Paris) 1989; 145: 151–152.

**Di Sabato F, Fusco BM, Pelaia P, Giacovazzo M. Hyperbaric oxygen therapy in cluster headache. Pain 1993; 52: 243–245.

Dodick DW, Campbell JK. Cluster Headache: Diagnosis, management and treatment. In: SD Silberstein, RB Lipton, DJ Delassio (eds), Wolff's headache and other head pain (7th edn). Oxford University Press, New York, 2001.

Eekers PJ, Koehler PJ. Naratriptan prophylactic treatment in cluster headache. Cephalalgia 2001; 21(1): 75–76.

Ekbom K. Nitroglycerin as a provocative agent in cluster headache. Arch Neurol 1968; 19: 487–493.

**Ekbom K. Prophylactic treatment of cluster headache with a new serotonin antagonist, BC 105. Acta Neurol Scand 1969; 45: 601–610.

Ekbom K. A clinical comparison of cluster headache and migraine. Acta Neurol Scand 1970; Suppl 41: 1.

* Ekbom K. Lithium for cluster headache: review of the literature and preliminary results of long-term treatment. Headache 1981; 21: 132–139.

Ekbom K, Paalzow L, Waldenlind E. Low biological availability of ergotamine tartrate after oral dosing in cluster headache. Cephalalgia 1981; 1(4): 203–207.

* Ekbom K, Krabbe AE, Paalzow G, Paalzow L, Tfelt-Hansen P, Waldenlind E. Optimal routes of administration of ergotamine tartrate in cluster headache patients. A pharmacokinetic study. Cephalalgia 1983; 3: 15–20.

*** Ekbom K, Monstad I, Prusinski A, Cole JA, Pilgrim AJ, Noronha D. Subcutaneous sumatriptan in the acute treatment of cluster headache: a dose comparison study. The Sumatriptan Cluster Headache Study Group. Acta Neurol Scand 1993; 88: 63–69.

* Ekbom K, Krabbe A, Micelli G, Prusinski A, Cole JA, Pilgrim AJ, Noronha D. Cluster headache attacks treated for up to three months with subcutaneous sumatriptan (6 mg). Sumatriptan Cluster Headache Long-term Study Group. Cephalalgia 1995; 15: 230–236.

*** El Amrani M, Massiou H, Bousser MG. A negative trial of sodium valproate in cluster headache: methodological issues. Cephalalgia 2002; 22: 205–208.

Evers S, Husstedt IW. Alternatives in drug treatment of chronic paroxysmal hemicrania. Headache 1996; 36: 429–432.

*** Fogan L. Treatment of cluster headache. A double-blind comparison of oxygen v air inhalation. Arch Neurol 1985; 42: 362–363.

* Forderreuther S, Mayer M, Straube A. Treatment of cluster headache with topiramate: effects and side-effects in five patients. Cephalalgia 2002; 22: 186–189.

Frishberg BM. Neuroimaging in presumed primary headache disorders. Semin Neurol 1997; 17: 373–382.

* Fusco BM, Marabini S, Maggi CA, Fiore G, Geppetti P. Preventative effect of repeated nasal applications of capsaicin in cluster headache. Pain 1994; 59: 321–325.

* Gabai IJ, Spierings EL. Prophylactic treatment of cluster headache with verapamil. Headache 1989; 29: 167–168.

* Gallagher RM, Mueller L, Ciervo CA. Analgesic use in cluster headache. Headache 1996; 36: 105–107.

Gawel MJ, Willinsky RA, Krajewski A. Reversal of cluster headache side following treatment of arteriovenous malformation. Headache 1989; 29: 45.

Goadsby PJ, Edvinsson L. Human in vivo evidence for trigeminovascular activation in cluster headache. Neuropeptide changes and effects of acute attacks therapies. Brain 1994; 117: 427–434.

Goadsby PJ, Lipton RB. A review of paroxysmal hemicranias, SUNCT syndrome and other short-lasting headaches with autonomic feature, including new cases. Brain 1997; 120: 193–209.

* Gobel H, Lindner V, Heinze A, Ribbat M, Deuschl G. Acute therapy for cluster headache with sumatriptan: findings of a one-year long-term study. Neurology 1998; 51: 908–911.

* Graff-Radford SB. SUNCT syndrome responsive to gabapentin (Neurontin). Cephalalgia 2000; 20(5): 515–751.

Hannerz J. Trigeminal neuralgia with chronic paroxysmal hemicrania: the CPH-tic syndrome. Cephalalgia 1993; 13(5): 361–364.

* Hannerz J, Linderoth B. Neurosurgical treatment of short-lasting, unilateral, neuralgiform hemicrania with conjunctival injection and tearing. Br J Neurosurg 2002; 16: 55–58.

* Hardebo JE. How cluster headache is explained as an intracavernous inflammatory process lesioning sympathetic fibers. Headache 1994; 34: 125–131.

*** Hardebo JE, Dahlof C. Sumatriptan nasal spray (20 mg/dose) in the acute treatment of cluster headache. Cephalalgia 1998; 18: 487–489.

Havelius U. A Horner-like syndrome and cluster headache. What comes first? Acta Ophthalmol Scand 2002; 79(4): 374–375.

* Hering R, Kuritzky A. Sodium valproate in the treatment of cluster headache: an open clinical trial. Cephalalgia 1989; 9: 195–198.

* Hering-Hanit R, Gadoth N. The use of baclofen in cluster headache. Curr Pain Headache Rep 2001; 5: 79–82.

Hochman MS. Chronic paroxysmal hemicrania. A new type of treatable headache. Am J Med 1981; 71: 169–170.

Horton BT. Histaminic cephalalgia: differential diagnosis and treatment. Mayo Clin Proc 1956; 31: 325–333.

Igarashi H, Sakai F. Natural history of cluster headache. Cephalalgia 1996; 16: 390–391.

Jerome A, Holroyd KA, Theofanous AG, Pingel JD, Lake AE, Saper JR. Cluster headache pain vs, other vascular headache pain: differences revealed with two approaches to the McGill Pain Questionnaire. Pain 1989; 34: 35–42.

* Kirkpatrick PJ, O'Brien MD, MacCabe JJ. Trigeminal nerve section for chronic migrainous neuralgia. Br J Neurosurg 1993; 7: 483–490.

* Kittrelle JP, Grouse DS, Seybold ME. Cluster headache. Local anesthetic abortive agents. Arch Neurol 1985; 42: 496–498.

Kudrow L. Physical and personality characteristics in cluster headache. Headache 1974; 13: 197–202.

Kudrow L. Plasma testosterone levels in cluster headache preliminary results. Headache 1976; 16: 28–31.

* Kudrow L. Lithium prophylaxis for chronic cluster headache. Headache 1977; 17: 15–18.

Kudrow L. Cluster Headaches: Mechanisms and Management. Oxford University Press, New York, 1980.

Kudrow L. Cluster headache. Clinical, mechanistic, and treatment aspects. Panminerva Med 1982; 24: 45–54.

Kudrow L. The cyclic relationship of natural illumination to cluster period frequency. Cephalalgia 1987; 7(Suppl 6): 76–78.

Kudrow L, Sutkus BJ. MMPI pattern specificity in primary headache disorders. Headache 1979; 19: 18–24.

Kudrow L, McGinty DJ, Phillips ER, Stevenson M. Sleep apnea in cluster headache. Cephalalgia 1984; 4: 33–38.

Lance JW, Anthony M. Migrainous neuralgia or cluster headache? J Neurol Sci 1971; 13: 401–414.

* Leandri M, Luzzani M, Cruccu G, Gottlieb A. Drug-resistant

cluster headache responding to gabapentin: a pilot study. Cephalalgia 2001; 21(7): 744–746.

Lee MS, Lessell S. Orbital myositis posing as cluster headache. Arch Neurol 2002; 59: 635–636.

Leira EC, Cruz-Flores S, Leacock RO, Abdulrauf SI. Sumatriptan can alleviate headaches due to carotid artery dissection. Headache 2001; 41(6): 590–591.

Leone M, Lucini V, D'Amico D, Moschiano F, Maltempo C, Fraschini F, Bussone G. Twenty-four-hour melatonin and cortisol plasma levels in relation to timing of cluster headache. Cephalalgia 1995; 15: 224–229.

**Leone M, D'Amico D, Moschiano F, Fraschini F, Bussone G. Melatonin versus placebo in the prophylaxis of cluster headache: a double-blind pilot study with parallel groups. Cephalalgia 1996; 16: 494–496.

*Leone M, Attanasio A, Grazzi L, Libro G, D'Amico D, Moschiano F, Bussone G. Transdermal clonidine in the prophylaxis of episodic cluster headache: an open study. Headache 1997; 37: 559–560.

*Leone M, Rigamonti A, Usai S, Damico D, Grazzi L, Bussone G. Two new SUNCT cases responsive to lamotrigine. Cephalalgia 2000; 20(9): 845–847.

***Leone M, D'Amico D, Frediani F, Moschiano F, Grazzi L, Attanasio A, Bussone G. Verapamil in the prophylaxis of episodic cluster headache: a double-blind study versus placebo. Neurology 2000; 54: 1382–1385.

Leone M, Russell MB, Rigamonti A, Attanasio A, Grazzi L, D'Amico D, Usai S, Bussone G. Increased familial risk of cluster headache. Neurology 2002; 56(9): 1233–1236.

*Leone M, Franzini A, Bussone G. Stereotactic stimulation of posterior hypothalamic gray matter in a patient with intractable cluster headache. NEJM 2002; 345: 1428–1429.

Levi R, Edman GV, Ekbom K, Waldenlind E. Episodic cluster headache. II: High tobacco and alcohol consumption in males. Headache 1992; 32: 184–187.

Loder E. Naratriptan in the prophylaxis of cluster headache. Headache 2002; 42: 56–57.

*Lovely TJ, Kotsiakis X, Jannetta PJ. The surgical management of chronic cluster headache. Headache 1998; 38(8): 590–594.

Manzoni GC. Male preponderance of cluster headache is progressively decreasing over the years. Headache 1997; 37: 588–589.

Manzoni GC. Cluster headache and lifestyle: remarks on a population of 374 male patients. Cephalalgia 1999; 19(2): 88–94.

Manzoni GC, Terzano MG, Bono G, Micieli G, Martucci N, Nappi G. Cluster headache — clinical findings in 180 patients. Cephalalgia 1983; 3: 21–30.

Manzoni et al., 1991. Manzoni GC, Micieli G, Granella F, Tassorelli C, Zanferrari C, Cavallini A. Cluster headache — course over ten years in 189 patients. Cephalalgia 1991; 11: 169–174.

**Marks DR, Rapoport A, Padla D, Weeks R, Rosum R, Sheftell F, Arrowsmith F. A double-blind placebo controlled trial of intranasal capsaicin for cluster headache. Cephalalgia 1993; 13: 114–116.

Matharu MJ, Goadsby PJ. Post-traumatic chronic paroxysmal hemicrania (CPH) with aura. Neurology 2002; 56(2): 273–275.

Matharu M, Goadsby PJ. Persistence of attacks of cluster headache after trigeminal nerve root section. Brain 2002; 125: 976–984.

*Mather PJ, Silberstein SD, Schulman EA, Hopkins MM. The treatment of cluster headache with repetitive intravenous dihydroergotamine. Headache 1991; 31: 525–532.

*Mathew NT. Clinical subtypes of cluster headache and response to lithium therapy. Headache 1978; 18: 27–29.

*Mathew NT, Hurt W. Percutaneous radiofrequency trigeminal gangliorhizolysis in intractable cluster headache. Headache 1988; 28: 328–331.

*Mathew NT, Kailasam J, Fischer A. Responsiveness to celecoxib in chronic paroxysmal hemicrania. Neurology 2000; 55: 316.

*Mauskop A, Altura BT, Cracco RQ, Altura BM. Intravenous magnesium sulfate relieves cluster headaches in patients with low serum ionized magnesium levels. Headache 1995; 35: 597–600.

May A, Bahra A, Buchel C, Frackowiak RSJ, Goadsby PJ. Hypothalamic activation in cluster headache attacks. Lancet 1998; 352: 275–278.

May A, Bahra A, Buchel C, Turner R, Goadsby PJ. Functional magnetic resonance imaging in spontaneous attacks of SUNCT: short-lasting neuralgiform headache with conjunctival injection and tearing. Ann Neurol 1999; 46(5): 791–794.

*Meyer JS, Hardenberg J. Clinical effectiveness of calcium entry blockers in prophylactic treatment of migraine and cluster headaches. Headache 1983; 23: 266–277.

***Monstad I, Krabbe A, Micieli G, Prusinski A, Cole J, Pilgrim A, Shevlin P. Preemptive oral treatment with sumatriptan during a cluster period. Headache 1995; 35: 607–613.

Monzillo PH, Sanvito WL, Da Costa AR. Cluster-tic syndrome: report of five new cases. Arq Neuropsiquiatr 2000; 58: 518–521.

Mosek A, Hering-Hanit R, Kuritzky A. New-onset cluster headache in middle age and elderly women. Cephalalgia 2001; 21: 198–200.

Moskowitz MA. Cluster headache: evidence for a pathophysiologic focus in the superior pericarotid cavernous sinus plexus. Headache 1988; 28: 584–586.

*Mueller L, Gallagher RM, Ciervo CA. Methylergonovine maleate as a cluster headache prophylactic: a study and review. Headache 1997; 37: 437–442.

Nappi G, Micieli G, Cavallini A, Zanferrari C, Sandrini G, Manzoni GC. Accompanying symptoms of cluster attacks: their relevance to the diagnostic criteria. Cephalalgia 1992; 12(3): 165–168.

*Newman LC. Effective management of ice pick pains, SUNCT, and episodic and chronic paroxysmal hemicrania. Curr Pain Headache Rep 2001; 5: 292–299.

Pareja J, Pareja J. Chronic paroxysmal hemicrania coexisting with migraine. Differential response to pharmacological treatment. Headache 1992; 32: 77–78.

Pareja JA, Sjaastad O. SUNCT syndrome. A clinical review. Headache 1997; 37(4): 195–202.

Pareja JA, Kruszewski P, Sjaastad O. SUNCT syndrome: trials of drugs and anesthetic blockades. Headache 1995; 35: 138–142.

Pareja JA, Shen JM, Kruszewski P, Caballero V, Pamo M, Sjaastad O. SUNCT syndrome: duration, frequency, and temporal distribution of attacks. Headache 1996; 36: 161–165.

Pareja JA, Kruszewski P, Sjaastad O. SUNCT syndrome. Diagnosis morbi. Shortlasting unilateral neuralgiform headache attacks, with conjunctival injection, tearing and rhinorrhoea. Neurologia 1997; 12(Suppl 5): 66–72.

*Pascual J, Peralta G, Sanchez U. Preventive effects of hyperbaric oxygen in cluster headache. Headache 1995; 35: 260–261.

Pearce JM. Chronic migrainous neuralgia Brain 1980; 103: 149–159.

*Peres MF, Rozen TD. Melatonin in the preventive treatment of cluster headache. Cephalalgia 2001; 21: 993–995.

Penarrocha M, Bandres A, Penarrocha MA, Bagan JV. Relationship between oral surgical and endodontic procedures and episodic cluster headache. Oral Surg Oral Med Oral Pathol Oral Radiol Endod 2001; 92(5): 499–502.

*Pieper DR, Dickerson J, Hassenbusch SJ. Percutaneous retrogasserian glycerol rhizolysis for treatment of chronic intractable cluster headaches: long term results. Neurosurgery 2001; 46: 363–370.

Pollmann W, Pfaffenrath V. Chronic paroxysmal hemicrania: the first possible bilateral case. Cephalalgia 1986; 6: 55–57.

Raeder JG. Paratrigeminal paralysis of oculo-pupillary sympathetic. Brain 1924; 47: 149–158.

Rapoport AM, Sheftell FD, Baskin SM. Chronic paroxysmal hemicrania — case report of the second known definite occurrence in a male. Cephalalgia 1981; 1: 67–69.

Raskin NH. On the origin of head pain. Headache 1988; 28: 254–257.

Reik L Jr. Cluster headache after head injury. Headache 1987; 27: 509–510.

Riess CM, Becker WJ, Robertson M. Episodic cluster headache in a community: clinical features and treatment. Can J Neurol Sci 1998; 25(2): 141–145.

*Robbins L. Intranasal lidocaine for cluster headache. Headache 1995; 35: 83–84.

*Rozen TD. Olanzapine as an abortive agent for cluster headache. Headache 2001; 41: 813–816.

Rozen TD, Niknam RM, Shechter AL, Young WB, Silberstein SD. Cluster
headache in women: clinical characteristics and comparison with cluster headache in men. J Neurol Neurosurg Psychiatry 2001; 70(5): 613–617.

Russell D, Storstein L. Chronic paroxysmal hemicrania: heart rate changes and ECG rhythm disturbances. A computerized analysis of 24 h ambulatory ECG recordings. Cephalalgia 1984; 4: 135–144.

Safar HA, Alanezi KH, Cina CS. Successful treatment of threatening limb loss ischemia of the upper limb caused by ergotamine. A case report and review of the literature. J Cardiovasc Surg (Torino) 2002; 43: 245–249.

*Sanders M, Zuurmond WWA. Efficacy of sphenopalatine ganglion blockade in 66 patients suffering from cluster headache: 12–70-month follow-up evaluation. J Neurosurg 1997; 87(6): 876–880.

***Saper JR, Klapper J, Mathew NT, Rapoport A, Phillips SB, Bernstein JE. Intranasal civamide for the treatment of episodic cluster headaches. Arch Neurol 2002; 59: 990–994.

*Savoldi F, Bono G, Manzoni GC, Micieli G, Lanfranchi M, Nappi G. Lithium salts in cluster headache treatment. Cephalalgia 1983; 3(Suppl 1): 79–84.

*Schuh-Hofer S, Reuter U, Kinze S, Einhaupl KM, Arnold G. Treatment of acute cluster headache with 20 mg sumatriptan nasal spray — an open pilot study. J Neurol 2002; 249: 94–99.

**Sicuteri F, Geppetti P, Marabini S, Lembeck F. Pain relief by somatostatin in attacks of cluster headache. Pain 1984; 18: 359–365.

Sjaastad O, Antonaci F. Chronic paroxysmal hemicrania: a case report. Long-lasting remission in the chronic stage. Cephalalgia 1987; 7: 203–205.

Sjaastad O, Dale I. Evidence for a new (?) treatable headache entity. Headache 1974; 14: 105–108.

Sjaastad O, Kruszewski P. Trigeminal neuralgia and 'SUNCT' syndrome: similarities and differences in the clinical pictures. An overview. Funct Neurol 1992; 7(2): 103–107.

Sjaastad O, Rinck P. Cluster headache: MRI studies of the cavernous sinus and the base of the brain. Headache 1990; 30: 350–351.

Sjaastad O, Shen JM, Stovner LJ, Elsas T. Cluster headache in identical twins. Headache 1993; 33: 214–217.

Sjaastad O, Pareja JA, Zukerman E, Jansen J, Kruszewski P. Trigeminal neuralgia. Clinical manifestations of first division involvement. Headache 1997; 37(6): 346–357.

Sjostrand C, Waldenlind E, Ekbom K. A follow-up study of 60 patients after an assumed first period of cluster headache. Cephalalgia 2000; 20: 653–657.

Sjostrand C, Giedratis V, Ekbom K, Waldenlind E, Hillert J. CACNA1A gene polymorphisms in cluster headache. Cephalalgia 2001; 21: 953–958.

Solomon GD, Skobieranda FG, Gragg LA. Does quality of life differ among headache diagnoses? Analysis using the medical outcomes study instrument. Headache 1994; 34: 143–147.

**Steiner TJ, Hering R, Couturier EG, Davies PT, Whitmarsh TE. Double-blind placebo controlled trial of lithium in episodic cluster headache. Cephalalgia 1997; 17: 673–675.

Sumatriptan Cluster Headache Study Group. Treatment of acute cluster headache with sumatriptan. The Sumatriptan Cluster Headache Study Group. N Engl J Med 1991; 325: 322–326.

*Taha JM, Tew JR. Long term results of radiofrequency rhizotomy in the treatment of cluster headache. Headache 1995; 35: 193–196.

*Tay BA, Ngan Kee WD, Chung DC. Gabapentin for the treatment and prophylaxis of cluster headache. Reg Anesth Pain Med 2001; 26: 373–375.

Tehindrazanarivelo AD, Visy JM, Bousser MG. Ipsilateral cluster headache and chronic paroxysmal hemicrania: two case reports. Cephalalgia 1992; 12(5): 318–320.

Tonon C, Guttmann S, Volpini M, Naccarato S, Cortelli P, D'Alessandro R. Prevalence and incidence of cluster headache in the Republic of San Marino. Neurology 2002; 58(9): 1407–1409.

Torelli P, Manzoni GC. What predicts evolution from episodic to chronic cluster headache? Curr Pain Headache Rep 2002; 6: 65–70.

Torelli P, Cologno D, Cademartiri C, Manzoni GC. Possible predictive factors in the evolution of episodic to chronic cluster headache. Headache 2000; 40: 798–808.

Turkewitz LJ, Wirth O, Dawson GA, Casaly JS. Cluster headache following head injury: a case report and review of the literature. Headache 1992; 32: 504–506.

Van Vliet JA, Bahra A, Martin V, Aurora SK, Mathew N, Goadsby PJ. Intranasal sumatriptan is effective in the treatment of acute cluster headache — a double-blind placebo controlled crossover study. Cephalalgia 2001; 21: 270.

Watson CP, Evans RJ. Chronic cluster headache — a review of 60 patients. Headache 1987; 27: 158–165.

*Wheeler SD, Carrazana EJ. Topiramate-treated cluster headache. Neurology 1999; 53: 234–236.

Wingerchuk A, Nyquist PA, Rodriguez M, Dodick DW. Extratrigeminal short-lasting unilateral neuralgiform headache with conjunctival injection and tearing (SUNCT): new pathophysiologic entity or variation on a theme? Cephalalgia 2000; 20: 127–129.

Zukerman E, Peres MF, Kaup AO, Monzillo PH, Costa AR. Chronic paroxysmal hemicrania-tic syndrome. Neurology 2000; 54(7): 1524–1526.

Assessment and Management of Orofacial Pain
Pain Research and Clinical Management, Vol. 14
Edited by J.M. Zakrzewska and S.D. Harrison
© *2002 Elsevier Science B.V. All rights reserved*

CHAPTER 13

Maxillary sinusitis

Sheelah D. Harrison [*]

Department of Oral and Maxillofacial Surgery, Eastman Dental Hospital, 256 Gray's Inn Road, London WC1X 8LD, UK

Objectives for this chapter:

This chapter will attempt to:
- define maxillary sinusitis
- describe how the clinical features of maxillary sinusitis have been determined
- list and evaluate the investigations used to differentiate between maxillary sinusitis and other conditions affecting the sinuses
- discuss the management of maxillary sinusitis in the light of the available evidence

1. Definition

The definition of acute maxillary sinusitis of the International Association for the Study of Pain (IASP) is "constant burning pain with zygomatic and dental tenderness from the inflammation of the maxillary sinus". The IASP acknowledges that there is also chronic sinusitis, but states that in chronic cases there may be no pain or only mild, diffuse discomfort from time to time (Merskey and Bogduk, 1994).

The International Headache Society (IHS) classification system (Olesen, 1988) groups all types (maxillary, frontal, ethmoid and sphenoid) of sinusitis together stating that the difference between them is merely anatomical location of the sinus and its specific headache. The pain from sinusitis is described as acute sinus headache. The diagnostic criteria are shown in Table 1.

---
[*] Tel.: +44-20-7915-1021; Fax: +44-20-7915-1259;
E-mail: sharrison@eastman.ucl.ac.uk

TABLE 1

KEY FACTS: maxillary sinusitis — diagnostic criteria as proposed by the IHS

- Purulent discharge in the nasal passage either spontaneous or by suction
- Pathological findings in one or more of the following tests
- X-ray examination
- Computerised tomography or magnetic resonance imaging
- Transillumination
- Simultaneous onset of headache and sinusitis
- Headache location
  - In acute maxillary sinusitis headache is located over the antral area and may radiate to the upper teeth or the forehead (other anatomical sites of sinusitis are also described)
- Headache disappears after treatment of acute sinusitis

2. Epidemiology

It is estimated that 0.5–5% of all upper respiratory tract infections will be complicated by maxillary sinusitis (Lindbaek et al., 1996a; Hickner et al., 2001). Both sexes are equally affected (Merskey and Bogduk, 1994), adults more than children. It is postulated that general practitioners overestimate the prevalence of maxillary sinusitis as they do not use strict diagnostic criteria (Lindbaek et al., 1996b). In the USA it is one of the ten most common diagnoses in outpatient medical settings and the fifth most common diagnosis for which antibiotics are prescribed (Hickner et al., 2001). The evidence here is poor and essentially that of expert opinion.

3. Aetiology

For normal sinus functioning the following three key elements are required: patent ostia, satisfactory functioning of the ciliary apparatus and appropriate quality of secretions. Retention of secretions within the sinus leads to sinusitis and may be due to obstruction of the ostia, change in function and number of cilia and overproduction or change in viscosity of the secretions.

Causes of acute sinus inflammation include allergy, infection, and local irritants. Symptoms due to allergy or irritants are more often recurrent, but are infrequently associated with purulent nasal discharge and frequently associated with itching, sneezing and following specific exposures. Infectious causes of sinusitis include respiratory viruses, fungi and bacteria. Fungal infections rarely occur in immunocompetent individuals. Acute sinusitis is most frequently caused by prolonged viral infection, and evidence of sinus inflammation in patients with a viral upper respiratory tract infection (the common cold) can be seen in 39% of sinus radiographs (Puhakka et al., 1998) and 87% of CT scans (Gwaltney et al., 1994). Viral and bacterial sinusitis are difficult to differentiate on clinical grounds (Hickner et al., 2001). It has been suggested that a diagnosis of bacterial sinusitis is reserved for those patients with symptoms lasting 7 days or more, despite evidence that bacterial infection can exist in 20% of patients with symptoms lasting less than 7 days. The most commonly implicated bacteria are *Streptococcus pneumoniae* and *Haemophilus influenzae*. The infection persists until the secretions drain from the sinuses.

4. Clinical features

Have a look at the three clinical cases in Table 2. The clinical features are summarised in Table 3.

Lindbaek et al. (1996a) assessed the methods for diagnosis of acute sinusitis in primary care. They analysed 27 factors and found that 4 were reliably related to a diagnosis of acute sinusitis. These were:

- complaint of purulent rhinorhea
- history of recovery from a nasal cold and then a worsening of symptoms
- finding of purulent secretions in the nasal cavity
- an ESR above 10 mm/h.

4.1. Bacterial or viral?

Several investigators have attempted to assess which signs and symptoms were helpful in distinguishing between viral and bacterial sinusitis. All of these have been criticised for using imperfect diagnostic standards; the gold standard diagnostic tool is that of aspiration of the purulent secretions which upon culture yields good growth (greater than 10^5 organisms per millilitre) of a likely respiratory pathogen. In all studies no single sign or symptom had strong diagnostic value, although some combinations gave more helpful results. Hickner et al. (2001) summarise the evidence and suggest that there is a higher likelihood of predicting bacterial infection in those patients with

- purulent nasal discharge
- maxillary tooth or facial pain (especially unilateral)
- unilateral maxillary sinus tenderness

- a worsening of symptoms after initial improvement

4.2. Examination

There will be tenderness over the affected cheek and occasionally some redness. Intra-orally the upper teeth on the affected area will be tender to percussion. The sinus will transilluminate if a torch is put in intra-orally.

Differential diagnosis must include dental causes as well as possible malignancy.

5. Investigations

Opacities, fluid levels and mucosal thickening can be visualised using maxillary sinus radiography or CT scanning. The use of these positive findings to predict a bacterial sinusitis is shown in Table 4.

The expert opinion given the findings in Table 4 is that sinus radiography is not recommended for routine cases (Hickner et al., 2001).

6. Management

Expert opinion is that the initial management should be with symptomatic treatment and reassurance, antibiotic therapy being reserved for those with

- moderately severe symptoms and acute bacterial sinusitis
- symptoms of more than 7 days
- maxillary pain of face or teeth
- purulent nasal secretions, or
- severe symptoms regardless of duration (Hickner et al., 2001)

6.1. Symptomatic treatments

There are numerous types of symptomatic treatments available. The agents include

- alpha-adrenergic agents
- proteolytic agents
- mucolytic agents
- antihistamines
- corticosteroids
- analgesics
- decongestants

The RCTs of these treatments have been inconclusive when assessing reduction of symptoms (Ryan, 1967; Seltzer, 1967; Taub, 1967; Lewison, 1970; Harris, 1971; Meltzer et al., 1993; Wiklund et al., 1994; Braun et al., 1997). (As summarised in Best Evidence in Further reading.) They have not been evaluated in treatment of acute maxillary sinusitis.

6.2. Antibiotics

A randomised, double-blind, placebo-controlled trial of antibiotic treatment of acute bacterial sinusitis with pre- and post-treatment cultures of sinus aspirates has not been performed. Most of the randomised controlled trials on the use of antibiotics can be found in the Cochrane database of clinical trials. Two meta-analyses have been published with similar conclusions:

- antibiotics are more effective than placebo in reducing/eliminating symptoms at 10–13 days
- the effect size is small
- most placebo patients improve without antibiotics (Williams et al., 1997; Zucher et al., 2002)

6.2.1. Penicillin and amoxycillin
Lindbaek et al. (1996b) carried out a randomised controlled trial in 130 adults with acute sinusitis and showed penicillin V and amoxycillin to be more effective than placebo but more adverse reactions were reported in the active treatment arm. Using CT scanning for diagnosis, improvement at 10 days was found in 56% patients following placebo, 82% following penicillin and 86% following amoxycillin therapy.

This conflicts with a later study that found that amoxycillin was not of value in these patients (Van

TABLE 2

Case studies

See if you can make a diagnosis or treatment plan for each of the patients. Please see Table 6 for the answers.

CASE 1

Name	MN
Age	69
Gender	male
Development of pain	constant over about 6 months, initially a lower level pain but increasing in severity with time
Character	aching and heavy, sometimes sharp and shooting
Site/radiation	right side of face
Severity	VAS 6.9/10 cm
Duration, periodicity	constant with intermittent severe episodes
Provoking factors	bending and lying down and touching the right cheek
Relieving factors	nil
Associated factors	bad taste
Medical history	late onset diabetes — diet controlled
Current medication	codydramol
Social factors	married, retired, does not smoke, drinks 3–4 glasses of wine per day
Examination	tender right maxilla, dysaesthesia and anaesthesia of right infraorbital nerve
Investigation	orthopantomogram — right maxillary antrum poorly defined; occipitomental radiograph — opaque right antrum with destruction of the lateral maxillary wall

CASE 2

Name	JG
Age	31
Gender	female
Development of pain	constant over last couple of days, worsening especially bad at night, unable to sleep
Character	ache and tender
Site/radiation	right side of face
Severity	VAS 5.1
Duration, periodicity	constant with intermittent severe episodes
Provoking factors	touching the area
Relieving factors	nil
Associated factors	bad taste in mouth/back of throat, upper teeth tender to bite on
Medical history	fit and well, allergic to penicillin
Current medication	oral contraceptive pill, paracetamol and nurofen
Social factors	single, French teacher, smokes 10–15 cigarettes per day, drinks 3–4 units of alcohol at weekends, some days
Examination	tender right maxilla, well restored dentition, maxillary premolars and molars tender to percussion, pain worsened upon leaning forward
Investigation	orthopantomogram — right maxillary antrum not clearly defined; occipitomental radiograph — right maxillary antrum has an (opaque) fluid level

Buchem et al., 1997). However, less specific diagnostic criteria were used (radiographic diagnosis).

In a randomised controlled trial Hayle et al. (1996) compared azithromycin to penicillin V and found no difference in efficacy or adverse effect profile but suggested that the shorter duration of treatment with azithromycin was an advantage.

6.2.2. Sulphonamides

A small randomised controlled trial compared the efficacy of trimethoprin-sulphamethoxazole used for

TABLE 2 *continued*

CASE 3	
Name	WM
Age	24
Gender	male
Development of pain	intermittent, over past 4 months; began 2 weeks after a tooth extraction; the socket had failed to heal and had left a 'hole' into the sinus; two attempts had been made to close this oro-antral fistula but the pain remained
Character	tender aching and heavy
Site/radiation	right side of face
Severity	VAS 6.2/10 cm
Duration, periodicity	intermittent severe episodes
Provoking factors	touching the area, bending and lying down
Relieving factors	inhalations
Associated factors	sometimes the face is red and slightly swollen on the right
Medical history	fit and well
Current medication	amoxycillin
Social factors	single, lives with parents and family, does not work, smokes 20 cigarettes a day, drinks a couple of pints of beer every day
Examination	tender right maxilla, well restored dentition, absent upper right first premolar granulation tissue in socket, communication with antrum detected with a blunt probe
Investigation	orthopantomogram — bony defect in antral floor in region of previously extracted tooth, cloudy right antrum; occipitomental radiograph — increased opacity of right maxillary antrum

3 or 10 days in adult men with acute maxillary sinusitis and concluded that a 3-day course was equally effective (Williams et al., 1995).

6.2.3. Brodimoprim

Rahlfs et al. (1996) did a meta-analysis of randomised controlled trials on the use of this drug as compared to amoxicillin, cefalexin, doxycycline and roxithromycin in acute sinusitis. They showed that brodimoprim once daily was more effective than amoxicillin but doxycycline produced fewer side effects.

6.2.4. Cephalosporin

Comparison of two cephalosporins in a randomised controlled trial showed no significant differences (Kohler et al., 1995)

6.2.5. Doxycycline

A placebo controlled randomised controlled trial was conducted in primary care and concluded that doxy-cline did not add to the effectiveness of nasal decongestants and inhalations in the resolution of facial pain and return to normal activities (Stalman et al., 1997).

Expert opinion concludes that if an antibiotic is required it should be the most narrow spectrum active against the most likely pathogens of *S. pneumoniae* and *H. influenzae*. Reviews of efficacy have failed to show that any antibiotic is superior to amoxycillin (Low et al., 1997) and this is therefore the drug of choice (Hickner et al., 2001).

7. Prognosis

Gwaltney et al. (1967) studied the natural history of sinusitis in an industrial population of young adults. The duration of illness was from 1 to 33 days, with a quarter of patients having symptoms lasting longer than 13 days, and most patients being well in 7–10 days. Serious complications of acute sinusitis such as

TABLE 3

Maxillary sinusitis: clinical features

Site	over the affected sinus, unilateral or bilateral
Radiation	to surrounding structures, upper teeth, forehead
Character	dull ache, boring, aching, tender, fullness
Severity	mild to moderate/severe
Duration	few days after upper respiratory tract infection or (less frequently) following dental infection or treatment of a maxillary molar or premolar
Periodicity	continuous for a few days, up to a week
Provoking factors	touching the area, biting on upper teeth, bending
Relieving factors	treatment with antibiotics or drainage of sinus, lying on the other side
Associated factors	purulent nasal discharge, sense of fullness over the cheek, radiographic evidence of a fluid level

TABLE 4

Ability of radiological findings to predict bacterial sinusitis (Hickner et al., 2001)

Finding	Specificity (%)	Range (%)
Complete opacification	85	76–91
Air–fluid level	80	71–87
Mucosal thickening	40–50	
Absence of all three	sensitivity of 90% in ruling out sinusitis	

TABLE 5

Summary for Chapter 13

- There is little good quality evidence concerning any aspect of acute maxillary sinusitis
- Diagnosis in routine cases can be made on clinical findings alone
- For most patients symptoms resolve with reassurance and symptomatic treatments
- Serious complications are rare

meningitis, brain abscess and periorbital cellulitis are rare, but there are no data available comparing those patients treated with antibiotics to those who were not. None of the treatment trials using a placebo reported a serious complication.

8. Summary

Table 5 provides a summary for this chapter.

Appendix A

Table 6 shows the answers to the cases in Table 2.

Appendix B. Further reading

(1) *www.acpjc.org* American College of Physicians Journal Club (Best Evidence on CD ROM). Annals of Internal Medicine.

(2) *www.annals.org* (These web sites provide good regularly updated evidence-based information on many areas of medicine; maxillary sinusitis (rhinosinusitis) is comprehensively covered.)

(3) The Cochrane Library should also be accessed for the latest updates.

TABLE 6

Answers to cases in Table 2

CASE 1

This case did not appear to be a straightforward acute (or chronic) sinusitis. The anaesthesia and dysaesthesia and associated shooting pain with touch are all worrying signs of nerve damage or involvement, most commonly associated with trauma (including surgery). No dental work/surgery had been undertaken in the previous year. In addition the apparent destruction of the lateral antral wall on the OM radiograph suggested pathology which was aggressive; the differential diagnosis would include: ameloblastoma, odontogenic myxoma, carcinoma of the antrum. A biopsy was undertaken which showed adenocarcinoma. The patient was seen in a joint oncology clinic and surgery was suggested (maxillectomy) for the patient.

CASE 2

When questioned further this patient recalled that she had suffered with 'flu' the previous week. The worsening of pain at night was almost certainly positional (as with bending forward). This appeared to be a classic case of post upper respiratory tract infection acute sinusitis. A number of treatment options were available, any prescribing would need to take into account the patients allergy and the use of the oral contraceptive pill. The available studies were discussed with the patient. It was imperative that she did not become pregnant. As there appeared to be conflicting evidence (in the literature) as to whether antibiotics would improve the pain or alter the clinical course of the disease the patient preferred not to have antibiotics prescribed, but would use inhalations to reduce the pain associated with the condition.

CASE 3

This patent had recurrent acute maxillary sinusitis associated with a chronic sinusitis. This devolved following a maxillary molar extraction and the subsequent development of an OAF. Two attempts at closure had been unsuccessful and the intermittent acute maxillary sinusitis resulted with associated facial swelling. He had been prescribed antibiotics and inhalations in the past which had been helpful. A third attempt at closing the OAF was successful and the cloudy appearance on the OM was no longer visible at 3 months post-op.

References

Marked as regards quality according to criteria set by author.

SR = systematic review or high quality review with methodology

* Poorer quality studies but only ones in the field, old style reviews.

** Cohort studies, high quality case series with controls.

*** Randomised controlled trials, high quality original studies.

** Braun JJ, Alabert JP, Michel FB, Quiniou M, Rat C, Cougnard J, et al. Adjunct effect of loratadine in the treatment of acute sinusitis in patients with allergic rhinitis. Allergy 1997: 52: 650–655.

Gwaltney JM, Jr, Hendley JO, Simon G, Jordan WS, Jr. Rhinovirus infections in an industrial population. II. Characteristics of illness and antibody response. JAMA 1967; 202: 494–500.

** Gwaltney JM, Jr, Phillips CD, Miller RD, Riker DK. Computed tomographic study of the common cold. N Engl J Med 1994; 330: 25–30.

*** Harris PG. A comparison of 'bisolvomycin' and oxytetracycline in the treatment of acute infective sinusitis. Practitioner 1971; 207: 813–817.

** Hayle R, Lingaas E, Hoivik HO, Odegard T. Efficacy and safety of azithromycin versus phenoxymethylpenicillin in the treatment of acute maxillary sinusitis. Eur J Clin Microbiol Infect Dis 1996; 15: 849–853.

** Hickner JM, Bartlett JG, Besser RE, Gonzales R, Hoffman JR, Sande MA. Principles of appropriate antibiotic use for acute rhinisinusitis in adults: Background. Ann Intern Med 2001; 134: 498–505.

** Kohler W, Schenk P, Hayle R, Lingaas E, Hoivik HO, Odegard T. Cephalosporin treatment of maxillary sinusitis. Laryngorhinootologie 1995; 74: 355–360.

*** Lewison E. Comparison of the effectiveness of topical and oral nasal decongestants. Eye Ear Nose Throat Mon 1970; 49: 16–18.

Lindbaek M, Hjortdahl P, Johnsen UL. Use of symptoms, signs, and blood tests to diagnose acute sinus infections in primary care: comparison with computed tomography. Fam Med 1996a; 28: 183–188.

*** Lindbaek M, Hjortdahl P, Johnsen UL. Randomised, double blind, placebo controlled trial of penicillin V and amoxycillin in treatment of acute sinus infections in adults. BMJ 1996b; 313: 325–329.

Low DE, Desrosiers M, McSherry J, Garber G, Williams JW, Jr, Remy H, Fenton RS, Forte V, Balter M, Rotstein C, Craft C, Dubois J, Harding, G, Schloss M, Miller M, McIvor RA, Davidson RJ. A practical guide for the diagnosis and treatment of acute sinusitis. CMAJ 1997; 156 (Suppl 6): S1–14.

*** Meltzer EO, Orgel HA, Backhaus JW, Busse WW, Druce HM, Metzger WJ, et al. Intranasal flunisolide spray as an adjunct to oral antibiotic therapy for sinusitis. J Allergy Clin Immunol 1993; 92: 812–823.

Merskey H, Bogduk N. Classification of Chronic Pain. Descriptions of Chronic Pain Syndromes and Definitions of Pain Terms. IASP Press, Seattle, WA, 1994.

Olesen J. Classification and diagnostic criteria for headache disorders, cranial neuralgias and facial pain. Cephalgia 1988; 8 (Suppl 7).

* Puhakka T, Makela MJ, Alanen A, Kallio T, Korsoff L, Arstila P, et al. Sinusitis in the common cold. J Allergy Clin Immunol 1998; 102: 403–408.

*** Rahlfs VW, Macciocchi A, Monti T. Brodimoprin in upper respiratory tract infections: two meta-analysis of randomised controlled clinical trials in acute sinusitis and otitis media. Clin Drug Invest 1996; 11: 65–76.

*** Ryan RE. A double-blind clinical evaluation of bromelains in the treatment of acute sinusitis. Headache 1967; 7: 13–17.

** Seltzer AP. Adjunctive use of bromelains in sinusitis: a controlled study. Eye Ear Nose Throat Mon 1967; 46: 1281–1288.

*** Stalman W, Van Essen GA, Van der Graaf Y, et al. The end of antibiotic treatment in adults with acute sinusitis-like complaints in general practice? A placebo-controlled double-blind randomised doxycycline trial. Br J Gen Pract 1997; 47: 794–799.

*** Taub SJ. The use of bromelains in sinusitis: a double-blind clinical evaluation. Eye Ear Nose Throat Mon 1967; 46: 361–462.

** Van Buchem L, Peeters M, Beaumont J, Knottnerus JA. Acute maxillary sinusitis in general practice: the relation between clinical picture and objective findings. Eur J Gen Pract 1995; 1: 155–160.

*** Van Buchem FL, Knotterus JA, Schrijnemaekers VJ, Peeters MF. Primary- care based randomised placebo-controlled trial of antibiotic treatment in acute maxillary sinusitis. Lancet 1997; 349: 683–687.

** Wiklund L, Stierna P, Berglund R, Westrin KM, Tonnesson M. The efficacy of oxymetazoline administered with a nasal bellows container and combined with oral phenoxymethyl-penicillin in the treatment of acute maxillary sinusitis. Acta Otolaryngol Suppl 1994; 515: 57–64.

Williams JW, Jr, Simel DL, Roberts L, Samsa GP. Clinical evaluation for sinusitis. Making the diagnosis by history and physical examination. Ann Intern Med 1992; 117: 705–710.

*** Williams JW, Holleman DR, Samsa GP, Simel DL. Randomised controlled trial of 3 vs. 10 days of trimethoprim/sulfamethoxazole for acute maxillary sinusitis. JAMA 1995; 273: 1015–1021.

SR Williams JW, Jr, Aguilar C, Makela M, Cornell J, Hollman D, Chiquette E, et al. Antibiotic therapy for acute sinusitis: a systematic literature review. In: Douglas R, Bridges-Webb C, Glasziou P, Lozano J, Steinhoff M, Wang E (eds) Acute Respiratory Infections Module of The Cochrane Database of Systematic Reviews. The Cochrane Library, Oxford, 1997 (updated software).

Zucher DR, Balk E, Engels E, Barza M, Lau J. Agency for Health Care Policy and Research Publication No. 99-E016: Evidence Report/Technology Assessment Number 9. Diagnosis and Treatment of Acute Bacterial Rhinosinusitis, 2002. Available at: *http://www.ahrq.gov/clinic/sinussum. htm.*

Assessment and Management of Orofacial Pain
Pain Research and Clinical Management, Vol. 14
Edited by J.M. Zakrzewska and S.D. Harrison
© *2002 Elsevier Science B.V. All rights reserved*

CHAPTER 14

Atypical facial pain and atypical odontalgia

Sheelah D. Harrison[*]

Department of Oral and Maxillofacial Surgery, Eastman Dental Hospital and University College London Hospitals Trust,
256 Gray's Inn Road, London WC1X 8LD, UK

Objectives for this chapter:

This chapter aims to:
- define atypical facial pain and atypical odontalgia
- explain why there is confusion concerning these two conditions in the literature
- describe the clinical features of atypical facial pain and atypical odontalgia
- discuss some management strategies that may be helpful in patients with either atypical facial pain or atypical odontalgia

---

1. Atypical facial pain

This diagnosis is controversial. While being widely accepted within Europe and Australasia, the existence of such a condition is debated and a definition for this is lacking in the IASP Chronic Pain Classification.

This condition is not frequently seen in non-specialist clinics and this factor must be taken into account when assessing the evidence presented. Consequently studies including large numbers of patients are not likely to be found (or indeed undertaken in the foreseeable future) and the evidence should not be adversely judged on this alone.

* Tel.: +44-20-7915-1021; Fax: +44-20-7915-1059;
E-mail: S. Harrison@eastman.ucl.ac.uk

1.1. Definition

The definition used is from the International Headache Society (Olesen, 1988), under the heading 'Facial pain not fulfilling criteria in groups 11 and 12, along with previously used terms Atypical facial pain and Atypical odontalgia'.

Description. Persistent facial pain that does not have the characteristics of the cranial neuralgias classified above and is not associated with physical signs or a demonstrable organic cause.

Diagnostic criteria. (A) Is present daily and persists for most or all of the day. (B) Is confined at onset to a limited area on one side of the face; may spread to the upper or lower jaws or a wider area of the face or neck; is deep and poorly localised. (C) Is not associated with sensory loss or other physical signs. (D) Laboratory investigations including X-ray of face and jaws do not demonstrate relevant abnormality.

Comment. Pain may be initiated by operation or injury to face, teeth or gums but persists without any demonstrable local cause.

Madland and Feinmann (2001) advocate the use of the term 'chronic facial pain' rather than 'atypical facial pain'.

1.2. Epidemiology

There is no epidemiological study investigating AFP. Most of the evidence presented here is of poor quality and essentially from respected authorities. In prospective cases series reported in the literature most patients are female (70–80%) and have a mean age of around 40–46 years (range 30–55) (Smith et al., 1969; Feinmann et al., 1984; Mock et al., 1985; Remick and Blasberg, 1985; Melzack et al., 1986; Pfaffenrath et al., 1993).

1.3. History

Atypical facial pain (AFP) was first described in 1924 by Frazier and Russell, who noted that 10–15% of patients with chronic facial pain had pain which differed in nature from trigeminal neuralgia. The pain was described by the patients as a deeply located throbbing or aching pain which involved bony areas of the face being continuous lasting from several hours to days. The pain was not restricted to the anatomical boundaries of trigeminal nerve branches and had no trigger points. A variety of accompanying symptoms have been described such as facial flushing, oedema, lacrimation, photophobia, blurred vision, salivation, nausea and vomiting. The pain appears to present more commonly in women (Feinmann and Harris, 1984a,b; Remick and Blasberg, 1985), and was originally described as a psychiatric diagnosis often in young professional women in whom hysterical, obsessional and anxiety traits have been detected (Engel, 1951; Lesse, 1956).

1.4. Aetiology

The aetiology is unknown. Numerous factors have been proposed by various experts in the field, but none have been validated by case control studies. These are mentioned below for interest.

The migraine-like features of AFP led Fay (1932) to propose a vascular aetiology. It was proposed that sympathetic stimulation of blood vessels resulted in a dimensional change resulting in pain. Treatment of AFP with vasoconstrictors has been investigated by Reik (1985) who found limited success. This would suggest that a more complex aetiology exists.

Lesse (1956) suggested that the condition was psychogenic in origin; this has since been reported by many investigators (Engel, 1951; Moore and Nally, 1975; Feinmann and Harris, 1984a,b; Remick and Blasberg, 1985), who have also suggested that emotional disturbance and psychological problems precede the pain history. There is no evidence to support these expert theories and may be based upon their own possibly biased clinic populations. Mock et al. (1985) report that the onset of pain is related to medical or dental treatment, trauma or an organic disorder in half of all patients, and it has been suggested that symptoms appear to worsen following surgical intervention (Frazier and Russell, 1924; Kuhner, 1988).

The vascular hypothesis for migraine has been questioned and a neurogenic aetiology has been proposed by Moskowitz (1992) involving neurogenic inflammation within the dura mater due to vasoactive neuropeptides (CGRP) release from sensory fibres within the blood vessels. It is proposed that similar mechanisms may operate in AFP. Both concepts involve actions upon 5-hydroxytryptamine (5-HT) receptors. The argument for involvement of 5-HT is strengthened by the known relief of AFP by tricyclic antidepressants which can act via inhibition of noradrenaline or 5-HT. The relationship does not appear, however, to be straightforward. Hampf (1989) found that given a single dose of a 5-HT antagonist 12 of 30 patients with AFP had increased pain. A double-blind crossover study of patients with AFP involving use of a selective 5-HT-like receptor agonist, sumatriptan, produced pain relief following administration of the drug, further implicating 5-HT in the aetiology of AFP (Harrison et al., 1997a).

1.5. Clinical features

There are no good studies comparing controls with patients. The evidence presented in this section will therefore be from those studies that are available, essentially from selected clinics, and perhaps representing biased populations, although most are prospective case series; they are essentially anecdotal. The data are summarised in Table 1.

1.6. Examination

By definition, no abnormal findings are usually detected, except pain upon palpation of the area; however, in some groups of patients 38–63% of patients have altered sensations (Mock et al., 1985; Pfaffenrath et al., 1993), an area of tenderness or increased temperature of the skin overlying the painful area (Friedman, 1995). Again there is no good level of evidence for the findings upon examination.

1.7. Investigations

As AFP is essentially a definition by exclusion, all investigations of the painful area should be 'normal'. Again there are no studies to support appropriate investigations in AFP. It is suggested that appropriate radiographs of the area of pain should be sufficient to confirm the diagnosis, given that the features are those given in the definition. Positive emission tomography has been used to attempt to show that differences can be found in patients with or without facial pain (Derbyshire et al., 1994). Currently the studies are still not conclusive.

Please read through the case studies in Table 2 and decide on diagnosis and management.

1.8. Management of AFP

Trigeminal neurectomy was apparently common treatment for AFP in the 19th century (McMurty, 1969) and it is still reported. Ziccardi et al. (1994) suggest that peripheral trigeminal nerve surgery does give improved outcomes in patients who do not have a history of psychiatric treatment.

Lascelles (1966) introduced the use of monoamine oxidase inhibitors for pain relief in patients with AFP, and in a placebo-controlled crossover trial of patients who suffered simultaneously with depression, showed marked improvement in those patients with a short pain history. Simple analgesics appear to be ineffective (Feinmann and Harris, 1984b). Many

---

TABLE 1

KEY FACTS: clinical features of atypical facial pain

Duration	2–21 years [1,2,3,4,8]
Periodicity	varies from constant daily pain (57–90% patients) to months that are pain free (17–35% of patients) [2,3,10]
Character	deep poorly localised pain, many pain words are used to describe the pain (here is only a selection): vicious, throbbing, stabbing, nagging, burning [1,3,5,6]
Site	usually unilateral, 14–19% of cases bilateral [2,3,4,10]
Radiation	in 83% [2], 74% [3] of cases
Severity	varies from mild to severe [7,8], VAS 6.7 ± 2.5 cm [11]
Provoking factors	stress [3,8], cold weather [3], chewing [3], head movements [3], life events [1,3,8]
Relieving factors	local warmth and pressure [3], medication [3,8]
Associated factors	may follow trauma/dental treatment to area [3,9], psychiatric conditions [1,4,8], altered sensations [2,3], lacrimation [10], facial swelling/flushing [3,10]
Psychological associations	psychological abnormalities [10], depression [1,3,4], psychiatric diagnosis [1,3,4], psychosis [1,3,4], hysteria [1]

[1] Smith et al., 1969; [2] Mock et al., 1985; [3] Pfaffenrath et al., 1993; [4] Remick and Blasberg, 1985; [5] Melzack et al., 1986; [6] Zakrzewska, 1995; [7] Seltzer et al., 1982; [8] Feinmann et al., 1984; [9] Olesen, 1988; [10] Rasmussen, 1990; [11] Vickers et al., 1998.

TABLE 2

Case study 1

Please read through these histories and decide on diagnosis and how you would manage them. See Table 8 for the answers.

CASE 1
Name	DB
Age	56
Gender	female
Development of pain	began over 10 years ago and has over time worsened with very painful episodes intermittently; has had many teeth removed, numerous surgical explorations of the area, various injections and drug therapies, some with limited success for brief periods during this time; has seen numerous specialists, had numerous radiographs, scans and no one has been able to give her a diagnosis
Character	sharp, lancinating, throbbing, aching, heavy
Site/radiation	right side of face and intraorally on the alveolar ridge and buccal mucosa in the area of previously extracted canines and premolars; it occasionally radiates to the whole side of the face and head
Severity	visual analogue scale (VAS) 6.7/10 cm
Duration, periodicity	continuous, can be worse later in the day, but no obvious pattern
Provoking factors	none known
Relieving factors	nil
Associated factors	none
Medical history	stomach ulcers, previous hysterectomy and thyroidectomy
Current medication	diazepam, zantac and thyroxine
Social factors	married 33 years; two grown-up children; does not work; does not smoke; drinks alcohol socially (less than 4 units per week)
Examination	tender over right parasymphyseal region and intraorally in right buccal mucosa and alveolus in canine to premolar region; edentulous; wears upper full denture only (lower too painful to wear)
Investigation	orthopantomogram — unremarkable

CASE 2
Name	SY
Age	29
Gender	female
Development of pain	spontaneous 2 years ago, no real change since that time, has taken over the counter medication which did not really help; seen by a specialist who advised her that there was no treatment for her pain and discharged her
Character	throbbing, aching, heavy, numbing, itching
Site/radiation	left cheek and side of face radiating towards the ear occasionally
Severity	VAS 5.9/10 cm
Duration, periodicity	constant, tends to be worse in cold weather
Provoking factors	touching the area, eating
Relieving factors	none
Associated factors	numbness of the cheek and occasional itching and tingling; headaches
Medical history	fit and well
Current medication	none
Social factors	single; lives in a shared house; architectural student; does not smoke, drinks alcohol on special occasions only
Examination	tender left maxilla and zygomatic prominence; dysaesthesia of left infra-orbital nerve distribution; intact dentition
Investigation	orthopantomogram — nil abnormal detected; occipitomental radiograph — nil abnormal detected

TABLE 2 *continued*

CASE 3	
Name	ED
Age	54
Gender	female
Development of pain	constant over about 5 years, recent exacerbation which has not settled as usual; has not taken any medication for it as it was not 'that bad'; saw a few specialists when the pain began; they found nothing wrong to account for the pain
Character	aching and heavy, sometimes throbbing and sharp
Site/radiation	right side of face
Severity	VAS 3.7/10 cm
Duration, periodicity	constant with intermittent severe episodes
Provoking factors	opening mouth, eating, chewing and touching the area
Relieving factors	nil
Associated factors	sometimes the area feels warm and appears reddened
Medical history	migraine
Current medication	'over the counter' migraine medication
Social factors	divorced, does not work, does not smoke, drinks a glass of wine per day
Examination	tender right maxilla; well restored dentition
Investigation	orthopantomogram — nil abnormal detected; occipitomental radiograph — nil abnormal detected

types of tricyclic and related antidepressants are currently prescribed, their efficacy being shown by various workers (Lascelles, 1966; Moore and Nally, 1975; Remick et al., 1983; Feinmann et al., 1984), in a variety of uncontrolled and controlled trials. Psychological disturbance and depression are reported to be common in this group of patients and psychiatric assessment and treatment is often required (Harris, 1974). It is suggested that this is a biased view based upon specialist clinic populations.

The use of antidepressants investigated in a controlled manner has only been undertaken by three investigating groups. Lascelles (1966) in a crossover trial using the mono-amine oxidase inhibitor (MAOI) phenelzine in 40 patients with AFP found an improvement of pain in 75% of the patients and an improvement in depression in 12 patients after one month. Dothiepin has also been found to be effective for treatment of AFP, at lower doses than that required for treatment of depression (Feinmann et al., 1984). A dose titration system was used in this RCT to obtain a pain-free state in 71% of patients at 9 weeks. It should be noted that 48% of patients receiving placebo were also pain-free at 9

weeks. Assessment of the second generation antidepressant fluoxetine was undertaken in a mixed group of chronic facial pain (CFP) patients, showing effectiveness of the drug in reducing pain (Harrison et al., 1997b) after treatment with the drug for three months. When the diagnosis of the individual patients was compared, data suggested that AFP was more effectively treated with fluoxetine than TMJ pain, although the number of patients with AFP was smaller and therefore gave larger confidence intervals (this may represent a larger variation in the effectiveness in pain score reduction between patients with fluoxetine use or may merely reflect low numbers of trial patients) (Harrison, 1998). The same data compare dothiepin and fluoxetine trials, showing that fluoxetine (over 12 weeks) may be more effective in AFP than dothiepin (over 9 weeks) in reducing pain severity.

The use of cognitive behaviour therapy was investigated in patients with AFP in the above-mentioned fluoxetine trial (Harrison et al., 1997b). No improvement of pain scores was found related to the CBT; however, an improvement in patients control (over their lives), interference (with their life) and distress

TABLE 3

KEY FACTS: management of atypical facial pain (AFP)

1. Establish and advise patients of diagnosis

2. Reassure and explain possible aetiological or exacerbating factors (if appropriate)

3. Empathise with patient

4. Consider (and discuss fully with the patient) management with either or both of: (i) antidepressant drugs if pain is a major problem for the patients; (ii) cognitive behaviour therapy (CBT) if other aspects of the patients' life are being adversely affected by the patients pain or if the patient is motivated to use a psychological approach to manage the pain

5. Review patient regularly with regard to symptoms, psychological status and ability to cope with the condition

was noted overall in CBT patients. The trial patients were of mixed diagnosis (TMJ pain and AFP/AO) and consequently it is difficult to interpret the results with regard to AFP patients. The data appear to suggest that CBT may be helpful in patients whose pain is affecting their ability to manage other aspects of their lives.

Management of atypical facial pain is summarised in Table 3.

Patients may benefit by being given jargon-free information as well as a graphic explanation of how their pain may have arisen. Please see Chapter 9 for further details including support groups.

1.9. Prognosis

No data exist on prognosis of AFP from epidemiological studies. Long-term follow-ups are lacking in most clinical drug trials. However, one of the previously mentioned trials did follow up patients for 4 years, with helpful results.

Long-term follow-up (4 years) of patients after initial treatment with dothiepin has shown that pain improvements can be maintained over time.

Attempts at withdrawal of the drug at 6 months, however, led to relapse and required reintroduction of dothiepin to control pain and it has been suggested that long-term symptom control may require long-term administration of the drug (Feinmann, 1993). If long-term use of dothiepin is undertaken it is possible to achieve a pain-free status in individual patients; over 80% were rendered pain-free in the study (Feinmann, 1993).

2. Atypical odontalgia

This is a variant of AFP, localised to the teeth or tooth which may be an identical condition to that of phantom tooth pain (Schnurr and Brooke, 1992).

2.1. Definition

Tooth pain not associated with lesions (atypical odontalgia, AO). Severe throbbing pain in the tooth without major pathology (IASP).

The International Headache Society uses the same definition as in atypical facial pain.

2.2. Explanatory definition

A continuous pain or severe discomfort in the teeth or in the tooth socket after an extraction, in the absence of any usual dental cause. The pain may be made worse by dental treatment and can move from tooth to tooth.

2.3. History

The term atypical odontalgia was originally described as "idiopathic periodontalgia" by Harris (1974), the more accurate description being introduced later by Rees and Harris (1978). The pain was described as a severe throbbing pain and continuous, usually starting in one quadrant, in clinically and radiologically sound teeth, and by hypersensitivity of the teeth to any stimulus, often being widespread and bilateral. It is reportedly frequently precipitated by local dental procedures, and the tooth is invariably extensively treated or extracted, giving only transient pain relief. The pain recurs within a few weeks in the site of the extraction or moves to another site. It is not unusual for whole quadrants to be rendered edentulous, and possible surgical investigations of the area begin. Spontaneous remissions may occur; these are usually short-lived, but can be permanent (Rees and Harris, 1978).

A large number of the patients report other bodily pains and have a history of depressive illness or have emotional or social stresses. The history of the condition was usually that of exacerbations and remissions relating to the patients psychological health or social circumstances.

2.4. Epidemiology

There are no epidemiological studies of this condition. The epidemiological studies that have been undertaken in the field of facial pain will almost certainly include this type of pain, but unfortunately the research methods (i.e. questionnaires without an examination of the patient) employed in the studies do not allow differentiation between the various types of facial pain.

2.5. Aetiology

The aetiology is unknown. Again there are no epidemiological studies, although several theories as to the origin of pain exist.

It has been suggested that the condition is a symptom of an underlying disorder of affect, associated with a temporary or permanent biochemical defect. Rees and Harris (1978) explained the pain according to the catecholamine hypothesis of affective disorders. This proposes that depression is associated with an absolute or relative deficiency of catecholamines, which when anecdotally induced by an antihypertensive drug in a female patient produced both depression and odontalgia. Treatment with an antidepressant (increasing noradrenaline availability) and withdrawal of the drug limiting noradrenaline availability alleviated the depression and the odontalgia.

It has also been suggested that the pain was due to a persistent vasodilatation in the microcirculation of the affected tissues secondary to the catecholamine activity impairment. The reported strong association of depression and migraine in these patients gave support to the theory. Support for the vasodilatation theory is found in a thermographic study of patients with atypical odontalgia, which found that the areas overlying the pain were warmer than unaffected areas (Gratt et al., 1989).

Marbach (1993a,b) suggests that there are many common features to both phantom limb pain and atypical odontalgia and as such atypical odontalgia is a deafferentation pain syndrome caused by pulpal amputation. This is supported by tooth pulp deafferentation studies in adult cats showing that central somatosensory pathways alter as a result of removal of the pulp (Hu and Sessle, 1989). However, this theory has a number of problems. Atypical odontalgia is frequently found in patients with apparently intact pulps, and pain is often the reason for the removal of the pulp and not just as a consequence of such treatment.

2.6. Clinical features

There again is little evidence except for that of expert opinion as to what the clinical features of this condition are. It is a condition seen mainly in adult females (Merskey and Bogduk, 1994). The key facts are summarised in Table 4.

2.7. Investigations

There are no specific investigations that are diagnosis-specific. This pain may be associated with teeth which are sound, restored, endodontically treated or extracted. Teeth which are clinically sound are vital and tender to thermal stimuli (Merskey and Bogduk, 1994). The pain can sometimes mimic cracked tooth syndrome (see Chapter 10 for details).

2.8. Management

Please read through the case study 2 in Table 5 and see if you can decide how to manage this patient.

TABLE 4

KEY FACTS: clinical features of atypical odontalgia (AO)

Duration	2 months to 20 years [2,3,4,5]
Periodicity	usually continuous, but may last from a few minutes to hours [1,2]
Character	severe throbbing [1,2], aching [1]
Site	teeth and gingivae [1,2,3,4,5]
Radiation	to other teeth [1,4,5]
Severity	varies from mild to severe [1,5]
Provoking factors	hot and cold [1], dental treatment [1,2,4], pressure on tooth [1]
Relieving factors	antidepressant drug therapy [1,2,4,5], counselling [1,4], avoidance of unnecessary pulp extirpations and extractions [1,2]
Associated factors	bruxism [1], hypersensitivity to heat and cold [1], emotional problems [1,2,3,4], anxiety or depression [2,3,4]; may be associated with hypotensive therapy [1]

[1] Merskey and Bogduk, 1994; [2] Rees and Harris, 1978; [3] Brooke, 1980; [4] Schnurr and Brooke, 1992; [5] Marbach, 1978.

TABLE 5

Case study 2

In addition to facial pain there are a number of management problems. How do you suggest these are approached? Please see Table 9 for the answers.

CASE 1

Name	HS
Age	49
Gender	female
Development of pain	constant over about 15 years; has been prescribed numerous types of medication for it which have not helped; has seen more specialists than she can remember since the pain began; she has had numerous dental treatments, teeth extracted and surgical explorations of the painful area; several 'brain scans' have been performed; nothing has been detected to account for the pain; The pain both prevents and disturbs sleep.
Character	aching and heavy, sometimes throbbing and sharp
Site/radiation	left side of top and bottom jaw radiating to front teeth and to head and eye
Severity	VAS 8.7/10 cm
Duration, periodicity	constant with intermittent severe episodes
Provoking factors	opening mouth, eating, chewing and touching the area
Relieving factors	nil
Associated factors	dental treatments in the past have relieved pain for short periods of time
Medical history	'under active thyroid'
Current medication	thyroxine
Social factors	married, three children of school age; helps husband in his work, does not smoke or drink alcohol
Examination	tender left maxilla and mandible; no teeth in upper and lower left quadrants; anterior upper and lower incisors tender to percussion; remaining teeth sound and unrestored
Investigation	periapical radiographs — Nil abnormal detected; orthopantomogram — nil abnormal detected; occipitomental radiograph — nil abnormal detected

Rees and Harris (1978) originally suggested that the management of atypical odontalgia should be with a slowly increasing dose of tricyclic antidepressant drugs, and if these fail to give adequate pain relief the use of a mono-amine oxidase inhibitor was suggested. It was suggested that patients resistant to both of these therapies should be referred for a psychiatric opinion. Marbach (1978) suggested a multiple treatment approach combining antidepressant, analgesic and antipsychotic drugs along with trigger point injections and exercises. There has been no successful long-term follow-up (Schnurr and Brooke, 1992) or controlled clinical trial to date of patients with atypical odontalgia. The evidence is thus anecdotal and further investigation is therefore required. The previously mentioned RCT of fluoxetine and CBT (Harrison et al., 1997b) included patients with AO, although mixed with other chronic facial pain patients. Data from the author indicated that the number of patients within the study with AO was so small that separate analysis of these patients was inappropriate.

2.9. Prognosis

Again there is no evidence above expert opinion concerning patients' symptoms and their development or regression over time. Many authors cite antidepressant drugs for use in managing patients symptoms (Marbach, 1978; Rees and Harris, 1978; Brooke, 1980; Schnurr and Brooke, 1992; Merskey and Bogduk, 1994).

It is suggested that if given in slowly increasing doses (initially tricyclic and then if ineffective MAOIs) they can be effective in giving complete pain relief or occasional brief mild attacks in 75% of cases over 3 months (Rees and Harris, 1978). The combined treatment approach suggested by Marbach (1978) gave 52% of patients an overall improvement of their condition.

The condition is very similar in many respects to atypical facial pain and thus the management is very similar. Key facts of AO management are however listed below in Table 6 for the sake of completeness.

TABLE 6

KEY FACTS: management of atypical odontalgia

1. Establish and advise patient of diagnosis

2. Reassure and explain possible aetiological or exacerbating factors (dental treatment)

3. Empathise with patient

4. Consider (and discuss fully with the patient) management with either or both of: (i) antidepressant drugs if pain is a major problem for the patients; (ii) CBT if other aspects of the patient's life are being adversely affected by the patient's pain or if the patient is motivated to use a psychological approach to manage the pain

5. Review patient regularly with regard to symptoms, psychological status and ability to cope with the condition

---

3. Summary

The chapter is summarised in Table 7. Tables 8 and 9 give the answers for the case studies in Tables 2 and 5, respectively.

TABLE 7

Summary of the chapter

- The diagnosis of atypical facial pain (AFP) remains controversial
- AFP presents as a poorly localised throbbing, nagging pain of varying severity which can be unilateral or bilateral and may be continuous
- Many patients with AFP have some form of psychological morbidity
- Examination and all investigations are normal
- Antidepressants and cognitive behaviour therapy may be helpful
- Atypical odontalgia may be a variant of AFP in that the pain is localised to teeth but otherwise has similar characteristics
- Management may be the same as for AFP but there is no good-quality evidence
- Patients need empathy and written information is helpful

TABLE 8

Answers to case histories in Table 2

CASE 1, DB

This patient had been diagnosed a number of years ago (according to our referral letter) as having AFP. She was, however, unaware of this and felt she was searching for the clinician who could diagnose her condition; it was only then that she felt she could have confidence in the clinician to treat her. The numerous surgical explorations and extractions she had undergone to no avail did not inspire confidence in her.

DB initially took part in the fluoxetine/cognitive therapy trial as she was keen to try any avenue to help her pain which occasionally was so severe she could not function. Over time and with further insight into her acute exacerbations of pain it became clear that the severe pain episodes were frequently following some traumatic incident or period of time. The cognitive therapy helped her become more aware of the stress connections and be able to monitor her status and develop and use several different coping strategies to deal more effectively with the situation both in the long and short term. Fluoxetine was helpful for the patient, but it exacerbated her stomach discomfort and did not aid her sleeping at night. The medication was changed to dothiepin; very quickly her sleeping patterns improved and more gradually her pain reduced as the dothiepin was titrated to a dose of 150 mg which rendered her pain-free for most of the time. After several months on dothiepin the drug was reduced to see if a maintenance dose was necessary. It was never possible to reduce the drug dose to less than 50 mg without reintroduction of the pain, and frequently large doses are needed to control symptoms. Over the years DB has learned how to effectively manage her own pain, the medication being prescribed by her own GMP and being taken in an appropriate dose to reduce pain to a minimum. Initially the GMP was unhappy to prescribe the drug; however, with communication developing over time and now maintained and DB still attending for review (six-monthly) at the hospital it is felt by all sides that self-management of the daily drug dosage is the most effective method of management. It is assumed that this patient will remain on dothiepin in the long term.

CASE 2, SY

This patient initially presented with dysaesthesia of the left infraorbital nerve with no obvious cause. Radiographs were normal and an MRI scan of the brain and brainstem was requested in order that intracranial pathology could be excluded. The MRI was 'normal' and a diagnosis of AFP was made. Some time later it emerged that the patient had been assaulted by a previous partner which had led initially to anaesthesia and then to dysaesthesia. At her initial visits she had been too embarrassed to mention this and did not realise that such signs had potentially serious ramifications. It appeared that this case of AFP had aetiology of traumatic origin. The patient was much reassured by being given a diagnosis. She felt that although the pain was severe at times she was able to cope well with it. She was not keen to take any medication for her pain partly for fear of being labelled as 'mad' by her partner/peers and partly because of a fear of side effects which may affect her ability to concentrate and study in an important year at college. She underwent cognitive behaviour therapy. She found that a specific relaxation technique was particularly useful with severe pain episodes and she also felt that CBT was useful in helping her cope with college and family stresses so that the pain did not get out of control.

CASE 3, ED

All investigations were normal. A diagnosis of AFP was made. The patient was not keen to take medication but decided that she would try fluoxetine to see if it was helpful whilst she was waiting for CBT. A number of different medications and their side-effect profile were discussed with the patient. She felt that other symptoms she would like to be helped with if at all possible were difficulty with sleeping and tiredness. She was not keen to put on any more weight. She took 20 mg of fluoxetine increasing to 40 mg, over a 4-month period. This had no measurable effect upon the facial pain but she felt that the frequency and severity of her migraine had reduced and she felt as if she had more energy. She discontinued the fluoxetine and started dothiepin, although her quality of sleep improved, her weight increased and she stopped taking the dothiepin. The CBT was very effective in enabling her to manage her stress effectively and she felt that as a consequence of this her frequency of migraine attacks remained low and she was more able to cope with constant low-level facial pain. She felt much more in control of her life as opposed to being limited by her symptoms of pain and tiredness and her sleep improved, and was able to start a college course. She still attends for review every 4–6 months and has had some CBT 'top up' sessions when she felt that she was not managing her symptoms as well she had previously been.

TABLE 9

Answers to the case study in Table 5

CASE 1, HS

This patient had atypical odontalgia. She attended requesting extraction of her upper and lower incisor teeth. She had visited numerous dentists, but all had refused to carry out her request. In her microfiched hospital notes there was evidence of one consultation with a consultant some 8 years previously and more recently two visits to the (dental) casualty department requesting extractions of premolars and molars. At each visit a diagnosis of AO was made and requests for extractions were refused. Eight years ago she had been prescribed phenalzine (MAOI) for several months with no effect upon pain. The medication was then changed to dothiepin, then amitriptyline, then nortriptyline, then motival, then motipress to no avail. She refused further changes in medication and was discharged back to the care of her GMP. In the intervening time between this and the previous consultation she managed to persuade several dentists to extract most of her left-sided teeth. She advised us that after each extraction she did have short-term (a few weeks) pain relief and she was convinced that there was a true 'dental' problem for each tooth extracted, as she was convinced (at this initial consultation) that her anterior teeth had a similar abscess or infection. The pain was occasionally so severe that she was not able to function and she felt her head would explode. A long time was spent reassuring this patient and explaining all that was known about AO. There were elements of the history that suggested she suffered from somatisation and she was seen by our Liaison Psychiatrist who confirmed this. Treatment continued with a combination of fluoxetine and CBT. The pain severity reduced only slightly; however, the patient found that she was less anxious and catastrophising less, thus reducing the frequency of the periods when she was unable to function at all. Medication was changed to dothiepin again but this made the patient too drowsy. The patient was again seen by the psychiatrist who prescribed lustral, but then changed back to fluoxetine as the patient felt that this was the most effective medication helping her to 'feel calm'. It was decided that further medication changes be avoided as they were likely to have a negative effect upon the patient. She remains very much unchanged, being reviewed every two months and reviewed occasionally by our psychiatrist. The main aim of our present management regime is to prevent her doing further harm with unnecessary dental extractions, whilst monitoring her somatisation and reducing her anxiety with the help of our liaison psychiatrist.

4. Further reading

The following provides overviews on orofacial pain.

(1) Madland G, Newton-John T, Feinmann C. Chronic idiopathic orofacial pain, I. What is the evidence base? Br Dent J 2001; 191: 22–24.

(2) Newton-John T, Madland G, Feinmann C. Chronic idiopathic orofacial pain, II. What can the general dental practitioner do? Br Dent J 2001; 191: 72–73

(3) Sharav Y, Orofacial pain. In: Wall P, Melzack R (eds) Textbook of Pain. Churchill Livingstone, London, 1999, pp. 711–737 (ISBN 0-443-06252-8).

References

Marked as regards quality according to criteria set by author.
* Poorer quality studies but only ones in the field, old style reviews.
** Cohort studies, high quality case series with controls.
*** Randomised controlled trials, high quality original studies.

Brooke RI. Atypical odontalgia. Br J Oral Surg 1980; 49: 196–199.

Engel GL. Primary atypical facial neuralgia: a hysterical conversion syndrome. Psychosom Med 1951; 13: 375–396.

** Derbyshire SW, Jones AK, Devani P, Friston KJ, Feinmann C, Harris M, Pearce S, Watson JD, Frackowiak RS. Cerebral responses to pain in patients with atypical facial pain measured by positron emission tomography. J Neurol Neurosurg Psychiatry 1994; 57: 1166–1172.

Fay T. Atypical facial neuralgia, a syndrome of vascular pain. Ann Otorhinolaryngol 1932; 41: 1030–1062.

* Feinmann, C. Long term outcome of facial pain treatment. J Psychosom Res 1993; 37: 1–7.

*** Feinmann C, Harris M. The diagnosis and management of psychogenic facial pain disorders. Clin Otololaryngol 1984a; 9: 199–201.

Feinmann C, Harris M. Psychogenic facial pain, Part I. The clinical presentation. Br Dent J 1984b; 156: 156–168.

*** Feinmann C, Harris M, Cawley R. Psychogenic facial pain: presentation and treatment. BMJ 1984; 288: 436–438.

Frazier CH, Russell EC. Neuralgia of the face. An analysis of 754 cases with relation to pain and other sensory phenomena before and after operation. Arch Neurol Psychiatry 1924; 11: 557–563.

Friedman MH. Atypical facial pain: the consistency of ipsilateral. Maxillary area tenderness and elevated temperature. J Am Dent Assoc 1995; 126: 855–860.

* Gratt BM, Sickles EA, Graff-Radford SB, Solberg WK. Electronic thermography in the diagnosis of atypical odontalgia: a pilot study. Oral Surg Oral Med Oral Pathol 1989; 68: 472–481.

Hampf G. Effect of serotonin antagonists on patients with atypical facial pain. J Craniomandibular Dis 1989; 3: 211–212.

Harris M. Psychogenic aspects of facial pain. Br Dent J 1974; 136: 199–202.

*** Harrison SD, Balawi SA, Feinmann C, Harris M. Atypical facial pain: a double blind placebo-controlled crossover pilot study of subcutaneous sumatriptan. Eur Neuropsychopharmacol 1997a; 7: 83–88.

*** Harrison S, Glover L, Feinmann C, Pearce S, Harris M. A comparison of antidepressant medication alone and in conjunction with cognitive behavioural therapy for chronic idiopathic facial pain. In: Jensen TS, Turner JA, Wiesenfeld-Hallin Z (eds) Proceedings of the 8th World Congress on Pain. Progress in Pain Research and Pain Management, Vol. 8, IASP Press, Seattle, WA, 1997b, pp. 663–672.

Harrison SD. Letter to the Editor. Pain 1998; 75: 160.

*** Hu JW, Sessle BJ. Effects of tooth pulp deafferentation on nociceptive and nonnociceptive neurons of the feline trigeminal subnucleus caudalis (medullary dorsal horn). J Neurophysiol 1989; 61: 1197–1206.

* Kuhner A. The value of destructive surgery of the trigeminal nerve in atypical facial pain. Neurochirurgia 1988; 31: 210–212.

** Lascelles RG. Atypical facial pain and depression. Br J Psychiatry 1966; 112: 651–659.

Lesse S. Atypical facial pain syndrome of psychogenic origin. J. Nerv Ment Dis 1956; 124: 341–363.

Madland G, Feinmann C. Chronic facial pain: a multidisciplinary problem. J Neurol Neurosurg Psychiatry 2001; 71: 716–719.

Marbach JJ. Phantom tooth pain. J Endocrinol 1978; 4: 362–372.

Marbach JJ. Is phantom tooth pain a deafferentation (neuropathic) syndrome? Part I. Evidence derived from the pathophysiology and treatment. Oral Surg Oral Med Oral Pathol 1993a; 75: 95–105.

Marbach JJ. Is phantom tooth pain a deafferentation (neuropathic) syndrome? Part II. Psychosocial considerations. Oral Surg Oral Med Oral Pathol 1993b; 75: 225–232.

McMurty JC. The history of medical and surgical interest in facial pain. Headache 1969; 9: 1–6.

** Melzack R, Terrence C, Fromm G, Amsel R. Trigeminal neuralgia and atypical facial pain: use of McGill Pain Questionnaire for discrimination and diagnosis. Pain 1986; 27: 297–302.

Merskey H, Bogduk N. Classification of Chronic Pain. Descriptions of Chronic Pain Syndromes and Definitions of Pain Terms. IASP Press, Seattle, WA, 1994.

Mock DS, Frydman W, Gordon AS. Atypical facial pain. A retrospective study. Oral Surg 1985; 59: 121–123.

Moore DS, Nally FF. Atypical facial pain an analysis of 100 patients with discussion. J Can Dent Assoc 1975; 7: 396–401.

Moskowitz MA. Neurogenic versus vascular mechanisms of sumatriptan and ergot alkaloids in migraine. Trends Pharmacol Sci 1992; 13: 307–311.

Olesen J. Classification and diagnostic criteria for headache disorders, cranial neuralgias and facial pain. Cephalgia 1988; 8 (Suppl 7).

** Pfaffenrath V, Rath M, Pollman W, Keeser W. Atypical facial pain — application of the IHS criteria in a clinical sample. Cephalalgia 1993; 13 (Suppl 12): 84–88.

Rasmussen P. Facial pain, II. A prospective survey of 1052 patients with a view of: character of the attacks, onset, course, and character of pain. Acta Neurochir 1990; 107: 121–128.

Rees RT, Harris M. Atypical odontalgia. Br J Oral Surg 1978; 16: 212–218.

Reik LR. Atypical facial pain. A reappraisal. Headache 1985; 25: 30–32.

Remick RA, Blasberg B. Psychiatric aspects of atypical facial pain. J Can Dent Assoc 1985; 51: 913–916.

Remick RH, Blasberg B, Barton JS, Campos PE, Miles JE. Ineffective dental and surgical treatment association with atypical facial pain. Oral Surg 1983; 55: 355–358.

Schnurr RF, Brooke RI. Atypical odontalgia. Update and comment on long term follow up. Oral Surg Oral Med Oral Pathol 1992; 73: 445–448.

Smith DP, Pilling LF, Pearson JS, Rushton JG, Goldstein NP, Gibilisco JA. A psychiatric study of atypical facial pain. J Can Med Assoc 1969; 100: 286–291.

* Seltzer S, Dewart D, Pollack RL, Jackson E. The effects of dietary tryptophan on chronic maxillofacial pain and experimental pain tolerance. J Psychiatr Res 1982; 17: 181–186.

Vickers ER, Cousins MJ, Woodhouse A. Pain description and severity of chronic orofacial pain conditions. Aust Dent J 1998; 43: 403–409.

Zakrzewska JM. Trigeminal Neuralgia, 1st edn. W.B. Saunders, London, 1995.

* Ziccardi VB, Janosky JE, Patterson GT, Jannetta PJ. Peripheral trigeminal nerve surgery for patients with atypical facial pain. J Craniomaxillofac Surg 1994; 22: 355–360.

Assessment and Management of Orofacial Pain
Pain Research and Clinical Management, Vol. 14
Edited by J.M. Zakrzewska and S.D. Harrison
© *2002 Elsevier Science B.V. All rights reserved*

CHAPTER 15

Trigeminal neuralgia

Joanna M. Zakrzewska[*]

Department of Clinical and Diagnostic Oral Sciences, Oral Medicine Unit, Dental Institute, Barts and the London Queen Mary's School of Medicine and Dentistry, Turner Street, London E1 2AD, UK

Objectives for this chapter:

This chapter will enable you to:
- Recognise the classical and atypical features of trigeminal neuralgia
- Order the correct investigations
- Manage a patient on drug therapy
- Decide when surgery may be indicated
- List the different surgical options available including their recurrence rates and complications
- Consider how to manage patients who develop a recurrence of pain after surgery
- Advise patients where they may access more information
- Develop your own protocol for managing patients with trigeminal neuralgia

1. Definitions

Trigeminal neuralgia is a neuropathic pain with distinct diagnostic criteria which are included in both the International Association for the Study of Pain (IASP) and International Headache Society (IHS) classification systems. See Table 1 for the definitions of trigeminal neuralgia by IASP and IHS.

Both the IASP and the IHS Classification recognise two forms of trigeminal neuralgia. Trigeminal neuralgia or tic douloureux (IASP Code 006.x8a and IHS Code 12.2.1) is trigeminal neuralgia of unknown aetiology. Secondary or symptomatic trigeminal neuralgia is related either to central nervous system lesions (tumour or aneurysm) or to local facial trauma

and is much rarer. Nurmikko and Eldridge (2001) suggest a condition of trigeminal neuropathy which they define as "painful or non-painful, is associated with a structural lesion or systemic disease or caused by severe arterial compression, usually from an ectatic basilar artery. It may be seen following direct trauma to the nerve, e.g. supra- and infraorbital neuralgias following facial fractures". They also include in this group patients who have developed dysaesthesia and anaesthesia dolorosa following neuro-destructive procedures. Most clinicians recognised that there is an atypical form of trigeminal neuralgia which is not as clear cut and which may be an overlap with atypical facial pain or may be pain that has progressed or changed. In this group may be included patients who have been labelled as having pre-trigeminal neuralgia or atypical trigeminal neuralgia. Nurmikko and Eldridge (2001) define this pain as atypical trigeminal neuralgia and this type of

* Tel. +44-20-7377-7053; Fax: +44-20-7377-7627;
E-mail: j.m.zakrzewska@qmul.ac.uk

TABLE 1

KEY FACTS: definitions of trigeminal neuralgia

IASP definition:

A sudden, usually unilateral, severe, brief, stabbing, recurrent pain in the distribution of one or more branches of the fifth cranial nerve

IHS definition:

Painful unilateral affliction of the face characterised by brief electric shock-like (lancinating) pains limited to the distribution of one or more divisions of the trigeminal nerve. Pain is commonly evoked by trivial stimuli including washing, shaving, smoking, talking and brushing the teeth but may also occur spontaneously. The pain is abrupt in onset and termination and may remit for varying periods.

IASP, International Association for the Study of Pain. IHS, International Headache Society.

pain is clearly identified in four studies describing surgical treatments (Szapiro et al., 1985; Yoon et al., 1999; Zakrzewska et al., 1999; Tyler-Kabara et al., 2002). Most clinical data contain a mixture of types with some reports differentiating between them.

2. Epidemiology

Zakrzewska and Hamlyn (1999) have done a systematic review of the epidemiology of trigeminal neuralgia and the main findings are summarised in Table 2.

TABLE 2

KEY FACTS: epidemiology of trigeminal neuralgia

- Trigeminal neuralgia is a rare condition

- The peak incidence is in 50–60 age group and it increases with age

- Women are more likely to get trigeminal neuralgia but it may be age-related

- At increased risk of developing trigeminal neuralgia are patients with multiple sclerosis and hypertension

Munoz et al. (1988) found a point prevalence 0.1% in a French village. Macdonald et al. (2000) assessed the incidence and lifetime prevalence of neurological disorders in a UK community-based study and found a lifetime prevalence of 0.7 (95% CI 0.4–1)/ 1000 for trigeminal neuralgia. Incidence data on trigeminal neuralgia have been collected in Rochester (USA) since 1945 and reports relating to these data have been published over a period of time. The crude annual incidence for women and men was 5.7 and 2.5 per 100,000, respectively, and incidence rates increased with age but not with sex. The annual incidence when age-adjusted to the 1980 USA population was 5.9 per 100,000 women and 3.4 per 100,000 men. The average annual incidence increased with age and was highest in those over 80 years of age when the figure was 25.9 per 100,000. It was higher in females than males for nearly all age groups; however, the highest average annual incidence rate was recorded in males aged over 80 years when the figure was 45.2 per 100,000. In a review of the world literature it was found that five Japanese and Chinese reports quoted a male predominance (Zakrzewska and Hamlyn, 1999). Macdonald et al. (2000) in a population of 100,230 patients in London reported an age- and sex-adjusted incidence rate per 100,000 a year of trigeminal neuralgia as 8 with 95% confidence interval (CI) of 4–13.

Familial history of trigeminal neuralgia has been reported and in most series no connections have been identified but there are a small cluster of patients who may have Charcot–Marie–Tooth Neuropathy (Coffey and Fromm, 1991).

The disease most frequently linked with trigeminal neuralgia is multiple sclerosis. Katusic et al. (1990) estimated that the relative risk was 20 (95% CI, 4.1–58.6). The timing of the two conditions is variable and has been reviewed extensively by Hooge and Redekop (1995) who included in their review patients attending a multiple sclerosis clinic. Hooge and Redekop found in their 1882 population of multiple sclerosis patients 35 (1.9%) that had trigeminal neuralgia. In 5 of them the trigeminal neuralgia was the first symptom appearing between 1 and 11 years after the diagnosis of multiple sclerosis whereas in 30 it was 3–28 years after the multiple sclerosis diagnosis. Two indicators they identified were younger age and a higher incidence of bilateral cases (14%).

Katusic et al. (1990) found 19 patients with hypertension in their series. The odds ratio for hypertension was 1.96 (95% confidence limits 1.2–3.1). Katusic et al. (1990) did not find a viral, seasonal or familial link.

Risk factors for trigeminal neuralgia have been assessed by Katusic et al. (1990) in their longitudinal cohort of patients and Rothman and Monson (1973a) assessed risk factors using a case control study. Rothman and Monson looked at the following variables: age at diagnosis, sex, religion (Catholic, Jewish), race, marital status, handedness, socioeconomic status, country of birth, distance from Massachusetts, alcohol consumption, cigarette smoking, coffee consumption, stroke or heart attack, gallstones, asthma, stomach ulcer, tonsillectomy, multiple sclerosis, cold sores and clinic at which first presented. Relative to controls trigeminal neuralgia patients smoked less, consumed less alcohol, had fewer tonsillectomies, were less likely to be Jewish and less likely to be immigrants.

3. Aetiology and pathophysiology

Determining the aetiology of trigeminal neuralgia has been difficult due to the lack of an animal model but over the years considerable progress has been made. A hypothesis for the mechanism of pain generation in trigeminal neuralgia has been put forward but more clinical evidence is needed to prove it. I will provide a summary of the findings and I suggest you read the recent articles by Devor et al. (2002) and Love and Coakham (2001) as well as Section 8.3 in Chapter 2 or in the overview article by Nurmikko and Eldridge (2001).

Most researchers will agree that the most likely site for the generation of trigeminal pain is in the nerve itself at the point called the root entry zone (REZ). This is a point at which the peripheral and central myelins of Schwann cells and astrocytes meet. This is a vital area as any changes here result in altered function of the whole neurone. There is clinical evidence to show that compression of the nerve at the REZ by blood vessels or tumours does occur. It has also been shown that plaques of demyelination such as seen in multiple sclerosis are found in this area. The subsequent nerve injury results in abnormal firing of the nerve which has led to the ignition hypothesis (Devor et al., 2002). The injured afferents become hyperexcitable and if the after-discharge becomes sufficiently large it results in a nociceptive signal being perceived as pain. It is further postulated that this constant barrage of impulses can eventually lead to central sensitisation and hence a change in the character of the pain to the more atypical type which has a continuous background element similar to other neuropathic pains.

This hypothesis allows us to explain why the various treatments all result in pain relief but it also suggests that surgical treatment should be carried out earlier rather than later. Evidence for this needs to be collected from clinical material where patients' pain and sensory changes have been carefully monitored over a longer period of time. Drug therapy attempts to reduce this hyperexcitability. Decompression of the nerve allows for return to normal function, prevents further damage and enables remyelination to occur. All the other surgical procedures result in destruction of the relevant fibres and so prevent pain being transmitted. These later treatments therefore all result in an element of sensory loss and may allow the process to continue. However, patients still get recurrences of pain even after decompression and negative findings on re-operation and this probably reflects the neuroplasticity of the nervous system.

4. Clinical features

Before reading the text on clinical features look through case studies in Table 3. See if you can come to a decision about the diagnosis. The measures used in the case studies are described in detail in Chapter 6.

TABLE 3

Case studies 1 and 2

List what you consider to be the key features of trigeminal neuralgia. Now read these two histories: do these patients have trigeminal neuralgia? How may you proceed in order to make a firmer diagnosis?

Case history 1

Name	DM
Age	57
Gender	Female
Development of pain	First episode of pain one and a half years ago, beginning suddenly. Lasted for several weeks and then no pain for nine months. Present episode of pain began 2 months ago after eating a meal.
Character/quality	Words from McGill pain questionnaire: quivering, shooting, stabbing, sharp, crushing, tingling, aching, tender, tiring, terrifying, killing, blinding, unbearable, piercing, tight, agonizing.
Site and radiation	Left mental area is the trigger point and the pain radiates up along the whole of the left mandibular branch occasionally radiating to the outer canthus of the eye.
Severity	The pain varies in severity from 9 cm on the visual analogue scale of 0–10 cm to an average of 4 cm. There are times when there is no pain.
Duration and periodicity	Each pain episode lasts a few seconds but there may be bouts of these pains many times a day. There may be no pain for a week or two. There is no pain at night and it does not wake at night.
Provoking factors	Eating, talking, attempting to put make up on her lower lip, washing lower part of the face.
Relieving factors	No activities.
Associated factors	Smoking makes the pain worse.
Use of medication	Responds to anticonvulsant drugs.
Effect of pain on life style	Has a considerable effect on her quality of life, took a week off work as could not do her job as a personal secretary.
Examination	No cranial nerve abnormalities and fully dentate with no dental disease.

Case history 2

Name	DW
Age	71
Gender	Female
Development of pain	Slowly developed first five years ago, there have been periods of weeks when there has been no pain.
Character/quality	Words from McGill pain questionnaire: quivering, jumping, pricking, sharp, gnawing, burning, stinging, aching, tender, tiring, wretched, annoying, piercing, numb, nagging.
Site and radiation	Right mandibular and maxillary region, always the same area, felt deep in the face.
Severity	On visual analogue scale of 0–10 cm, at its worst 6 cm, mean of 3 cm, pain may go completely.
Duration and periodicity	Each burst of pain lasts a few seconds, and then these may repeat in episodes every few hours. There have been periods of weeks of complete pain relief.
Provoking factors	Eating and brushing the teeth starts up pain.
Relieving factors	Only drugs help.
Associated factors	Some neck pain but no other pain or disturbances.
Effect of pain on life style	Unable to socialise as much as would like, no evidence of anxiety or depression on Hospital and Anxiety Scale.
Examination	No gross abnormalities, partial denture wearer.

Please see the end of the chapter for the answers in Table 44.

TABLE 4

Characteristics of trigeminal neuralgia as determined from studies whose major purpose is to describe the signs and symptoms of trigeminal neuralgia

Feature	No. Pts.	Characteristics	Reference
Site	155	R 56%; L 38%; B 4%	Rushton and Macdonald, 1957
	75	R 57%; L 40%; B 1%	Katusic et al., 1990
	229	R 64%; L 34%; B 2%; deep pain 45%, superficial 35%, mixed 20%	Rasmussen, 1991a [a]
	126	R 64%; L 36%; B 0%	Bowsher, 2000
Radiation	229	Most in division; outside face 6%	Rasmussen, 1991a [a]
Character	43	Flashing, terrifying, blinding and torturing (% not given) using MPQ	Melzack et al., 1986 [a]
	229	Shooting/cutting 95%, dull 1.7%, smarting-burning 1.7%, pricking/sticking 1.3%	Rasmussen, 1990a [a]
	95	Sharp 69%, shooting 63%, unbearable 51%, stabbing 47%, exhausting 47%, tender 33%, terrifying 34%, torturing 30%, using MPQ	Zakrzewska, 1995 [a]
	31	Shooting and exhausting 68%, sharp, piercing 58%, throbbing, tender 50%, aching, tiring 30%, wretched 20%, nagging 10%, using MPQ	Zakrzewska et al., 1999 [a]
	102	Sharp 67%, stabbing 51%, shooting 43%, searing 38%, burning 7%, using MPQ	Bowsher, 2000
Severity	31	Moderate, PRI 35.6 ± 11.5, NWC mean 12.5 ± 3.56, using MPQ	Zakrzewska et al., 1999 [a]
	102	PRI 30.9 ± 9.6, NWC mean 10.5 ± 3.4, using MPQ, in 59 new patients on VAS 9.5 ± 10	Bowsher, 2000
Onset of pain	109	Patients relate it to dental treatment or disease 22%, started acutely 55%	Rasmussen, 1990a [a]
	126	Memorable onset 86.5, 27% first consulted a dentist	
Duration	109	Less 1 yr 15%; 1–5 yrs 43%; 5–10 yrs 23%; 10–20 yrs 13%; 20–30 yrs 4%; progressive 37%	Rasmussen, 1990b [a]
	44	Less than 2 yrs 7%; 2–4 yrs 23%; over 4 yrs 70%	Weddington and Blazer, 1936 [a]
	75	Number of attacks per year 21%	Katusic et al., 1990
Periodicity	229	Pain-free periods in 73%: years 6%, months 36%, weeks 16%, days 16%, constant 23%; pain during day 71%, at night 18%, seasonal variation 31%	Rasmussen, 1990a, 1991b [a]
	75	Mean time of episode of pain is 116 days range 1–1462, second episode of pain within 5 years 65%	Katusic et al., 1990
Provoking factors	229	Provoking factor 96%: chewing talking 76%, touching 65%, trigger zone 50%, cold 48%, heat 1%, head movements, bed rest 2%, stooping, abdominal contraction 1%, dentures 0.4%, psychological factors 2%	Rasmussen, 1991b [a]
	72	Chewing/eating 74%, touch 74%, talking 65%, movement 60%, wind/cold 51%, emotional stress 38%, sexual activity 32%, heat 5%, trigger points 97%	Bowsher, 2000
Relieving factors	72	Warmth 18%, rest 7%, nothing 65%	Bowsher, 2000
Associated factors	229	Lacrimation 31%, rhinorrhoea 9%, salivation 7%, swelling and flashing 5%, migranoid features 0.4%	Rasmussen, 1991b
	126	No relief from carbamazepine 19%	Bowsher, 2000
	229	Psychological abnormalities 4%	Rasmussen, 1991b [a]
	31	Depression mild/moderate 51%, anxiety mild/moderate 49%	Zakrzewska et al., 1999 [a]

TABLE 4 *continued*

Feature	No. Pts.	Characteristics	Reference
Signs	25	60% at least one abnormal measure of sensation on the affected side, tactile and warm sensation, pinprick and heat pain no change	Nurmikko, 1991 [a]
	28	Perception thresholds for touch, warmth and coolness raised, normal for pinprick and hot pain	Bowsher et al., 1997 [a]

R, right; L, left; B, bilateral; MPQ, McGill Pain Questionnaire; PRI, pain rating index; NWC, number words chosen; VAS, visual analogue scale 0–10 cm.

[a] Reports using some form of control, i.e. other form of facial pain, although Bowsher (2001) surveyed 126 patients not all patients completed the required questions and they were also divided whether they had previous surgery (54) or not (72).

Richardson et al. (2000) suggest that the validity of the clinical manifestations should be considered under five headings which are discussed in Chapter 8. I attempted to apply these criteria to trigeminal neuralgia and found that not all are fulfilled. This is because there are no case control studies to validate the characteristics and so assess how reproducible these features are when different clinicians take the history (Zakrzewska, 2002a). I have done a systematic review of all studies to assess the current criteria and the findings are summarised in Table 4.

Clinicians are all agreed that there are patients whose histories fulfil all the criteria listed in Table 5, but this is not true of all patients. The history may be modified by a number of factors: progression over time, change related to medical or surgical intervention and psychological factors.

4.1. Character

There is overall agreement that the pain of trigeminal neuralgia has a sharp quick quality to it. This is clearly shown when using the McGill pain questionnaire to elicit the character of the pain as shown in Table 4. Szapiro et al. (1985) reported that in 26/70 of their pre-surgical patients there was a background pain that was not always just dull and aching but at times throbbing and burning and of considerable intensity. They suggest that this could indicate some element of dysaesthesia even in patients who have not been operated on. In their patients those with back-

TABLE 5

KEY FACTS: features of trigeminal neuralgia as proposed by the International Headache Society (IHS)

A. Paroxysmal attacks of facial or frontal pain which last a few seconds to less than 2 minutes

B. Pain has at least 4 of the following characteristics:
   1. Distribution along one or more divisions of the trigeminal nerve
   2. Sudden, intense sharp, superficial, stabbing or burning in quality
   3. Pain intensity severe
   4. Precipitation from trigger areas, or by certain daily activities such as eating, talking, washing the face or cleaning the teeth
   5. Between paroxysms the patient is entirely asymptomatic

C. No neurological deficit

D. Attacks are stereotyped in the individual patient

E. Exclusion of other causes of facial pain by history, physical examination and special investigation when necessary

ground pain were more likely to have pain in two or three divisions, a sensory deficit in two or three divisions, be female and on exploration of the posterior fossa have the least advanced compression and for it to be in the region of the posterior superior area.

Nurmikko and Eldridge (2001) describe the pain in their atypical trigeminal neuralgia patients as having additional features of burning and smarting and they report it as being less severe. Those with trigeminal neuropathy also have shooting pain but in addition describe their pain as dull, smarting and of steady duration.

4.2. Periodicity, timing, duration, onset

Trigeminal neuralgia is paroxysmal and there are periods of complete freedom from pain. Penman (1968) made a distinction between (a) 'paroxysms' or short periods when pain is continuous, (b) 'runs' when there are only brief periods of relief between paroxysms, (c) 'bouts' when there are longer periods of pain relief but some pain can still occur, and (d) 'remissions' when there is no pain at all. The paroxysms of pain last for only a few minutes or even seconds but outlast the provoking stimulus.

Each attack of pain reaches maximum intensity fairly rapidly, and then becomes stable before finally subsiding (Kugelberg and Lindblom, 1959). The pain spreads rapidly at the beginning of the attack and then recedes more slowly. The attack is followed by a refractory period whose length is related to the intensity and duration of the pain and not to the stimulus. Attacks that occur within the refractory period are of decreased duration and intensity (Kugelberg and Lindblom, 1959). Bowsher (2000) reported that there was no clear consensus whether subsequent attacks of pain after a pain remission period were longer.

It has remained difficult to determine the frequency and length of remissions and relapses. Katusic et al. (1990) in their epidemiological survey of 75 patients used Kaplan–Meier life table methodology to estimate frequency of pain episodes and they predicted that 65% of patients would have the second episode of pain within 5 years and 77% within 10 years. Age did not correlate with timing of the next episode. Rushton and Macdonald (1957) reported that in 155 patients with trigeminal neuralgia 78 (50%) had one or more remissions for 6 months or longer and 38 (25%) had them for over 12 months. They also showed that patients who had the longest remission periods were least likely to want to have surgery. It must be remembered that at the

time carbamazepine was not yet being used and the surgical techniques used were either very short-lived (avulsions, or alcohol) or major surgery with high complication rates. Anecdotally, I have also found that patients with good pain control on medication and periods of pain relief are less willing to undergo surgery (Zakrzewska and Patsalos, 2002). Without using any statistical analysis Rushton and Macdonald (1957) suggest that time of onset of disease, first presentation and duration of the longest pain-free interval could be used to predict the future course of the condition. They make a very important observation that no treatment can be deemed successful until it has given pain relief for over one year. Rothman and Monson (1973b) found that the 10 year survival from the onset of trigeminal neuralgia to death in their cohort of patients with trigeminal neuralgia was 46% compared with the expected rate of 39% thus suggesting that trigeminal neuralgia does not shorten life span.

By definition it is obvious that the paroxysmal nature of trigeminal neuralgia cannot be ascertained on its first presentation and so it is sufficient to fulfil the other criteria put forward by the IHS in order to make the diagnosis. When relapses occur the pain is usually paroxysmal. Szapiro et al. (1985) noted that of their 70 patients 44 (65%) had only paroxysmal pain whereas the others also had a background of permanent pain.

Trigeminal neuropathy pain is constant with some pain-free intervals and no refractory periods and progresses slowly (Nurmikko and Eldridge, 2001).

Many patients link the onset of their trigeminal neuralgia with some form of dental treatment and this is a recurring theme in the neurosurgical data and one that I have heard from patients attending trigeminal neuralgia support group meetings. Tew and Taha (1995) state that in their 2000 patients one third had unnecessary dental extractions and 4% of patients linked the onset of their trigeminal neuralgia to dental extractions. Garvan and Siegfried (1983) in their cohort of 140 patients with trigeminal neuralgia reported that 67 patients had a total of 680 teeth extracted. Bowsher (2000) analysing 120 patients with trigeminal neuralgia attending a specialist pain clinic reported that 27% of patients first attended a dentist. Rushton and Macdonald (1957) writing before the days of any effective treatments pointed out that 39 out of their 155 patients (25%) had dental extractions and in 17 of them (10%) relief of pain for periods up to four years was achieved.

Bowsher (2000) and Tyler-Kabara et al. (2002) point out that most patients remember vividly their first attack, 86.5% and 93% respectively. Tyler-Kabara et al. (2002) in their retrospective review of 2264 patients undergoing microvascular decompression, also state that the atypical types of trigeminal neuralgia are less likely to have a memorable first attack (38.5%) and that memorable onset is a prognostic factor for improved outcomes.

4.3. Site and radiation

Most series describe the site of pain according to the anatomy of the trigeminal nerve. Henderson (1967) preferred to describe the site of pain not in terms of divisions, but of 'zones'. Pain is either in the mouth-to-ear zone (ear, upper and lower gums) or in the nose-to-orbit zone (eye, nose, cheek). He was able to assign all but 5% of 650 patients to one or other of these groups: 33% nose-to-orbit and 62% mouth-to-ear. In the remaining 5% of patients, the pain moved from one zone to the next at some stage. Bowsher (2000) points out that careful questioning of patients does suggest that although the pain is experienced intra-orally it is felt in the gingival area rather than in the tooth itself.

The predominant side of involvement is the right although a review of the literature did show some slight variation (Zakrzewska and Hamlyn, 1999) and there does not appear to be a link with handedness, age or gender (Rothman and Wepsic, 1974). From Table 4 you can see that a small percentage of patients have bilateral trigeminal neuralgia. Rushton and Macdonald (1957) in their review of 155 patients found seven patients with bilateral pain and in none had both sides started simultaneously. The interval between onset of pain in the two sides varied from 3 to 24 years. Pollack et al. (1988) reported on 35 patients who were undergoing microvascular decom-

pression for trigeminal neuralgia who had bilateral pain. They compared their characteristics to 664 patients with unilateral trigeminal neuralgia who were undergoing surgery. Patients with bilateral symptoms did not vary in respect of gender, age, duration of symptoms from the unilateral cases. However there was a higher incidence of family history, hypertension and more cranial nerve dysfunction. Only one of their patients was found to subsequently have multiple sclerosis. In their series no patient had single first division symptoms and the majority had involvement of second and third divisions. In 77% of patients pain began on the right side and only 3% had pain beginning simultaneously on both sides. The average time prior to onset of pain on the other side was 8.9 ± 7.3 years. Tacconi and Miles (2000) in their 16 patients with bilateral trigeminal neuralgia had one patient in whom the pain began at the same time. Two patients had MS and two had familial Charcot–Marie–Tooth disease. Surgical outcomes were poorer on these patients.

There is no evidence from cohort studies that shows how number of divisions involved changes with time. Rothman and Beckman (1974) using case controls showed in 500 patients that those with lower facial involvement were younger and tended to be male.

Bederson and Wilson (1989) when analysing their surgical cases noted that longer duration of symptoms correlated with more involved divisions but there were no control data available. In the patients undergoing cryotherapy it was noted that in 38% patients pain recurrence correlated with migration of pain to another nerve branch (Zakrzewska and Nally, 1988) whereas in patients who had a previous radiofrequency rhizotomy the pain returned to a different division in 19% (Bowsher, 2000). Szapiro et al. (1985) noted that patients with less typical pain were more likely to have pain in more than one division.

4.4. Severity

The pain of trigeminal neuralgia can be suicidal (Harris, 1926) and those of you who have witnessed these acute episodes will be in no doubt as to the potential severity of the pain. Egan et al. (2001) report a patient who committed suicide after radiofrequency thermorhizotomy which not only did not relieve his pain but also left him blind. The patient also had bilateral pain which was successfully controlled on the other side. One of our patients with bilateral trigeminal neuralgia and severe dysaesthesia after radiofrequency thermorhizotomy also committed suicide (unreported). The McGill pain questionnaire shows that both sensory and affective elements are high (see Table 4). Up to 60% of patients report that the pain increases with severity after the first attack (Bowsher, 2000).

4.5. Provoking and relieving factors

One of the diagnostic criteria for trigeminal neuralgia is that it is light touch provoked. Henderson (1967) suggested that stress may be a provoking factor and Bowsher (2000) reported it in over 35% of their patients. The stimuli can be mechanical (76%) or thermal (60%) and Bowsher (2000) also reports six patients who had extratrigeminal triggers, e.g. noise, lights, and sweets. In two thirds of patients no relieving factors are reported and only 7% are helped by rest and relaxation (Bowsher, 2000). Many suggest that the response to carbamazepine can be taken as evidence that the correct diagnosis has been made but from RCTs and case reports between 20 and 30% of patients may not have a positive response (McQuay et al., 1995; Bowsher, 2000).

4.6. Associated factors

Patients with trigeminal neuralgia typically have trigger areas which when touched provoke pain but this is not found in patients with trigeminal neuropathy who have large areas which are allodynic (Nurmikko and Eldridge, 2001). Patients in severe pain will be reluctant for anyone to touch their face and have a characteristic pain behaviour pattern (Nurmikko and Eldridge, 2001). Bowsher (2000) argues that the trigger points of trigeminal neuralgia are the same as allodynia but the lack of background pain makes this

feature more noticeable. Tyler-Kabara et al. (2002) suggest that the presence of trigger points is a good predictor of good outcome after microvascular decompression.

Vasodilation and swelling has been reported in patients with severe pain (Nurmikko et al., 2000). This finding is potentially significant as it provides evidence that during a paroxysmal attack a response is obtained from antidromic invasion of the cutaneous endings of certain C-nociceptors.

Patients with trigeminal neuralgia may have hemifacial spasm and in the series from Pittsburgh they found that a higher percentage of patients with vertebrobasilar artery compression were likely to have both these complaints, 5/31 (15%) vs. 8/1373 (0.6%) (Linskey et al., 1994).

Most reports indicate that patients are rarely affected by pain at night and Bowsher (2000) has reported that flexing of the head forward brings on an attack of pain. It has been argued that this is evidence that compression of the trigeminal nerve is more likely to occur in the upright position.

Neither the IHS nor IASP descriptions provide any indication of the effect trigeminal neuralgia has on patients' quality of life and psychosocial functioning which may be diagnostic for this condition. Bowsher (2000) reported that 72% of their patients reported severe disturbance in daily living. These are often the chief factors I take into consideration when opting to proceed to surgical management.

Gordon and Hitchcock (1983) assessed personality and illness behaviour in patients with facial pain. They divided the patients into those with trigeminal neuralgia and those with other facial pain including temporo-mandibular joint pain (TMJ). Patients with trigeminal neuralgia (32) were more likely to deny non-pain problems, were less irritable and less convinced that there was a physical cause for their pain than all the other facial pain patients. No data are available on the severity of pain, the duration and periodicity of the pain at the time that these assessments were made.

Marbach and Lund (1981) reported that in 89 trigeminal neuralgia patients (non-pain controls used) depression correlated with pain severity, number of symptoms and help seeking behaviour whereas anhedonia did not.

I use the Hospital Anxiety and Depression Scale (see Chapter 6 for further details) on all my patients. Using this measure I have shown that patients have considerable depression and anxiety prior to surgery and that depression improves after successful surgery (Zakrzewska and Thomas, 1993; Zakrzewska et al., 1999).

4.7. Findings on examination

As shown in Table 4 several studies have shown that sophisticated sensory testing picks up some sensory changes but not in all modalities. The sensory loss can be in a small area round the trigger point and too subtle for the patient to notice. Szapiro et al. (1985) during their analysis of cases for microvascular decompression found 17 patients to have a sensory deficit preoperative despite not having had any previous surgery. Seven of these were in patients with only paroxysmal pain and ten in those with added background pain. They further correlated this with operative findings and did not find increased compression in those who had preoperative sensory loss. Bergenheim et al. (1997) tested 37 patients prior to surgery and found on clinical examination that 7 had reduced sensation to cotton wool (1 totally impaired), 7 had impaired pin prick sensation (2 totally impaired) and the corneal reflex was diminished in 1 and totally absent in 1 patient. Eide and Stubhaug (1998) showed in 14 non-surgically treated patients that gross neurological testing only showed reduced sensation in one patient but on sensitive testing they showed that all patients showed progressive increase in pain intensity and after-sensation in the trigger areas and that surgery resulted in a reversal of these features of temporal summation. It is important to repeat neurological examinations at intervals as changes may occur indicating that there is a secondary cause of trigeminal neuralgia (see section below). These sensory changes may be indicative of more extensive nerve changes but there are few carefully controlled studies using independent observers to correlate clinical findings, operative findings and outcomes.

4.8. Clinical features in secondary trigeminal neuralgia

Secondary causes of trigeminal neuralgia include benign or malignant tumours of the posterior fossa or multiple sclerosis and these may present later in the disease process. Cheng et al. (1993) in their review of facial pain patients seen at the Mayo clinic (1976–1990) identified 2972 patients with trigeminal neuralgia of whom 296 (10%) had tumours. Of these 296 patients only 58 (2%) had classical trigeminal neuralgia with no objective motor or sensory deficit but they were younger than the average patient with idiopathic trigeminal neuralgia. However 27 (47%) proceeded to develop neurological signs which resulted in further investigations mainly by CT which led to a diagnosis on average 6.3 years after presentation with trigeminal neuralgia. Radiological assessment had not been done in 78% of patients at the onset although this is now changing with the more extensive use of magnetic resonance imaging (MRI). The neurological signs detected were not just of the trigeminal nerve but were found in other cranial nerves or centrally. Although many of these patients responded initially to treatment both medical and surgical, all suffered relapses. Most of the tumours were meningiomas of the posterior fossa. A review of 136 patients with middle and posterior fossa tumours by Puca et al. (1995) showed that 33% of patients presented with classical trigeminal neuralgia. To further complicate the clinical picture it is not unusual for patients to have 2 possible secondary causes. Meaney et al. (1995b) demonstrated that 7 patients with multiple sclerosis and trigeminal neuralgia had either tumours or vascular compression on magnetic image resonance scanning in addition to plaques of multiple sclerosis and Broggi et al. (1999) have also reported compression in patients with trigeminal neuralgia and multiple sclerosis.

Compression of the trigeminal nerve can also occur intraorally and the most common area is the mental region where trauma or loss of alveolar bone after tooth extraction leads to the mental nerve being at risk of compression from dentures.

Careful recordings of the clinical features of trigeminal neuralgia are essential and will not only affect medical management but may have considerable effect on outcomes after surgery. Two prospective (Szapiro et al., 1985; Zakrzewska et al., 1999) and one retrospective study (Tyler-Kabara et al., 2002) have shown that outcomes after surgery are affected by initial diagnosis.

Now, having read all the scientific data, take some time to read some of the poems in Table 6 which were written by patients with trigeminal neuralgia or their spouses at the suggestion of the committee

TABLE 6

Poems written by patients or their spouses about their trigeminal neuralgia

Poem 1

TIC DOULOUREUX

The Serpent comes
Fork tongued and unctuous
It slithers down the ganglion
Fang flickering, nerve licking
Where and when to strike?

You have become my Demon
I know you for what you do
But I know not who you are
Or from where you come
Why do you mean me harm?

Can we be friends?
Can I make peace with you?
Can I succour you, without pain?
Have you needs greater than mine?
Must I give my life for you?

I grow weary
The torment strengthens
We die together
Unless I can find an end
Then, where will you be?

Without me, you are nothing!
And, if by blade or potion
Must I be rid of you, so let it be
For, there is not room for two
And I am taking charge

Roger Levy

TABLE 6 *continued*

Poem 2

TO MY DEAR HUSBAND

T.N.
It's the only pain
That can be seen
It's the only pain
That seems so mean

I see your pain
In your face
Then back to normal
Without a trace

Never knowing . . . when the next pain
Will come
I feel so helpless . . .
I feel so dumb

Want to help
But don't know how
Afraid to touch
Your cheek or brow

I'm here for you. . .
Take my hand
You know beside you. . .
I'll always stand

If I could take your
Pain away
I'd do it now. . .
This very day!

Just know I care. . .
Though I can't feel. . .
The pain you have
I know is real!

Judy 10.21.98

Poem 3

Hey, Dr. Edmonds
I'm back again today
Won't you please do something
And make this pain go away
It has hurt all night
It has hurt all day
I don't think I can stand this pain
For another single day

For years this has been my story
Each time I go, it is the same
Yes, that tooth no, that tooth
They all hurt just the same

TABLE 6 *continued*

Now take these pills
Puree your food
And pray this pain just goes away

Oh the horror of this pain
The ice pick stabs again
The quickness of the pain
Has come and gone again
Sometimes it will last forever
And I think that I might die
At other times it is a burning
Sometimes just a twitch
My face may sometimes quiver
This you hope no-one will see
It may feel like Novocain
That is beginning to wear off
What a weird feeling
There has been no shot at all

Now it is time to eat
Then brush those teeth
Here comes great fear again
So I bow my head and pray my prayer
God take this pain from me

Oh please not this pain
Then comes the worst of all
Pain like this I never knew existed
It invades the face it is here to stay
Oh please – make this pain go away
The blade of the knife is carving
The pain is so fierce
And now I see my face
As one of Jack-o-Lantern
It hurts so bad
I just want to die
The tears flow down my face
In my heart I ask
Please let this pain pass

This has been by story
For so many years
Then one day a light appears
And these words I hear
Trigeminal Neuralgia
Please tell me what that means

Betty Price

of the US Trigeminal Neuralgia Association. How well they express the pain and its effects. I have found them wonderful teaching material and they help other patients describe their pain.

5. Investigations

There are no investigations that can be used to validate the clinical findings and which could be used as a gold standard. The key investigations are shown in Table 7.

5.1. Psychosocial assessment

Some form of measure of the pain helps the clinician both in terms of diagnosis and treatment and these have been described in Chapter 6. The long McGill pain questionnaire, which is multidimensional, has been used to distinguish between trigeminal neuralgia and atypical facial pain (Melzack et al., 1986). I use it for all my patients who have sufficient command of the English language. Other quality of life, psychosocial or daily activities measures are used to gain improved insight on the disability caused by the condition and to evaluate treatment outcomes. Daily diaries are a way of gaining further diagnostic and treatment outcome data. All have been described in Chapter 6. I think it is quality of life issues that play a crucial role in patients' decision making processes and in their satisfaction after their chosen treatment. The use of psychosocial measures to report outcome after treatments have only been reported by ourselves (Zakrzewska et al., 1999; Zakrzewska and Patsalos, 2002).

5.2. Haematological and biochemical investigations

All patients for medical management of trigeminal neuralgia should have some baseline haematological and biochemical investigations performed so you can evaluate whether side effects to therapy are related to biochemical or haematological effects. Investigations should include haemoglobin with a full blood count, red cell, folate and B_{12} estimation, urea and

TABLE 7

KEY FACTS: investigations in patients with trigeminal neuralgia

Investigation	Indication
Pain, psychosocial and quality of life assessment	All patients to measure disease and illness
Haemoglobin, red cell folate and serum B12	Need to be monitored if on carbamazepine, phenytoin
Clotting and bleeding screen	Prior to surgical procedures
Urea and electrolytes, liver function tests	Monitoring for patients on drug therapy
Dental radiographs	If a dental cause is suspected
CT	To exclude tumours
MRI	To evaluate presence of compression, multiple sclerosis

electrolytes as well as liver function tests including gamma GT. These are further discussed in Chapter 7. Further tests may be indicated in patients undergoing surgical procedures especially to ensure there are no haemoglobinopathies.

5.3. Sensory testing, auditory testing, speech discrimination

Sensory testing using special equipment is not done routinely at present but these have showed that patients do have increased temperature and tactile thresholds (Nurmikko, 1991; Bowsher et al., 1997; Eide and Stubhaug, 1998). Sophisticated sensory testing should be considered in patients with non-classical features or changing symptoms.

Audiometry and speech discrimination is not done routinely but this may be necessary if you are trying to assess how frequent hearing loss is after posterior fossa surgery and whether it has been induced by the surgery. Auditory-evoked potentials are measured during microvascular decompression to reduce trauma to the eighth nerve as discussed in Chapter 9.

5.4. Radiological investigations

In patients suspected of also having a dental cause of pain, intraoral radiographs and rotational tomograms of the upper and lower jaws are required. These should be evaluated either by a dentist or a dental radiologist. Further details can be found in Chapter 7.

Computer tomography (CT) scans are useful for picking up tumours but the most important investigations used in patients with trigeminal neuralgia are magnetic resonance imaging (MRI) and 3D fast-inflow steady state precision (FISP). The MRI can determine if there are any benign or malignant lesions present or plaques of multiple sclerosis. Neurosurgeons will also gain information on the presence or absence of vessels in contact with the trigeminal nerve and this will help them to determine how to explore the area. It has now become fairly standard practise to perform an MRI and FISP prior to performing a microvascular decompression.

The axial MRI T2 weighted fast spin echo sequences are used routinely for assessing head and neck pathology and will pick up structural lesions such as tumours and multiple sclerosis. Enhanced T1-W sequences will give improved sensitivity for small tumours and meningeal disease, gadolinium being the contrast agent.

In order to assess the relationship of vessels with the trigeminal nerve, sequences which are more sensitive to flow have been utilised, e.g. MRA, 3D flash-inflow with steady state precision (FISP), MP-RAGE or constructive interference in steady state three-dimensional Fourier transformation MRI (CISS). Arterial contacts are easier to detect than venous ones for which contrast medium may be required (Majoie et al., 1997). A number of centres suggest that if negative scans are obtained after FISP then contrast medium should be used in order to see if there are

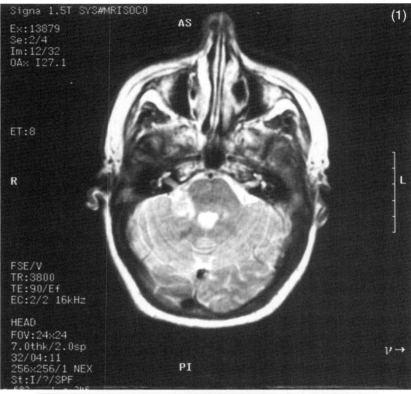

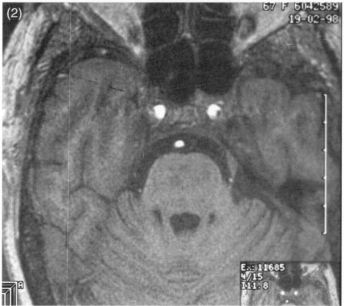

Fig. 1. MRI scans courtesy of Dr. Jane Evanson Consultant Neuroradiologist Case 1 MRI shows a demyelinating plaque in the right middle cerebellar peduncle. Case 2 MP-RAGE image shows a vessel deforming the left trigeminal nerve just beyond the root entry zone (axial). Case 3 MRI shows a vessel touching the right trigeminal nerve (coronal).

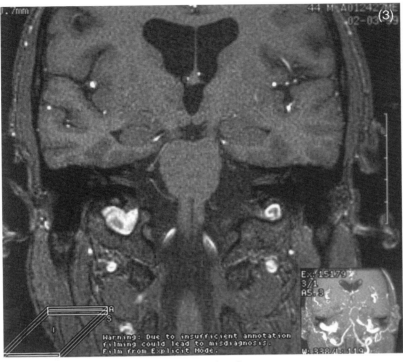

Fig. 1 *continued*

vascular contacts (Zakrzewska, 2002a). Majoie et al. (1997) showed that when using MP-RAGE venous contacts were more likely to be found. Chang et al. (2000b) showed that more compressions were found on operation than predicted on MRI and this may be because the MRI is not sensitive enough for small vessels.

It is important to ensure that not just the root entry zone (REZ) but also the pontine and cisternal areas are assessed and that both coronal and axial images are evaluated. Masur et al. (1995) suggests that contact in itself is not valid as these are found in many asymptomatic nerves but that compression or dislocation of the nerve needs to be identified as these are the ones that are positive on surgical procedures. More than one contact vessel may be found and in these cases compression during surgical procedures is more commonly found.

A review of the neuroradiological literature shows that the criteria necessary to evaluate a diagnostic test as suggested by Jaeschke et al. (1994a,b) are not fulfilled in many cases. Often the interpretation of the MRI has not been done by two blinded neuroradiologists on patients with and without trigeminal neuralgia and the findings have not been then correlated with surgical findings and clinical outcomes. The data that is available has been summarised in my paper on this topic (Zakrzewska, 2002a). Examples of MRI are shown in Fig. 1.

6. Medical management

Many patients are frustrated by the lack of recognition of trigeminal neuralgia and many undergo extensive dental treatment before a diagnosis is made (Tew and Taha, 1995; Bowsher, 2000). Although initial management is relatively easy, long-term management can be difficult as it often depends on the specialist they consult. Patients themselves remain undecided about the types of treatment they could have (Zakrzewska, 2001).

All patients will begin with drug therapy. The clinician has to make a decision about choice of drug and dosage. Please work through the case study in Table 8 first and see if you can make a decision about treatment.

Patients who are diagnosed as having trigeminal neuralgia need to be started on drug therapy which is known to be effective. If you provide careful written instructions and tell the patients that they are in control adherence will be increased as shown in Chapter 9 on management. Before considering individual drugs I will discuss some principles of medical management.

6.1. Starting drug therapy

- Reassess the medical history including current drugs and past experience of drugs in the light of proposed drug therapy (if new, patient will most probably be carbamazepine)

- Do some baseline screening tests as indicated in Section 5.2., in particular, patients who are going to be put on carbamazepine or oxcarbazepine are at risk of hyponatraemia if taking diuretics

- Measure pain intensity, character and quality of life and establish which ones will be used for outcome measures

- Obtain consent to treatment which includes; warning that all the drugs used cause side effects, they are not curative but palliative, do not cause addiction and tolerance is unlikely (it is likely that the disease itself becomes more severe)

- Choose not only the drug but also its formulation, e.g. tablets, suspension, retard (slow release)

- Explain the importance of keeping a daily pain diary and how it can be used to establish the

---

TABLE 8

Case 3

Please read through case history 1 in Table 3 under the diagnosis section. What drug/s would you prescribe, what dose, what instructions would you give your patients, what side effects would you warn them about, how would you assess outcome, when would you next see the patient?

Case 3

This patient has tried carbamazepine but developed a rash which resolved on discontinuation of the drug. The patient had a good response to the drug and is keen to continue medical therapy. What would you prescribe?

Name	LD
Age	42
Gender	Female
Development of pain	First developed pain four years ago but has had months of pain relief.
Character/quality	Words from McGill pain questionnaire: throbbing, shooting, stabbing, sharp, gnawing, hot, tingling, aching, tender, tiring, frightful, vicious, unbearable, penetrating and dreadful.
Site and radiation	Right maxillary division involved with a trigger area over infraorbital foramen.
Severity	The pain is severe. On the visual analogue scale of 0–10 cm, the pain on average is 8 cm and at maximum it reaches 9 cm.
Duration and periodicity	Each stab of pain lasts a few seconds but she gets pain hourly. Does not interrupt sleep. Has had long periods of remission.
Provoking factors	Eating, talking, brushing her teeth, washing her face.
Relieving factors	Rest, drugs
Associated factors	None
Use of medication	Carbamazepine resulted in a rash.
Effect of pain on life style	Has had to take time off work during acute phases
Examination	No cranial nerve abnormalities, full dentition, no dental problems.

Please see the end of the chapter for the answer in Table 45.

correct dose and efficacy of the drugs

- Give some written material explaining the use of the drug stressing that the patient has ultimate control
- Use slow dose escalation and ensure patient understands that fewer side effects are likely if this is done; I tend to do a dosage rise every three days
- Frequency and timing of dosages depend on the pharmacokinetics of the drugs you are using; e.g. baclofen has a short half-life and so needs to be given more frequently than lamotrigine which has a long half-life
- Make an estimate of adherence to treatment and overall understanding of the condition; crucial to ensure that patients understand that the drugs they are going to be using are not standard analgesic with a time-limited effect
- Arrange for regular review and emergency number to call

6.2. Reviewing patients on drug therapy

- Assess how much and how often the drug is being taken, this is most effectively done by discussing the pain diary with the patient
- Make a global estimate of the effectiveness of the drug both in terms of pain relief and side effects
- Perform further assessment of pain outcomes, e.g. Brief Pain Inventory. Hospital Anxiety and Depression Scale, McGill Pain Questionnaire, long or short (see Chapter 6 on assessment for the use of these)
- Do blood tests to check for any side effects that the patient has not reported and which are known to occur
- Consider further use of the same drug at the same, higher or lower dosage, adding on other drugs or change of drug
- Consider the gradual withdrawal of the drug if pain control has been achieved and a period of remission has occurred
- Consider referral for neurosurgical opinion including performance of MRI if pain continues
- Always be on the alert for changing signs and symptoms, e.g. multiple sclerosis, tumour and be

prepared to reconsider the diagnosis, e.g. idiopathic facial pain, dental causes, cluster headache
- Take patient's wishes into consideration and ensure patient feels in control
- Patients on medical management must be kept under regular review while taking medication

6.3. Overview of drugs used

Over the years a wide range of drugs have been used for trigeminal neuralgia but it was not until the introduction of phenytoin in 1942 and then carbamazepine in 1962 that significant progress began to be made in medical management of patients with trigeminal neuralgia. The groups of drugs used for managing trigeminal neuralgia include ion channel blockers such as phenytoin, carbamazepine, lamotrigine, gabapentin and GABA-B agonists such as baclofen. All the drugs try to reduce neuronal hyperexcitability either peripherally or centrally. A further overview of their mode of action can be found in Chapter 9 on management.

Due to the rarity of the condition and the difficulty of designing trials that take into account the natural pain remission periods there are few high quality randomised controlled trial in this area. Some of the problems encountered when doing trials are discussed below.

- Choice of patients for the trials may influence result. Use of patients who have fulfilled all the diagnostic criteria is essential but it is also important to assess specific symptoms, e.g. shooting pain or dull ache and severity.
- Age of the patients may influence outcome.
- Duration of the condition may affect results. It is known that pain relief periods are longer initially and that with time the pain-free intervals decrease. We have shown that oxcarbazepine became less effective with time, not because it was not achieving the same serum concentrations but because the disease itself had become more severe as shown on the outcome measures we used (Zakrzewska and Patsalos, 2002).
- Standardised outcome measures have not been

agreed upon although several trialists have attempted to measure several parameters in order to improve evaluations. Quality of life is as essential to measure as pain relief.

- Intention to treat analysis, i.e. include even patients who have dropped out of trials, have not been done in older trials.
- Placebos are difficult to justify due to the severity of the pain which has resulted in the use of either crossover trials or trials in which the new drug or placebo is added on the current sub-optimal therapy. Placebos which reproduce the side effects of the drug being tested have also been used to try and reduce bias (Gilron et al., 2000).
- Carbamazepine is used in most trials as the crossover drug and this poses problems as the autoinduction effect of carbamazepine can take 3 weeks to disappear. It also interacts with many drugs.
- Size of trials. Randomised controlled trials have been done with 341 patients with the largest involving 77 and the smallest 3 patients. Few centres have enough patients to enter into trials of sufficient size to show a significant treatment effect.

Drugs evaluated in randomised controlled trials are baclofen, carbamazepine, dextromethorphan, lamotrigine, pimozide, proparcaine eye drops, tizanidine, tocainide, topiramate. For most of these drugs therefore there are available numbers needed to treat for effective pain control (NNT) as well as numbers needed to harm, i.e. side effects or adverse effects in excess to those seen with placebo (NNH). As Sindrup and Jensen (1999) point out, the comparison of NNTs is only really valid if the optimal dose intervals are compared to the corresponding NNH. Some drug dosages cannot be raised to their maximum pain efficacy levels due to unacceptable side effects.

Not all the drugs which will be mentioned are available in all countries and in some there are restrictions on their use such that some of the drugs have not been licensed for use in trigeminal neuralgia, e.g. oxcarbazepine in the UK.

Given the narrow mechanism of action of some of the drugs and the examples from epilepsy it would

seem logical to use several drugs at once. Although there are some trials which have evaluated new drugs while keeping patients on sub-optimal doses of other anticonvulsants (Fromm et al., 1984; Zakrzewska et al., 1997), polytherapy has never been compared with monotherapy.

There are several reviews which have not only assessed the evidence for the efficacy of the drugs in trigeminal neuralgia but also provide pharmacokinetic, metabolic and drug interactive data and these have been marked in the references (McQuay et al., 1995; Sindrup and Jensen, 1999; Jensen, 2002; McQuay, 2002). My short, updated overview here is based on a chapter from my book on trigeminal neuralgia (Patsalos, 1995) and pharmacological data from Martindale. Updates on randomised controlled trails are to be found in the 'Cochrane Library' (Wiffen et al., 2000) and in 'Clinical Evidence' (Zakrzewska, 2002b). When prescribing any drug you *must* check the latest information in a current pharmacopoeia which in the UK would be the British National Formulary or MIMS.

The first drugs to be discussed will be those that have been evaluated in randomised controlled trials (listed alphabetically) and the three levels of recommendation will be used as described in Chapter 9, table 9. These drugs are shown in Table 9.

6.4. Baclofen

This drug has been used in spasticity and other neurological conditions since 1972 but Fromm et al. (1980) introduced it for use in trigeminal neuralgia in 1980.

Pharmacokinetics

Baclofen is easily absorbed by mouth and its peak concentration is reached between 3 and 8 hours. It is excreted largely unchanged by the kidneys and it has a serum half-life of 3–4 hours.

Side effects

Its main side effects are ataxia, lethargy, fatigue, nausea and vomiting. Care must be taken when stopping the drug as any rapid withdrawal can precipitate a seizure, hallucinations, anxiety and tachycardia.

Drug interactions

No major drug interactions and it will not alter the serum concentration of other drugs that may be used for control of trigeminal neuralgia.

Antineuralgic effects and use

As well as reporting a pilot study Fromm et al. (1984) have reported its use in a randomised controlled trial as shown in Table 14. It seems to have an excellent NNT. This may be related to the fact that it has a low side effect profile and hence the dosages can be made high. It has also been used as an adjunct to carbamazepine and phenytoin and Fromm et al. (1984) suggest that its efficacy is greatest when used in this way. The racemic form, which is the only one commercially available, seems to be less effective than the L form. I begin with 5–10 mg three times daily depending on the weight of the patient. I then recommend raising the dose by 10 mg every three days till a maintenance dose of 50–60 mg is achieved. In severe attacks daily dosage of up to 80 mg may be needed. If pain control is not fully established I will maintain the daily dose at 60 mg and add in carbamazepine 600 mg daily or phenytoin 300 mg daily. The drug needs to be withdrawn over a 3–4 week period. It is important that the drug is taken frequently even on a four-times-a-day schedule due to its short half-life.

6.5. Carbamazepine

Carbamazepine is a tricyclic imipramine first synthesised in 1961 and introduced for treatment of trigeminal neuralgia by Blom (1962).

Pharmacokinetics

Carbamazepine is slowly but nearly completely absorbed when taken orally within 2–8 hours. Its absorption is erratic and this is in part related to its poor water solubility and hence influenced by other stomach contents. It is bound to proteins and distributed throughout the body. Serum concentrations of carbamazepine vary not only across individuals but even within the same individual. Its epoxide metabolite has been shown to have antineuralgic effects and it may also contribute to the side effects. The elimination half-life changes in chronic use from being 20–40 hours initially to 11–27 hours and this is further altered if the patient is also taking phenytoin. Carbamazepine undergoes autoinduction and even heteroinduction by other drugs which could account for its varying neurotoxic side effects. Using retard (slow release) formulations may help to reduce the variations in serum concentrations and so allow for higher dosage schedules without a concomitant rise of side effects. This process of autoinduction usually takes around 3–5 weeks and this accounts in part for the loss of effectiveness of pain control after a few weeks use.

Side effects

All patients will report some side effects on this drug but these will vary depending on age, rapidity with which the drug is introduced as well as dosing schedules. A list of these is to be found in all pharmacopoeias. Most of the side effects are minor and reversible. Hypersensitivity may develop in 5–10% of patients and there are individual case reports of severe Steven–Johnson syndrome cases. Carbamazepine-induced folic acid deficiency as well as megaloblastic anaemia have been reported often enough to warrant regular monitoring, especially in the initial year of treatment. Carbamazepine has an antidiuretic effect and it can cause water retention in patients with cardiac problems, the elderly and those on higher doses.

Drug interactions

These are very common and it is mandatory to check these when prescribing carbamazepine for any patient already on other drugs. Carbamazepine may inhibit or enhance the potential of other drugs and this is especially important in patients taking warfarin. Patients taking warfarin will need to go for regular testing and this is a group of patients in whom I do not recommend changing dosage schemes.

Antineuralgic effects and use

Randomised controlled trials and as well as clinical use provide ample evidence that this is a highly effective drug for the control of the sharp, shooting pain of trigeminal neuralgia. Many neurosurgeons consider it a diagnostic drug and use a patient's response to it as being indicative that the patient has

TABLE 9

KEY FACTS: randomised, double blind, placebo-controlled trials of drugs used in trigeminal neuralgia

Type of trial (no treated)	Active drug daily dosage	Other arm	Duration of trial	Number improved NNT (95% CI)	Side effects/withdrawals, no. of side effects in reports, NNH (95% CI)	Comments/recommendation	References
Controlled trials, cross-over (10)	Baclofen (Lioresal) 50–80 mg	Placebo	2 weeks	7/10 active, 1/10 placebo; NNT 1.4 (1–2.6)	Ataxia, lethargy, fatigue, nausea, vomiting 1/10	In some cases baclofen used as an add on. Slow withdrawal as may cause seizures and hallucinations A	Fromm et al., 1984
Controlled trial, cross-over (15)	L-Baclofen 6–12 mg	Racemic baclofen 60 mg	2 weeks	9/15 L baclofen, 6/15 racemic 2 (1–4)	Dizziness, confusion, lethargy 6/15 on racemic, 1/15 L-baclofen	L-baclofen not available commercially C	Fromm and Terrence, 1987
3 Randomised controlled trials, cross-over (178)	Carbamazepine (Tegretol) 400 mg–2.4 g	Placebo	8 weeks–46 months	178/315 active, 41/224 placebo (same patients entered several times during sequential trial), NNT 2.6 (2.2–3.3)	Side effects: ataxia, dizziness, diplopia, lethargy 71/150 NNH = 3.4 (2.5–5.2); withdrawal 6/114 NNH = 24 (13–110)	Reduced white cell count, hyponatraemia higher doses, folate deficiency in prolonged use A	McQuay et al., 1995; trials included Campbell et al., 1966, Killian and Fromm, 1968, Nicol, 1969
Randomised controlled trial, cross-over (3)	Dextromethorphan 120–920 mg	Lorazepam 0.24–1.84 mg	6 weeks	0/2 more pain on active drug but wide fluctuations	1 withdrew due to poor pain control; 2 non-trigeminal neuralgia patients withdrew, 1 sedation, 1 rash on placebo; all had mild side effects: cognitive impairment, dizziness and ataxia	Part of a trial to assess use in all forms of facial neuralgia C	Gilron et al., 2000
Randomised controlled trial, cross-over (14)	Lamotrigine (Lamactal) 200–400 mg	Placebo	4 weeks	10/13 active, 8/14 placebo; NNT 2.1 (1.3–6.1)	Dizziness, drowsiness, constipation, ataxia, diplopia, irritability 7/14 active and placebo; withdrawal 1 due to poor pain control	Rapid dose escalation increases incidence of rashes. All patients were on some other anticonvulsant A	Zakrzewska et al., 1997

Randomised controlled trial, cross-over (48)	Pimozide (Orap) (4–12 mg)	Carbamazepine 300–1200 mg	24 weeks	48/48 pimozide, 28/48 carbamazepine; NNT 3 (2–3)	Extrapyramidal, e.g. tremor, rigidity, memory 40/48 pimozide, 22/48 carbamazepine NNH 3 (2–6)	Side effects too severe to recommend routine use including sudden death C	Lechin et al., 1989
Randomised controlled trial, parallel (47)	Proparcaine hydrochloride; 2 drops of 0.5% solution	Placebo	30 days	6/25 active, 5/22 placebo NS	None reported	Toxic keratopathy in long-term use C	Kondziolka et al., 1994a
Randomised controlled trial, parallel (12)	Tizanidine 6–18 mg	Carbamazepine up to 900 mg	3 weeks	1/6 tizanidine, 4/6 carbamazepine NS	2 withdrew due to poor pain control	Effect is short lasting C	Vilming et al., 1986
Randomised controlled trial, cross-over (12)	Tocainide Tonocar 60 mg/kg	Carbamazepine variable	2 weeks	8/12 tocainide; 9/12 carbamazepine NS	Nausea, paraesthesia, 2/12; withdrawal rash 1/12	Risk of aplastic anaemia precludes its routine use C	Lindstrom and Lindblom, 1987
Randomised controlled trial, cross-over (3)	Topiramate 75–600 mg	Placebo	12 weeks	0/3 NS	Irritability, cognitive gastrointestinal fatigue 3/3	May provide some reduction in pain but trial was very small C	Gilron et al., 2001

NNT, number needed to treat; NS, not significant; NNH, number needed to harm; for level of recommendation see Table 9 in Chapter 9.

TABLE 10

Example of dosage schedule (in mg) for carbamazepine (Tegretol) as given to patients

Daily dosage	Day	Morning	Lunch time	Afternoon	Night time
200	1–3	100			100
300	4–6	100	100		100
400	7–9	100	100	100	100
500	10–12	200	100	100	100
600	13–15	200	100	100	200
700	16–18	200	200	100	200
800	19–21	200	200	200	200

- You do not need to go up the full scale and you can do the changes more slowly.
- The amount of drug you need is related to your body weight and age so you may start at a different point in the scale.
- Stop at the point at which you get good control of pain and few side effects.
- You should take it 30–60 minutes before eating or engaging in an activity that will involve touching your face so that you have improved pain control.
- After three to four weeks you may need a further adjustment as your liver gets used to handling the drug.
- When stopping the drug you need to go down in the same way.

Carbamazepine retard

You may also be given a retard form of this drug which is a special form that releases the drug more slowly than the usual form. This is especially good to use at night as it ensures that you have a good level of drug in your blood throughout the night. Sometimes it is also prescribed for use during the day to cut down on the number of times you need to take your drugs especially if your pain has stabilised.

trigeminal neuralgia. Attempts have been made to set therapeutic serum concentrations for pain control but due to its highly variable serum concentrations this has not proven to be useful. Table 10 is an example of a leaflet that we provide in our clinic for patients due to start on carbamazepine. In some patients we will commence with a 300 mg daily regimen.

6.6. Dextromethorphan

Dextromethorphan is an antagonist of NMDA and in the laboratory has been shown to be effective in nerve injuries. It was first evaluated in neuralgic facial pain in 2000.

Pharmocokinetics

It is rapidly absorbed, metabolised by the liver and excreted unchanged in the urine.

Side effects

Rare, occasionally dizziness and gastrointestinal disturbances.

Drug interactions

Will interact with especially MAOIs but need to beware of antidepressant drugs and antiarrhythmics.

Antineuralgic effects and use

It has been evaluated in a group of 19 patients with facial neuralgias of which 3 had trigeminal neuralgia (Gilron et al., 2000). This was a randomised controlled trial in which lorazepam was used as a placebo as it has similar side effects to dextromethorphan. One of the patients withdrew, as he did not get adequate pain relief. Overall in the other two patients there was no change although the pattern in terms of frequency of attacks was altered. More trials with larger numbers would be needed to prove its effectiveness.

6.7. Lamotrigine

Lamotrigine became available for clinical use in epilepsy in 1991. In the UK it is not licensed for use in trigeminal neuralgia at the current time.

Pharmacokinetics

Lamotrigine is well and quickly absorbed after oral ingestion and peak blood concentrations are reached in 2–3 hours. About 60% binds to protein and it is extensively metabolised and over 60% is excreted as a glucuronide. Its approximate half-life is 24 hours longer in the elderly.

Side effects

In line with other anticonvulsants, side effects, especially neurological ones, are common. The most common cause for withdrawals has been the development of a rash. Many of them are probably not true allergies but related to rapid dose escalation. There have been reports of Steven–Johnson syndrome. It does not cause hyponatraemia or other biochemical or haematological effects.

Drug interactions

Lamotrigine does not necessitate alteration in dose of other anticonvulsants and there are no contraindications for its use with other commonly used drugs.

Antineuralgic effects and use

As well as case reports a small randomised controlled trial when it was used as an add on medication showed lamotrigine to be an effective drug. Due to its potential to cause a rash dose escalation must be slow and so it is not the drug of choice in an acute severe attack but more to maintain pain control.

6.8. Pimozide

Pimozide is a dopaminergic-blocking agent. There are two reports of its use in trigeminal neuralgia.

Pharmacokinetics

After oral ingestion, about half the drug is absorbed and peak concentrations are reached after 4–12 hours but these are subject-variable. It is metabolised in the liver and is excreted both through faeces and urine, metabolised or unchanged. It has a long half-life, 55 hours, but can be much longer in some patients.

Side effects

Extrapyramidal side effects are very common and there is a case report of a death with this drug. Its use is contraindicated in patients with a history of arrhythmias.

Drug interactions

Due to its cardiac effects it must not be used with cardioactive or antipsychotic drugs or any that affect electrolyte balance.

Antineuralgic effects and use

Although in a randomised controlled trial pimozide was found to be effective for trigeminal neuralgia its adverse reactions make it unacceptable as a routine drug. It has been recommended that all patients should have an ECG before starting treatment with it.

6.9. Proparcaine hydrochloride eye drops

Topical analgesic eye drops were discovered by chance to have caused relief of trigeminal neuralgia when used for an ophthalmic examination in a patient with trigeminal neuralgia in 1991.

Pharmacokinetics

This is a local anaesthetic with short duration of action. The speed of onset and duration of action depends on site of administration.

Side effects

Repeated use can lead to toxic keratopathy.

Drug interactions

None have been reported when used in this form.

Antineuralgic effects and use

Use of local anaesthesia has been previously reported in the form of an injection into the trigger area and some success had been reported in the use of lidocaine in cluster headaches. The initial case reports including 60 patients seemed to suggest that this could be an effective treatment in patients with trigeminal neuralgia in the first division (Spaziante et al., 1992; Vassilouthis, 1994). It was postulated that some might even be absorbed and so act centrally. However, when subject to a randomised controlled trial the eye drops were found to be no more effective than placebo and this is probably related to the fact that topically the drug cannot exert any appreciable central activity (Kondziolka et al., 1994a). It may have some use in the short-term control of an acute attack.

6.10. Tizanidine

This is an imidazole derivative with analgesic and muscle relaxant properties first reported in the use of trigeminal neuralgia in 1986.

Pharmacokinetics

Tizanidine is absorbed from the gastrointestinal tract and peak concentrations are reached within 1–2 hours. It undergoes first pass metabolism in the liver and is excreted via the urine as inactive metabolite. It is eliminated within 2–4 hours.

Side effects

It can cause drowsiness, fatigue, dizziness, dry mouth, gastrointestinal disturbances, hypotension.

Altered liver enzymes and acute hepatitis have been reported and so liver function monitoring tests are important. The side effects are dose-related.

Drug interactions

It interacts with a wide range of drugs including antihypertensive, cardiac drugs and phenytoin.

Antineuralgic effects and use

When used in a randomised controlled trial with carbamazepine in the other arm, tizanidine proved to be less effective than carbamazepine in pain control and 2 out of 12 patients withdrew due to poor pain control (Vilming et al., 1986).

6.11. Tocainide

Tocainide is a derivative of lidocaine and was first reported in patients with trigeminal neuralgia in 1984.

Pharmacokinetics

It is rapidly and completely absorbed after oral ingestion and is metabolised into a number of products but up to half may be excreted via the urine unchanged. Its plasma elimination half-life is between 12 and 15 hours.

Side effects

Although in the trials the side effects were not a major problem subsequently there have been reported deaths due to aplastic anaemia. It causes CNS and gastrointestinal as well as cardiac side effects. It has been virtually withdrawn for use except in life threatening cardiac arrhythmias.

Drug interactions

It should not be used with lidocaine and interacts with antibacterials and histamine receptor antagonists.

Antineuralgic effects and use

A small study involving 12 patients showed that it had antineuralgic effects but it was no greater than that of carbamazepine and yet it had serious side effects (Lindstrom and Lindblom, 1987). The drug has no place in the management of trigeminal neuralgia.

6.12. Topiramate

Topiramate is a relatively new anticonvulsant, whose use in trigeminal neuralgia was first reported in 2000.

Pharmacokinetics

It is easily absorbed from the gastrointestinal tract and reaches peak concentrations within 2 hours. About 50% of it is metabolised in the liver and the rest is excreted unchanged through the urine. Its mean plasma elimination half-life time is 21 hours and a steady state will not normally be achieved for 10–15 days. Its pharmacokinetics will be affected by other anti-epileptic drugs (AED).

Side effects

The usual CNS side effects occur, i.e. ataxia, impaired concentration, confusion, and dizziness. It needs to be used with care in patients with hepatic or renal impairment, as it has been associated with renal calculi formation and liver failure.

Drug interactions

There are complex interactions with other AEDs, which can be unpredictable. It also has an effect on cardiac glycosides and oral contraceptives.

Antineuralgic effects and use

Zvartau-Hind et al. (2000) first reported its successful use in 6 patients with multiple sclerosis who also had trigeminal neuralgia. It was subsequently used in a very small randomised controlled trial which failed to show any benefit (Gilron et al., 2001).

6.13. Drugs evaluated in case studies

A vast number of drugs have been reported for use in trigeminal neuralgia and a list of these can be found in Table 11.

Table 12 contains more detailed results for another six drugs that have been reported as being helpful in the management of trigeminal neuralgia as well as case studies of drugs reported in trials. These are poor quality studies often using inadequate outcome data. Some of the drugs will possibly be evaluated in the future but others will probably never be the subject of randomised controlled trials. I mention them here not to encourage you to use them

TABLE 11

Drugs used in trigeminal neuralgia

Drug	Class	Mechanism of action	Type of evaluation
Baclofen	Muscle relaxant GABA receptor agonist	Enhances GABA	RCT, case studies
Capsaicin cream	Anti-substance P	Ion channel blockers, local depletion of substance P	Case studies
Carbamazepine	AED	Ion channel blockers, enhances GABA	RCT
Clonazepam	Benzodiazepam	Enhances GABA	Case studies
Dextramethorphan	NMDA receptor antagonist	Blocks NMDA receptors	RCT
Gabapentin	AED	Ion channel blockers, blocks calcium channels, enhances GABA	Case studies
Lamotrigine	AED	Ion channel blockers	RCT
Mexiltetine	Antiarrhythmic	Ion channel blockers	Case studies
Oxcarbazepine	AED	Ion channel blockers, enhances GABA	Case studies, cohort
Phenytoin	AED	Ion channel blockers	Case studies
Pimozide	Dopamine receptor antagonist		RCT
Proparcaine eye drops	Local anaesthetic	Ion channel blockers	RCT
Tizanidine	Muscle relaxant	Alpha adrenoceptor agonist	RCT
Tocainidine	Local anaesthetic	Ion channel blockers	RCT
Topiramate	AED	Blocks non-NMDA glutamate receptors, enhances GABA	RCT
Tramadol	Narcotic analgesic	Inhibits norephedrine and serotonin reuptake	Case studies
Valproic acid	AED	Ion channel blockers, enhances GABA	Case studies

AED, anti-epileptic drug; RCT, randomised controlled trial.

as first line drugs but to give you an idea of the level of evidence on which their use is based. Some of the drugs have been evaluated in randomised controlled trials in other neuropathic pains and hence their use has been extrapolated to use in trigeminal neuralgia. The use of anticonvulsant drugs (antiepileptic drugs = AED) in neuropathic pain has recently been reviewed by Jensen (2002) and his data are used in the discussions on individual drugs.

Until recently the most commonly used alternative drug was phenytoin. This drug has complex pharmacokinetics with very variable effects across individuals. Its bioavailability and absorption is widely different between formulations. Its saturation kinetics mean that over 300 mg daily dose a small increase in dosage can result in a disproportionately large increase in serum concentration and hence unexpected side effects. It is excreted through the liver and also depletes folic acid so it is important to check folic acid levels when used long term. It is often used when patients develop an allergy to carbamazepine. Phenytoin is also a hepatic inducing drug so its drug interactions are similar to carbamazepine. Until the introduction of some of the newer AED phenytoin was the only other option to use if a patient was allergic to carbamazepine and also as an add on drug if pain control became difficult. Randomised controlled trials have been done in diabetic neuropathy where it was shown to be more effective than placebo. Its intravenous form, fosphenytoin, has been shown to be useful in controlling an acute attack (McCleane, 1999; Cheshire, 2001). When using the oral preparation I tend to use no more than 300 mg daily, which gives me little flexibility, and I have not used its intravenous form.

Clonazepam was first used in 1975. Maximum blood levels are achieved rapidly and it has a half-life of 1–2 days. Four case reports have reported

TABLE 12

Drugs used for trigeminal neuralgia case reports with no controls, grade of recommendation for these studies is C (see table 9 in Chapter 9)

No each report	Drug daily dosage	Outcome reported in each study	Side effects/withdrawals (no of side effects in reports)	Comments	References
2 reports (50, 16, 10)	Baclofen (Lioresal) 50–80 mg	37/50; 9/16 excellent or good; 5/10 excellent or good	Ataxia, lethargy, fatigue, nausea, vomiting (6/50, 1/16, nil)	Slow dose reduction, Desai used it as add on with valproic acid	Fromm et al., 1984; results of the open trial Steardo et al., 1984, Desai et al., 1991
2 reports (12, 5)	Capsaicin (Zostrix) 3 g for 21–28 days	6/12 complete, 4/12 partial; 4/12 relapses; 1/5 partial, 4/5 nil or little	Burning sensation (NS)	Rub on the skin, temporary relief in majority, avoid contact with the eye	Fusco and Alessandri, 1992, Epstein and Marcoe, 1994
4 reports (5, 19, 25, 14)	Clonazepam (Rivotril, klonopin) 2–8 mg	5/7 good result; 13/19 excellent or good; 10/25 excellent; 6/25 good; 64% complete/partial	Lethargy, fatigue, dizziness, personality change (5/5, 4/19, 22/25)	Drowsiness is very severe and dose related; thromocytopenia can occur	Caccia, 1975; Chandra, 1976; Court and Kase, 1976; Smirne and Scarlato, 1977
4 reports (2, 7, 13, 11)	Gabapentin (Neurontin) 1200–3600 mg	2/2; 6/7 excellent; 1/7 partial; 4/13 excellent; 5/13 good; 10/11 excellent	Ataxia, dizziness, drowsiness, nausea, headache, oedema of the feet (0, 0, 0, 0)	Khan's patients had multiple sclerosis and 1 year follow up; Solaro et al., used with low dose carbamazepine or lamotrigine	Sist et al., 1997; Khan, 1998; Valzania et al., 1998; Solaro et al., 2000
2 reports (20, 4)	Lamotrigine (Lamactal) 200–400 mg	16/20 excellent; 4/20 partial; 4/4 excellent	Dizziness, drowsiness, constipation, ataxia, diplopia, irritability (7/13, 1/20, 0/4)	Rapid dose escalation increases incidence of rashes	Lunardi et al., 1997, Canavero et al., 1995
4 reports (13, 15, 21, 24)	Oxcarbazepine (Trileptal) 300–1200 mg	13/13 excellent or good ; 16/21 excellent or good; 13/24 excellent/ good/fair; 15/15 excellent short term	Ataxia, dizziness, diplopia, lethargy which may be related to hyponatraemia (1/13, 10/21, 6/24, 13/15)	Side effects less severe than with carbamazepine, hyponatraemia is dose dependent	Farago, 1987; Remillard, 1994; Royal et al., 2001; Zakrzewska and Patsalos, 2002
2 reports (60, 15)	Proparcaine hydrochloride 2 drops of 0.5% solution	24/60 good; 17/60 nil; 9/60; 10 lost to follow up; 13/15	nil	Toxic keratopathy in long-term use; short lasting even if given repeatedly	Spaziante et al., 1992; Vassilouthis, 1994
2 reports (4, 20, 5)	Phenytoin (Epanutin) 200–300 mg	4/4 excellent; 8/20 excellent; 6/20 partial; 4/5 excellent; 1/5 partial	Ataxia, lethargy, nausea, headache, behavioural changes (1/4, NS, NS)	Folate deficiency in prolonged use, gingival hypertrophy, can be used intravenously for immediate effect	Iannone et al., 1958; Braham and Saia, 1960; Chinitz et al., 1966

TABLE 12 *continued*

No each report	Drug daily dosage	Outcome reported in each study	Side effects/with-drawals (no of side effects in reports)	Comments	References
2 reports (20, 10)	Valproic acid (Epilim, depakote) 600–2000 mg	9/20 excellent/good; 4/20 good if used with other drugs; 3/20 no response; 4/10 excellent/good; 6/10 poor but if used as add on 10/10 good	Irritability, restlessness, tremor, confusion, nausea (1/20, NS)	Rash and with prolonged use alopecia, weight gain, increase efficacy with baclofen	Peiris et al., 1980; Desai et al., 1991

NS – not stated.

excellent or good results in over 60% of patients. Drowsiness, which is dose-related, is a major problem however. This can be reduced if the dosage schedule is made more frequent.

Valproic acid was first used in trigeminal neuralgia in 1980. It is rapidly absorbed reaching peak levels within 2 hours and its half-life is relatively short, 6–17 hours. It does not exhibit a linear relationship between dose and serum concentration which accounts for the occurrence of side effects at peak concentrations. It is eliminated through the liver but does not induce the liver enzymes. Its main side effects are tremor, weight gain and hair loss, all of which are reversible on cessation. It has few drug interactions but it does interact with carbamazepine and phenytoin. It tends to be used by neurologists as they use it for epilepsy. An attempt was made to do a randomised controlled trial using valproate on its own or in combination with other drugs but the best results were obtained when a mixture of drugs was used (Desai et al., 1991). The small case reports suggest that it is an effective drug but there have been no randomised controlled trials for its use in any neuropathic pains. I have no personal experience of its use.

Oxcarbazepine, a daughter drug of carbamazepine with fewer side effects, was introduced many years ago in some countries but only recently has become available in the UK. A 300 mg dose is equipotent to 200 mg of carbamazepine. It is well absorbed and peak levels are reached within 2 hours. It is rapidly broken down to its pharmacologically active form which is then excreted through the kidneys. Its major advantage over carbamazepine is its lack of hepatic enzyme reduction which means fewer drug interactions. As it is related to carbamazepine cross-sensitivity with carbamazepine needs to be considered when considering using it in patients allergic to carbamazepine. It has a similar side effects profile to other antiepileptic drugs (AED) with less severe ones than carbamazepine. Hyponatraemia which is dose-related means that serum electrolyte levels need to be measured when doses are high. It has not been reported in randomised controlled trials in any neuropathic pain although it has been evaluated in epilepsy. Again, it is inferred that it would be useful in trigeminal neuralgia as it is so closely related to carbamazepine. In case reports it appears to be effective at controlling the pain of trigeminal neuralgia. We have recently reported a long follow up study on its use and showed that it was initially very effective but lost its effect, not because of the development of tolerance but because of progression of disease (Zakrzewska and Patsalos, 2002). I find the drug easier to use than carbamazepine and its improved safety profile makes it a better option than carbamazepine. It is unfortunate that it will probably not be evaluated in a randomised controlled trial because it has been available for many years. It is used extensively in the Scandinavian countries where it

TABLE 13

Example of dosage (in mg) schedule for oxcabazepine (Trileptal) as given to patients

Daily dosage	Day	Morning	Lunch time	Afternoon	Night time
600	1–3	300			300
900	4–14	300	300		300
1200	15–21	300	300	300	300
1500	22–28	300	300	300	600

If this is the first time you are taking this drug please read the additional leaflet the doctor gives you. You do not need to go up the full scale. Stop at the point at which you get good control of pain and few side effects. If you are replacing your carbamazepine with oxcarbazepine, substitute one dose of 200 mg carbamazepine for 300 mg oxcarbazepine every three days until the change over is complete.

TABLE 14

Example of dosage (mg) schedule for gabapentin (neurontin) as given to patients

Daily dose	Day	Capsules/tablets to be taken		
		Morning	Midday	Evening
300	1	0	0	300
600	2	300	0	300
900	3	300	300	300
1200	4	300	300	600
1500	5	600	300	600
1800	6	600	600	600
2000	7–14	600	600	800
2200	15–21	800	600	800
2400	22–28	800	800	800

You do not need to go up the full scale. Stop at the stage that good pain control has been achieved. Most patients use a range between 1200 and 1800 mg daily.

has been available for a long time. A dosage schedule is shown in Table 13 and I also give patients details on how to change over from carbamazepine to oxcarbazepine.

Topical treatments are used from time to time and Table 12 shows two products: capsaicin cream and proparcaine eye drops. The latter when tested in a randomised controlled trial failed to live up to expectations. These are only intended to give short-term relief before other drugs begin to have an effect. Capsaicin has been shown to be helpful in post-herpetic neuralgia.

The latest drug available for general use is gabapentin which has been shown to be effective in the management of post-herpetic neuralgia and so by inference has come to be used in trigeminal neuralgia. There are small case reports of poor quality of its use in trigeminal neuralgia and yet it is widely used in clinical practice. A trial is being conducted currently on its use in intractable pain patients. It causes fewer side effects than many other AEDs and has a better safety profile. I use it in clinical practice as a second line drug when patients cannot tolerate higher doses of carbamazepine. Table 14 shows the schedules I use.

From the current data, I have tried to summarise in Table 15 some of the advantages and disadvantages of the drugs that are used in the UK on a regular basis.

An overall summary of the use of drugs in trigeminal neuralgia is shown in Table 16.

7. Surgical management

For those of you who like a historical review of surgery for trigeminal neuralgia I would recommend an article by Wilkins (1999) which includes a range of very elegant drawings and a comprehensive list of references. I will only deal with surgical techniques that are in current use.

7.1. Indications for change to surgical management and timing of surgery

When to change patients from drug therapy to surgical treatments remains a difficult decision, especially if pain control and side effects are acceptable (see Section 4.2). Work through the following cases in Table 17 and try to make some decisions about treatment.

TABLE 15

Advantages and disadvantages of drugs currently being used for trigeminal neuralgia

Drug	Advantages	Disadvantages
Baclofen	Wide dosage range possible	Needs to be started and reduced slowly
	Few side effects	Needs to be taken on a three or four times a day schedule
	No major drug interactions	Monitor renal function in long-term use
	Can be used if patient allergic to other antineuralgic drugs	
	Can use as add on therapy	
Carbamazepine	Highly effective rapid pain control	All patients will have side effects
	Wide dosage range which enables a range of dosage schemes	Potent drug interactions
	Variety of formulations	Induces liver enzymes
		Allergy develops in 7%
		Regular blood tests needed
Lamotrigine	Can be used in the elderly	Its use as monotherapy has not been assessed
	Does not interact with common drugs	Rapid dose escalation leads to rashes so not suitable for acute pain control
	Effective if used twice daily	Side effects noted in most patients
	Tolerable side effects	
Clonazepam	May be effective	Not been evaluated in a randomised controlled trial
		Side effects very common with drowsiness being a major problem and enhanced by alcohol
		Regular blood tests especially liver function
		Must not be withdrawn rapidly
Gabapentin	May be effective as shown in other neuropathic pains	Not been evaluated in randomised controlled trial
	Fewer side effects than other AEDs so well tolerated	Needs to be started and reduced slowly
	No major drug interactions	Expensive
Phenytoin	May be effective	Little variation in dosage range
	Long history of use	Regular blood tests needed
	Appears to work synergistically with carbamazepine	Drug interactions especially anti-diabetic drugs
		Need to consider folic acid replacement if used long term
Oxcarbazepine	Effective in short term as shown in long-term cohort studies	Not evaluated in randomised controlled trial
	Fewer side effects than carbamazepine	Dose-related hyponatraemia
	Few drug interactions than carbamazepine	Patients allergic to carbamazepine may exhibit cross sensitivity
Valproic acid	May be effective	Not evaluated in randomised controlled trial
	Side effects as with other AED	Can cause hepatic failure so regular monitoring required

AED, anti-epileptic drug.

Current studies offer little help to the clinician and patient facing the decision of when to opt for surgery. It is likely that there are a number of factors involved in trying to predict prognosis, optimal time for surgery and response to treatment. These would include age at onset, frequency and duration

TABLE 16

KEY FACTS: medical management of trigeminal neuralgia

- Carbamazepine remains the current gold standard and so patients should be started on this drug.

- If side effects of carbamazepine are intolerable or pain control insufficient consider change or addition of baclofen or lamotrigine.

- Oxcarbazepine, a daughter drug of carbamazepine, has not been evaluated in RCTs but has been shown to be effective in longitudinal studies.

- Gabapentin has been shown to be effective in other types of neuropathic pain and has the best profile in terms of side effects.

- Dextromethorphan, pimozide, tocianide, tizanide, topiramate have been evaluated in RCTs but are either ineffective or have unacceptable side effects.

- The evidence for use of phenytoin, clonazepam, valproate and other topical agents is poor.

- New drugs are being introduced and it is essential that they are evaluated in randomised controlled trials which need to be multicentre to increase their size and hence provide meaningful results.

RCT, randomised controlled trial.

of pain episodes as well as severity and number of divisions involved. Although data from microvascular compression series suggest that shorter duration of symptoms (less than 8 years, see Table 30) results in a better prognosis, this has not been validated. The hypothesised pathophysiology of trigeminal neuralgia also points in the direction of early rather than late surgery. However no reports specify how the onset date was established nor do they make any attempt to characterise the patients in terms of severity of symptoms, number of remissions and the length of these periods. Katusic et al. (1990) showed that the attacks of pain do tend to get worse and Bowsher (2000) in his 126 patients found that 90% reported that the frequency of attacks increased with time. Rushton and Macdonald (1957) reporting prior to effective treatments being available suggest that patients with longer pain-free intervals are more likely to have a good prognosis. Garvan and Siegfried

(1983) recommend that any patient who has taken over 3000 tablets and who still needs drug therapy should be considered for surgery even if pain control has been achieved. The only long-term cohort data currently available are presented in a small study that we carried out in a group of 15 patients who had become intractable to conventional medication and yet did not want surgery (Zakrzewska and Patsalos, 2002). We showed that periods of pain remission were variable and not all patients experienced them. The severity of the pain did increase with time and led to 12 patients ultimately undergoing surgery (2 died while on drug therapy and one remains well controlled on drugs). Eight of the patients did admit that they should have undergone surgery earlier. The cohort however was very small and much larger national studies are needed to confirm these data.

Apart from two studies (Miles et al., 1997; Zakrzewska et al., 1999) no other surgical studies have been found which report the intensity of the pain and consequent disability of patients prior to undergoing surgery. Given that the outcome measure is pain relief and improved quality of life it seems naïve to just assume that all patients who have surgery have severe pain and that it will be relieved by surgery. The use of medication as a criterion for partial or complete relief of pain although useful is not sufficient and you need to measure at least two parameters to ensure valid outcome measures (McQuay, 2002). Patients may be taking medication because of fear of return of pain rather than because of actual pain (Hasegawa et al., 2002). I consider it essential that detailed records are kept on all patients and find it surprising that a surgeon writes in a chapter on surgical management of trigeminal neuralgia "sufficiently detailed assessments of recurrence of pain are not available for construction of Kaplan–Meier plots" (Young et al., 1998). Only by careful objective audit of all our patients will we gain insight into how best to manage this condition.

7.1.1. What do you need to know before making a decision about surgery?

All patients would like the surgeon to be honest about the advice they give and to take time to explain

TABLE 17

Case studies 4 and 5

Read through the following 2 cases. Should these patients be referred for surgery now or later? On what criteria are you basing your judgment?

Case 4

Name	IR
Age	48
Gender	Female
Development of pain	Facial pain initially felt like toothache as it began after a dental extraction
Character/quality	Words from McGill pain questionnaire: sharp, shooting, electric, hot, fearful, intense
Site and radiation	Right infraorbital and mental areas only felt deep in the tissue pain, may radiate to ophthalmic division but does not start from there
Severity	On the visual analogue scale 0–10 cm, at its worst 9 cm, mean 7 cm and may go completely
Duration and periodicity	Each stab of pain last for seconds but she is getting attacks every few hours. The pain began 4 years ago and there have been months when she has been pain-free. It does not disturb sleep.
Provoking factors	Eating, brushing teeth and washing her face provoke pain
Relieving factors	Currently only carbamazepine helps
Associated factors	No other pains reported
Use of medication	Carbamazepine is effective in large doses, 800 mg and above daily but results in severe tiredness and difficulty doing her job

Case 5

Name	JQ
Age	49
Gender	Male
Development of pain	Pain initially was felt only intraorally near the teeth on the right side
Character/quality	Words from McGill pain questionnaire: sharp, shooting, tiring, troublesome, penetrating
Site and radiation	Right maxillary and mandibular branches mainly, pain is intra-orally
Severity	On number rating scale worse is 4/5, mean is 2/5 and may have no pain
Duration and periodicity	Pain present for the last three years, initially months pain-free now weeks when pain-free and stops all medication
Provoking factors	Eating, shaving, stress
Relieving factors	Carbamazepine, relaxation
Associated factors	No other pain reported
Use of medication	Carbamazepine in dosage of 600 mg to 300 mg daily, currently controlled on 300 mg daily
Effect of pain on life style	At the present time can cope with the pain not resulting in any anxiety or depression and side effects are not troublesome
Investigations	MRI suggests compression of the trigeminal nerve

Please see answers at the end of the chapter in Table 45

things. Written information in a format that is jargon-free is greatly appreciated and this has even led to patients publishing their own book on the topic (Striking Back, see Further reading). Below are some questions I have been asked by my own patients or those attending meetings and which I feel should be answered by all surgeons who consider that patients have a right to fully informed consent.

- What are the results from this unit and how do they compare with others?
- Have you checked that I really have got trigeminal neuralgia?
- What types of surgical procedures are available and what are the indications for each of them?
- What are the recurrence rates? If I am having the operation for the first time? For the second time?

- What are the complications, especially serious ones, and how would they affect my quality of life? Which ones are likely to be permanent? Which are transient? How long would the transient ones last? How will you help me cope with them?
- How are recurrences dealt with?
- Is there any way you can predict how I will respond to treatment?
- Will I need to take medication after the operation? If yes, for how long?
- Will I be free of pain immediately?
- How often will I be reviewed?
- Does this unit offer a range of different treatments?
- How many operations of each type do you do annually?
- Does somebody have a special interest in this condition in this unit?
- Do you run a joint clinic involving surgeons, physicians, psychologist?

Patient support groups can offer more advice although this can be biased.

Further details on these groups are provided in Chapter 9 on management. Some details on how to evaluate them are also provided.

Read through Case 6 in Table 18 and try to make up your mind on what this patient chose.

7.2. Overview of how the evidence for surgical management has been compiled

The literature on trigeminal neuralgia is large but apart from a handful of studies in the field of peripheral surgery and one in gamma knife surgery there have been no randomised controlled trials and so all the studies are of the cohort type. The vast majority of the data is retrospective, written by experts and very rarely with an independent observer and so constitutes the lowest level of evidence. Reviewing the studies one is struck by the vastly varying data that is available and how the studies have been quoted and results compared (Zakrzewska and Lopez, submitted). Hamlyn (1999) in his book states that he found

1400 articles on surgical management of trigeminal neuralgia and yet he selected only 86 articles on microvascular decompression that he considered fulfilled his basic criteria.

There is no internationally agreed format for the reporting of these results and yet the need for such a format has been highlighted (Hamlyn, 1999). It can be solved as has been shown by the publication of the CONSORT guidelines for reporting of randomised controlled trials as discussed in more detail in Chapter 9 on management. With this in mind I decided to use some clear-cut criteria to select studies used to compare results of pain relief times and complications. The results are described in our paper and a summary is provided below (Zakrzewska and Lopez, submitted). Thirteen experts set the standard to which all retrieved studies were subjected. The criteria used and how the best studies scored are shown in Table 19

Of the 277 studies identified 219 were scored. The maximum score was 15 and was achieved by only 5 studies, the mean score was 8.5 and only 70 (32%) studies reached the set standard. Recurrence rates can only be compared if they are all reporting pain outcomes at the same time points and are only valid if they include all patients even those lost to follow up and those who have not developed recurrent pain. Therefore only studies using actuarial methodology which could be used to do a meta-analysis were used. Only 30 (14%) such studies were identified. How the different groups of studies scored is shown in Table 20.

Complications are quoted from other studies with high scores. I looked at all the complications in the poor scoring studies to see if the rate of complications was different and there did not appear to be any significant differences. Sweet (1990) did this when looking at studies dealing with radiofrequency thermorhizotomy (RFT) and found no significant differences. Mortality and major morbidity is reported in most studies and all studies were used for this data.

As Lunsford (commenting on the paper by Taha and Tew, 1996) points out, authors can be selective about the choice of studies used in their reviews

TABLE 18

Case study 6

Please read this patient's case history. What type of surgery would you recommend? What criteria are you using to make your choice?

Name	DH
Age	61
Gender	Male
Development of pain	18 months ago had first attack of pain which came under control with carbamazepine 1600 mg. He was referred to a neurosurgeon but when he went for his appointment his pain had abated and he declined surgery. He went into total pain remission for 3 months and has now represented with severe pain.
Character/quality	Sharp, shooting, stabbing, fearful, unbearable. He chose 19 words on the McGill Pain Questionnaire.
Site and radiation	All three divisions on right side, previously had only involved second division.
Severity	Visual analogue scale, 8–10 cm; McGill Pain rating index 34
Duration and periodicity	Last for seconds with very few periods of no pain
Provoking factors	Light touch provoked, cannot eat, talk
Relieving factors	Drugs only
Associated factors	Redness of the face and swelling
Use of medication	Carbamazepine 1600 mg daily, gabapentin 1500 mg daily
Effect of pain on life style	Brief Pain Inventory quality of life score 6–9 on all parameters (max score 10); Hospital Anxiety and Depression Scale: anxiety 10, depression 10 (>8 significant)
Medical history	Fit and no current medication other than his trigeminal neuralgia treatment
Investigations	MRI suggests compression of the trigeminal nerve at the infero-lateral aspect, no tumour

Please see the end of the chapter, Table 47, for the answer.

and only use those that fit their conclusions. To avoid bias in choice of studies the literature was searched by an independent body (BMA as part of an article on treatment of trigeminal neuralgia for 'Clinical Evidence'). The methodology they use is described in their publication or on the web (*www.clinicalevidence*.com). To this list I added all the references I had accumulated over the years and from literature listed in papers. All foreign literature was included. There is a large body of literature in Japanese and Chinese including some large series but the quality is extremely poor and none of the studies scored highly on my criteria. As an example, I would like to quote an abstract from a conference proceeding published in J Neurol Neurosurg Psychiatry (Fukushima, 1990). Fukushima in this abstract reports his results on ten years experience of MVD which includes 1620 patients with trigeminal neuralgia (the largest series in the world at that time). I have tried to find a definitive study by this team from

Tokyo as a follow up to this abstract and have failed. I personally spoke to him at the conference and tried to ascertain how he followed up patients and was told that patients were encouraged to write in once a year.

I will refer to a chapter written by Sweet and Poletti (1995) in which they report on their own personal survey they did among some 200 neurosurgeons. They wrote to their colleagues asking for details of their operative complications when treating patients with trigeminal neuralgia. Of these, 140 replied which covered 91 units not just ones in the US. The details of the survey are poor but they do highlight how major morbidity and mortality occur and remain unreported. More mortalities were reported by them than recorded in all the published data. I have found all the same mortality data in the studies that were reported by Sweet and Poletti (1995). Sweet also wrote a chapter on his analysis of the literature in Rovit et al.'s book (1990) on trigeminal neuralgia.

TABLE 19

Criteria used for inclusion of papers in review of surgical management of trigeminal neuralgia and how 50% of the top studies scored

Criterion	Data present		Data absent	Unable to ascertain
	no.	(%)		
Number of patients	50	(100)		
Prospective study	17	(34)	33	
Independent observer	13	(26)	29	7
Diagnostic criteria stated	36	(72)	14	
Mixed cases but can differentiate in analysis, e.g. tumour, MS, atypical	30	(60)	11	8
Age at operation or at onset disease	49	(98)	1	
Gender	48	(96)	2	
Side/division	41	(82)	9	
Length of disease prior to operation	37	(74)	12	
Number having previous surgery	40	(80)	7	3
Results reported in relation to previous surgery	32	(64)	15	3
Pre-op. measure of pain or assessment	1	(2)	48	
Pre-op. sensory assessment	17	(34)	33	
Definition of recurrence/success	42	(84)	8	
Length of follow up, range	49	(98)	1	
Length of follow up, mean	44	(88)	5	1
Withdrawals/dropouts accounted for	35	(70)	13	2
Description of operative findings	47	(94)	3	
How was outcome/reported	50	(100)		
Kaplan–Meier analysis/yearly outcome	32	(64)	18	
Mortality	47	(94)		3
Report complications outside V area	44	(88)	6	
Report complications within V area	50	(100)		
Report of pre-operative complications	38	(76)	13	
Definition of terms, e.g. sensory loss	19	(38)	31	
Psychological morbidity	2	(4)	48	
Quality of life assessment	3	(6)	49	
Economic costs	2	(4)	48	
Questionnaire/interview	32	(64)	18	

Those in italics are the ones used to score the quality of the study.

Even using these criteria it is difficult to be sure that all the relevant studies have been identified and selected. It is also difficult to establish if we are comparing like with like as data on the following items are often unavailable:

- diagnostic criteria
- differentiation between idiopathic trigeminal neuralgia and other types
- basic data sets such as age at onset, site, length of time of disease, age at operation, previous treatments
- severity of condition based on some measurements of pain
- analysis of data depending on type of trigeminal neuralgia and previous surgery
- operative data
- skill of surgeon
- patients lost to follow up and details of how they may differ from the other patients
- definitions, e.g. recurrence of pain, failure of treatment, sensory changes

TABLE 20

Results of systematic review of papers describing pain outcomes and complications on surgical management of trigeminal neuralgia using the criteria shown in Table 19 up to December 2001

Procedure	Total studies	Repeat studies	Other studies	Studies scored	Total patients	Studies reaching standard (%)	Studies used for pain outcome (%)	Number of patients used pain outcome (%)	Score: mean ± SD
Peripheral	46	9	3	34	4,287	19 (56)	3 (9)	284	6.9 ± 3.4
RFT	77	4	2	71	15,438	17 (24)	9 (13)	2,678	7.7 ± 2.9
PRG	38	4	2	31	4,238	12 (39)	9 (19)	497	8.4 ± 3.2
Balloon	21	2	1	19	2,454	3 (16)	1 (5)	50	7.0 ± 2.7
MVD	75	10	11	53	6,952	15 (28)	9 (17)	2,241	8.9 ± 3.1
GKS	23	6	6	11	843	4 (36)	2 (18)	157	10.4 ± 3
Total	**277**	**35**	**25**	**219**	**34,212**	**70 (32)**	**30 (14)**	**5,907 (17)**	**8.5**

RFT, radiofrequency thermorhizotomy; PRG, percutaneous glycerol rhizotomy; Balloon, balloon microcompression; MVD, microvascular decompression; GKS, gamma knife surgery.
Repeat studies: reported same data.
Other studies, dealt either with complications or recurrences only. Total patients, number of patients involved in all the studies; Studies reaching standard, number of studies which scored at or above standard set; studies used for pain outcomes, these include only those with actuarial data; Score, mean score reached on criteria defined in Table 19, maximum score 15 — peripheral techniques had to score 7 and above to be selected, if 10 and above had been used as the cut off only 7 would have been selected.

- outcome data: some divide patients into three groups only, i.e. excellent, partial relief, no relief, whereas others may put patients into five categories
- criteria for partial relief vary but are often defined as use of regular medication
- recurrence in some series is only reported if a patient has to undergo repeat surgery, in others it is any pain report
- details of follow up time and numbers of patients available in each follow up group
- Kaplan–Meier actuarial analysis
- reporting complications in relation to time
- reports of patients own assessment of outcome
- quality of life assessments
- economic factors

Szapiro et al. (1985) have pointed out how important the character and timing of the pain are in the analysis and yet there is only one other study that has analysed its data based on the character of the pain which has been obtained using a valid measure such as the McGill Pain Questionnaire (Zakrzewska et al., 1999). Two other studies have attempted to show that their patients could be divided into typical and atypical trigeminal neuralgia (Yoon et al., 1999; Tyler-Kabara et al., 2002) based on character and timing but they use retrospective methods and provide no details of how their data were validated.

North et al. (1990) showed how recurrence rates varied depending on whether a recurrence was defined as any return of pain even if controlled by medication or whether it was defined as a recurrence only if repeat surgery was needed. Recurrences should also be reported for first procedures and not based on a cumulative result where patients may have had a number of procedures done before becoming pain-free. Data should be given separately on those who have had more than one procedure to render them pain-free. Recurrence rates may vary if the patient has had previous surgery or secondary trigeminal neuralgia so this should be stated. Kaplan–Meier methodology enables all patients to be included in the analysis whether they have been lost to follow up, died or have not had a recurrence of pain. Unfortunately, even with some reports using actuarial methodology, patients who failed to respond to treatment at the onset are excluded whereas they should be included; beware of the graphs that show 100% results at the start.

The tables below will summarise the current result.

In most review articles on surgery each of the different types of surgery are dealt with individually. I thought it may be useful for readers to be able to compare the results of each procedure more easily if they are all reported under the following headings:

- Definition of the procedure and the presumed mechanism of action
- Selection of patients for each of the procedures
- Description of the operative technique
- Recurrence of pain on a yearly basis
- Prognostic factors for outcome
- Complications
- Management of recurrences
- Indications and contraindications for each procedure

Surgery for trigeminal neuralgia is done at three levels and some procedures are more invasive than others. Only microvascular decompression can be said to be a non-destructive procedure whereas all other forms of surgery are destructive and aim to reduce transmission of painful stimuli. This, therefore, results in loss of sensation over a varying part of the trigeminal nerve.

7.3. Definitions of surgical procedures and proposed mechanism of action

7.3.1. Peripheral surgery
Peripheral surgery aims to identify individual nerve branches that are acting as triggers and delivering treatment directly at that site. They all rely on some form of damage to the nerve be it mechanical, chemical or thermal. The treatments have included cryotherapy, laser, neurectomy, alcohol, radiofrequency, acupuncture or removal of necrotising

cavitation lesions. Most of the procedures aim to destroy peripheral nerve fibres although more central changes are likely as a result of these interventions. It was hoped that some of the agents used would be more selective and hence result in less sensory loss, e.g. cryotherapy and the area of loss would be smaller than after treatments at the level of the Gasserian ganglion.

Ratner et al. (1979) proposed that cavities developed in the alveolar bone after dental extractions and that many of them were infected or showed chronic inflammatory changes or abnormal osteoid tissues and that their removal led to diminution of the symptoms of trigeminal neuralgia. These cavities are always found in areas where teeth have been extracted months or years ago and many are not visible on examination or X-ray. The cavities are enclosed by bone or they may be empty. This procedure has been termed NICO, necrotising cavitational osteonecrosis. In total, 11 articles describing this procedure have been identified but none of them fulfil the criteria mentioned above. There has also been one published abstract of some work on cadaver material, which showed that bony cavities did not appear to be unique to trigeminal neuralgia or atypical facial pain (Graff-Radford et al., 1988).

7.3.2. Surgery at the Gasserian ganglion
Surgery at the level of the Gasserian ganglion until recently was the most frequently used treatment. The procedure involves reaching the Gasserian ganglion by insertion of a needle through the foramen ovale under radiographic control and then destroying all or parts of the nerve fibres either pre-ganglionically or post-ganglionically. Initially the agents used, e.g. alcohol, were nonselective and although good pain relief was obtained it was at the risk of inducing not just sensory loss but also dysaesthesia. Procedures currently done at this level include percutaneous radiofrequency rhizotomy (lysis) or thermocoagulation (RFT), percutaneous glycerol rhizolysis (rhizotomy) (PGR) or microcompression.

Electrocoagulation of the trigeminal nerve was first done by Kirschner in the 1930s but the uncontrolled use of heat led to severe side effects and this procedure did not gain widespread acceptance till it was modified by Sweet in the 1970s. The procedure of RFT relies on selective destruction of nerve fibres by an electric current. Tactile sensations mediated by A alpha fibres and A beta fibres are preserved whilst fibres carrying nociceptive sensation (A delta and C fibres) are destroyed. The temperature and time which are used can be altered in order to cause more or less sensory loss.

In PGR the Gasserian ganglion is bathed in glycerol, a mild neurolytic agent, and its exact mechanism of action has been investigated by a variety of workers and is summarised by Linderoth and Hakanson (1995) in their chapter on this technique. It is known that diluted solutions are not suitable and pure sterile anhydrous glycerol must be used. This was a chance finding by Hakanson who noted that injection of glycerol and tantalum powder (being used to mark the cistern prior to Gamma knife use) produced pain relief. It was thought that it would produce less sensory loss than RFT and yet give equally satisfactory pain relief periods. Altering the technique slightly allows sparing or inclusion of the 1st or 3rd divisions.

In the 1950s it was found that decompression of the nerve at the Gasserian ganglion level, especially if nerve injury occurred, seems to result in pain relief. It led to the development of microcompression of the trigeminal nerve at the point of its division. This procedure results in an uncontrolled compression of all fibres especially the large myelinated fibres.

Less sensory loss and preservation of corneal reflex can be achieved but often at the expense of shorter pain relief periods.

7.3.3. Posterior fossa

Microvascular decompression (MVD) and partial rhizotomy (PSR). The earliest operations and those often carried out if no compression is found is a rhizotomy or partial rhizotomy which aims to only cut some of the trigeminal nerve fibres. Microvascular decompression (MVD) aims to decompress the trigeminal nerve from vessels or tumours that may be in contact with it without causing damage to the nerve. The rationale behind this operation lies in the hypothesis that vessels or tumours compressing the trigeminal nerve result in areas of demyelination and resultant ephaptic transmission or reverberating circuits. Even if grooving is commoner in patients with trigeminal neuralgia than controls this still does not prove that this is the sole mechanism by which trigeminal neuralgia occurs (Hamlyn, 1999). Some other intrinsic factor is probably also involved as this would explain why not all patients with trigeminal neuralgia are found to have compression. The area particularly vulnerable to this compression is the root entry zone which is a cone-shaped junction between central and peripheral myelin in the main sensory root of the trigeminal nerve located approx. 3 mm from the pons. It needs to be clearly defined as not all compressions are found in this area and some are found more laterally (Hamlyn, 1999). Some compressions can now be visualised on MRIs but as discussed earlier the evidence is still not of high quality.

Gamma knife surgery (GKS) — radiosurgery. The relatively new method of stereotactic surgery using the gamma knife enables lesions of the trigeminal nerve to be made in the posterior fossa without the need to do an open procedure as it relies on high quality magnetic resonance imaging. The Leksell gamma knife represents the newest technique being used in the search for an ideal treatment for trigeminal neuralgia. Using 201 separate precisely directed sources (^{60}Co) gamma radiation is delivered in a hemispheric way to a preselected target. The precise location of the target is achieved by the stereotactic guidance and hence the name stereotactic radiosurgery. It is a non-invasive method and therefore potentially available to every patient, however medically unfit. The equipment needed is very expensive and at present there is limited availability.

Mechanism of action. Radiosurgery, i.e. the use of a radiation beam to perform noninvasive procedures has been used since Laskell introduced it in 1950. Its mechanism of action has not been entirely clarified. Radiation results in both acute and delayed changes in the targeted tissues. Clinical reports record a considerable latent period (up to 15 months) before maximum pain relief is obtained and maximum sensory loss is noticed (Young et al., 1998; Maesawa et al., 2001). It was hypothesised that irradiation of the trigeminal nerve would block ephaptic transmission but not normal axonal conduction and so its effects would be selective (Regis et al., 1995). It, however, seems logical to assume that any biological treatment be it chemical, thermal, mechanical or irradiation will affect the integrity of the whole trigeminal nerve and both myelinated and non-myelinated fibres will be damaged. It is being currently debated whether different types of fibres have different radiosensitivity. There remains controversy about the relative radiosensitivity of different cranial nerves and some believe that sensory nerves are more sensitive than motor ones. To date, clinical reports have reported sensory changes in up to 17% of patients but there is only one case report of motor involvement in the form of jaw clenching in a patient who received repeat surgery to a total of 160 Gy and which produced post-treatment enhancement on MRI (Hochman, 1998). The extent of this damage may be related both to the dose of irradiation and the area irradiated.

Animal work on irradiated nerves has shown that axonal degeneration and oedema affect all nerve fibres at doses of 80 Gy and necrosis is observed at six months when nerves receive doses of 100 Gy radiation (Kondziolka et al., 2000). These findings are supported by reports that patients who develop some loss of sensation (evidence of axonal damage) have a longer pain-free period than those without (Rogers et al., 2000; Pollock et al., 2001). Sensory loss is more likely to occur in those patients with higher doses of irradiation (Pollock et al., 2001) and those in whom the length of irradiated nerve is longer (Flickinger et al., 2001). It has further been suggested that patients with multiple sclerosis may be more radiation-sensitive because of their impaired ability to reverse the changes of radiation and Friedman et al. (2001) postulate this as a reason why they only saw post-treatment enhancements on their MRIs in patients who had multiple sclerosis. Vascular changes may also occur as Maher and Pollock (2000) report the presence of atheromatous

changes in blood vessels after 90 Gy irradiation which was found on MVD 10 months later. This was not a consistent finding as no such changes were found in 3 other patients who underwent MVD after failure of gamma knife surgery. Maesawa et al. (2001) postulate that recurrences may be due to incorporation of new afferent fibres, further aberrant axonal conduction or additional afferent propagation.

It is now appreciated that the exact location of the lesions may have a significant bearing on outcomes both in terms of pain relief and complications. It has been postulated that the portion of the trigeminal nerve closer to the brain stem (the so called root entry zone REZ) is myelinated by oligodendrocytes as compared to the distal retro-Gasserian portion which is myelinated by Schwann cells. The former are considered to be more radiosensitive. However, this needs to be weighed up against the fact that irradiating in the REZ inevitably leads to some irradiation of the brain stem. Urgosik et al. (1998) suggest that some brain stem function change needs to occur as well as axonal damage if results are to be improved. Irradiation of the retro-Gasserian portion avoids the brain stem and so theoretically larger doses could be used (Rand, 1997).

When initially used in trigeminal neuralgia the irradiation was aimed at the Gasserian ganglion and retro-Gasserian portion of the trigeminal nerve rather than the root entry zone (Regis et al., 1995; Rand, 1997). The results were not encouraging and did not appear to offer any advantage over other techniques. It was decided that results may be more reliable if the beam was to be directed more at the root entry zone with the brain stem receiving up to 20% of the dose as this was considered the site of compression. It was also necessary to consider patients with secondary trigeminal neuralgia, i.e. due to tumours whose tumour position dictated the position of the beam (Young et al., 1997). Thus, dosage, imaging methods, position and outcome measures needed to be addressed and this was initially done through a multicentre study which enabled rapid collection of data (Kondziolka et al., 1996). Nicol et al. (2000) reported improved results with 90 Gy but increased risk of sensory changes. Later, the position and length of irradiated nerve was determined in one of the first randomised controlled trials in neurosurgery for trigeminal neuralgia (Flickinger et al., 2001). When patients are irradiated for tumours, 3 month postoperative MRIs are performed to assess the accuracy of the target selection. This has also been done with patients undergoing therapy for trigeminal neuralgia but the MRI images have not been found to correlate with clinical outcome and so this follow up is not advocated (Friedman et al., 2001). The dosage needs to be low enough not to cause any post-treatment lesions that result in sensory changes and which could be visualised on MRI.

Factors to consider when reading reports on GKS. When trying to determine such important technical factors and assess their effect on both pain relief and complications the number of variables must be kept as low as possible. Unfortunately, due to the relatively small numbers of patients currently being offered this form of treatment and the lack of what I perceive as continued collaboration between centres, many reports include in their series a mixed group of patients. The diagnostic criteria are often missing, only one study differentiated between patients with paroxysmal pain and those with background pain. Not a single report states how many of the included patients fulfilled all the diagnostic criteria as suggested by the International Headache Association and only one report includes some form of preoperative pain assessment which, however, is not an internationally validated scale.

In the series by Maesawa et al. (2001) 220 patients have been reported but these include patients who have had one or two isocentres used, dose variations of 60–90 Gy and variable follow up times. Patients who are reported with a very short follow up may not have experienced all the delayed effects of radiation before being included. It is for this reason that Brisman (2000) excluded patients who had not been followed up for a minimum of 6 months. In the series of Pollock et al. (2001) evaluating the effect of two dosage levels, the length of follow up is short and different in the two groups and some patients are included who have been followed up for a mere 2 months, they may not have

had time to develop maximum pain relief or to develop sensory loss and bias is introduced into the results. The patient characteristics are variable in that some have had previous surgery, others are new cases and some have preoperative sensory changes. If sensory changes are to be evaluated it is important that these are assessed preoperatively. At this stage it may be important to do this very carefully and Urgosik et al. (1998) have measured blink reflex, a variety of sensory parameters and motor function using EMG both preoperatively and at six monthly intervals later. The question also needs to be posed as to how clinically significant is an added sensory loss to a patient who already has some decreased sensation. I would expect a patient with no previous sensory loss to be more aware of a reduction in sensation than one who already has some numbness. Urgosik et al. (1998) have shown that some patients are not aware of sensory changes found on formal testing. It has been reported that patients who already have a pre existing numbness are at higher risk of developing further paraesthesia and ultimately a dysaesthesia that comes to affect the quality of life (Maesawa et al., 2001). As well as the technical variations the study population is variable. Previous surgery must inevitably have some effect not only physiologically but also psychologically on patients and it is therefore essential for the analysis to take this into account. Data in the MVD literature suggest that outcome may be affected by length of disease and this therefore also needs to be considered. New techniques ideally should be used in those patients who present with the most classical features and not in those who have failed other treatments possibly due to incorrect diagnosis.

I remain concerned about the currently short follow up of most studies knowing that long-term effects of radiation-induced neuropathies is a distinct possibility. What evidence do we have that secondary tumours do not occur or that vascular changes such as atheromatous plaques do not occur? What would be the effect of atheromatous plaques in the superior cerebellar artery, the one most likely to be affected and which is most often associated with compression? How confident can a patient be that the exact area is treated given that it is difficult to be accurate when you want to reach a small area and keep the dose matrix small. Errors of a few millimetres could mean inaccurate targets. Clarification is needed on how to deal with recurrences. High quality control is essential and how this will be achieved in a reliable, unbiased way needs to be addressed.

It has been suggested that GKS costs 3.5 greater than a percutaneous procedure, but 40% less than a microvascular decompression procedure (Young et al., 1997) but this does not take in long-term costs such as repeated procedures, dealing with complications, etc.

7.4. Selection of patients for different surgical procedures

Although there are some selection criteria by which patients are offered different treatments most patients are eligible for all techniques and it is factors other than those mentioned below that are of consequence. All patients with cardiac disease are at risk and this probably explains some of the mortalities. Browne (1985) describes a fatal myocardial infarction in a patient who as well as trigeminal neuralgia had a dull, aching pain in his mandible which was thought in retrospect to be cardiac in origin.

7.4.1. Peripheral techniques
As most of these procedures are done under local anaesthesia the medical condition of the patients is not crucial. Care, however, needs to be taken if patients have a haemoglobinopathy or are taking anticoagulant drugs as surgery could result in haematoma formation. Patients can be seen in out-patients and do not need a hospital admission. Only short-term relief of pain is likely.

7.4.2. Gasserian ganglion surgery
Some of the procedures require a patient to have a general anaesthetic, others can be done under heavy sedation. As a needle has to be passed through the foramen ovale for RFT and PGR, patients with any tendency to bleed should not be considered for these techniques. Blood pressure also tends to rise

during these procedures and this should be taken into account (Sweet et al., 1985).

Selection for RFT

- Patients need to be co-operative during the procedure
- Patients with reduced vision should not be offered RFT in case they should develop corneal anaesthesia and possible eye complications
- Patients must be ready to accept sensory loss
- Patients who want some control over the amount of sensory loss
- Suitable for elderly patients but not for those with possible haemoglobinopathies
- Suitable for patients with multiple sclerosis
- Patients who do not want an MVD

Selection for PGR

- More acceptable to patients who are afraid of sensory loss and anaesthesia dolorosa as it causes less sensory loss than that predicted after RFT
- Can be done on most patients despite them being medically compromised as a general anaesthetic is not required
- Patients can have a general anaesthetic if they wish
- Avoid the procedure in patients with a possible allergy/adverse reaction to contrast medium or iodine
- Patients undergoing glycerol injections may not have an immediate result and need to be warned
- Patients ready to accept higher recurrence rates than for other procedures
- Patients who do not wish to have an MVD

Selection for microcompression

- Patients should have a CT scan and MRI to rule out ectatic vertebral or basilar artery as there is a suggestion that these patients do less well. A submental vertex view is used to predict patients whose foramen ovale may be difficult to visualise or may be too small to allow penetration by a 14-gauge needle.

- It is important to do an ECG to identify patients who may be at risk of arrhythmias.
- Patients who have first division pain and in whom corneal anaesthesia needs to be avoided and who do not wish to have an MVD may find this a good alternative.
- Patients who have contralateral masseteric muscle weakness should not have the procedure as most patients sustain short-term masseteric weakness on the operated side.
- Elderly patients tolerate the procedure well as only a short anaesthetic is required.
- Can be done in patients taking warfarin although it should be stopped preoperatively as there is a lesser risk of intracranial haemorrhage than with other Gasserian ganglion procedures as the needle does not penetrate intracranially.
- Patients with multiple sclerosis (MS) are eligible.

7.4.3. Posterior fossa surgery

Selection for microvascular decompression/partial rhizotomy

- As these procedures are classified as major neuro-surgical procedures patients need to be medically fit.
- Initially, patients over the age of 65 years were not considered good candidates but with improved anaesthetic techniques the medical condition rather than age of the patient should be taken into account. Ogungbo et al. (2000) in their small series of 62 patients showed that there were no significant differences in peri-operative mortality and morbidity in patients over 65 years of age. Their one death, however, was in an elderly patient who had a myocardial infarct two weeks after surgery.
- Meaney et al. (1995b), Broggi et al. (2000) and Ferroli et al. (2002) included patients with MS if MRI does not show any demyelinating plaques in the root entry zone, pontine tract and nuclei. They have found that these patients also had compressive lesions and although the numbers were small they did not consider their outcome to be worse than others.

- Partial rhizotomy is often done if patients are found not to have a compression and so patients need to be warned that they may have some sensory loss.
- As hearing loss is a well known complication it is important to stress this especially to patients who are musicians, others dependent on hearing, or who may already be deaf on the contralateral side.

7.4.4. Selection for gamma knife surgery

- As this technique does not require any major surgery almost all patients are eligible. Due to the low invasive nature of this procedure and no necessity for a general anaesthetic, patients who are medically compromised and/or very elderly remain eligible for the procedure.
- Patients who do not want an invasive procedure may find this technique an acceptable alternative.
- MRIs are used in the plotting of the fields and so patients who are not eligible for MRIs may be excluded. These will include patients with metal prosthesis/implants and those who suffer from severe claustrophobia (see Chapter 7, Investigations, for further discussion of these problems).
- Patient needs to be able to lie flat and still for around one hour so this may exclude patients with cardiac failure.
- The finding of a compression on MRI does not exclude a patient from this procedure. This is one of the few procedures that are probably suited to patients with haemoglobinopathies.
- Patients need to be aware that results may not be immediate, the latency varies as shown in Table 21 below (not mentioned in all reports) and although pain relief may be obtained early, maximum pain relief may not be achieved for many months. This may be a major problem in patients who are already on high drug dosage.
- Patients need to be warned that they may need to be on medication after treatment indefinitely if they only get a 'good' result.
- Sensory loss also can occur and may be delayed up to 2 years.

TABLE 21

Time before pain relief obtained after gamma knife surgery GKS as reported in the literature

Reference	Range of onset of pain relief	Median or mean onset of pain relief	% Relief at 6 months	Range of time for maximum pain relief
Young et al., 1997, 1998	1–120 days	Mean 14 days	14 days mean	
Urgosik et al., 1998	1 day–8 months	2 months median, 2.8 months mean		
Flickering et al., 2001	3 months median			1 week to 17 months
Nicol et al., 2000	1–82 days	3 weeks median		
Rogers et al., 2000	1–192 days	15 days median		0–253 days with median of 63 days
Friedman et al., 2001	3 weeks–3 months			
Maesawa et al., 2001	2–33 months	2 months median	81 ± 2.6%	6–33 months with median 2 months

- Patients need to be warned that radiation is culminative.
- The procedure is only available in a few centres and is very expensive.

7.5. Operative techniques

These are summarised here as it is important that anyone explaining the surgical treatments can give patients an idea of what surgery involves. For those of you who want more details I provide some references at the end which have more operative details. It is useful to look at illustrations of these techniques and these can be found in neurosurgical textbooks on operative techniques.

7.5.1. Peripheral techniques

The majority of these can be done under local anaesthesia in all ages and often irrespective of medical problems. They result in short-term pain relief and have few complications. Very clear anatomical diagrams of the location of all the branches of the trigeminal nerve can be found in Murali (1990).

Neurectomy. This is probably one of the oldest techniques used and there are several old reports of large series of patients undergoing these procedures. The trigger nerve branch is first identified by the use of a local anaesthetic. This also gives the patient an idea of the area of numbness they would expect to

be left with after the procedure. Then under local anaesthesia the peripheral nerve is exposed utilising an intraoral route wherever possible so that no scars will be left. The nerve is then severed (Mason, 1972; Murali and Rovit, 1996). Some surgeons have reported early re-growth of the nerve and so suggest obliterating the foramen through which the nerve emerges. This has involved either sealing the foramen with wax or packing with fatty tissues or wood chips. Mason (1972) suggests that this gives superior results.

Alcohol injections. These are mainly given at the level of peripheral branches but have involved lesions as far as the Gasserian ganglion and nerve blocks. Absolute alcohol 0.75–1 ml is injected after the trigger branch has been identified with the use of local anaesthesia (Horrax and Poppen, 1935; Grant, 1936).

Streptomycin. This technique is one of the very few that has been subject to randomised controlled trials. The involved branch is identified by the use of local anaesthesia and then streptomycin 1 g with lignocaine is injected. The injections need to be given once weekly over a period of 5 weeks (Stajcic et al., 1990; Bittar and Graff-Radford, 1993).

Phenol. Once the involved branch is identified and local anaesthesia inserted then 10% phenol in glycerol is injected. The total amount used varies between 0.5 and 1.5 ml (Wilkinson, 1999).

Glycerol. After giving a local anaesthetic to localise the trigger area 0.5–1.5 ml of sterile glycerol is injected into the trigger area (Erdem and Alkan, 2001).

Cryotherapy. The trigger nerve branch or branches are exposed using as far as possible intra oral incisions. A cryoprobe is then applied using temperatures varying from −30°C to −70°C for two or three freeze–thaw cycles each lasting 2 minutes (Politis et al., 1988; Barnard, 1989; Zakrzewska and Thomas, 1993).

Laser. Only one report has been identified using this technique. Walker et al. (1988) used a helium–neon laser and applied it on the face for 20 seconds. This was repeated three times a week for 10 weeks.

Peripheral radiofrequency rhizotomy. This technique is the same as when performed at the Gasserian ganglion level and lesions at temperatures of 70°C are made for 2–3 minutes (Gregg and Small, 1986).

Acupuncture. This technique has been reported by Shuhan et al. (1991) who used it on 1500 patients. They perform acupuncture as a course of ten sessions. The ten sessions are based on daily or alternate daily treatments. If the first course is not successful a further one can be done 3–5 days later. On average patients needed 26 sessions but the range was large (10–84).

Jaw bone cavity removal NICO. As it is difficult to locate these on radiographs, the patient is asked to point to the trigger areas and then a local anaesthetic is given to try to eliminate the pain and hence find the cavity. A mucoperiosteal flap is raised intraorally and the area is curetted out carefully and then may be packed with gauze soaked in tetracycline. This is repacked regularly until granulation tissue forms. For a month prior to the procedure and for a month after all pain has gone the patients are put on antibiotics (Ratner et al., 1979).

7.5.2. Gasserian ganglion surgery

Some of these procedures require a full general anaesthetic (microcompression) whereas others can be done under sedation using agents such as fentanyl. Penetration of the foramen ovale by a needle gauge 14 or under is the most difficult part of the procedure

and the point at which patients may experience pain and cardiovascular incidences. I quote some texts in the references which give precise details of the landmarks used for a successful penetration. Fluoroscopy techniques are essential to ensure accurate localisation of the Gasserian ganglion and Meckel's cave. Some patients may stay overnight but patients can often be discharged on the same day.

Vladyka and Subrt (1989) describe an instrument they have devised which enables them not only to do all three procedures using the same instrument but also to change technique during the procedure.

Percutaneous radiofrequency rhizolysis (thermocoagulation, RFT). The full technique is well described by Taha and Tew (1999) with diagrams to illustrate the various stages of the procedure.

(1) The patient is given a short acting anaesthetic (methohexital) intermittently. Atropine may be given as a premedication to reduce the possibility of bradycardia.

(2) The procedure has to be done in a room with facilities for fluoroscopic monitoring.

(3) The patient is positioned in the supine position.

(4) A 20 gauge needle of 100 mm length is introduced through the cheek using well established landmarks as described by Hartel in the early 1900s. It is very important to ensure that the needle does not penetrate the oral mucosa as the needle becomes contaminated and spreads infection resulting in bacterial meningitis.

(5) Prior to inserting the needle through the foramen ovale a further bolus of methohexital is given as bradycardia can occur when penetrating the foramen ovale. Patients will often also wince at this moment.

(6) Localisation of the needle now needs to be verified by fluoroscopy. The aim is to ensure that the needle lies in the retro-Gasserian area. Once the stylet is removed free flow of CSF is often seen. Flow of CSF does not equate with correct placement as CSF can be obtained from other places. If any blood vessel has been punctured inadvertently then blood will flow

through the cannula. Puncture of the carotid artery has been recorded in several studies.

(7) Once precise localisation has been achieved the electrode is inserted. This electrode can either be curved or straight. The cannula has previously been calibrated in 1 mm increments to allow its precise localisation depending on the number of divisions to be treated. It is at this point that patients are woken so that they can verify whether the correct area is being stimulated. The patients are asked to indicate whether the area of paraesthesia equates with the distribution of the pain. The stimulation can normally be achieved using low temperatures such as 40°C. There are now newer techniques available that monitor evoked potentials during the procedure and so may obviate the need to wake the patient.

(8) Once the desired effect has been achieved a further bolus of anaesthesia is given during the lesion generation. Lesions are made at temperatures from 60°C to 90°C in cycles of 45–90 seconds. Many operators note an area of flushing in the division being treated.

(9) The patient is then woken and sensory testing carried out. Further lesioning can then take place until the appropriate sensory loss has been achieved. The aim is to reduce the sensory loss to a minimum.

(10) The patients are then observed for a further 15 minutes before returning to the ward from which they are discharged the following day. Before discharge the extent of sensory loss needs to be established. Patients who are found to have loss or reduction of corneal reflex must be warned about eye care, given safety glasses and possible artificial tears. They should be asked to seek an ophthalmological opinion should the eye become red in appearance. If the muscles of mastication have been compromised the patient should be advised to eat a soft diet and do some jaw exercises for two weeks. The medication is slowly stopped.

Taha and Tew (1999) have shown that they have fewer complications when using the curved electrode without any compromise of pain relief. It is important to ensure that the needle is placed in the retro-Gasserian position to ensure maximum pain relief with reduced sensory loss.

Percutaneous retro-Gasserian glycerol rhizolysis (PRG). The exact techniques used for this procedure are well described by Linderoth and Hakanson (1995), Jho and Lunsford (1997) and Apfelbaum (1999) and several variations have been introduced over the years but none of them have been evaluated under controlled conditions.

(1) Patients are premedicated and a local anaesthetic is used for needle penetration. Patients can be given intravenous sedation with fentanyl. Later a brief anaesthetic using methohexital can be used if necessary (anxious patient). ECG and pulse oximetry is important as penetration of the foramen ovale can result in either hypertension or hypotension with bradycardia. Further bradycardia can occur during injection with glycerol (Jho and Lunsford, 1997). General anaesthesia can be used although it makes the technique more complicated.

(2) Use of a C arm fluoroscopic unit is necessary throughout the procedure.

(3) Patient is initially placed in the supine position and careful positioning is important as shown in the texts on techniques. Later the patient is brought up into a sitting position if cisternography is performed.

(4) A thin needle 18 gauge or smaller is introduced through the cheek, being careful not to breach the oral mucosa and guided into position by use of fluoroscopy. Exact details are provided in the above texts. Correct placement of the needle is very important and aims to enter the trigeminal cistern in such a way that the preganglionic trigeminal rootlets become bathed in the glycerol. Passing the needle through the foramen ovale does not guarantee entry into the trigeminal cistern. The needle may need to penetrate further if divisions 1 and 2 are to be

treated. Egress of CSF increases the chances of a successful outcome.

(5) The correct placement of the needle and the size of the cistern can be estimated by injecting a known amount of contrast medium and ascertaining the amount it takes to achieve a cup shape. It is important to remember that a certain volume of contrast medium needs to be injected before it is visualised on X-ray. Some operators do not do cisternography for one or more of the following reasons: increases the cost of the procedure; increases chance of needle moving out of position while it is draining; need to change patient position

(6) If cisternography has been used it is important to remove the contrast medium and this can be done by flushing with sterile saline. Contrast medium can be left if seeking to avoid the third division and wishing to affect the first division.

(7) The position of the needle must be checked again if cisternography has been used before the glycerol is injected with the patient in the sitting position. Placement of the glycerol outside Meckel's cave increases the chances of sensory change. It is important to ensure that the glycerol is sterile to minimise the risk of meningitis and the anhydrous form seems to be the most satisfactory. Volumes injected range from 0.25 to 0.4 ml. More than this and there is a risk of overfilling the cistern. Some will also add a small amount of tantalum dust so that the cistern can be visualised at a later date. Sweet and Poletti (1985) have recommended incremental injection of glycerol until some sensory loss has been achieved which means the patient has to co-operate. Sahni et al. (1990) has suggested that this method not only leads to increased numbers having sensory deficits but also increases the chances of recurrence. Arias (1986) suggests that after a injection of 0.05 ml of glycerol the patient should be asked whether they get focal paraesthesia with or without trigeminal pain. Some selectivity of which fibres are affected can be achieved by a variety of manoeuvres mainly related to changes in flexion of the head (Linderoth and Hakanson, 1995).

(8) After the injection the flow of CSF should be checked as this will confirm that dislocation of the needle has not occurred.

(9) It is important to leave the patient in the sitting position for 2–3 hours after the procedure to avoid leakage of the glycerol out of the cistern.

(10) Patients can be kept in overnight to ensure that no complications develop and this is recommended in elderly patients.

(11) Pain relief may not be immediate, it can be delayed for 5–7 days so it is important that medication is continued till the patient is pain-free.

Slettebo et al. (1993) showed that supposed technical failures (no egress of CSF, abnormal cistern, poor drainage) did not necessary correlate with poor outcomes as he had seven of these cases and five patients had a good result.

Percutaneous Gasserian ganglion balloon compression (micropression). The technique is well described by Brown and Gouda (1999) in a special supplement on trigeminal neuralgia in 'Techniques of Neurosurgery'.

(1) A general anaesthetic is used and the procedure must be done in a room with access to radiography as a C arm intensifier fluoroscope is required.

(2) The procedure lasts 30–60 minutes.

(3) Patient is placed either in the semi-sitting or supine position.

(4) Significant drops in blood pressure and heart rate occur at the time needle (larger than used in other techniques) is inserted into the foramen ovale or balloon catheter advanced and inflated. A case of asystole has been reported (Belber and Rak, 1987) and so it is crucial to monitor arterial blood pressure and heart rate. Either intravenous atropine must be available or as Brown and Gouda (1999) suggest, a non-invasive temporary pacemaker which responds rapidly to changes can be used. It is possible to

block this response completely but then a useful sign as to when the nerve has been engaged is lost.

(5) The needle is inserted through a point in the cheek using a No 14 needle or a liver biopsy needle. Fluoroscopy is used to guide the needle into position.

(6) Often at the point the needle touches the emerging nerve bradycardia occurs (called the pain reflex). It is crucial not to push the needle through the foramen ovale.

(7) A No 14 Fogarty balloon catheter without its stylet is then advanced through the needle. It is advanced beyond the needle in the aim of locating it in the posterior fossa. The balloon is fully distended if it begins to protrude posteriorly through the entrance to Meckel's cave. In doing this it should assume a pear shape. If not advanced far enough it will miss V_3 fibres.

(8) Compression should be achieved with 0.7 ml distention, intraluminal pressure is approx. 1200 to 1500 mmHg. If distended too much the balloon may burst, over distension leads to severe numbness and 4th nerve palsy. There have been no trials to estimate the optimal pressure to use or the duration of compression.

(9) Compression with the appropriate pear shape is maintained for one to one and a half minutes although longer times have been recorded. The duration of compression does relate to sensory loss. If the balloon is well inflated you will often at this stage get bradycardia and this is considered a good sign.

(10) The balloon is deflated and everything is withdrawn.

(11) Pressure maintained at puncture site for 5 min.

(12) Patient may be discharged the next day.

(13) May get delay in pain relief of a few days.

7.5.3. Posterior fossa surgery
Microvasuclar decompression (MVD)

The following summary of the procedure of microvascular decompression (MVD) is based largely on a study by McLaughlin et al. (1999) which is based on observations after 4400 operations. There are many other texts and books that describe variations of this technique and these are pointed out in the references at the end of the chapter and trainee neurosurgeons are encouraged to read these in greater detail. In performing this operation three major complications need to be avoided and careful attention to detail can reduce this as McLaughlin et al. (1999) have shown by analysing their early and late postoperative complication data. The three major complications are:

- Cerebellar injury
- Hearing loss
- CSF leak

Patient information prior to surgery is crucial and it is preferable for this to be available in a written format. An example of one of these is given in Appendix A. Most surgeons warn patients that if no compression is found a partial rhizotomy will be done. The patient therefore needs to be aware that they may have sensory changes after surgery because a PSR rather than an MVD was done (Aksik, 1993).

The position of the patient is crucial for correct exposure, the lateral position is used with the patients head placed at the foot of the operating table to enable the surgeon to have more room. The head is secured with a three point fixation device after intubation. The patient is carefully taped in the correct position.

Earlier operations were generally carried out with the patient in the sitting position. Sindou et al. (1990) compared 60 cases each using the two different positions and found that the lying position was faster, enabled smaller exposure and resulted in fewer complications. Aksik (1993) reported similar findings.

Surgical incision. The aim is to minimise the length of the incision but at the same time to allow adequate exposure for the burr hole. The position and size of this incision is dependent on the size and thickness of the patient's neck.

Bone removal. Before opening the dura it is essential to identify the junction of the transverse and the sigmoid sinus, this may involve some partial removal of mastoid air cells. These air cells need to be immediately protected with wax or muscle after exposure to reduce ear complications (Coakham, 2000).

Expose the trigeminal nerve. One of the most intricate steps of the procedure is the exposure of the cerebello pontine angle. Once the dura is sutured back an operating microscope with a 250 mm objective lens is brought into the operating field. Draining CSF helps to expose this area and reduces the amount of traction that may be necessary. At all stages very gentle traction should be applied. Ogungbo et al. (2000) report that less traction is required in elderly patients due to atrophy and that this therefore reduces the risk of postoperative complications. Veins must be very carefully pared away and coagulated and it is essential to have excellent haemostasis at all stages. Sindou et al. (1991) and Coakham (2000) suggest preserving the superior petrosal vein so that it can later be used as a support for the mobilised superior cerebellar artery (SICA). It may also protect the cerebellum from swelling or infarction.

Look for the compression. It is important to bear in mind that the dorsal route entry zone can be very variable in length and can extend fairly distally. Several reports stress the importance of exploring the full length of the nerve and Hamlyn and King (1992) have reported that of 33 cases, 11 compressions were found beyond the root entry zone (REZ). The use of a small angled fibrescope to inspect the whole area may be useful adjunct to the microscope (Coakham, 2000). Vessels may be found behind an exostosis of the petrous bone or behind the sensory root. Any arachnoid should be careful dissected off. Kondo (1997) advocates straightening of the axis of the trigeminal nerve by resecting the surrounding arachnoid membrane. The commonest vessel involved is the rostroventral superior cerebellar artery loop (see end of this section for further details).

The use of brain stem evoked potentials is advocated in order to reduce damage to the auditory nerve. If these potentials begin to decline this may be due to tethering of arachnoid between the seventh and eighth nerve complex. Careful removal to relieve the tension on the cochlear nerve may be required. Potentials may also change during the procedure due to retraction, a few millimetres can make all the difference and this needs to be monitored continually. Brain-evoked potentials may also change during closure of the dura, it is essential then to go back in and access the area as there may be tension on the nerve from either the Teflon pad or any other displaced vessels which could have occurred during CSF replacement. It has also been noted that small amounts of blood or cold irrigation of the cochlear nerve may affect these potentials. Kondo (1997) suggests that hearing problems can also be reduced if retraction of the cerebellum is limited to 5 minutes.

Decompressive materials. Decompression can be done in a variety of ways using a range of materials. There have been no controlled trials to assess the effectiveness of different materials. The materials used have ranged from resorbable ones such as muscle, autologous dura, hard materials such as Ivalon (polyvinyl alcohol foam), Dacron, to softer materials such as gelatine sponge, Surgicel and Teflon in a variety of forms: shredded felt, tapes and woollen slings and glue. Reports on reoperations have shown that resorbable materials tend to cause adhesions, are lost and so lead to recompression (Rath et al., 1996). Teflon felt can cause adhesions and granulomas but it tends to remain in place (Cho et al., 1994; Coakham, 2000) as does Ivalon sponges (Goya et al., 1990). Sindou et al. (1991) have suggested that improved results are obtained if the offending artery is dislodged from the nerve by pulling with small tapes of Teflon (2 mm wide, 4 cm in length) passed round the vessel and maintained in position by a rectangular piece of Dacron suspended by superior petrosal vein. Fukushima (1990), Sindou et al. (1991), Kondo (1997) and Coakham (2000) stress that they avoid any contact of the nerve with any decompressant as Teflon has been reported to cause compression in its own right (Cho et al., 1994). McLaughlin et al. (1999) suggest the use of shredded Teflon and illustrate how it is placed. Linskey et al. (1994) report that mobilisation of the vertebral artery or basilar artery can be very difficult and an aneurysmal cuff clip may need to be used or glues. More manipulations are likely and hence more complications.

Veins are difficult to decompress and so these are often coagulated. If no compressing vessels are found most surgeons will then proceed to do a partial rhizotomy. By careful sectioning sensory loss can be reduced to a partial lower facial sensory loss.

Closure. Complete and effective haemostasis is essential to prevent cerebellar injury. McLaughlin et al. (1999) advocate the use of the valsalva procedure to check that the dura is watertight. Coakham (2000) suggests use of muscle to plug any deficiencies. It is again repeated after fascial closure to ensure no CSF leak is present. It is important to wax the mastoid air cells again. McLaughlin et al. (1999) advocate placing cellulose and gel foam over the durotomy and to perform the cranioplasty with glue or a wire mesh. Fascial closure needs to be watertight.

Postoperative care. Monitoring of blood pressure is crucial and McLaughlin et al. (1999) will also use invasive arterial pressure monitoring to ensure that the blood pressure does not rise above 160 mmHg. To reduce blood pressures, nausea and vomiting must be carefully controlled with use of drugs. Patients can be mobilised after one day and discharged within 48 to 72 hours. Frontal and incisional pain is expected but should be controllable with mild narcotics. If mild narcotics fail to control the pain then investigations need to be done to rule out haemorrhage or a CFS leak with the use of a CT Scan. Medication can be tailed off slowly.

Compression. There is relatively good evidence to suggest that compression of the trigeminal nerve by a vessel is not normal although up to 16–40% of non-trigeminal neuralgia patients may exhibit contact between a blood vessel and the nerve but no grooving or distortion of the nerve is found (Hamlyn and King, 1992). The vessels involved in order of frequency are:

superior cerebellar artery (SCA)
anterior inferior cerebellar artery
basilar artery
superior petrosal vein
inferior petrosal vein
petrosal vein

It is considered that compression by an artery is likely to be more significant than by a vein although Aksik (1993) suggests that venous compression can be significant. The presence of compression or contact between vessels and the trigeminal nerve is not always easy to establish and many neurosurgeons do not define their criteria and some change their views with increasing experience (Piatt and Wilkins, 1984). Compression by the vertebrobasilar artery may be more complex resulting in the trigeminal nerve being sandwiched between the vertebrobasilar artery and SCA. Linskey et al. (1994) suggest a modified approach to these patients which is possible because MRI will often predict this occurrence.

A range of descriptions is used to describe the relationship between the vessels and the nerve. Piatt and Wilkins (1984) have three categories of relationships: distortion, wedging (artery is wedged into the crevice between anteriosuperior border of the fifth nerve root and the pons) and contact. Grooving or distortion of the nerve once the vessel has been lifted off is considered by most to indicate compression. Sun et al. (1994) also describe the direction of the compression, its exact site and if the contact is apparent (obvious vascular grooving or distortion) or mild compression where contact is seen but there is no grooving or distortion. Sun et al. (1994) assessed the level of compression in relation to duration of symptoms and found more definite compression in those who had trigeminal neuralgia for over five years 29/37 vs. 11/24 under five years of trigeminal neuralgia. However, they did also find that mild compression was found in patients with 10 year histories.

Hamlyn (1999), based on his anatomical and clinical work, proposes the following definitions which he considers to be feasible when using an operating microscope with binocular vision "vessels are, or are not, in contact; they either do, or do not, lie within half of their diameter from the brain stem or nerve; and there either is, or is not, a groove left after the vessel is dissected free."

Lovely and Jannetta (1997) performed an anatomical analysis of vascular compression based on pain distribution and did not find a correlation. They postulated that the distribution of pain is related to the place at which the vessel impinges on the nerve or where the demyelination has occurred. Goya et al. (1990), however, in their small series of 33 patients suggest that the direction of compression does relate to involved division and this can therefore be useful when operating. Szapiro et al. (1985) showed that sensory deficit preoperatively did occur in some patients but was not correlated with degree of compression and was commoner in patients with paroxysmal and dull background pain. Miles et al. (1997) on the other hand found no sensory loss in 19 virgin cases preoperatively and although some changes were noted postoperatively these were all reversed by one year and yet all the patients continued to be free of pain. These findings do suggest that in contrast to all other procedures, sensory loss after MVD does not lead to improved outcome and may even lead to burning, aching pains (Barker et al., 1997). Compression has been looked at as a prognostic factor and this is shown in Table 30.

Reduction of complications. Using careful techniques with evoked potentials during operation as highlighted above. Aksik (1993) suggests regular use of antibiotics to avoid meningitis. Klun (1992) has shown that experience of the surgeon is an important factor in reduction of complications. Sweet and Poletti's (1995) review of complications from 140 neurosurgeons (total surveyed 200) also support this observation.

Partial rhizotomy (PSR). This procedure is initially the same as MVD but if no compression is found many neurosurgeons will go on to do a partial rhizotomy. It is important that the surgeon identifies the orientation of the oval shaped sensory root so as to avoid making the rhizotomy through the motor fibres. The section closest to the pons is taken. The amount of section taken depends on the distribution of the pain. A one half section is taken for third division pain and a two thirds section for second division pain. This method ensures that some sensory sensation is preserved especially light touch.

Gamma knife surgery (GKS)
It is important to have a high quality assurance programme in operation. More technical details on this technique can be found in Kondziolka et al. (1997).

Frame fitting. A stereotactic frame is fitted on the head often using local anaesthesia (e.g. sedation midazolam 1–2 mg and analgesia fentanyl 50–100 µg). Friedman et al. (2001) also give 10 mg of intravenous dexamethasone prior to placement of the frame and then 6 hourly for the first 24 hours.

Localisation of the trigeminal nerve. This is best done using stereotactic MRIs but CT can be used in those patients who have implanted metallic foreign bodies or those who do not have easy access to an MRI machine. Contrast-enhanced short repetition time sequences and axial volume acquisitions of 512×216 matrices divided into 1 mm slices are done. Previous surgery can make this more difficult and additional axial long time relaxation time MRI images are done. In patients who have had Teflon the image can mimic a meningioma and in patients who have sensory loss due to previous surgery the nerve may be atrophic and so difficult to find (Kondziolka et al., 1997).

Computer dose planning. The isocentre is positioned on the axial and coronal MR images over the trigeminal root such that the 40% or 50% isodose line is tangential to the pontine surface (Young et al., 1997) which aims to treat about 4 mm of the nerve approximately 2 to 4 mm anterior to the junction of the nerve and brain stem. A 4 mm collimator secondary helmet is used. Except for one study a single isocentre is used. It was then thought that the recurrence rate could be improved on by exposing a longer length of the affected trigeminal nerve and so two isocentres were used. One was placed close to the root entry zone and the other 3–5 mm further down so that the mean length of the trigeminal nerve was $5.4 + 0.4$ mm for one and $8.7 + 1.1$ mm for the two isocentres (Flickinger et al., 2001). The dose used has varied from 28 to 90 Gy and Kondziolka et al. (1997) and Young et al. (1997) estimate that the amount delivered to the adjacent pontine surface is about 14–21 Gy. Doses between 80 and 90 Gy are used in patients with recurrences (Kondziolka et al., 1997). When treatment is planned for tumours the dose is calculated based on tumour volume and proximity to radiosensitive structures.

Treatment. This can be delivered over periods varying from 20 to 50 minutes (Kondziolka et al., 1997; Friedman et al., 2001). It is not known whether the dose rate is important for outcomes (Kondziolka et al., 1997).

Completion of treatment. The frame is removed and the patient hospitalised overnight although some may be discharged home at the end of the day. The whole procedure takes around three hours.

Postoperative management. Medication needs to be continued for at least 3–4 days and tapering down should only begin once pain relief is being achieved. Delays of up to 120 days have been noted but the mean is 14 days. Postoperative MRI s are not used routinely (Friedman et al., 2001). As complications can theoretically occur up to 2 years after treatment regular long-term follow up is important.

7.6. Outcome on pain relief

7.6.1. General remarks on recurrence rates

Trigeminal neuralgia is one of the few neuropathic pains in which 100% pain relief can be obtained. In general, you can say that the more central the surgery the longer is the time to recurrence likely to be and this is seen in Fig. 2. The results for different forms of surgery are shown in greater detail in the next series of tables. These are based on the best quality studies. The greatest number of recurrences occurs in the first two years. There continues to be a gradual decline in patients who remain pain-free but it is smallest in the MVD group. The data for all procedures seems to suggest that the rate of decline changes over time.

Patients who are medically unfit are more likely to be offered peripheral techniques and this may affect results. There is conflicting evidence as to whether previous surgery affects future treatments. Some patients may prefer to have a reversible procedure like cryotherapy initially to assess how they cope with sensory changes. Other patients want long

lasting pain relief and make the decision to have microvascular decompression despite the risks. When I asked a group of 200 patients attending a support group meeting how long a pain relief period they were looking for, given that a permanent cure could not be guaranteed, they suggested a minimum of five years. This would therefore preclude any peripheral therapies and even some of the Gasserian ganglion options.

Oturai et al. (1996) report a patient satisfaction survey among their patients who underwent peripheral alcohol injections, neurectomy or RFT. From their initial cohort of 383, 67 were lost to follow up of which 52 had died. The questionnaire and follow up telephone interviews was sent to 316 and gave a response rate of 288 (91%). The non-responders tended to be older and had had a wider range of treatments at the time of the questionnaire. At the time of the questionnaire 91 (49%) reported no pain, 62 (33%) less pain, 14 (8%) unchanged pain and 18 (10%) more pain. Of those reporting pain, 9 (5%) said it was continuous, 73 (40%) had attacks of pain and 12 (6%) had a mixture of both. The frequency of pain attacks was daily 36 (20%), weekly 15 (8%), monthly 16 (8%). They also asked about quality of life as affected by the complications and found that 36% were unaffected by them, 51% were slightly or severely affected by them and 13% reported a marked effect. We also showed in patients undergoing RFT that quality of life was affected either slightly or markedly by sensory loss in over 60% of patients and it did not drop off significantly after time (Zakrzewska and Thomas, 1993; Zakrzewska et al., 1999).

7.6.2. Peripheral surgery results

The results from all the better quality studies are shown in Table 22. In several of them actuarial analysis was possible due to provision of sufficient data. The results are also shown in Fig. 2 where it can be seen that the results are very poor in comparison to other surgical techniques. The mean time to a recurrence is 9–18 months and it is interesting to note how consistent these changes are in all the techniques. The RCT trial of streptomycin by Staj-

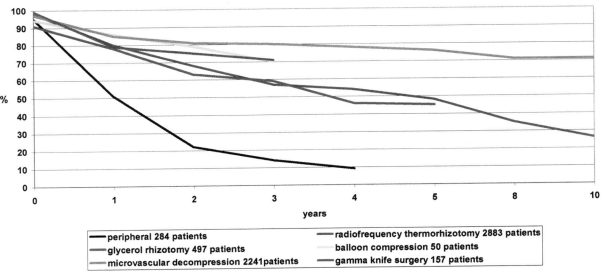

Fig. 2. Probability of being pain-free after surgery for trigeminal neuralgia based on a review of the literature, from studies using actuarial methodology.

cic et al. (1990) showed that initially more patients responded to the streptomycin injections than lignocaine alone but at 30 weeks this effect was lost. Bittar and Graff-Radford (1993) showed no effects even in the initial follow up time. Erdem and Alkan (2001) claimed that in their group of 157 patients, 64% were still pain-free at 1 year and that the mean time to recurrence was 2–3 years. If you look at the patient data you will see that the patients had a very short history of trigeminal neuralgia and it could be that these patients were going through a period of remission and this then resulted in these good results. My own experience with glycerol reported in Fardy et al.'s (1994) study was very poor. The small RCT on the use of laser reports very good results but only short-term (10 weeks) results are given.

7.6.3. Gasserian ganglion surgery results
RFT
The number of patients likely to be pain-free at any one time point is shown in Table 23 and in Fig. 3. In the general overview of all procedures as shown in Fig. 2, RFT would appear to offer better results than PRG but these results have not been statistically analysed and this may not be a real trend. Technical

failures or complete lack of pain relief does occur but is not reported by all and this may be because they are excluded from the analysis.

Taha et al.'s (1995) meticulous attention to detail has resulted in the best results of any reported series as seen in Fig. 3 and their results are comparable to the MVD results whereas others are much lower with Tronnier et al. (2001) reporting high recurrence rates. In their 15 year follow up of 154 patients, Taha et al. (1995) showed that the rate of recurrence was higher in those with mild analgesia as opposed to deep analgesia and this is also reflected in the data from Tronnier et al. (2001) who specifically say they reduce the lesioning time in order not to get sensory loss. Tew and Taha (1995) acknowledge that in some patients who do not wish to have significant analgesia, less sensory loss can be achieved but patients need to accept that recurrence of pain will be earlier.

Taha et al. (1995) showed that patients were very satisfied with the results and reported outcomes at 14 years as: 77% excellent, 18% good, 2% fair, 2% poor, the last 4% poor and fair satisfaction were due to complications. In our prospective study we inferred patient satisfaction with treatment from a

TABLE 22
Randomised controlled trials and cohort studies of peripheral treatments for trigeminal neuralgia, recommendation grade for all these C (see table 9 in Chapter 9)

Intervention	Number patients/procedures	Mean and (range) of follow up in years	% Pain-free one year	Median/mean time to recurrence years	Complications	Reference
Cryotherapy, 70°C	10 patients	0.80 (0.25–1.1)	61	Mean 0.9	Mild analgesia, postoperative swelling	Politis et al., 1988
Cryotherapy, 30°C	26 patients	2	25	Mean 0.8 ± 0.5	Nil	Barnard, 1989
Cryotherapy, 70°C	145 patients	3.7 ± 2	27[a]	Median 0.75–1.2 depending on nerve	Sensory loss locally 37%, eating problems 14%, taking anticonvulsants 49%	Zakrzewska and Thomas, 1993
Streptomycin 1 g/lidocaine weekly for 5 weeks versus lidocaine RCT	17 patients	(0.5–2.5)	35[a] for streptomycin and lidocaine and 38 for lidocaine	Mean 0.9, median 0.4 for streptomycin, mean 0.8 for lidocaine	None	Stajcic et al., 1990
Streptomycin 1 g/lidocaine injections weekly for 5 weeks versus lidocaine cross-over RCT	20 patients	11 weeks	Not applicable	Not applicable	Swelling at site of injections, painful injection	Bittar and Graff-Radford, 1993
Glycerol 0.5–1.5 ml into nerve endings	157 patients	Minimum 4 years	64	2–3 years	Mild dysaesthesia 14, haematomas local	Erdem and Alkan, 2001
Alcohol 1 ml	68 patients, 413 procedures	0.2–3	52[a]	Median 1.2	Pain on administration, oedema, sensory loss over area of injection	Fardy et al., 1994
Alcohol 0.75 ml	185 patients, 331 injections	Unknown	Unable to tell	Mean 0.9–1.4	Ulceration in the mouth 1%, transient diplopia 7%, VII palsy 0.5%	Grant, 1936
Alcohol	468 patients, 600 injections	(0.75–8)	Unable to tell	Mean 0.75–1.4	Haematomas, diplopia 0.3%	Horrax and Poppen, 1935
Alcohol	45 patients	8 (3–14)	25[a]	Median 0.2	Hypaesthesia 21%, paraesthesia 11%, eye complications 4%, dysaesthesia 6%, taking anticonvulsants 69%	Oturai et al., 1996
Neurectomy	53 patients	7 (1–16)	25[a]	Median 0.2	Hypaesthesia 40%, paraesthesia 20%, eye complications 8%, dysaesthesia 5%, taking anticonvulsants 72%	Oturai et al., 1996
Neurectomy	36 patients, 47 procedures	(1–4)	64	Overall mean 1.9	Oedema and bruising	Mason, 1972

TABLE 22 *continued*

Intervention	Number patients/procedures	Mean and (range) of follow up in years	% Pain-free one year	Median/mean time to recurrence years	Complications	Reference
Neurectomy	40 patients	2 (2–10)	85 at 2 years	No mean	Oedema, mild dysaesthesia 5%	Murali and Rovit, 1996
Neurectomy	26 patients	(1–15)	82	Mean 1.9	Anticonvulsants needed by some	Freemont and Millac, 1981
Peripheral radiofrequency thermocoagulation 70°C for 2–3 min	71 patients	1.5 (0.25–5)	78	Mean 2.7, median 1.4	Mild analgesia in all, trismus postoperative, minor haematoma	Gregg and Small, 1986
Phenol injection 10% in glycerol 0.5–1 ml	18 patients	2 (0–3)	50 [a]	Median 1, mean 1.6	Mild sensory loss, taking anticonvulsants 44%	Wilkinson, 1999
Acupuncture every day or other for ten times, then another course 3/4 days later	1500 patients	1 (1–6)	46	Not possible to calculate	Difficulty opening mouth 6%	Shuhan et al., 1991
Laser three times a week for 10 weeks RCT	35 patients	10 weeks	Unable to ascertain	Significant improvement if had high baseline of pain, no numbers given	Nil	Walker et al., 1988

RTC – Randomised controlled trial.
[a] Kaplan–Meier analysis.

TABLE 23

Cohort studies reporting pain outcomes in 4995 patients with trigeminal neuralgia who underwent percutaneous radiofrequency thermorhizotomy (thermolysis), grade of recommendation B (see table 9 in Chapter 9)

No. of patients	Mean (range) follow up years	Lost to follow up	Operative features	Technical failures/immediate failures (%)	% Pain free			Median/mean time to recurrence years	Reference
					1 year	2 years	5 years		
78	4.6	Died 4, lost 5	No details	Technical 6 (8), immediate 15 (19)	68	46	35	NA	Burchiel et al., 1981
96	5(1–8)	Died 14, lost 10	Little detail no temperature	Technical failure 6 (6)	90[a]	87[a]	52[a]	Median 6	Latchaw et al., 1983
400	4.5 (1–6)	NA	60°C, 90 s repeated	Technical 11 (3)	NA	NA	NA	Overall recurrence 9.4%	Schvarcz, 1982
1000	9.3 (5–14)	NA	65–70°C, 60 s repeat until analgesia	Failure 52 (5)	NA	NA	At 3 years 82	NA	Broggi et al., 1999
124	3.7 (1–6)	NA	No details	Failures 15 (12)	85[a]	74[a]	63[a]	NA	Ischia et al., 1990a,b
265	3.7 (3–3.75)	Died 21 (8), lost 58 (22)	70–80°C for 300 s	Failures 5 (2)	63[a]	47[a]	20[a]	Median 2, mean 3	Zakrzewska and Thomas, 1993
154	14 (5–15)	Died 19, lost 35	Other paper straight probe	Failure 1 (0.6)	96[a]	94[a]	85[a]	25%[a] recurrence at 14 years, median 2.9 if only mild hypalgesia	Taha and Tew, 1996
185	8(1–15)	Lost 67 from total of 383 pts.[b]	Nil	NA	68[a]	63[a]	50[a]	Median 6, 75 (49) recurrence	Oturia, 1996
500	9(2–12)	NA	Curved electrode	Failure (2) 12	NA	NA	NA	20% no time period stated	Taha and Tew, 1996
81	(6–11)	NA	60–90°C for 90–450 s		65[a]	49[a]	37[a]	Median 2	Yoon et al., 1999
48	2.5 ± 1 (0.6–4.7)	Died 2, lost 5	70–80°C, 300 s	0	90[a] TN, 80[a] ATN	65[a] TN, 80[a] ATN	4[a] years, 65[a] TN, 55[a] ATN	Mean 3.3 TN, 3 ATN, median 4.3	Zakrzewska et al., 1999
258	3.2 (1–6.5)	Nil	60°C for 60 s raise up to 8°C for 60 s curved/straight	Failures 34 (14)	NA	NA	NA	NA	Mathews and Scrivani, 2000
1600	5.8 (1–25)	NA	55–70°C	Failures 163 (2.4)	0	93[a]	58[a] (10 yrs 50)	1216 (76) needed only one treatment	Kanpolat and Savas, 2001
206	10.9	26 lost	70–75°C, 60–90 s	NA	64[a]	46[a]	21[a]	Median 1.75	Tronnier et al., 2001
2883					**80[a]**	**68[a]**	**48[a]**	**Totals only Kaplan–Meier**	

NA, not available; TN, trigeminal neuralgia; ATN, atypical trigeminal neuralgia.
[a] Kaplan–Meier analysis.
[b] Oturai reported on three different techniques.

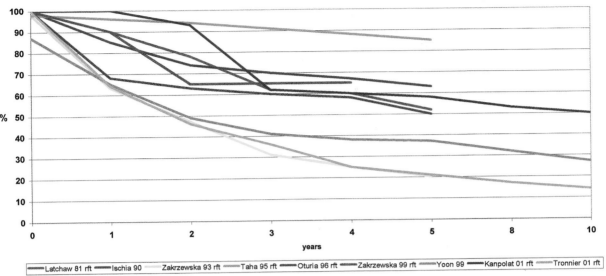

Fig. 3. Probability of being pain-free after radiofrequency thermorhizotomy based on a review of the literature, from studies using actuarial methodology.

yearly questionnaire that asked patients whether they wished to have repeated surgery (Zakrzewska et al., 1999). There was little change over time and over 90% of patients were prepared to undergo a repeat RFT if necessary but patients with atypical trigeminal neuralgia who had less pain relief and more complications were less sure whether they would want to undergo the treatment a second time (12% no, 43% unsure).

The importance of clear diagnostic criteria has again been shown to be important in this technique. In our small cohort of 48 patients followed up for three years we carefully classified patients into those with classical trigeminal neuralgia and those with atypical trigeminal neuralgia, i.e. a background pain, and have shown that those with classical pain had better results (Zakrzewska et al., 1999). Further evidence for this can be seen in earlier data we published on 265 procedures (Zakrzewska and Thomas, 1993) which were done by the same surgeon but patient selection was not as meticulous and at three years only 31% of patients were likely to be pain-free as compared to 65% in my later study. We also showed that depression and, less so, anxiety (measured using the Hospital Anxiety and Depression

Scale) are reduced after successful RFT. Yoon et al. (1999) also had a poorer outcomes in patients with atypical trigeminal neuralgia but the data were analysed retrospectively and little details are given as the criteria used to assign patients to the two groups.

PRG

The number of patients estimated to be pain-free at any one year is shown in Table 24 and Fig. 4 where only data from Kaplan–Meier analysis is used. When looked at in comparison with other procedures of the Gasserian ganglion, Fig. 2, the recurrence rates appear to be the highest. No statistical tests have been done as there is too much variation in the quality of the data. North et al. (1990) show how recurrence rates change depending on which end points are used, use of medication or need for re-operation. No trials have been done to assess the value of doing cisternography. This is impossible to do from the reported studies as the results are too disparate. These high recurrence rates have led some clinicians to abandon this type of surgery. Multiple sclerosis does not appear to affect recurrence rates (Kondziolka et al., 1994b; Bergenheim and Hariz, 1995).

TABLE 24

Cohort studies reporting pain outcomes in 1363 patients with trigeminal neuralgia who underwent percutaneous retro-Gasserian glycerol rhizotomy (PRG), grade of recommendation B (see table 9 of Chapter 9)

No. of patients	Mean (range) follow up years	Lost to follow up	Operative features	Technical failures/immediate failures (%)	% Pain-free			Median/mean time to recurrence years	Reference
					1 year	2 years	5 years		
552	4 (1–6)	83 (15%)	No cisternography, 0.2–0.3 ml glycerol	NA	All 72, no previous surgery 96, previous surgery 76	60 all	18 all	NA	Saini, 1987
162	2.5 (0.5–5.6)	NA	Cisternography on early ones and V1 pain only 0.1–0.2 ml glycerol	Failures 16 (10)	85	76, previous surgery increased recurrence	NA	NA	Young et al., 1998
60	1 (0.25–3.75)	Died 3, lost 3	Cisternography glycerol 0.15–0.25 ml	Failures 12 (20)	TN 67[a], MS 25	45[a]	NA	Median 1.5[a]	Burchiel et al., 1988
112	3.5 (0.1–5.5)	NA	Cisternography, 0.4–0.5 ml glycerol	Failures 11 (9.8)	89[a]	80[a]	74[a]	NA	Ischia et al., 1990a,b
85	3 (0.5–4.5)	NA	No cisternography, incremental glycerol 0.3–0.4 ml	NA	60[a] control with drugs, 68 if repeat surgery	57[a] control with drugs, 52 if repeat surgery	NA	Median 2[a] no drugs, median 3[a] with drugs, repeat median 1	North et al., 1990
58	Median 1.4 (0.5–4.5)	Lost 4	Cisternography, 0.3–0.5 ml glycerol	Technical failures 5 (7)	No hypaesthesia 88[a], hypaesthesia 25[a]	No hypaesthesia 45[a]	NA	Overall median 1.4, median 0.6 if hypaesthesia, if no hypaesthesia 1.6	Sahni et al., 1990
122	2 (0.1–8)	NA	Cisternography 0.2–0.35 ml glycerol	Technical failures 8 (6.6)	78[a]	76[a]	59[a]	NA	Steiger, 1991
60	6.5 median 4.5 (4.5–9)	Died 10	Cisternography, 0.15–0.7 ml, average 0.3 ml	Technical 8 (13) but proceeded, failures 4 (7)	87[a]	75[a]	45[a]	Median 4[a], in MS patients all recurred 1.4–5 years	Slettebo et al., 1993
99	(1–12)	None	Cisternography mean 0.26 ml range 0.2–0.35	Failures 3 (4)	76[a], recurrence rate highest previous glycerol	NA	NA	NA	Bergenheim and Hariz, 1995
53 all MS	Median 3 (0.5–10)	Lost 4	Cisternography, 0.15–0.3 ml anhydrous glycerol with tantalum	Abnormal cisterns in 11 (20)	NA	NA	NA	29 (59) median 3 years	Kondziolka et al., 1994a,b
768					63[a]	45[a]		**Totals only Kaplan Meier**	

TN, trigeminal neuralgia; NA, data not available.
[a] Kaplan–Meier analysis.

TABLE 25

Cohort studies reporting pain outcomes in 294 patients with trigeminal neuralgia who underwent balloon microcompression of the Gasserian ganglion, grade of recommendation B (see table 9 in Chapter 9)

No. patients	Mean and (range) of follow up in years	Lost to follow up	Operative notes	Technical failures/ immediate failures	% Pain-free			Median/mean time to recurrence years	Reference
					1 year	2 years	4–5 years		
100	6 (1–10)	8 died, 3 lost	Mean compression 5–7 min, balloon vol. 0.7–1 ml	Technical 2 (4), failures 4 (4)	95	NA	40 based on 61 patients at 5 yrs	NA	Lichtor and Mullan, 1990
144	3 (0.5–4.5)	5 died, 4 lost	Mean compression 1 min, balloon vol. 0.7–1 ml	Technical 3 (2), failures 9 (6)	100	94	NA	NA	Lobato et al., 1990
50	3 (1–7)	NA	Mean compression 1–3 min, balloon vol. 0.7–0.75	Failures 3 (6)	86[a]	79[a]	NA	Mean 1.6	Brown et al., 1993

[a] Kaplan–Meier analysis; NA, data not available.

Percutaneous balloon microcompression
There are only two studies that report longer-term outcomes and there is only one report which uses Kaplan–Meier analysis which is illustrated in Fig. 2. The report recording the largest number of procedures (496) contains insufficient data (Skirving and Dan, 2001). The results are shown in Table 25. When compared to other Gasserian ganglion data the results appear promising but these are based on a very small number of patients. Technical failures are not uncommon and are shown in Table 25.

7.6.4. Posterior fossa
There are little data on partial rhizotomies and no Kaplan–Meier analysis. Most of the data are included in the MVD data.

Table 26 below and Figs. 2 and 5 included only those studies using actuarial methodology which enables yearly data to be compared and fulfilling the criteria used above.

Patients said to have excellent pain relief are those who are on no medication and have no pain. Results labelled as good often include patients who have either had some minor episodes of pain not requiring surgical treatment or who have to take medication to gain complete pain relief. Some studies present their data in individual categories and others combine all their categories. Two studies, by Piatt and Wilkins (1984) and Bederson and Wilson (1989), contain patients who have had partial rhizotomies (21 and 86, respectively) as Bederson and Wilson (1989) showed that recurrence rates were no different in those patients having PSR compared to MVD. Broggi et al. (2000) showed that 79% patients who had trigeminal neuralgia for less than 7 years would be likely to be pain-free at five years whereas this fell to 63% in those who had a longer duration of pain. Barker et al. (1996) showed that the rate of recurrence changes over time being 2% at 5 years but becoming 1% by ten years. The highest rate of recurrences is in the first year. Pollack et al.'s (1988) data are on patients who had bilateral trigeminal neuralgia. Patients who have bilateral trigeminal neuralgia or who have a second operation do not have such good results. Tacconi and Miles (2000) also reported that in their

16 bilateral cases only 4 had good long-term relief. They advocate doing immediate bilateral MVDs in patients who have simultaneous bilateral pain. Depression and anxiety as measured on the Hospital Anxiety and Depression Scale is low after MVD (Zakrzewska and Thomas, 1993).

Patients with MS undergoing posterior fossa surgery. Resnick et al. (1996) reported 5 cases and in their cases patients who had both an MVD and PSR did better than patients with just MVD. Broggi et al. (1999) reported on 15 patients with MS in whom they did MVD. One patient needed another MVD in 10 months. Seven had complete relief, two partial relief and six experienced a recurrence. The mean time to recurrence was 13.5 months but the overall follow up was only for a mean of 2 years.

GKS
Data on GKS are complicated to report in that maximum benefits may not occur for up to six months. This has meant that some have excluded patients from their analysis unless they have been followed up for a minimum of 6 months (Brisman, 2000) whereas others have included patients with follow up as short as 2 months (Pollock et al., 2001). Many of the GKS studies divide outcome up into four groups (Flickering et al., 2001; Maesawa et al., 2001):

- Excellent, relief with no medication
- Good, relief but with the use of medication or occasional pain requiring no medication
- Fair, over 50% improvement but needing medication
- Fail, no improvement or less than 50% improvement after treatment

Rogers et al. (2000) have broken down the last category into those with some pain that is not adequately controlled with medication and those with severe pain and no relief whereas Young et al. (1997, 1998) and Brisman (2000) use only three categories.

Not all the reports can be used for evaluation of recurrence rates. As only those that could give yearly figures are used, authors were contacted in order to gain additional data but the information has not been forthcoming. Table 27 summarises the number of pa-

TABLE 26

Cohort studies reporting pain outcomes in 2506 patients with trigeminal neuralgia who underwent microvascular decompression MVD, grade of recommendation B (see table 9 in Chapter 9)

No. pts.	Mean (range) follow up years	Lost to follow up	Immediate failures	% Pain-free									Reference
				1 year			5 years			10 years			
				E	G	C	E	G	C	E	G	C	
104	5 (NA)	died 5, lost 8	2			83		85	71				Piatt and Wilkins, 1984[a]
41	8.5 (7.5–11.5)	died 2	2	90		95	74		88				Burchiel et al., 1988[a]
35[b]	6.2 (0.3–12)	NA		70	84	82			66			60	Pollack et al., 1988[a]
10[b]	6.2 (0.3–12)	NA			100				78				Pollack et al., 1988[a]
252	5 (0.5–16)	NA	13			88			84				Bederson and Wilson, 1989[a]
147	NA (0.3–6.3)	died 2	0			NA			NA			NA	Aksik, 1993
94	4.8 (NA)	died 18, lost 6	3	87			75			59			Cutbush and Atkinson, 1994[a]
61	6.1–10.5	died 6, lost NA	3			88			85				Sun et al., 1994[a]
94	6.5 (1.8–12)	died 2, lost 1	1									65	Walchenbach et al., 1994
133	5.3 (0.5–15)	died 14	NA	83	91	87	77		81	74	85	80	Mendoza and Illingworth, 1995[a]
1185	Median 6.2	121	24	75	9	84	74		78	64		70	Barker et al., 1996[a]
132[c]	NA	NA		62		57	48		52	42		47	Barker et al., 1996[a]
25	Median 3.3 (0.5–5.5)	none	2										Slettebo and Eide, 1997
146	3.2 (1–7)	7	11	78			73						Broggi et al., 1999[a]
225	10.9 (NA)	lost 26	0			82			70			85	Tronnier et al., 2001[a]
2231			**means:**	**82**		**85**	**75**		**74**	**67**		**70**	**Totals only[a]**

E, excellent results, no medication; G, good results but some minor recurrence, use of medication; C, combined good and excellent; NA, not available.

[a] Kaplan–Meier analysis.

[b] Pollack et al. (1988) did 45 operations on 35 patients and the results on 10 patients who had bilateral procedures are reported separately.

[c] Repeat operations.

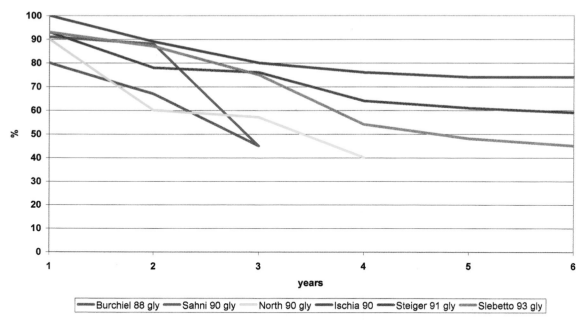

Fig. 4. Probability of being pain-free after percutaneous glycerol rhizotomy based on a review of the literature, from studies using actuarial methodology.

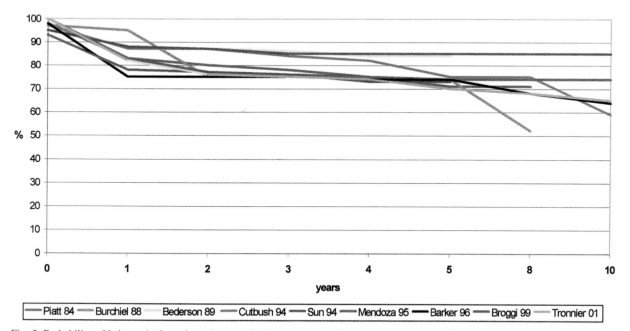

Fig. 5. Probability of being pain-free after microvascular decompression based on a review of the literature, from studies using actuarial methodology.

TABLE 27

Time to recurrence of pain after GKS

Reference	Total number of cases	Total number reported as failed or recurrence (number failed)	Mean/median time to recurrence
Young et al., 1998	110	13 (2 failed)	25.5 ± 3 months if previous surgery – mean 33.4 ± 3 months no prior surgery – mean
Pollock et al., 2001	68	32 (4 failed)	NA
Maesawa et al., 2001	220	30	15.4 months mean
Brisman, 2000	126	21 (? failed)	NA
Nicol et al., 2000	42	2 (0 failed)	NA
Rogers et al., 2000	54	11 (2 failed)	6.7 months median
Flickering et al., 2001	87	45 (15 failed)	12 months median
Urgosik et al., 1998	41	8	All within 15 months

tients who have failed to get a response or have had a recurrence. It is important to be aware that the period of time over which the results are reported is variable and so they cannot be compared but it does provide some clues as to the likely time for recurrence.

Table 28 is based on those series who analysed their data using actuarial methodology or where the data at one year could be used as the median follow up time. The actuarial data are also shown in Fig. 2 but are based on two studies only. Overall, the results are not as good as for other procedures but the only long-term data at 5 years contain patients who had lower dose radiations of 60 Gy and formed a very variable group.

Nicol et al. (2000) used 90 Gy and concluded that this was an effective dose to use and only caused minimal side effects, loss of sensation, whereas Maesawa et al. (2001) rarely used doses of 90 Gy but did not report their complications in relation to dosage. Pollock et al. (2001) in their comparison of dosages concluded that doses no more than 80 Gy should be used. Young et al. (1998) used doses of 70–80 Gy and suggested that previous surgery may affect recurrence rates although statistically this was not found. GKS has been reported in the use of tumour-related surgery where it appears to be effective but as would be expected, progression of tumour may lead to recurrence of pain (Regis et al., 1995; Chang et al., 2000a; Pollock et al., 2001).

7.7. Prognostic factors for recurrence rates

There are several studies that analyse their results in terms of factors that may affect long-term outcome but some of these are conflicting. This could be due to some of the factors mentioned above, i.e. lack of diagnostic criteria and including mixed cases, length of follow up, definition of recurrence, lost to follow up cases. Each of the different procedures will be discussed where data are available.

7.7.1. Prognosticators for RFT

There are two studies that have looked at prognostic factors using actuarial data (Latchaw et al., 1983; Yoon et al., 1999). Both studies found that classical trigeminal neuralgia cases did better and I also found that classical trigeminal neuralgia patients did better in terms of both pain-free intervals and complications (Zakrzewska et al., 1999). Most would suggest that sensory loss increases the chances of a longer pain-free period. Duration of disease, response to medication, age, presence of multiple sclerosis made no difference to outcome (Latchaw et al., 1983; Yoon et al., 1999). Yoon et al. (1999) showed that prior surgery other than RFT was a poor prognostic sign and multiple division pain was probably also a poor prognostic factor.

TABLE 28

Cohort studies reporting pain outcomes in 614 patients with trigeminal neuralgia who underwent gamma knife surgery, grade of recommendation C (see table 9 in Chapter 9)

No. patients	Mean (range) follow up	Lost to follow up	Failures	% Pain-free 1 year E	G	C	2 years E	G	C	5 years E	G	C	Reference
72 no prior surgery	1 (0.3–4)	NA	2			88			79				Young et al., 1998[a]
38 prior surgery													
88	2.2 median (0.1–3)	1	15		79	59			69			NA	Flickinger et al., 2001[a]
54	1 median (0.4–2.2)	0	2			median			64[b]				Rogers et al., 2000[a]
85 no previous surgery	2 (0.5–6.5)	NA	0	70 ± 5			70.4 ± 5			33.3 ± 14[c]			Maesawa et al., 2001[a]
220 includes all above	2 (0.5–6.5)	NA	0	63.6 ± 3		75.8 ± 3	59.2 ± 4		71.3 ± 3	37.7 ± 16[c]		55.8 ± 9[c]	Maesawa et al., 2001[a]
292						**82**			**75**			**58**	**Totals[a] only**

E, excellent results, no medication; G, using medication, over 50% relief; C, combined excellent and good; NA, not available.
[a] Kaplan–Meier analysis.
[b] Results at 2.5 years.
[c] Patients treated with low doses.

7.7.2. Prognosticators for PRG

Some of the principal factors affecting recurrences are summarised in Table 29. There is considerable discrepancy between the results and, again, it is related to small numbers and lack of clear criteria for recording of these. The type of glycerol used can affect results and has led to the use of the anhydrous form. Previous peripheral treatment made no difference to the outcomes but craniotomy and neurolysis may make a difference. Patients with multidivisional pain had better results than those with single division pain in contrast to the RFT patients. The amount of sensory loss was a significant predictor, the more sensory loss the more likely a low recurrence rate was found. In those patients with no sensory loss at 5 years no patient was still pain-free (Latchaw et al., 1983).

7.7.3. Prognosticators for balloon microcompression

Given the small numbers reported and the lack of Kaplan–Meier analysis there are no reliable data on prognostic factors. As in all procedures, it is important to ensure that only patients with trigeminal neuralgia are selected. This is especially true in this

TABLE 29

Factors which may affect recurrence rates after PRG

Factor	Good outcome	Poor outcome	No difference to outcome
Classical trigeminal neuralgia	North et al. (1990)		
Background pain			Slettebo et al. (1993)
Female	North et al. (1990)	Slettebo et al. (1993) (trend)	Steiger (1991)
Age younger	North et al. (1990)	Steiger (1991) (trend)	Slettebo et al. (1993), Bergenheim and Hariz (1995)
Division	Steiger (1991) trend for left	North et al. (1990)	Slettebo et al. (1993)
Side		North et al. (1990)	
Multiple sclerosis		Slettebo et al. (1993) trend but only if bilateral	Bergenheim and Hariz (1995)
Shorter duration of symptoms	North et al. (1990)		Slettebo et al. (1993), Bergenheim and Hariz (1995), Steiger (1991)
Good response to medical treatment	North et al. (1990)		
No preoperative sensory loss	Steiger (1991)		
Amount of glycerol			Bergenheim and Hariz (1995)
CSF flow at time of surgery	North et al. (1990)		
Suboptimal injection		Burchiel et al. (1988)	Slettebo et al. (1993)
Previous treatment different		Sahni et al. (1987), Slettebo et al. (1993) (may)	
Repeat surgery		Bergenheim and Hariz (1995)	
Sensory loss	Burchiel et al. (1988), Steiger (1991) trend: Slettebo et al. (1993), Bergenheim and Hariz (1995)	Sahni et al. (1987)	

Slettebo et al. (1993), Bergenheim and Hariz (1995), Steiger (1991) factors differ slightly depending whether assessing initial success or long term. The data in the tables relate to long-term results.

procedure as patients with atypical trigeminal neuralgia may already have some sensory changes prior to having the procedure and are then at increased risk from dysaesthesia.

7.7.4. Prognosticators for MVD

These are based only on reports that used actuarial methods and are included in Table 30. Szapiro et al. (1985) stress the importance of dividing the pa-

tients into two groups before doing any analysis, i.e. those who have only paroxysmal pain and those who have paroxysmal and background pain as this was a major predictor for outcome. When they did their further analysis on the separate groups they had very small numbers and so did not get statistical significance. They found more compression in those with pure pain and were unable to explain why patients with mixed pain did not show a correlation between

TABLE 30

Factors which may affect recurrence rates after MVD

Features	Good outcome	Poor outcome	No difference
Classical features	Szapiro et al., 1985		
Background pain		Szapiro et al., 1985	
Female		Bederson and Wilson, 1989; Barker et al., 1996	Steiger, 1991; Mendoza and Illingworth, 1995; Broggi et al., 2000
Age younger			Steiger, 1991; Sun et al., 1994
Division	Single division but only mixed pain, Szapiro et al., 1985		Bederson and Wilson, 1989; Steiger, 1991; Sun et al., 1994; Barker et al., 1996 (bilateral cases)
Side			Sun et al., 1994
Age at onset	Over 53 years, Bederson and Wilson, 1989	Less than 35 years, Mendoza and Illingworth, 1995	
Shorter duration of symptoms	Bederson and Wilson, 1989 best if 4 years and compression found. Barker et al., 1996 > 8 years. If >7 years Broggi et al., 2000		Piatt and Wilkins, 1984 if arterial contact, Steiger, 1991; Sun et al., 1994; Mendoza and Illingworth, 1995
Type of compression	Piatt and Wilkins, 1984 if distortion and wedging. Definite only Mendoza and Illingworth, 1995	For major recurrence no arterial compression, Burchiel et al., 1988. Venous and arterial	Arterial compression 1 or 2 vessels, degree of compression, Sun et al., 1994; Broggi et al., 2000
Venous compression		Burchiel et al., 1988; Piatt and Wilkins, 1984; Sun et al., 1994; Barker et al., 1996; and background pain Szapiro et al., 1985	
Immediate response to surgery	Barker et al., 1996		
Previous treatment different		Only minor recurrences, Burchiel et al., 1988. If mixed pain and sensory loss: Szapiro et al., 1985; Bederson and Wilson, 1989; Mendoza and Illingworth, 1995	If arterial contact, Piatt and Wilkins, 1984. Major recurrence only: Burchiel et al., 1988; Steiger, 1991; Sun et al., 1994; Barker et al., 1996; Broggi et al., 2000
Repeat surgery		Barker et al., 1996	
Sensory loss		If preoperative Szapiro et al., 1985; Steiger, 1991	Burchiel et al., 1988
Arterial hypertension			Broggi et al., 2000
Type of material used for decompression		If use resorbable material, Szapiro et al., 1985	

sensory loss and degree of compression. They were also at a loss to explain why, despite decompressing a definite compression, patients still reported background pain. They suggest that when doing analysis for prognosis the following factors should be analysed: type of pain, distribution of pain and any preoperative sensory changes. Some of these issues will only be resolved if data are collected prospectively, combined from many centres and collected independently of the surgeon. A very important factor is the timing of the operation. According to two studies, patients should be encouraged to have an operation within 8 years of developing trigeminal neuralgia but four other studies did not find early treatment to correlate with long-term success. Again this will not be resolved until clear criteria are laid down for what constitutes the first symptoms. This should be achievable given that over 85% of patients remember their first attack (Bowsher, 2000).

7.7.5. Prognosticators for GKS

The factors that have been looked for are summarised in Table 31.

Rogers et al. (2000) in their series of 54 patients reported that of the 22 patients who stop medication after therapy only one had a recurrence whereas in the 30 who continued with drug therapy 10 had a recurrence. This was a statistically significant result.

Side, type of division, duration of disease, previous good response to medication have not been looked at as prognostic factors. Young et al. (1998) report that one patient did not get relief of pain for 18 months which also coincided with sensory loss. From the above data it appears that there remains considerable debate as to whether sensory loss is important for improved outcome.

7.8. Complications and their management

The most serious complication reported after any surgery is the death of a patient, which given the fact that trigeminal neuralgia does not affect overall life expectancy, must be taken seriously and explained to all patients. The highest number of mortalities has been reported after MVD and some of them relate

directly to the surgery. These are discussed in greater detail in Section 7.8.3. Deaths have been reported after other procedures some of which may be related to the specific procedure being done, e.g. needle penetrating too far but others occur after any type of surgery, e.g. pulmonary embolus, myocardial infarct. Still others may be related to the patient's cardiac condition or the presence of a tumour. I would therefore argue that some patients are at higher risk of mortality even before the start of an operation.

Some reports have classified their complications as major or minor. There is a lack of uniformity about this form of reporting and the criteria for inclusion to the groups is not specified. It has therefore not been possible to do this for this report. You also need to remember that one patient may have several complications and some studies therefore give an overall figure for how many patients had complications whereas others do not specify this and it is not possible to extract the data from the given figures.

Overall complications and their lack of occurrence are shown in Fig. 6. More specific complications are shown in Fig. 7 and the relative risk of developing a complication after different types of surgery are shown in Fig. 8. Complications can be divided into those that:

- occur peri-operatively of which some result in long-term sequelae, e.g. CVA after an intracranial haemorrhage but most are transient and include CSF leaks, herpes, cardiac, respiratory and medical complications, wound infections and meningitis
- relate to cranial nerves 4, 6 and 7 most of which are transient, i.e. one to six months
- relate to the 8th cranial nerve which can be mild and transient or can result in permanent effects
- relate to the 5th cranial nerve, some may be permanent others may be transient such as motor paresis or temporary hearing problems due to paresis of the tympani muscles
- eye problems which are mainly related to loss of corneal reflex

Sensory loss is not shown as a complication on Fig. 7 as it is very high after all Gasserian ganglion

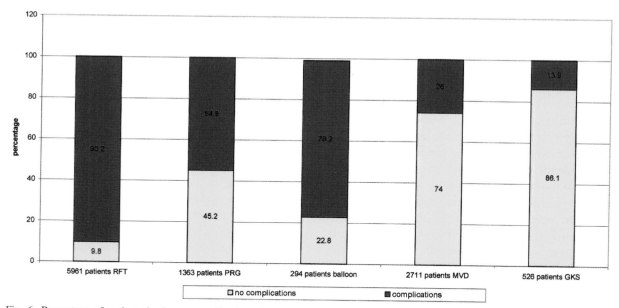

Fig. 6. Percentage of patients having a complication after surgery for trigeminal neuralgia based on review of the literature. RFT, radiofrequency thermorhizotomy; PRG, percutaneous glycerol rhizotomy; MVD, microvascular decompression; GKS, gamma knife surgery.

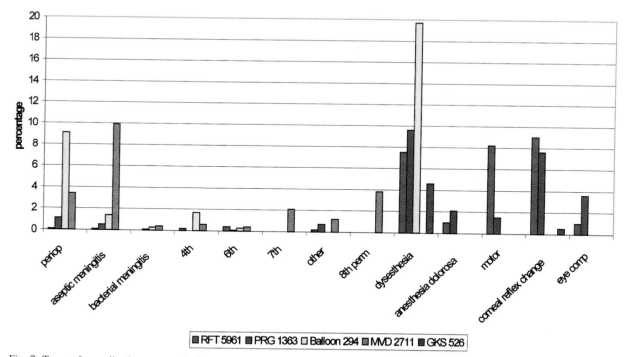

Fig. 7. Types of complications reported after surgery for trigeminal neuralgia based on a review of the literature. RFT, radiofrequency thermorhizotomy; PRG, percutaneous glycerol rhizotomy; MVD, microvascular decompression; GKS, gamma knife surgery; periop, peri-operative complications; 4th 6th 7th, cranial nerves; 8th perm, damage to 8th cranial nerve which does not recover; dysaesthesia, any unpleasant sensory changes over the face; motor, paresis of the motor component of the trigeminal nerve; corneal reflex change, either reduced or lost — eye complications such as keratitis.

TABLE 31

Factors which may affect recurrence rates after GKS

Features	Good outcome	Poor outcome	No difference
Classical trigeminal neuralgia	Young et al., 1998; Rogers et al., 2000		
Background pain		Maesawa et al., 2001	
Female			Kondziolka et al., 1997; Young et al., 1998; Rogers et al., 2000
Age younger	Flickinger et al., 2001		Kondziolka et al., 1997; Young et al., 1998; Rogers et al., 2000
Division	First and single Brisman, 2000, any single Rogers et al., 2000		
Multiple sclerosis			Rogers et al., 2000
Preoperative sensory loss		Maesawa et al., 2001	
Position of isocentre	Brisman, 2000 improved when use REZ		
Better initial response	Rogers et al., 2000		
Previous treatment different		Maesawa et al., 2001; Young et al., 1998; Flickinger et al., 2001	Kondziolka et al., 1997
Sensory loss post op	Rogers et al., 2000; Pollock et al., 2001	Pollock et al., 2001	Kondziolka et al., 1997
Poor visualisation of nerve			Kondziolka et al., 1997; Flickinger et al., 2001
Dose over 70 Gy	Kondziolka et al., 1996; Pollock et al., 2001		
Number of isocentres			No difference for pain relief but increases complication, Flickinger et al., 2001

procedures and is considered essential after procedures such as RFT. Overall sensory loss is reported as occurring in the following percentage of cases: 62% after RFT, 38% after balloon microcompression, 28.6% after PRG, 2.8% after MVD and 8.7% after GKS. More details can be found under each of the procedures. These are probably under-reported; Saini (1987) in his series of 552 PRG procedures reports no sensory loss. It could be that they assume that this is an expected result after this procedure and so do not report it, as verified by Professor Kanapolat when I asked him to comment on this in his series of 1600 RFT procedures (Kanpolat and Savas, 2001). Very few studies define what they mean by dysaes-

thesia and some classify it as mild and severe but this can again affect the numbers reported. The rates of development of dysaesthesia, anaesthesia dolorosa have been shown to be highest in those procedures that result in nerve destruction. Some of these resolve over time whereas others necessitate treatment with antidepressant drugs. Except in the rare case of the loss of an eye or the need for a tarsorrhaphy most eye complications are in the form of a single episode of keratitis.

Fig. 8 attempts to show the relative contribution to complications made by each of the different procedures and it highlights the difference in the type of sensory complications after different destructive pro-

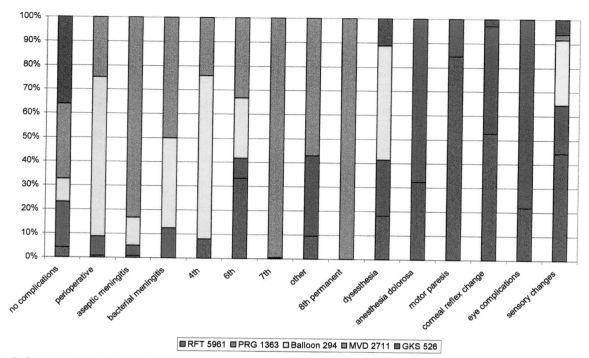

Fig. 8. Percentage contribution of each technique to the complications. RFT, radiofrequency thermorhizotomy; PRG, percutaneous glycerol rhizotomy; MVD, microvascular decompression; GKS, gamma knife surgery. The first column shows the proportion of patients having different types of surgeries who have no complications. Periop, peri-operative complications; 4th 6th 7th, cranial nerves; 8th perm, damage to 8th cranial nerve which does not recover; dysaesthesia, any unpleasant sensory changes over the face; motor, paresis of the motor component of the trigeminal nerve; corneal reflex change, either reduced or lost — eye complications such as keratitis.

cedures and the relative risk of developing a hearing problem after MVD which remains virtually unique to this procedure. The few recorded after Gasserian ganglion surgery relate not to 8th nerve damage but to 5th nerve damage of the tensor tympani and or tensor veli palatini muscles. If sensory loss is included as a complication then only 10% of patients undergoing RFT have no complication whereas 74% of patients undergoing a MVD are likely to have no complications, 45% of patients undergoing PRG and 23% of those having balloon compression, as shown in Fig. 6. Fig. 9 illustrates a patient's view point.

The management of complications after surgery has been the topic of one of my chapters in my book on trigeminal neuralgia and I will cover some of the managements of the complications in the next sections (Zakrzewska, 1995, see further reading).

7.8.1. Complications after peripheral surgery

The complications from these procedures are summarised in Table 22 which reported on pain-free intervals. The only procedure that reported no complications was laser therapy.

- Peripheral surgery causes relatively few complications outside the trigeminal nerve but eye complications can occur due to inadvertent injections. Alcohol injections have been reported by Grant (1936) to cause diplopia, 7% and facial palsy, 0.5%. Fardy et al. (1994) also reported 3 major complications after alcohol injection. In one patient skin necrosis round the ala of the nose required skin grafting, a sequestrum from the mandible had to be removed and diplopia occurred after injection of the superior alveolar nerve.

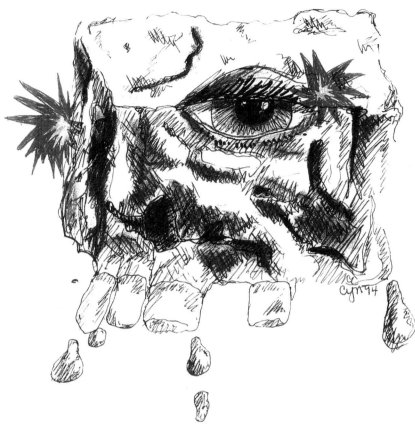

Fig. 9. Picture drawn by a patient who had a recurrence of trigeminal neuralgia after a radiofrequency thermorhizotomy which had left her with anaesthesia dolorosa.

- Most procedures result in some local oedema and haematoma formation. The injections are all painful to give even if initially local anaesthetic is used. All procedures requiring direct access to the nerve such as cryotherapy and neurectomy can result in local infections as after any minor surgical procedure.
- An area of sensory loss and in some cases, dysaesthesia is also reported after these procedures although the area is less extensive than after Gasserian ganglion surgery and so less effect on overall satisfaction is reported. It is more often reported after injections with alcohol and neurectomies than after cryotherapy.
- Many reports also state that up to 50% of patients may need to continue to take anticonvulsants al-

though often in smaller doses that cause fewer side effects.
- Difficulty in mouth opening due possibly to masseteric spasms is reported after acupuncture in up to 6% of patients and in a small number having peripheral radiofrequency thermorhizotomy.

7.8.2. Complications after Gasserian ganglion surgery

Very few peri-operative complications have been reported and yet Sweet (1990) notes that there are significant hypotensive and bradycardic episodes during placement of the needle. ECG monitoring is common and the placement of temporary pacemakers during balloon compression is considered important as it cuts down on complications (Brown and

Gouda, 1999). The presence of abnormal anatomic features can also lead to puncture of the wrong foramen as well as penetration of the inferior orbital fissure (Sweet, 1990).

Eye complications are difficult to compare between the different Gasserian ganglion procedures as selection of patients may have occurred. Patients with first division pain are often not offered RFT and a higher proportion of these patients may have balloon compression.

Complications after RFT

The complication rates after RFT are shown in Table 32. Overall, from the studies selected 90% of patients will have complications, this drops to 28% if you exclude sensory loss. You need to bear in mind that some patients may have several complications and by inference there may be more patients who have no complications. Fewer complications tend to be reported from the larger centres (Sweet and Poletti's, 1995). Sweet (1990) describes a wide range of serious complications ranging from death to intracranial haemorrhages leading to hemiparesis and aphasia; infections, eye loss can occur but is not reported. This is often due to intracranial or subarachnoid arterial haemorrhages and intracerebral haematomas often on the opposite side. Sweet's (1990) review of the literature suggests that complications were no different from units reporting under or over 450 procedures and so suggesting that technical skill for this procedure was not essential. He provides extensive details of all the complications. Overall, RFT has the second highest rate of complications but this needs to be weighed up carefully as many of those after RFT are relatively minor. However, Latchaw et al. (1983) reported complications in 75% of their patients.

- Several mortalities have been reported. Sweet and Poletti (1995) reported 13 deaths most due to intracranial haemorrhage from their informal survey some of which had not been reported. One mortality from an intracranial haemorrhage occurred in a patient who had previously had an astrocytoma removed and radiotherapy (Mittal and Thomas, 1986). Nugent and Berry (1974) report a death

in a patient from bilateral pneumonia after an unsuccessful RFT and another patient who had a myocardial infarct when leaving hospital (Nugent, 1997). Brandt and Wittkamp (1983) report a death after a cerebral abscess but it is not possible to ascertain whether it occurred after RFT using the Sweet method or the older technique of uncontrolled thermocoagulation. Gocer et al. (1997) report a death in a 44 year old woman 17 days after the procedure from a subdural empyema (*Staph. aureus* infection). They thought it was secondary to bacterial meningitis due to penetration of the oral mucosa with the needle.

- Of the Gasserian ganglion surgeries meningitis is least likely to occur after this procedure.

- Few peri-operative complications are reported and there is a very low incidence of complications outside the trigeminal nerve. Most of them result in transient diplopia. Carotid-cavernous fistulae have been reported (see Table 32).

- It can probably be said that in order to obtain lasting pain relief after RFT some sensory loss must be obtained. This is probably the reason why sensory loss is not mentioned in some of the reports on complications shown in Table 32 as it is considered normal. Tew and Taha (1995) suggest that this can be reduced using the curved electrode. Sensory loss may be restricted to the area in which the pain was present or may be both in the area and outside the pain area which Kanpolat and Savas (2001) refer to as non-selective pain control. They reported that 68% of their patients had selective pain control whereas in the rest sensory loss was outwith the pain area. Latchaw et al. (1983) also report similar results. For best results dense hypalgesia but not analgesia in the affected division/s is needed as the rate of dysaesthesia is related to depth of analgesia. Dysaesthesia affects the satisfaction rates (Taha et al., 1995) and I would postulate that the area involved could also contribute to this. It is difficult to compare the rates of dysaesthesia between different reports as few give their criteria. Taha et al. (1995) clearly define dysaesthesia and divide it into a mildly disturbing sensation or a major dis-

TABLE 32

Cohort studies reporting complications in 5961 patients with trigeminal neuralgia who underwent percutaneous radiofrequency thermorhizotomy (thermolysis) (RFT)

No. pts.	Complications peri-operative	Meningitis	Complications outside area of V	Sensory loss (%)	Dysaesthesia (%)	Anaesthesia dolorosa (%)	Motor paresis (%)	Change corneal reflex (%)	Eye problems (%)	Other complications	Reference
78	NA	NA	1 reduced hearing	Mild all	11 (14)	3 (4)	NA	NA	Decreased vision 2 (3)	Frostbite in analgesic area 1	Burchiel et al., 1981
96	0	NA	0	Substantial 29 (29), moderate 53 (53)	Mild 12 (12). Severe 13 (13).	1 (1)	5 (5)	39 (39)	3 (3)	72 patients had a complication	Latchaw et al., 1983
400	NA	NA	0 Diplopia transient 5	All	0	1 (0.3)	0	14 (4)	0	Vasomotor rhinitis 1	Schvarcz, 1982
1000	NA			NA	52 (52)	15 (15)	105 (10.5)	197 (19.7)	6 (6) lost sight 1		Broggi et al., 1999
124	1	1	6th: 1	20 (16)	3 (2.4)	4 (3.2)	4 (3.2)	7 (6)	2 (1.6)	Hearing 4	Ischia et al., 1990a
265	Epilepsy # arm	NA	6th, 2. 8th, 1. 5th, 6th and 7th, 1.	135 (51)	15 (6)	14 (8)	2 (0.8)	Loss reduced 16 (19)	10 (6)	Facial pain 65 (37). Decreased anxiety and depression.	Zakrzewska and Thomas, 1993; Mittal and Thomas, 1986 [a]
154	0	0	0	Total 66 (46) 47. Dense 61 (42) 43. Mild 17 (12) 10.	31 (24)	0	22 (15%); at one year 3 (2)	Loss 8 (5.1). Reduced 21 (13.6).	3 (1.9)	TMJ surgery for joint dysfunction 1	Taha and Tew, 1996 [b]
185	NA	NA	NA	Dense 43 (23). Mild 78 (42).	7 (4)	NA	NA	Tearing, reduced sensation, pain 20 (11)		65% reported some complications	Oturai et al., 1996
500	0	0	0	490 (98)	Mild 45 (9). Severe 10 (2).	1 (0.2)	35 (7)	Loss 15 (3)	0		Taha and Tew, 1996; curved electrode
700	Herpes 36 (3)	Aseptic 2 (0.2)	3rd, 1 (0.1). 4th, 6 (0.5). 6th, 7 (0.6).	All	Minor 154 (22). Major 35 (5).	11 (1.6)	168 (24)	56 (8)	14 (2)	Carotid-cavernous fistula 1 (0.1)	Taha and Tew, 1999; straight electrode
81 48	0 0	0 0	2 (8) TN. 1 (6) ATN.	24 (96) TN. 14 (94) ATN.	20 (25) 2 (8) TN. (25) ATN.	0 0	4 (5) 2 (8) TN. 4 (25) ATN.	12 (15) NA	2 (2.5) 2 (8) TN. 4 (25) ATN.	Hearing 1 1 (4) TN. 2 (16) ATN do not want repeat surgery.	Yoon et al., 1999 Zakrzewska et al., 1999 [c]
258	0	Aseptic 2 (0.8)	0	0	21 (8)	5 (2)	74 (28.8) transient	Loss 8 (3)	Keratitis 2 (0.8)		Mathews and Scrivani, 2000
1600	CSF leak 2, carotid cavernous fistula 1	Aseptic 1 (0.06)	4th, 11. 3rd overall (0.75) permanent in 2 (0.1).	All mild	16 (1)	12 (0.8)	48 (3) paresis. 18 (1) paralysis.	Loss 91 (5.7)	Keratitis 10 (0.8)		Kanpolat and Savas, 2001
206	NA	NA	NA	2 (0.9)	NA	NA	NA	NA	NA		Tronnier et al., 2001
5961	4 (0.1)	6 (0.1)	41 (0.7)	3732 (62)	450 (7.5)	67 (1.1)	494 (8.2)	539 (9)	60 (1.0)	Total complications 90.2%	

[a] Mittal and Thomas report one mortality; see text for details.

[b] Taha and Tew (1996) report their complications at 15 years in 100 patients; TMJ, temporo-mandibular joint; 3rd to 8th, cranial nerve palsies; most are reported as transient.

[c] Zakrzewska et al. (1999) report their complications at 3 years in 41 patients based on a questionnaire; yearly data are available; two groups: TN, classical trigeminal neuralgia; ATN, atypical trigeminal neuralgia.

turbing sensation, enough to need medication and they suggest that older patients are more liable to get this complication (Tew and Taha, 1995). They define anaesthesia dolorosa as a constant burning. Although the incidence of anaesthesia dolorosa is highest after RFT (up to 15% in some) the incidence of dysaesthesia is the lowest of the three Gasserian ganglion surgeries. These complications are very much under the control of the operator and the operator has more control over the amount of sensory loss induced by these procedures than after the other Gasserian procedures. Their incidence will, therefore, vary and will link with recurrence rates as Latchaw et al. (1983) showed when at 5 years, those with no sensory loss had all had a recurrence whereas those with deep analgesia had 74% chance of being pain-free. Some patients will need treatment and antidepressants appear to be the drugs of choice. Coping strategies are going to play an important role in helping patients come to terms with these complications.

- Reduction or loss of corneal reflex is around 8% and is as high as found in PRG. The comparison may not be valid as patient selection could bias the results. Patients with first division pain are often not offered RFT and PRG is suggested due to initial reports that suggested that corneal reflex loss did not occur with PRG. Eye problems such as keratitis are rare but one patient is reported as losing his sight due to severe neuroparalytic keratitis (Broggi et al., 1999). Sweet and Poletti (1995) report 4 cases of blindness due to cranial nerve damage. Egan et al. (2001) report three cases of monocular blindness and their search of the literature revealed 7 more cases. One of the patients reported by Egan et al. (2001) committed suicide postoperatively and a postmortem was done which showed optic nerve damage due to stylet misdirection.

- Transient masseteric problems, around 7% are reported similar to those after microcompression but are probably under-reported. These can lead to difficulty in eating and wearing dentures as we showed in our studies (Zakrzewska and Thomas,

1993; Zakrzewska et al., 1999). Patients may be embarrassed about eating in public and so quality of life can be compromised. It is important to explain to patients that they need to be careful when eating and that they do not need new dentures.

- We have reported that up to 37% of patients may report facial pain other than trigeminal neuralgia and this is higher in patients with atypical trigeminal neuralgia (Zakrzewska et al., 1999). It can be postulated that some of the facial pain post-surgery reported by Oturai et al. (1996) is also not trigeminal neuralgia as the drugs the patients used to control it included analgesics and antidepressants with only 47% taking anticonvulsants. It may also be postulated that the procedure may uncover other pain. Strategies for general management of facial pain as described in Chapter 9 may be needed for these patients rather than to offer further surgery. I, therefore, consider it crucial to take a careful pain history when patients return with pain after surgery.

- There is a significant reduction in the number of patients who report depressive symptoms as picked up on a Hospital Anxiety and Depression Scale (see Chapter 6) after surgery and anxiety is also significantly reduced (Zakrzewska et al., 1999).

Complications after PRG

Complications after this procedure are shown in Table 33; only the best quality studies are utilised and in these 55% of patients have complications. Other studies do not report any other major complications.

- Two mortalities have been reported. Hakanson (1981) reported a patient who had a pulmonary embolus one week after procedure but this may not be due to the technique itself but a general complication to be expected after any type of surgery. Jho and Lunsford (1997) report a fatal myocardial infarct 30 minutes after the procedure.

- Peri-operatively, venous bleeding or cheek haematomas are reported by many.

- Both aseptic and bacterial meningitis has been

TABLE 33

Cohort studies reporting complications in 1363 patients with trigeminal neuralgia who underwent percutaneous retro-Gasserian glycerol rhizotomy (PRG)

No. of pts.	Complications peri-operative (%)	Meningitis	Complications outside area of V (%)	Sensory loss (%)	Dysaesthesia (%)	Anaesthesia dolorosa (%)	Motor paresis (%)	Change in corneal reflex (%)	Eye problems	Reference
552	Herpes 15 (2.7)	NA	0	NA	61 (11)	26 (4.7) had previous surgery	16 (2.8) recovered 3–4 months	23 (4)	23 (4)	Saini, 1987
162	Haematoma 1, ocular pain 1, herpes 61 (37.6)	Bacterial 1	0	Mild 117 (71) in 49 only in affected division. Dense 20 (12.3)	Mild 15 (9.2). Severe 5 (3.1).	0	NA	Loss 3 (1.8). Reduced 5 (3.1).	0	Young et al., 1998
60	Herpes 3 (5). Headache 7 (12).	Bacterial 1	Vertigo 1 (2). Tinnitus 3 (5). Rhinorrhoea 5 (8).	Mild 43 (72)	6 (10)	NA	NA	Loss 4 (7). Reduced 9 (15).	1	Burchiel et al., 1988
112	0	0	0	Mild 27 (26)	20 (20)	0	0	Loss 1 (1). Reduced 1 (1).	0	Ischia et al., 1990a
85	Bleeding and oedema at injection site 4 (4.7)	NA	Transient diplopia 1 (1)	Hypaesthesia 3 (4)	Mild 3 (4). Transient.	0	NA	Loss 2 (3). Reduced 3 (4).	0	North et al., 1990
58	NA	NA	NA	Hypaesthesia 22 (37). Dense 6 (10).	NA	NA	NA	0	0	Sahni et al., 1990
122 / 60	0 Venous bleeding	0 Aseptic 1	6th, 1 transient / 0	62 (51) / 17 patients with no pre-op. loss 6. 21 no previous surgery, 11 new sensory loss.	9 (7) / 8 (13)	0 / 2 (3)	5 (4) / NA	Reduced 19 (16) No previous surgery. Reduced 5/21, previous surgery 17/37 but 9 present pre-op.	0 Keratitis 1 (2). Conjunctivitis 25 (41).	Steiger, 1991 Slettebo et al., 1993[a]
99	NA	NA	NA	Light touch loss 54%, reducing to 42% at 3/12. Pin-prick 55%, reducing to 44% at 3/12.	6 (6), all one prior treatment	1 (1), prior RFT	NA	Loss in 5 reduced to 4 all but one treatment before. Reduced reflex 26 reducing to 24.	0	Bergenheim and Hariz, 1995[b]
53[c]	Herpes 10 (18.5)	0	0	Total analgesia 1 (2). Dense 5 (10). Mild 12 (12).	NA	NA	NA	NA	NA	Kondziolka et al., 1994b
1363	**117 (8.5)**	**3 (0.2)**	**11 (0.8)**	**385 (28.2)**	**133 (9.8)**	**29 (2.1)**	**21 (1.5)**	**104 (7.6)**	**50 (3.6)**	**Total complications 54.8%**

[a] Results based on follow-up questionnaire median 7 years postoperatively.
[b] Sensory testing done clinically and with instruments, two mortalities have been reported — see text for details.
[c] Patients all had multiple sclerosis; 6th cranial nerve palsy, RFT radiofrequency thermorhizotomy.

reported. They necessitate a lumbar puncture in order to culture the CSF and some will require treatment with antibiotics and the aseptic ones with steroids. The aseptic form may be due to the contrast medium or overfilling of the cistern whereas the bacterial one may be due to penetration of the oral mucosa during needle insertion (Linderoth and Hakanson, 1995).

- Cranial nerve complications other than the 5th are very rare. North et al. (1990) and Steiger (1991) both report one case each of transient 6th cranial nerve palsy and transient vertigo and tinnitus have been reported (Burchiel et al., 1988).

- Herpes labialis has been reported in up to a third of patients but this figure is probably inaccurate as some may consider the complication too minor to report and it often happens after the patient has been discharged. It is speculated that it may increase the tendency to development of dysaesthesia (Linderoth and Hakanson, 1995).

- Sensory loss, anaesthesia dolorosa and change in corneal reflex are the major reported complications after PRG. Bergenheim et al. (1991) looked at sensory loss one month and three months after surgery and correlated it with recurrence rates at one year in 54 patients. There was a tendency for higher recurrence rates in patients with mild or no sensory loss. They showed an increased risk of developing dysaesthesia if patients had had previous surgery but it was not related to whether they had sensory loss prior to the procedure. Sensory loss did not correlate with quantity of glycerol used, preoperative dose of carbamazepine, age or duration of disease, presence of multiple sclerosis. Sweet and Poletti (1985) injected glycerol incrementally until some sensory loss was obtained in 77 patients. Dysaesthesia was reported in 28 (37%) patients in whom it was mild in 16 (21%) but 9 (12%) needed medication and in 3 it was a major source of distress. It needs to be noted that 27 had had previous RFT and details are provided of how many had changes preoperatively. The highest number of cases of anaesthesia dolorosa has been reported by Saini (1987) who does not use cisternography prior to injection. The other

cases have all occurred in patients who had prior surgery.

- Post-treatment patients are noted to sometimes complain of periodic itchiness of the eye as well as change in flow of tears. This, as well as reduced corneal reflex, may contribute to the development of conjunctivitis reported in up to 40% (25/60) of patients (Slettebo et al., 1993).

- Sweet and Poletti (1985) reported that of 77 patients 14 had decreased corneal sensation, 7 lost their corneal reflex but it returned in 4 and 1 patient did not show corneal loss until some days after surgery. Bergenheim et al. (1991) also reported 2 patients with deterioration of corneal reflex after 3 months. There does not appear to be any increased risk of corneal anaesthesia after recurrent surgery (Bergenheim and Hariz, 1995). The type of glycerol used may affect sensory disturbance as it depends on the amount of arachnoiditis that it induces, as it is this that reduces the size of the cistern.

- Motor paresis of the masticatory muscles is rarely reported.

Complications after microcompression

The complications reported in the higher quality studies are shown in Table 34. Similar complications are noted in the poor quality studies but these could represent under-reporting. The largest series of 496 patients from Australia provides too little detail to be included in this review (Skirving and Dan, 2001).

- Two mortalities have been reported (Spaziante et al., 1988; Abdennebi et al., 1997). The case reported by Spaziante et al. (1988) resulted in a subarachnoid haemorrhage, in a patient who had an enlarged trigeminal cistern which was punctured by the needle. The progressive hydrocephalus which occurred required several shunts and the patient died of a shunt infection. The other was due to the metal introducer part of the cannula penetrating the skull and resulting in a haematoma and the patient died 10 days postoperatively (Abdennebi et al., 1997).

- Peri-operative complications most frequently encountered are due to bleeding with haematoma

TABLE 34

Cohort studies reporting complications in 294 patients with trigeminal neuralgia who underwent balloon compression of the Gasserian ganglion

No. of patients	Complications peri-operatively (%)	Meningitis	Complications outside area of V (%)	Sensory loss (%)	Dysaesthesia (%)	Motor paresis (%)	Change in corneal reflex (%)	Reference
100	NA	NA	4th, 1 (1) transient	Most but 17 (17) persisted	Mild 12 (12). Severe 4 (4).	Common for 3 months	NA	Lichtor and Mullan, 1990
144	Venous bleeding 16 (11). Arterial bleeding 4 (3). Rise in BP 5 (4). Cheek haematoma 4 (3). Headaches, herpes 16 (11). 0	Bacterial 1, aseptic 1	4th, 4 (3) transient	All initially after 1 year 58 (40). Preoperative 86 (60) normal sensation.	Mild 28 (19). Severe 4 (3).	All initially 1 year 17 (12)	Transient in all	Lobato et al., 1990
50	0	Aseptic 3	6th, 1 transient nerve palsy	Mild 37 (74). Dense 1 (2).	10 (20)	Many resolved 1 year	0	Brown et al., 1993
294	**27 (9.2)**	**5 (1.7)**	**6 (2.0)**	**113 (38.4)**	**58 (19.7)**	**18 (6.1)**	**0**	**Total complications 76.2%**

No eye problems, anaesthesia dolorosa reported. 4th cranial nerve palsy, 5th cranial nerve palsy. NA, data not available. Two mortalities have been reported — see text for details.

formation on the cheek. Balloons may burst but do not always result in complications (Sweet, 1990).

- Aseptic meningitis thought to be due to small haematoma results in headache, fever, nuchal rigidity, altered mental state within 6 hours and usually resolves in 48 hours. It does, however, necessitate a lumbar puncture.

- Temporary 6th nerve palsy has been reported (Brown et al., 1993). Sweet (1990) reports a personal communication about blindness in the ipsilateral eye due to optic atrophy.

- Herpes labialis is common in patients who have had previous herpes and some consider it a good sign as it indicates that nerve damage has occurred.

- The procedure aims to cause numbness without dysaesthesia but as Table 34 indicates, dysaesthesia does occur and can be severe but as yet no cases of anaesthesia dolorosa have been reported.

- A very small number of cases have been reported with transient reduction of corneal reflex but there are no reports of keratitis or other eye problems and this is lower than after other Gasserian ganglion procedures.

- Motor weakness especially of the pterygoid is invariable for up to 3 months and is reported in most studies and is more frequent than after other Gasserian ganglion procedures. Patients need to be warned that eating may be difficult and that dribbling may be a problem. Patients may do better if they eat a soft diet that requires less chewing and hence risk of biting the inside of their cheeks.

- Patients may complain of otalgia or buzzing noises due to weakness of tensor tympani muscles (Brown and Gouda, 1999).

7.8.3. Complications after MVD

With over 8000 procedures being reported in the literature it is now possible to gain a much better picture of the types and rates of complications. Complications as reported in the best quality studies are shown in Table 35 and in Figs. 6–8 and overall 26% of patients are reported as having complications. A review of the poorer quality studies shows similar types of complications but fewer of them 12.5% (370/2958). I suspect that some series collect their data more meticulously and so report in greater detail all their complications, including such relatively minor ones as herpes infections. Others only report the more major ones. Yet if we are to obtain fully informed consent from our patients we need to be able to give them substantial information on complications and how these change over time. Some reports stress that complications are transient but few give any indication of the length of this transient period. The only reports that give details of change of complications over time are those reporting specifically on hearing changes and sensory features. Not a single study reports all their complications at different time periods. Some reports classify complications as major or minor but none specify what criteria they use to place these into these categories. I consider that it is only the patient who can decide whether a complication is major or minor as they need to judge their quality of life after the procedure. Reports of complications can also be found in studies involving posterior fossa surgery for hemifacial spasm. This appears to be a more frequent problem in Japan than anywhere else and large series are reported from that country (Hamlyn, 1999). Hanakita and Kondo (1988) report serious complications including 2 deaths in their series of 278 posterior fossa surgery procedures but all occurred in patients with hemifacial spasm. The surgical approach is slightly different and hence may account for the higher complication rate.

Attention to detail during the operation including the use of auditory evoked potentials as well as surgical experience does affect the number of complications. Modifications have been introduced which appear to have further reduced complications. Broggi et al. (2000) quote their complication rate for the first 50 cases using a wider surgical technique and then a mini approach for 146 cases and show a marked difference in complication rates, especially hearing, CSF rhinorrhoea, transient numbness and diplopia as seen in Table 35. This is also noted overall in the studies with earlier reports having higher numbers of complications.

TABLE 35

Cohort studies reporting complications in 2711 patients with trigeminal neuralgia who underwent microvascular decompression MVD

No. pts.	Mortality	Aseptic meningitis	Bacterial meningitis	CSF	I	H	PE	Ataxia	Herpes	4th	5th	6th	7th	8th trans	8th perm	Other complications	Reference
147	2	27	2	2									17	18	3	Occipital neuralgia 16	Aksik, 1993
1336	2	225	5	20	2	4			16	13	22	2	12	18	16	Pseudomeningocele 1. Oedema/hydrocephalus 6.	Barker et al., 1996[a]
246	0	11	1	6			2[b]		5		5		8	1	7	Steroid confusion 8. Headaches 8. Oedema/hydrocephalus 3.	Bederson and Wilson, 1989
146	0			3	1	1					6		1		3	Hearing loss only audiometry 8	Broggi et al., 1999
50	0			9							10		2		5		Broggi et al., 1999[c]
41	1					1					5						Burchiel et al., 1988
94	1						1	3			4		3		7	Lateral medullary syndrome 1	Cutbush and Atkinson, 1994
133	1	1		2	2		1			3	1		4	2		Otitis media 1, wound infection 1	Mendoza and Illingworth, 1995
104	1	3		2		2	1	4			11		2		15	Pseudomeningocele 1, GI bleed 1, wound laceration 1, drug reaction 1	Piatt and Wilkins, 1984
45	0			1			1	1			5		1		3		Pollack et al., 1988
25	0										2					Dizziness and anosmia 1	Slettebo and Eide, 1997
61	0			3					6	1	4	1	2	3	1	Vertigo and tinnitus 8	Sun et al., 1994
225	3							1	7				3	18			Tronnier et al., 2001
58	0	1	1	3	1		1						2			GI bleed 1, MI 1. Oedema/hydrocephalus 2.	Walchenbach et al., 1994
2711	11 / **0.41**	268 / **9.9**	9 / **0.4**	51 / **1.9**	6 / **0.2**	8 / **0.3**	6 / **0.2**	9 / **0.34**	34 / **1.3**	17 / **0.6**	75 / **2.8**	9 / **0.4**	57 / **2.1**	42 / **1.5**	60 / **2.2**	Total number / % **Total complications 26**	

CFS, CFS leaks; I, cerebellar infarcts; H, haematomas; PE, pulmonary embolus; MI, myocardial infarct; GI, gastrointestinal; 4th, 5th, 6th, 7th, 8th cranial nerve palsies/dysfunctions; trans, transient; perm, permanent.

[a] Barker includes re-operations,
[b] Deep vein thrombosis.
[c] Broggi 50 first operations.

Mortality. Early reports quoted a 1 to 0.9% mortality rate for this operation. This has now dropped and in the total literature of over 5000 reported cases which quote their mortality data there have been 26 deaths giving a percentage of 0.46. If we look just at the top studies then the mortality rate is 0.41% and in the poorer reports it is 0.5%.

Most common causes of death are either cerebellar infarcts or haemorrhage, more likely to occur in patients with tumours as shown in Table 36. One death was related to a large air embolism which occurred in a patient that was being operated on in the sitting position which has now been discarded (Klun, 1992). The cardiac causes occur one to two weeks later. Nineteen causes of death were intracranial, the others were due to events at distant sites (Table 36).

Peri-operative complications. The most common complication is that of an aseptic meningitis and can occur in up to 11% of patients. Cerebellar infarct and haematomas which are not lethal but could leave patients with a significant disability such as ataxia, hemiparesis are also reported. Some of these patients needed to be re-explored. Other complications are those associated with any neurosurgical operation and are not specific to posterior fossa surgery. Focal seizures have been reported by Apfelbaum (1984) in 4 patients and he also reports that 13 patients had some form of medical complication. Headaches, postoperative nausea and vomiting, wound infections, postoperative confusion, myocardial infarcts, pulmonary emboli, pulmonary oedema and gastrointestinal bleeds are reported and I suspect some of these are underreported because they are considered nonspecific.

Herpes is reported by some but not others. Klun (1992) reports that half his patients having MVDs and all his patients undergoing PSR had postoperative herpes and he relates this to the degree of manipulation of the nerve. The numbers of patients developing herpes postoperatively has led to a randomised controlled trial to assess the value of giving patients a preoperative injection of interferon. This was done in a group of 55 patients and surprisingly interferon, rather than inhibiting herpes infections, appeared to enhance them (Ho et al., 1984).

Complications involving cranial nerves except the 8th. Many of the complications involving the 5th, 6th and 7th cranial nerves are transient and the percentages of reported complications are low. Complications within the trigeminal nerve are low compared to the Gasserian ganglion procedures and are either mild sensory loss or, at the most, dysaesthesia but with no reports of anaesthesia dolorosa. Many of these sensory changes may have been present preoperatively as few reports give preoperative details of sensory loss and some are as a result of doing a partial rhizotomy. Other sensory changes may be too mild to pick up on gross testing. Miles et al. (1997) and Bergenheim et al. (1997) performed in-depth sensory testing on 19 and 37 patients pre- and post-surgery. They found that up to 30% of patients may have some deficits postoperatively but this is reduced with time. Bergenheim et al. (1997) found that at mean follow up of 3.5 years only 5 patients had some sensory changes. They also reported that of the three patients who had a recurrence of pain, two had elevated sensory thresholds but no sensory disturbance on clinical testing. More complications especially in relation to the trigeminal nerve are found in patients who have had a PSR although they tend to have fewer hearing problems (Bederson and Wilson, 1989). Linskey et al. (1994) suggest that patients with vertebrobasilar artery compression are more likely to have sensory complications than patients with other compressions due to the need for manipulation.

Hearing complications. The most serious and frequent complication after MVD is a hearing loss. Hearing loss is reported as transient, permanent and either complete or partial. Some also distinguish between hearing loss that is picked up on audiometry and not reported by the patient. It is also difficult to be sure how many were really post-surgery as these were not measured preoperatively. Very few centres report that they do audiometry preoperatively so the accuracy of the postoperative findings must be questioned. Some studies also report on positional vertigo and ataxia which may be related to the 8th nerve damage as well as transient middle ear effusions or otitis media which is picked up on

TABLE 36

Causes of 27 reported deaths after MVD

Cause	CVA	Cerebellar infarct	Cerebellar haemorrhage	Distant causes
Number	2	12	5	2 pulmonary emboli, 1 pneumonia, 3 myocardial infarcts, 1 gastrointestinal bleed

immediate postoperative audiometric tests (Moller and Moller, 1989). Hearing complications occur less frequently if auditory evoked potentials (BAEPs) are performed during surgery (Kakizawa et al., 1990; Barker et al., 1996; Broggi et al., 1999). Moller and Moller (1989) suggest that intra-operative monitoring of BAEPs will not only result in fewer cases of hearing loss but will also inform the surgeon as to which particular manipulation is likely to cause alterations to the potentials. Sindou and Mertens (1993) have modified their procedure in such a way that they no longer consider it important to measure BAEPs routinely.

Fritz et al. (1988) performed audiometry on 21 patients pre- and post-MVD and found that 5 patients developed a hearing loss postoperatively. Middle ear effusions occur probably due to lack of application of bone wax to the mastoid air cells. Fuse and Moller (1996) reported a case of delayed hearing loss three years after a MVD and on re-operation for recurrence of pain noted scar tissue and progressive atrophy of the auditory nerve. Although very rare, other examples have been reported (Kuchta et al., 1998).

7.8.4. Complications after GKS

No peri-operative complications or deaths have been reported. In contrast to all other surgical treatments complications after gamma knife surgery may be delayed for months or even years and so it is crucial that these patients are carefully followed up and questioned about developed of late complications.

All reports acknowledge that the major complication after radiosurgery is the development of sensory loss and the data is shown in Table 37. In the largest series with the longest follow up, 17 (7.7%) of patients developed paraesthesia which took a median

of 8 months to develop (Maesawa et al., 2001). In the one randomised controlled trial Flickinger et al. (2001) showed that estimated sensory loss at 2 years was 32.5% with those treated with two isocentres (longer nerve length treated) and 16.8% in those with one isocentre when doses of 75 Gy were used. Young et al. (1997, 1998) report changes at 2.5 to 18 months but in their series, having preoperative sensory changes increased the risk of sensory changes. In their series one patient developed deafferentation pain but this was a patient who had had a prior MVD and had atypical dull pain. She had also been treated with two isocentres. Sensory loss may be dose-related. Pollock et al. (2001) reported that up to 32% of patients had bothersome facial dysaesthesia after doses of 90 Gy and Nicol et al. (2000) using 90 Gy as a one treatment, also reported 7/42 patients developed sensory changes. Hasegawa et al. (2002) reported more patients developing sensory loss after re-operation.

Nicol et al. (2000) using 90 Gy reported 4 cases of taste change or alteration, in 2 this was complete and in 2 it was partial. Formal testing showed that 2 modalities of taste had been lost. No details are provided of timing or progress of these changes. Hochman (1998) reported jaw clenching in a patient exposed to a total of 160 Gy but Rogers et al. (2000) reported using a dose of 150 Gy with no sequel and Nicol et al. (2000) repeated a 90 Gy dose to two patients with recurrences and noted no changes.

Corneal reflex has been noted to be decreased in 3 patients receiving radiation at 90 Gy (Pollock et al., 2001). Kondziolka et al. (1997) showed no correlation of the following with sensory change: age, multiple sclerosis, dose, gamma knife model, nerve identification.

TABLE 37

Cohort studies reporting complications in 526 patients with trigeminal neuralgia who underwent Gamma Knife surgery (GKS)

Total number patients (preoperative sensory loss)	Number sensory loss no prior loss (prior loss)	Number dysaesthesia	Corneal reflex decreased	Time scale	Reference
49 (33)	3 (all)	0			Urgosik et al., 1998
110 (?)	3	0		6–18 months	Young et al., 1998
126		4 (2 prior surgery? sensory changes) + 1 after repeat GKS		3–18 months	Brisman, 2000
42	7 (all)	0			Nicol et al., 2000
54 (17 pre-op.)	5/37 (0/17)	0			Rogers et al., 2000
88 (37)	11	9 mild, 1 severe (pre-op. sensory loss		Up to 2 years	Flickinger et al., 2001
220 (80 pre-operative)	17 (all)	1 post-MVD using 2 isocentres		Median 8 months, range 1–19 months	Maesawa et al., 2001
72 (42) but data not analysed this way	27/41 treated 90 Gy, 6/27 at 70 Gy	13 treated 90 Gy, 1 treated 70 Gy	3 on dose of 90 Gy		Pollock et al., 2001
526	**46 (8.7)**	**24 (4.6)**	**3 (0.5)**		**Total complications 13.9%**

No reported mortality; peri-operative complications; complications outside 5th cranial nerve, anaesthesia dolorosa or motor paresis. In totals row excluded patients with prior sensory loss. MVD, microvascular decompression.

Maher and Pollock (2000) reported in one patient having an MVD after radiosurgery (dose 90 Gy) evidence of atheromatous plaques. However, three other cases who had MVD after gamma knife surgery did not have these changes and no other series have so far reported these changes. These however need to be looked for as radiosurgery is used for vascular lesions and so is known to cause vascular changes although these may be dose-related.

No reports mention any psychological problems that the patients may have encountered during MRI scanning which could impact on the treatment. A systematic review by Melendez and McCrank (1993) indicated that up to 30% of patients having an MRI may suffer from anxiety related reactions. This can be allayed most effectively by the use of patient information which also contains some hints on psychological preparation, the use of music, prone position, and presence of relative and distracting thoughts. In severe cases sedation may be needed.

7.9. Management of recurrences

It would seem to me that it is fairly crucial to determine whether any report of facial pain after surgery is a recurrence of trigeminal neuralgia or some other pain. It would also be useful to know whether the recurrent pain has the same features in terms of intensity, character and quality of life as preoperatively. Unfortunately, no data like this are currently variable. Pain recurrence or failure of the procedure is the major concern of patients. There are some guidelines on how to manage these patients in the literature. How would you proceed? Read through the next case in Table 38 and try to come to a decision.

As Table 39 shows, most patients tend to have a repeat of the same surgery that they initially had unless there is a contraindication for its repeat. The results after surgery are variable as indicated. Oturai et al. (1996) showed that in their 316 patients 72%

TABLE 38

Case history 7

This patient has returned in pain after surgery. What are you going to do in the short and long term?

Name	JQ
Age	41
Gender	Male
Development of pain and previous history	First developed pain in 1984 and by 1989 pain was very severe affecting right maxillary division, classical features and on 1200 mg daily dose of carbamazepine was not getting pain control and unacceptable side effects. He had a radiofrequency thermocoagulation which rendered him pain-free and resulted in slight loss of sensation over the second and third division but no loss of corneal reflex. In October 2000 presents with a five month history of pain.
Character/quality	Describes his pain as sharp and shooting.
Site and radiation	Pain is in the right ophthalmic and maxillary division and radiates up to the top of the head. No intra-oral pain.
Severity	On visual analogue scale pain at its worse is 10 cm, average 2 cm but can be nil.
Duration and periodicity	The pain lasts for seconds but he may get several bouts in a few minutes and then it goes for days with no pain.
Provoking factors	Washing and brushing his hair, cold wind.
Relieving factors	Only drugs.
Associated factors	Notices some facial oedema under the eye and facial redness at time of worse pain. Altered sensation right side of face.
Use of medication	Controlled on carbamazepine 1600 mg daily and gabapentin 300 mg daily.
Effect of pain on life style	Currently the pain has had a mild effect on his life. He has had to change his duties at the post office. He was delivering letters on foot but found the cold winds started up his pain; now doing deliveries in the van. From his previous surgery he is aware that a repeat radiofrequency thermocoagulation would result in corneal anaesthesia, something that would make his job difficult.

Please see Table 48 for the answer.

had one form of surgery, 19% two and 9% had more than two different types of surgery. There is relatively little good quality data on patients who have had recurrent surgery. The numbers in each centre are probably fairly low and so multicentre studies would be needed to provide some better data.

7.9.1. Management of recurrences after peripheral surgery

Many patients will undergo repeat procedures and this can be seen in the reported numbers, e.g. 68 patients underwent 413 alcohol injections (Fardy et al., 1994). The results from repeat procedures appear to be similar as we showed in our cryotherapy data and patients will undergo a large number of repeat procedures (Zakrzewska and Nally, 1988).

7.9.2. Management of recurrences after Gasserian ganglion surgery

RFT. Only Latchaw et al. (1983) have given accurate data on recurrence rates after repeat surgery and these were comparable to those after the initial procedure. The complication rate is the same at 70% after a second procedure and in 3 patients having 4 RFTs there were no complications.

PRG. It is not advisable for re-injection within 3–4 weeks as you may still get some response. In repeat procedures the cistern is often not as clearly outlined and this has resulted in the injection of tantalum at the initial procedure to help in relocation of the cistern. If no CSF exits after placement of the needle it is important to do cisternography. Some arachnoiditis may have been induced by the glycerol so

TABLE 39

Reported management of recurrences after surgery for all procedures

Initial procedure	Total number of patients	Number of recurrences (%)	Management of recurrences	Reference
RFT	78	25 (32)	repeat RFT 12, MVD 10, neurectomy 3	Burchiel et al., 1981
RFT	96	48 (50)	repeat RFT 30, MVD 8, peripheral 2, drug therapy 26	Latchaw et al., 1983
RFT	124	35 (28)	repeat RFT 16, PRG 14, drug therapy 5	Ischia et al., 1990a,b
RFT	1000	181 (18)	drug therapy 15, repeat RFT 160, other surgery 6	Broggi et al., 1999
RFT	265	59 (22)	repeat RFT 59	Zakrzewska and Thomas, 1993
RFT	154	33 (21)	drug therapy or nil 10, MVD 7, repeat RFT 16	Taha and Tew, 1996
RFT	185	75 (40)	NA	Oturia, 1996
RFT	81	46 (57)	repeat RFT 35, MVD 10, PRG 3, peripheral 4, tumour 1 (14 patients needed more than 1 treatment)	Yoon et al., 1999
RFT	258	68 (26)	drug therapy 37, repeat RFT 31	Mathews and Scrivani, 2000
RFT	1600	480 (30)	drug therapy 96, repeat RFT 384	Kanpolat and Savas, 2001
PRG	552		all repeated up to three times, RFT in 18	Saini, 1987
PRG	162	44 (27)	drug therapy 14, repeat PRG 10, RFT 16, MVD 4	Young et al., 1998
PRG	112	23 (20)	repeat PRG 8, balloon 1, drug therapy 14	Ischia et al., 1990a,b
PRG	85	47 (55)	repeat PRG 24, MVD 9, RFT 8	North et al., 1990
PRG	122	28 (23)	drugs 13, repeat PRG 15	Steiger, 1991
PRG	60	28 (47)	drug therapy 10, surgery 18, repeat PRG, alcohol, MVD compression	Slettebo et al., 1993
PRG	53 all MS	28 (53)	repeat PRG 16, other surgery 12	Kondziolka et al., 1994a,b
Balloon	100	17 (17)	drug therapy 10, repeat microcompression 3, MVD 4	Lichtor and Mullan, 1990
Balloon	144	13 (9)	drug therapy 1, repeat microcompression 11, RFT 1	Lobato et al., 1990
Balloon	50	8 (16)	repeat microcompression 8	Brown et al., 1993
MVD	147	13 (9)	repeat MVD 2, rest NA	Aksik, 1993
MVD	1185	282 (24)	MVD 132, 34% drug therapy, 20% ablative surgery, 22% ablative surgery, drug therapy	Barker et al., 1996
MVD	252	31 (12)	drug therapy 11, MVD 2, PSR 18	Bederson and Wilson, 1989
MVD	146	39 (27)	repeat MVD 7, rest NA	Broggi et al., 1999
MVD	41	17 (41)	drug therapy 6, repeat MVD 4	Burchiel et al., 1988
MVD	94	17 (18)	no treatment 7, others NA	Cutbush and Atkinson, 1994
MVD	104	24 (23)	repeat MVD/PSR 6, rest NA	Piatt and Wilkins, 1984
MVD	45	9 (20)	drug therapy 4, PSR 1, rest Gasserian ganglion surgery	Pollack et al., 1988
MVD	25	4 (16)	PRG 1, rest NA	Slettebo and Eide, 1997
MVD	61	10 (16)	drug therapy 3, repeat MVD 2	Sun et al., 1994
GKS	41	8 (20)	no details	Urgosik et al., 1998
GKS	110	13 (12)	GKS 7, rest not specified	Young et al., 1998
GKS	54	11 (20)	not specified	Rogers et al., 2000
GKS	87	30 (34)	GKS 9, MVD 3, PRG 7, RFT 7, Alcohol 2, drugs 8	Flickinger et al., 2001
GKS	126	21 (17)	not specified	Brisman, 2000
GKS	42	2 (5)	GKS 2	Nicol et al., 2000
GKS	68	32 (47)	GKS 7, PRG 9, MVD 3, alcohol 1, drugs 12	Pollock et al., 2001
GKS	220	31 (14)	other forms of surgery not specified	Maesawa et al., 2001

MVD, microvascular decompression; RFT, radiofrequency thermocoagulation (rhizotomy); PRG, percutaneous glycerol rhizotomy; Balloon, balloon microcompression; PSR, partial sensory rhizotomy; GKS, gamma knife surgery.

reducing the size of the cistern (Rappaport and Gomori, 1988). It is important to ensure that the needle is placed in the part of the cistern where all the nerve fibres are concentrated. The risk of increased sensory loss and development of dysaesthesia is increased but appears to be higher if patients had a prior RFT (Bergenheim and Hariz, 1995).

Microcompression. Most patients will have a repeat procedure and Abdennebi et al. (1995) report patients having up to three repeat procedures. Similar results seem to be obtained (Brown and Gouda, 1999).

7.9.3. Management of recurrences after MVD

Recurrences are treated medically, with a repeat of the same surgery or with different surgery. None of the reports give any indication of the intensity or character of this recurrent pain but many imply that patients with less severe pain recurrences are managed medically. All the reports on recurrences have been considered as most series are small but the overall quality of the reports is poor. Only Barker et al. (1996) report their recurrence data using actuarial data and these have been included in Table 26 on results of MVD.

Jannetta and Bissonette (1985) provide details on re-operative techniques. Liao et al. (1997) suggested using the same scar and craniotomy but a fresh dural edge. Reasons for recurrences have been postulated to be due to continuing elongation of vessels, change in arterial position due to aging, recanalisation of divided veins, missed compressions or changes to the implants. However, many reoperations show negative findings as summarised in Table 40. Barker et al. (1996) do not report negative explorations but record a high number of small unidentified veins and arteries. In an older report based on 51 patients from the same group resorption of muscle implants is reported as is one negative exploration and one tumour (Jannetta and Bissonette, 1985). If no compression or other cause for recurrence is found partial rhizotomies or neurolysis is performed and if the implant had induced a reaction it was not used again. Jannetta and Bissonette (1985) point out that Ivalon sponge can become a compressive force in its own right and

so has led to them no longer using it. On the other hand Yamaki et al. (1992) use muscle or dura as they consider it the most natural product. However, in 2 of their cases they found that it had slipped or was not adequate and in a further 2 it had induced fibrosis and adhesions. Kureshi and Wilkins (1998) reported that 5 out of 23 implants showed scarring and were themselves now compressing the nerve. The scarred implant could only be dissected away safely in one patient and in the rest they performed partial rhizotomies.

The findings at re-operation are shown in Table 40. Rath et al. (1996) showed that if patients had had a prior ablative procedure the results on re-operation were worse than if they had only had an MVD previously. Barker et al. (1996) operated on 10% within 30 days of first operation, 58% within 2 years. They reported that if patients got immediate relief of pain it was more likely that the success would be sustained. Barker et al. (1996) showed that their re-operation recurrence rates were higher than those undergoing their first operation whereas Bederson and Wilson (1989) reported an improved outcome in their 20 patients. Cho et al. (1994) reported on 30 re-operations and had 21 recurrences within 1 year and a further 10 later. Poor prognosis was noted in those with negative exploration and arterial compression (Table 40).

Most reports show an increased number of complications after re-operation. Rath et al. (1996) reported complications in 11/16 patients with two serious ones: haemorrhage leading to a stroke and death after 6 months and another developing a mental disorder and hearing loss. This is similar to Barker et al. (1996) who also reported more cranial nerve complications, 1 brain infarct and 27 cases of aseptic meningitis. Kureshi and Wilkins (1998) reported that 7 out of their 23 cases had complications, 3 had hearing loss but 3 losses of corneal reflex were due to the partial rhizotomy that was done. There is insufficient evidence to make a decision as to whether patients should be undergoing a second procedure or whether they should opt for a procedure at the level of the Gasserian ganglion.

TABLE 40

Findings at re-operation for MVD

References	No. re-operated/ original number	Negative exploration	Compression new or old	Slippage/ resorption	Arachnoiditis/ adhesions	Procedure	Overall results
Piatt and Wilkins, 1984	6/104	6				4 PSR	3 good result
Bederson and Wilson, 1989	20/246	17	1 vascular contact		2 adhesions	18 PSR, 2 MVD	15 pain-free at 4 years
Klun, 1992	10/220	6	3 vessels found	1 muscle resorbed		6 PSR, 4 MVD	7 did well
Yamaki et al., 1992	7/60	1	2	2 resorbed or inadequate muscle	2 adhesions	6 MVD	2 complete remissions, 3 recurrences, 2 no relief
Cho et al., 1994	31/400	16	7 arterial, 4 venous		4 Teflon adhesions	16 PSR, 15 MVD	11/16 PSR pain-free, 10/15 MVD pain-free
Rath et al., 1996	16/135	7	9 new compressions	resorbed prosthesis, 5 slipped	extensive adhesions	7 PSR, 9 neurolysis, MVD	11 pain-free, 38% morbidity
Barker et al., 1996; Jannetta and Bissonette, 1985	132/1185	1	higher % veins and small arteries	5		1 tumour	high recurrence, 11 sensory loss, 2 facial palsy
Liao et al., 1997	5/80		3 compressions new		2 adhesions Teflon		4 complete relief, 1 partial, 9–48 months follow-up
Kureshi and Wilkins, 1998	23/331	16	1 artery, 1 bony ridge		5 scarred implant	16 PSR	15 complete relief, 6 partial, 2 nil
Broggi et al., 2000	7/146		2 missed, 2 new venous, 2 mixture of new/old		1		4 complete relief, 3 partial relief

7.9.4. Management of recurrences after GKS

In contrast to other surgical techniques where management of recurrences is discussed very few reports provide information on how patients who have failed or developed recurrent pain after GKS are managed. Some have repeat gamma knife surgery (Nicol et al., 2000) but most others have either other procedures or drugs alone. In 1997, Kondziolka suggested that the area irradiated could be changed to reduce the complication effects. The Pittsburgh group have reported that when carrying out a second procedure they overlap part of the field but aim to avoid irradiating the brain stem (Hasegawa et al., 2002). Friedman et al. (2001) also postulate that re-treatment should be directed at the retro-Gasserian portion rather than the REZ in order to reduce brain stem irradiation.

Pollock et al. (2001) have reported the treatment of recurrences. In their 100 patients 26 recurrences occurred and of these 10 underwent repeat gamma knife surgery using a range of doses 70–120 Gy. The others had the following procedures: MVD, 4; peripheral alcohol injections, 3; glycerol at the Gasserian ganglion level, 3. Those who had had significant reduction in their pain after the first procedure did achieve pain relief the second time, 9/10 with one recurrence at 3 months. However 6 were left with sensory loss (3 were present preoperatively) and 2 with dysaesthesia. Young et al. (1998) re-treated 7 patients using doses of 35 Gy but they give no outcome data. Hasegawa et al. (2002) retreated 31 patients using mean doses of 74 Gy and of these 13 achieved excellent results. Three experienced sensory loss after the second procedure. The dosage used did not make a difference to the recurrence rates.

More sensitive MRI scans may in the future pick up consistent identifiable enhancing lesions, which

TABLE 41

KEY FACTS: surgical management of trigeminal neuralgia; quality of surgical data is poor, most is retrospective and few use actuarial data to analyse recurrence rates; level of evidence C

Procedure	% Probability of being pain-free	Mortality	Morbidity
Peripheral neurectomy, cryotherapy, alcohol, injection, acupuncture	2 years — 22	Nil	Low, sensory loss, transient haematoma, oedema
Radiofrequency thermorhizotomy (RFT)	2 years — 68 5 years — 48	Low	62% sensory loss and 25% other complications mainly relating to trigeminal nerve, dysaesthesia, anaesthesia dolorosa, eye problems, masseteric problems
Percutaneous glycerol rhizotomy (PRG)	2 years — 63 5 years — 45	Low	28% sensory loss and 27% other complications mainly relating to trigeminal nerve, dysaesthesia, anaesthesia dolorosa, eye problems, masseteric problems
Balloon microcompression	2 years — 79 5 years — no data	Low	38% sensory loss and 38% other complications mainly relating to trigeminal nerve, dysaesthesia, eye problems, masseteric problems
Microvascular decompression (MVD)	2 years — 81 5 years — 76 10 years— 71	0.5%	Overall 75% no complications, complications 14% peri-operative complications, 5% transient cranial nerve 4th, 6th, 8th dysfunction, 2.2% permanent deafness, 3% sensory loss
Gamma knife surgery (GKS)	2 years — 75 5 years — 58	Nil	12% sensory loss up to 2 years post-treatment

could influence decisions about re-treatment. As yet no correlation between postoperative MRI findings and clinical features have been reported.

7.10. Indicators for different surgical procedures

Data is still very limited and these criteria may change as more cases are reported from different centres. I consider it essential that results are audited by an external body which collects uniform data from all centres. Using multiple centres and standardised outcome measures will enable some of the questions to be answered fairly quickly and in a less biased way.

7.10.1. Indicators for use of peripheral surgery

Advantages:

- Elderly and medically unfit can be treated
- Immediate results and most can be done in the dental office
- Least invasive of all surgical procedures
- Relatively small area of sensory loss and no anaesthesia dolorosa
- No mortality

Disadvantages:

- Very high recurrence rate, most within the year
- Can only be done if there is a very discrete trigger area
- Many patients need to continue to take drugs

- High incidence of transient side effects
- Sensory loss occurs and some cases of dysaesthesia have been reported

7.10.2. Indicators for use of Gasserian ganglion surgery: RFT, PRG, microcompression

Advantages of RFT:

- Safe in medically compromised patients
- Does not require a very skilled surgeon
- Highly specific and can avoid other branches
- Can vary amount of sensory loss
- Immediate pain relief
- Low mortality
- Relatively low recurrence rate
- Few complications outside trigeminal area

Disadvantages of RFT:

- Patients with haemoglobinopathies not suitable
- Co-operative patient needed — patients anxious about their ability to give accurate response
- Expensive equipment
- Tedious to do as need to keep waking the patient
- Mortality has been reported
- Sensory loss inevitable
- Risk of anaesthesia dolorosa
- Risk of corneal damage, need to wear safety glasses
- Risk of masseteric dysfunction

Advantages of PRG:

- Suitable for the elderly
- More suitable for patients with first division pain
- Can use sedation or general anaesthesia for the procedure
- Easier to carry out than RFT
- No sophisticated machinery required so is one of the cheapest procedures
- Not necessary to do intra-operative sensory testing so causing less anxiety
- Lower mortality and morbidity than after RFT
- Less risk of anaesthesia dolorosa and eye problems than after RFT
- Few problems outside trigeminal area
- Easy to repeat

Disadvantages of PRG:

- Cannot use in patients with sensitivity to contrast medium
- Very technique sensitive so needs a skilled operator
- Higher recurrence rate than other Gasserian ganglion procedures
- May have a delay before get pain relief
- Glycerol does induce arachnoiditis and this could lead to long-term problems
- Difficult to do repeat procedures

Advantages of microcompression:

- Suitable for most elderly as less likely to cause intracranial bleeding as needle not advanced all the way
- Although it requires a general anaesthetic it is a quick one
- Does not cause pain and anxiety while doing procedure as there is no need to wake the patient during the procedure
- Less experienced surgeon than for RFT as there is no need to be selective as all fibres get the same amount of compression
- Very low mortality
- Few complications outside trigeminal area
- No reports of anaesthesia dolorosa
- Less likely to cause loss of corneal reflex than other Gasserian ganglion procedures so useful for patients with first division pain

Disadvantages of microcompression:

- Not suitable in patients who have arrhythmias due to risk of bradycardia.
- Requires general anaesthetic with intubation.
- Recurrence rate as high as for any Gasserian ganglion procedure and higher than posterior fossa.
- Masseteric weakness can be a problem especially if patients are trying to control their dentures. Patients with contralateral masseteric weakness should not undergo the procedure.
- Sensory loss is inevitable and can be a problem in patients who already have some sensory loss.

7.10.3. Indicators for use of posterior fossa surgery: MVD, GKS

Advantages of MVD:

- Longest pain-free intervals
- Few patients will need a further surgical procedure
- Small percentage of patients will have complications
- Most complications are transient
- Risk of sensory loss is very small
- No anaesthesia dolorosa or keratitis

Disadvantages of MVD:

- Mortality rate of 0.5%
- Expert surgeons required
- Need to be fit enough to undergo a surgical procedure with a full general anaesthetic
- Requires longest hospital stay
- Risk of strokes or infarcts higher than with other procedures
- Permanent hearing loss in up to 3% of patients
- Initially expensive procedure

Advantages of GKS:

- Can be done on medically unfit patients and elderly
- Suitable for patients with acromegaly or other bony disorders which make entry through foramen ovale difficult
- No general anaesthesia needed
- Noninvasive with no peri-operative complications
- Rapid return to normal life
- Few complications
- Especially useful for first division as no keratitis
- At the most requires one overnight stay
- Can be done on patients who have had previous surgery although results may not be as good
- Can possibly be repeated

Disadvantages of GKS:

- Patients who are claustrophobic may not tolerate the treatment
- Not suitable for patients who cannot lie flat, e.g. some cardiac patients or stay still
- Currently still lack long-term results
- Current five year data are poor but may be related to early use of low doses
- Need to continue medication after treatment for months or in some cases indefinitely
- Can take over 6 months to get maximum pain relief
- Difficult to decide when treatment has failed and what treatment should be used next
- Side effects in the form of sensory loss can occur months after treatment
- Other side effects may have not yet become apparent, e.g. vascular or increased risk of cancer
- Patients with preoperative sensory loss may be at increased risk of developing troublesome anaesthesia dolorosa
- Although not reported I postulate that anxiety may be high even post-treatment due to delayed effects and fear of the unknown
- Concerns remain about the long-term effect of radiation
- Availability is poor, costs much higher than Gasserian ganglion

8. Algorithms on management

Based on the review of literature and my own clinical experience the following algorithm (Fig. 10) is one that can be used to determine treatment planning. As more evidence becomes available so this will change and need updating. Guidelines for managing trigeminal neuralgia in the primary care sector have been developed and can be accessed on the Prodigy scheme for GPs website www.Prodigy.nhs.uk.

However at the end of the day you need to remember that each patient is an individual and the treatment must be patient-centred. You must ensure that you manage the patient in a biopsychosocial way and not purely a biomedical way. The effect trigeminal neuralgia has on the patient's life and how your proposed treatment will impact on this must be the key facts to consider when negotiating management proposals. All the above information will give you the framework but it must fit the

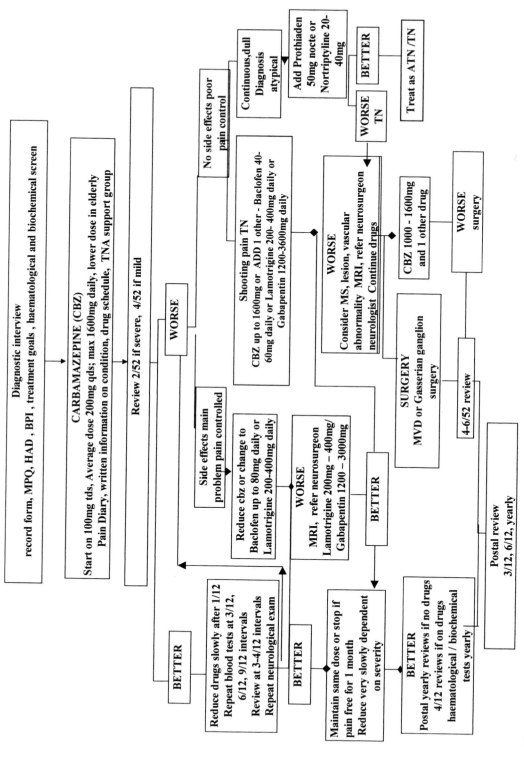

Fig. 10. Algorithm of management of trigeminal neuralgia. At each assessment: (1) measure pain, e.g. McGill pain questionnaire, long or short, VAS; (2) measure psychological effects, e.g. hospital anxiety and depression scale (HAD), brief pain inventory. At each visit give patient pain diary and drug dosage schedule. Record details on special forms. TNA, trigeminal neuralgia association; cbz, carbamazepine; ATN, atypical trigeminal neuralgia; TN, trigeminal neuralgia; MS, multiple sclerosis; MRI, magnetic resonance imaging; MVD, microvascular decompression. → represents several visits.

requirements of the individual patient as discussed in Chapter 9.

9. Patient information and support

Patients with trigeminal neuralgia become expert patients and can teach many health care professionals a thing or two. There are at least two national organisations (US and UK) run by patients with trigeminal neuralgia who provide support and information to patients with this condition.

All patients should have written jargon-free information about the different treatment modalities that are available. In Appendix A (Fig. 11) you will find an example of a patient information leaflet. In Chapter 9 I discuss some of the issues involved in giving patients information and assessing its quality. The appendix in Chapter 9 lists the addresses of the different support groups and their internet sites. For the patient with trigeminal neuralgia there are now many sources of information ranging from locally produced leaflets to national and international booklets and even a book called Striking Back (see Appendix A Fig. 12 for book cover). This latter is written by a patient with the help of a neurosurgeon and has attempted to be as free of bias as possible. The internet remains a very important source of information and both the US and the UK support groups have their own web sites which link to other sites which may be of value. Both these organisations also organise meetings at which patients can exchange news and to which specialists are invited. Not only do the specialists provide information but their views and results can be challenged by the consumers. I have found it extremely useful to attend meetings run by patients as it gives me real insight into what the patients are facing and it helps us to treat patients in a biopsychosocial way as compared to a biomedical way. These meetings are a wonderful forum for exchange of ideas and for surveys and it was just at such a meeting that I conducted a survey into patients' views of treatment (Zakrzewska, 2001). It is also an opportunity for health care professionals to meet and discuss a variety of issues among themselves.

Although as yet not formally assessed the trigeminal neuralgia support groups appear to provide a wealth of information, enable patients to meet each other without the need for a health care professional and can influence national research institutes (Kitt et al., 2000). The poems in Table 42 provide some biased evidence for the value of such support groups.

10. Future research

Following a consensus conference at the National Institute of Health Kitt et al. (2000) outline the research needs for trigeminal neuralgia. There is a need for research into basic neurophysiology to explain the pathophysiology of the condition and also to look at mechanisms for drug action. Epidemiological research would give further data on prevalence and incidence world wide and may indicate some high risk groups and risk factors as well as determine prognosis. Impact of the disease and its economic costs could be determined. Careful case control studies may better elucidate the features of trigeminal neuralgia over time and determine whether atypical trigeminal neuralgia and trigeminal neuropathy are distinct entities or part of the spectrum of the same disease. It would also enable better comparisons between studies, e.g. surgical outcomes as all would be using the same criteria, and differences between the study groups could be identified.

Even if surgery is shown to be the best treatment there will always be patients who wish to be treated medically. The medical management of trigeminal neuralgia would be greatly improved if there was a generally agreed template for the conduct of randomised controlled trials as has been proposed by clinicians managing patients with cluster headaches. This template could then be applied to all emerging drugs in several centres at once.

Longitudinal cohort surgical studies which use a range of objectively assessed outcomes including quality of life measures and monitored by external observers on an international basis are essential if we are to answer questions quickly and provide patients with evidence-based answers. As the evidence seems

TABLE 42

Poems submitted by patients telling of their experience at managing their pain and the value of support groups

Poem 1
ACRONYM

*T*rigger points
*R*are nerve disorder
*I*nformation — Trigeminal Neuralgia Association
*G*amma knife stereotactic radiosurgery
*E*xacerbations and remissions
*M*agnetic resonance imaging
*I*nvasive microvascular decompression
*N*on-invasive balloon compression
*A*nti-convulsant medication — tegretol
*L*ightning — shock-like attacks

*N*eurologists, neurosurgeon
E-mail *Tna@scionline.net*
*U*tilize computer TNA 'home page'
*R*adiofrequency rhizotomy
*A*lternative therapies
*L*ancinating pain
*G*lycerol rhizotomy
*I*nternet Worldwide Web *http://neurosurgery*, mgh.edu/tna/#services
*A*rtery and vein compression

Peggy Ruther, Central N.J. Support Group

Poem 2
Ode to a tic

Quick as lightning one day it began,
with a cool breeze after the rain.

You suffered alone in pain and confusion,
it almost drove you insane.

You searched alone in silent frustration,
and looked for a reason in vain.

It was such a relief when you first found out,
your pain really did have a name.

Trigeminal neuralgia, tic douloureux,
you tried to pronounce it in vain.

Then lo and behold, a support group you found,
with people that all shared your pain.

Information was learned, medications tried,
and the tic you started to tame.

Things improved for a while, you started to smile,
then back with a vengeance it came.

Your group rallied round you with love and support,
and agreed "the tic's back again!"

Successful surgeries were told, doctors names shared,
even Dr Jannetta of fame.

The decision was made, and hope returned,
so to the hospital you came.

When you woke, a big headache you had,
but behold, no tic did remain.

The journey was long, your problem was solved,
and now you have your life back again.

Terah Biszantz

Poem 3
T.N.

Trigeminal neuralgia
Is as fierce as its name
And no one has quite figured out
From which origin, it came.

It isn't a lion
Of that I'm quite sure,
But what to do with it,
Or how, it to cure.

It's puzzling at the least.
It's a challenge by far
And to many people
Causes, quite a jar.

Whether talking or eating
Or standing in a breeze,
Why sometimes it's caused
By no less than a sneeze

Some have tried glycerol
And others the O.R.,
Some tried the Gamma knife.
What's your cure for that bear?

We try to make light of it,
But it's no laughing matter.
Sometimes it can make you
As mad as a hauteur.

"To learn to live with it"
I've heard some people say
Is better than surgery
On any old day.

Guess we're the same
In one way or another,
For we've tried many things
To get of this bother!
If the medicine doesn't work
And you stumble around,
Take courage my friend
As many others have found

That getting together
At least once a month
Helps those who want info
To get a whole bunch.

So don't get discouraged
Keep faith for today.
Maybe soon a cure will be found
To take it away.

Veverly J. Van Hoven
San Diego Support Group

TABLE 43

Summary for this chapter

- Trigeminal neuralgia is a sudden, usually unilateral, severe, brief, stabbing, recurrent pain in the distribution of one or more branches of the fifth cranial nerve provoked by light touch.

- The diagnostic criteria of trigeminal neuralgia have not been formally validated but those of the International Headache Society are of sufficient quality to be used in trials.

- There are now a wide variety of drugs available for management of trigeminal neuralgia but only some have been evaluated in randomized controlled trials. The current gold standard remains carbamazepine despite its considerable side effects.

- The majority of patients will suffer from side effects when on medical therapy, especially if higher dosages are used.

- Evidence for surgical management of trigeminal neuralgia is mainly based on retrospective data with lack of clarification of the diagnostic criteria used and the vast majority of the data is of poor quality.

- Except for microvascular decompression all other surgical procedures are neurodestructive.

- Surgery at the periphery includes neurectomies, cryotherapy, laser, radiofrequency thermorhizotomy and a variety of injections including streptomycin, alcohol, glycerol and phenol. The mean time to recurrence of pain is in the order of 1 year.

- Surgery at the level of the Gasserian ganglion includes radiofrequency thermorhizotomy, glycerol rhizotomy, microcompression and a mean time to recurrence is 4 years.

- Gamma knife surgery is a non-invasive procedure that irradiates the trigeminal nerve in the posterior fossa and early data suggest a mean recurrence rate of 2 years.

- Microvascular decompression of the trigeminal nerve in the posterior fossa is the most invasive procedure but at 10 years 70% of patients may still be pain-free.

- All surgery apart from peripheral procedures carry a potential for mortality but it is highest in microvascular decompression. Mortality rates for microvascular decompression have fallen to 0.5%.

- All forms of surgery have a potential for complications, many of which are irreversible. The more peripheral the surgery, the less likelihood there is of a serious complication.

- The major complication of all surgeries except microvascular decompression is sensory loss and in some forms of surgery it is considered essential for good results and so 96% of patients will have a complication.

- Microvascular decompression has the highest level of peri-operative complications many of which are transient and the most common permanent complication is hearing loss in 2% of patients; 76% of patients will have no complications.

- Surgery should be performed in specialised units as these centres have consistently better outcomes.

- Results of surgery should be centrally monitored by independent observers.

- Patients need information and contact with other patients in order to make decisions about treatment.

- Patients need to be more actively involved in research in this area and their satisfaction with treatments must be included in any evaluations.

to be increasing that the cause of trigeminal neuralgia is a compression of the nerve more accurate studies are needed to provide the clinical evidence. A way needs to be found of classifying accurately and reliably the level of compression found at MVD and then linking these findings to the clinical features including sensory changes, characteristics of the pain and its duration. The role of MRI and other newer techniques need to be further evaluated to provide the neurosurgeons with more accurate and reliable preoperative data. It would be useful to have better evidence to decide when surgery should be performed. If, as Burchiel and Slavin (2000) hypothesise the condition gets progressively worse and more intractable then patients should be encouraged to choose surgery earlier rather than later.

National and even international guidelines on management of trigeminal neuralgia could be produced both for the primary care and secondary care sectors which would ensure more consistent care for these patients.

Patients need help with making decisions about drug therapy, about the timing of surgery and then the type of surgery that would best suit them. Decision analysis needs to be done to enable patients to have a more systematic way of achieving optimal care. I would like to see this as a computer-run programme that patients can access with the help of a health care professional.

11. Conclusion

Once accurately diagnosed the patient with trigeminal neuralgia has a variety of treatment options available ranging from medical to surgical. Remember that patients with trigeminal neuralgia have chronic pain and need the same psychosocial approach to their management as other chronic pain patients. Each patient must be seen as a whole and treatment has to be tailored to the individual patient and this means that a variety of treatment modalities may need to be used. Table 43 provides a summary of the whole chapter.

Appendix A

Figs. 11 and 12

Appendix B. Further reading

B.1. Textbooks on trigeminal neuralgia or surgical techniques

(1) Fromm GH (ed). The Medical and Surgical Management of Trigeminal Neuralgia. Futura Publishing Company, New York, 1987, ISBN 0-87993-303-8.
(2) Rovit RL, Murali R, Jannetta PJ (eds). Trigeminal Neuralgia. Williams and Wilkins, Baltimore, MD, 1990, ISBN 0-683-07393-1.
(3) Zakrzewska JM. Trigeminal Neuralgia. W.B. Saunders, London, 1995, ISBN 0-7020-1696-9.
(4) Fromm GH, Sessle BJ (eds). Trigeminal Neu-

TABLE 44

Answers to cases in Table 3

Answer case 1
This patient presents with all the characteristic features of trigeminal neuralgia as suggested by the IHS classification. Assessing patient's response to standard drug therapy can be used as a diagnostic tool given that there are no other investigations with greater specificity and sensitivity. The patient responded well to management with carbamazepine. There are no clear criteria as to when patients should undergo further investigations such as MRI, or be assessed for a possible diagnosis of multiple sclerosis.

Answer case 2
This patient does present with many of the classical features of trigeminal neuralgia. Its distribution, periodicity and provoking factors fulfil the criteria suggested by the IHS classification. However, when assessing the words the patient is using on the McGill pain questionnaire some words are not those associated with trigeminal neuralgia, e.g. nagging, aching, gnawing. Does this patient have trigeminal neuralgia with overlying stress-related pain or is it what some clinicians suggest a atypical trigeminal neuralgia? The sharp element of the pain did respond to anticonvulsant pain therapies. Based on this history the patient underwent radiofrequency thermocoagulation at the level of the Gasserian ganglion as she did not feel that the drug therapy gave her sufficient pain relief. Three months postoperatively the patient reported great improvement and described some of her residual continuous pain as flickering, stinging, taut, annoying and numb.

Trigeminal Neuralgia

What is trigeminal neuralgia?

Trigeminal Neuralgia is a condition that affects one of the large nerves in your head, called the trigeminal nerve. It is characterised by a sudden, severe, electric shock-like or stabbing pain typically felt on one side of your jaw or cheek. It may also feel like toothache and be felt inside your mouth rather than outside. It is more common in women than in men and usually affects people aged 50 and older.

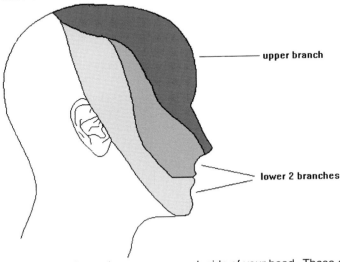

There are twelve major nerves on each side of your head. These are called cranial nerves. Each one has a different function. The trigeminal nerve is the fifth cranial nerve. It is responsible for sending impulses of touch, pain, pressure, and temperature to your brain, from your face and mouth. They also supply the muscles that help you to eat. Although you have two trigeminal nerves, almost always only one of them is affected, in trigeminal neuralgia.

There are three main branches of the trigeminal nerve. The area that each branch receives signals from is shaded on the diagram. In trigeminal neuralgia it is typically one or both of the lower two branches that are affected.

The pain is typically described as a sudden electric shock-like or jabbing, stabbing pain that suddenly comes and goes, but that may be repeated as a salvo or volley. The pain attacks may come and go throughout the day and last for days, weeks or months at a time, and may then disappear for months or years.

Various actions may trigger the pain:

- lightly touching the skin on the side of your face;
- eating;
- talking;
- tooth brushing;
- cold air on your face.

The pain can be severe and disabling, sometimes preventing washing or shaving the affected side or applying makeup. Some sufferers may stop eating during these periods because they fear they might trigger a painful attack. You may be unable to brush your teeth on that side. if the pain is left untreated or is unmanageable, weight loss and other complications could result.

Fig. 11. Example page from Dr Online information for GPs to give to patients.

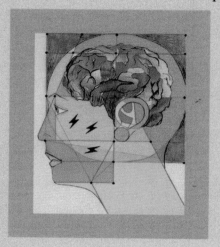

striking Back!

THE TRIGEMINAL NEURALGIA HANDBOOK

A layman's guide
to understanding and treating
what is often called the world's worst pain.

by

George Weigel

and

Kenneth F. Casey, M.D.

Foreword by Peter J. Jannetta, M.D.

 The Trigeminal Neuralgia Association

Fig. 12. Book cover of Striking Back, a book written for patients with trigeminal neuralgia.

TABLE 45

Answers to case studies in Table 8

Read through medical treatment.

Answer case 1
The current literature reviews on medical management of trigeminal neuralgia suggest that the most effective drug in up to 70% of patients is carbamazepine. The first drug of choice should therefore be carbamazepine (CBZ). It needs to be started at a low dose and gradually increased over the course of a few weeks. The level of pain and the weight of the patient will dictate the initial dosage. The initial dose may vary from 100 mg twice daily to 200 mg twice a day. A 100 or 200 mg rise in dose should be made no more than every three days. The drug is best taken four times a day. A retard formulation is useful especially for taking at night so serum drug levels remain reasonably high overnight. Taken at least half an hour before food so the drug is effective when trying to do light touch provoked activities. CBZ has the potential for significant side effects and drug interactions. Do some baseline investigations, HB, WBC, U and E, LFT. Side effects: drowsiness, tiredness, difficulty concentrating, ataxia, disturbed vision. Give patient a pain diary to record pain severity and its relief, possible side effects and drug dosages. Stress importance of bringing the completed diary to the next appointment. Review the patient in three weeks. Check level of pain on a visual analogue scale, assess quality of life on scale such as HAD or brief pain inventory.

Answer case 3
Baclofen has been used successfully in trigeminal neuralgia but it is not as useful in very severe cases. Lamotrigine has been shown to have antineuralgic effects but the only RCT was one using as an add on medication to CBZ. It could be used in this patient, but dose escalation will have to be slow to prevent a rash developing. Other drugs which have been assessed in RCTs have either been ineffective or have had side effects that outweigh the benefits. Oxcarbazepine, although not used in an RCT, has been reported in long-term studies and shown to have good initial effects. Each 200 mg dose of CBZ is replaced by 300 mg oxcarbazepine. This 'daughter' drug of CBZ does not cause autoinduction and hence drug interactions are lower. There is cross-sensitivity between the drugs and so some patients may have an allergy to both. This patient managed well on oxcarbazepine for over 4 years before requiring surgery, and was one reported in our paper on long-term use of oxcarbazepine (Zakrzewska and Patsalos, 2002). The other drug that could be used would be gabapentin not assessed in an RCT for trigeminal neuralgia but used in other neuropathic pains.

TABLE 46

Answers to case studies 4 and 5 in Table 17

It remains unclear as to when patients should have surgical rather than medical management. Several years ago most clinicians would suggest that patients should remain on medical treatment until pain control becomes difficult or side effects are intolerable. However, results from surgery, especially microvascular decompression, are suggesting that surgical treatment should be an earlier option as the long-term results are better if patients are operated on within 8 years of onset of trigeminal neuralgia (see prognostic factors). A recent survey among patients with trigeminal neuralgia has shown that patients remain undecided about treatment options even after they have had both surgical and medical treatments.

Mrs. IR (case 4) has got pain that significantly interferes with her life and so is keen to have surgery. She went to a consultation with a neurosurgeon and although ready to have surgery, is now unsure whether she should opt for microvascular decompression or radiofrequency thermocoagulation. She is concerned about the risk of side effects of the microvascular decompression given that she has a young family but is keen on a long-term solution. Mrs. IR has decided to discuss things with other patients from the Trigeminal Neuralgia Association support group to see if she can make a decision. She is currently well controlled on medication which makes it harder for her to decide.

Mr. JQ (case 5) has a classical history of trigeminal neuralgia suggestive of progression but currently it is not affecting the quality of his life. He has evidence of a compression, has a clear medical history and so would seem to be a good candidate for microvascular decompression. He went to see a neurosurgeon but decided against any surgery until his pain becomes more severe. Although the current evidence would suggest that he would benefit from surgery, the patient must make the decision himself.

There are no evidence-based criteria for making the decision. Factors I take into consideration are listed in the section below the case study. Some patients find the prospect of major surgery very daunting and it is not until they have enjoyed some time free from all pain and medication that they appreciate the benefits. However, the risks remain and patients need help with decision making.

TABLE 47

Answer to case study 6 in Table 18

Mr. DH has the classical features of trigeminal neuralgia. He had thought that as his trigeminal neuralgia had gone into remission after his first visit to the neurosurgeon he would be pain-free for a long time. He did not expect this severe attack so quickly. He was totally incapacitated by this second attack. He is fit and well and has not had ablative surgery before. There was a short history and so it would seem that the best treatment would be an MVD. If he had surgery at the Gasserian ganglion level he would also do well but if he had a recurrence a few years later he may no longer be medically fit enough to have an MVD. He chose to have an MVD and had an excellent result. See also Section 7.10.

TABLE 48

Answer to case study 7 in Table 38

At present Mr. JR is well controlled and feels that his pain has started to reduce. This, however, could be due to his medication rather than a natural period of remission. Mr. JR is relatively young and has a clear medical history. He responded well to surgery before but it is obvious that radiofrequency thermocoagulation is not the procedure of choice given the current location of the pain. He will either have to consider having a microvascular decompression, a glycerol rhizotomy or a balloon microcompression at the level of the Gasserian ganglion. There is no easy answer and the patient again has to make the decision.

ralgia: Current Concepts Regarding Pathogenesis and Treatment. Heinemann Medical Books, 1990, ISBN 0409901261.

(5) Hamlyn PJ. Neurovascular Compression of the Cranial Nerves in Neurological and Systematic Disease. Elsevier, Amsterdam, 1999, ISBN 0-444 82977 6.

(6) Coakham HB. The microsurgical treatment of trigeminal neuralgia, hemifacial spasm and glossopharyngeal neuralgia. In: Robertson JT, Coakham HB, Robertson JH (eds). Cranial Base Surgery. Churchill Livingstone, London, 2000, ISBN 0443056854.

(7) Weigel G, Casey KF. Striking Back. The trigeminal neuralgia handbook. The Trigeminal Neuralgia Association, Barnegat Light – patient handbook, 2000, ISBN 0-9672393-0-3.

B.2. Classifications

(8) Anonymous. Classification and diagnostic criteria for headache disorders, cranial neuralgias and facial pain. Headache Classification Committee of the International Headache Society. Cephalalgia 1988; 8(Suppl 7): 1–96.

(9) Merskey H, Bogduk N. Classification of Chronic Pain. Descriptors of Chronic Pain Syndromes and Definitions of Pain Terms. IASP Press, Seattle, WA, 1994.

B.3. Evidence-based medicine references

(10) Jaeschke R, Guyatt G, Sackett DL. Users' guides to the medical literature. III. How to use an article about a diagnostic test. A. Are the results of the study valid? Evidence-Based Medicine Working Group. JAMA 1994a: 271: 389–391.

(11) Jaeschke R, Guyatt GH, Sackett DL. Users' guides to the medical literature. III. How to use an article about a diagnostic test. B. What are the results and will they help me in caring for my patients? The Evidence-Based Medicine Working Group. JAMA 1994b; 271: 703–707.

(12) Richardson WS, Wilson MC, Williams JW Jr, Moyer VA, Naylor CD. Users' guides to the medical literature: XXIV. How to use an article on the clinical manifestations of disease. Evidence-Based Medicine Working Group. JAMA 2000; 284: 869–875.

References

Marked as regards quality according to criteria set by author.
SR = systematic review or high quality review with methodology
* Poorer quality studies but only ones in the field.
** Cohort studies, high quality case series.
*** Randomised controlled trials, high quality original studies.

* Abdennebi B, Bouatta F, Chitti M, Bougatene B. Percutaneous balloon compression of the Gasserian ganglion in trigeminal neuralgia. Long-term results in 150 cases. Acta Neurochir (Wien) 1995; 136: 72–74.

* Abdennebi B, Mahfouf L, Nedjahi T. Long-term results of percutaneous compression of the gasserian ganglion in trigeminal neuralgia (series of 200 patients). Stereotact Funct Neurosurg 1997; 68: 190–195.

* Aksik I. Microneural decompression operations in the treatment of some forms of cranial rhizopathy. Acta Neurochir (Wien) 1993; 125: 64–74.

* Apfelbaum RI. Surgery for tic douloureux. Clin Neurosurg 1984; 31: 351–368.

* Apfelbaum RI. 1999; Glycerol trigeminal neurolysis. Tech Neurosurg 5: 225–231.

* Arias MJ. Percutaneous retrogasserian glycerol rhizotomy for trigeminal neuralgia. A prospective study of 100 cases. J Neurosurg 1986; 65: 32–36.

* Barker, FG II, Jannetta PJ, Bissonette DJ, Larkins MV, Jho HD. The long-term outcome of microvascular decompression for trigeminal neuralgia. N Engl J Med 1996; 334: 1077–1083.

* Barker, FG II, Jannetta PJ, Bissonette DJ, Jho HD. Trigeminal numbness and tic relief after microvascular decompression for typical trigeminal neuralgia. Neurosurgery 1997; 40: 39–45.

* Barnard D. Cryoanalgesia in the management of paroxysmal trigeminal neuralgia. Hosp Dent (Tokyo) 1989; 1: 58–60.

* Bederson JB, Wilson CB. Evaluation of microvascular decompression and partial sensory rhizotomy in 252 cases of trigeminal neuralgia. J Neurosurg 1989; 71: 359–367.

* Belber CJ, Rak RA. Balloon compression rhizolysis in the surgical management of trigeminal neuralgia. Neurosurgery 1987; 20: 908–913.

* Bergenheim AT, Hariz MI. Influence of previous treatment on outcome after glycerol rhizotomy for trigeminal neuralgia. Neurosurgery 1995; 36: 303–309; discussion 309–310.

* Bergenheim AT, Hariz MI, Laitinen LV. Selectivity of retrogasserian glycerol rhizotomy in the treatment of trigeminal neuralgia. Stereotact Funct Neurosurg 1991; 56: 159–165.

* Bergenheim AT, Shamsgovara P, Ridderheim PA. Microvascular decompression for trigeminal neuralgia: no relation between sensory disturbance and outcome. Stereotact Funct Neurosurg 1997; 68: 200–206.

* Bittar GT, Graff-Radford SB. The effects of streptomycin/lidocaine block on trigeminal neuralgia: a double blind crossover placebo controlled study. Headache 1993; 33: 155–160.

* Blom S. Trigeminal neuralgia. Its treatment with a new anticonvulsant drug (G32883). Lancet 1962; I: 839–840.

* Bowsher D. Trigeminal neuralgia: a symptomatic study of 126 successive patients with and without previous interventions. Pain Clin 2000; 12: 93–101.

* Bowsher D, Miles JB, Haggett CE, Eldridge PR. Trigeminal neuralgia: a quantitative sensory perception threshold study in patients who had not undergone previous invasive procedures. J Neurosurg 1997; 86: 190–192.

* Braham J, Saia A. Phenytoin in the treatment of trigeminal and other neuralgias. Lancet 1960; 2: 892–893.

* Brandt F, Wittkamp P. [Late results of thermocoagulation in Gasser's ganglion in tic douloureux]. Neurochirurgia (Stuttg) 1983; 26: 133–135.

* Brisman R. Gamma knife radiosurgery for primary management for trigeminal neuralgia. J Neurosurg 2000; 93(Suppl 3): 159–161.

* Broggi G, Ferroli P, Franzini A, Pluderi M, La Mantia L, Milanese C. Role of microvascular decompression in trigeminal neuralgia and multiple sclerosis. Lancet 1999; 354: 1878–1879.

* Broggi G, Ferroli P, Franzini A, Servello D, Dones I. Microvascular decompression for trigeminal neuralgia: comments on a series of 250 cases, including 10 patients with multiple sclerosis. J Neurol Neurosurg Psychiatry 2000; 68: 59–64.

* Brown JA, Gouda JJ. Percutaneous balloon compression treatment for trigeminal neuralgia. Tech Neurosurg 1999; 5: 232–238.

* Brown JA, McDaniel MD, Weaver MT. Percutaneous trigeminal nerve compression for treatment of trigeminal neuralgia: results in 50 patients. Neurosurgery 1993; 32: 570–573.

* Browne L. Radiofrequency lesioning of the trigeminal ganglion for the treatment of trigeminal neuralgia. Ir Med J 1985; 78(3): 68–71.

Burchiel KJ, Slavin KV. On the natural history of trigeminal neuralgia. Neurosurgery 2000; 46(1): 152–154.

* Burchiel KJ, Steege TD, Howe JF, Loeser JD. Comparison of percutaneous radiofrequency gangliolysis and microvascular decompression for the surgical management of tic douloureux. Neurosurgery 1981; 9(2): 111–119.

* Burchiel KJ, Clarke H, Haglund M, Loeser JD. Long-term efficacy of microvascular decompression in trigeminal neuralgia. J Neurosurg 1988; 69(1): 35–38.

* Caccia MR. Clonazepam in facial neuralgia and cluster headache. Clinical and electrophysiological study. Eur Neurol 1975; 13: 560–563.

*** Campbell FG, Graham JG, Zilkha KJ. Clinical trial of carbamazepine (Tegretol) in trigeminal neuralgia. J Neurol Neurosurg Psychiatry 1966; 29: 265–267.

* Canavero S, Bonicalzi V, Ferroli P, Zeme S, Montalenti E, Benna P. Lamotrigine control of idiopathic trigeminal neuralgia [letter]. J Neurol Neurosurg Psychiatry 1995; 59: 646.

* Chandra B. The use of clonazepam in the treatment of tic douloureux (a preliminary report). Proc Aust Assoc Neurol 1976; 13: 119–122.

* Chang JW, Chang JH, Park YG, Chung SS. Gamma knife radiosurgery for idiopathic and secondary trigeminal neuralgia. J Neurosurg 2000a; 93(Suppl 3): 147–151.

* Chang JW, Chang JH, Park YG, Chung SS. Microvascular de-

compression in trigeminal neuralgia: a correlation of three-dimensional time-of-flight magnetic resonance angiography and surgical findings. Stereotact Funct Neurosurg 2000b; 74: 167–174.

* Cheng TM, Cascino TL, Onofrio BM. Comprehensive study of diagnosis and treatment of trigeminal neuralgia secondary to tumors. Neurology 1993; 43: 2298–2302.

* Cheshire WP. Fosphenytoin: an intravenous option for the management of acute trigeminal neuralgia crisis. J Pain Symptom Manage 2001; 21: 506–510.

* Chinitz A, Seelinger DF, Greenhouse AH. Anticonvulsant therapy in trigeminal neuralgia. Am J Med Sci 1966; 252: 62–67.

* Cho DY, Chang CG, Wang YC, Wang FH, Shen CC, Yang DY. Repeat operations in failed microvascular decompression for trigeminal neuralgia. Neurosurgery 1994; 35: 665–669; discussion 669–670.

* Coffey RJ, Fromm GH. Familial trigeminal neuralgia and Charcot–Marie–Tooth neuropathy. Report of two families and review. [Review] [31 refs]. Surg Neurol 1991; 35: 49–53.

* Court JE, Kase CS. Treatment of tic douloureux with a new anticonvulsant (clonazepam). J Neurol Neurosurg Psychiatry 1976; 39: 297–299.

* Crooks DA, Miles JB. Trigeminal neuralgia due to vascular compression in multiple sclerosis — post-mortem findings. Br J Neurosurg 1996; 10: 85–88.

* Cutbush K, Atkinson RL. Treatment of trigeminal neuralgia by posterior fossa microvascular decompression. Aust N Z J Surg 1994; 64(3): 173–176.

** Desai N, Shah K, Gandhi I. Baclofen sodium valporate combination in carbamazepine resistant trigeminal neuralgia — a double blind clinical trial Cephalalgia 1991; 11: 321–322.

* Devor M, Amir R, Rappaport ZH. Pathophysiology of trigeminal neuralgia: the ignition hypothesis. Clin J Pain 2002; 18: 4–13.

* Egan RA, Pless M, Shults WT. Monocular blindness as a complication of trigeminal radiofrequency rhizotomy. Am J Ophthalmol 2001; 131: 237–240.

* Eide PK, Stubhaug A. Relief of trigeminal neuralgia after percutaneous retrogasserian glycerol rhizolysis is dependent on normalization of abnormal temporal summation of pain, without general impairment of sensory perception. Neurosurgery 1998; 43: 462–472.

* Epstein JB, Marcoe JH. Topical application of capsaicin for treatment of oral neuropathic pain and trigeminal neuralgia. Oral Surg Oral Med Oral Pathol 1994; 77: 135–140.

* Erdem E, Alkan A. Peripheral glycerol injections in the treatment of idiopathic trigeminal neuralgia: retrospective analysis of 157 cases. J Oral Maxillofac Surg 2001; 59: 1176–1180.

* Farago F. Trigeminal neuralgia: its treatment with two new carbamazepine analogues. Eur Neurol 1987; 26: 73–83.

* Fardy MJ, Patton DW. Complications associated with peripheral alcohol injections in the management of trigeminal neuralgia. Br J Oral Maxillofac Surg 1994; 32: 387–391.

* Fardy MJ, Zakrzewska JM, Patton DW. Peripheral surgical

techniques for the management of trigeminal neuralgia — alcohol and glycerol injections. Acta Neurochir (Wien) 1994; 129: 181–184; discussion 185.

* Ferroli P, Franzini A, Farina L, La Mantia L, Broggi G. Does the presence of a pontine trigeminal lesion represent an absolute contraindication for microvascular decompression in drug resistant trigeminal neuralgia? J Neurol Neurosurg Psychiatry 2002; 72: 122–123.

*** Flickinger JC, Pollock BE, Kondziolka D, Phuong LK, Foote RL, Stafford SL, Lunsford LD. Does increased nerve length within the treatment volume improve trigeminal neuralgia radiosurgery? A prospective double-blind, randomized study. Int J Radiat Oncol Biol Phys 2001; 51: 449–454.

* Freemont AJ, Millac P. 1981; The place of peripheral neurectomy in the management of trigeminal neuralgia. Postgrad Med J 57: 75–76.

* Friedman DP, Morales RE, Goldman HW. Role of enhanced MRI in the follow-up of patients with medically refractory trigeminal neuralgia undergoing stereotactic radiosurgery using the gamma knife: initial experience. J Comput Assist Tomogr 2001; 25: 727–732.

* Fritz W, Schafer J, Klein HJ. Hearing loss after microvascular decompression for trigeminal neuralgia. J Neurosurg 1988; 69: 367–370.

** Fromm GH, Terrence CF. Comparison of L-baclofen and racemic baclofen in trigeminal neuralgia. Neurology 1987; 37: 1725–1728.

* Fromm GH, Terrence CF, Chattha AS, Glass JD. Baclofen in trigeminal neuralgia: its effect on the spinal trigeminal nucleus: a pilot study. Arch Neurol 1980; 37: 768–771.

*** Fromm GH, Terrence CF, Chattha AS. Baclofen in the treatment of trigeminal neuralgia: double-blind study and long-term follow-up. Ann Neurol 1984; 15: 240–244.

* Fukushima T. Microvascular decompression for hemifacial spasm and trigeminal neuralgia. J Neurol Neurosurg Psychiatry 1990; 53: 811.

* Fusco BM, Alessandri M. Analgesic effect of capsaicin in idiopathic trigeminal neuralgia. Anesth Analg 1992; 74: 375–377.

* Fuse T, Moller MB. Delayed and progressive hearing loss after microvascular decompression of cranial nerves. Ann Otol Rhinol Laryngol 1996; 105: 158–161.

Garvan NJ, Siegfried J. Trigeminal neuralgia — earlier referral for surgery. Postgr Med J 1983; 59(693): 435–437.

*** Gilron I, Booher SL, Rowan MS, Smoller MS, Max MB. A randomized, controlled trial of high-dose dextromethorphan in facial neuralgias. Neurology 2000; 55: 964–971.

*** Gilron I, Booher SL, Rowan JS, Max MB. Topiramate in trigeminal neuralgia: a randomized, placebo-controlled multiple crossover pilot study. Clin Neuropharmacol 2001; 24: 109–112.

* Gocer AI, Cetinalp E, Tuna M, Gezercan Y, Ildan F. Fatal complication of the percutaneous radiofrequency trigeminal rhizotomy, Acta Neurochir 1997; 139(4): 373–374.

* Gordon A, Hitchcock ER. Illness behaviour and personality in intractable facial pain syndromes. Pain 1983; 17: 267–276.

* Goya T, Wakisaka S, Kinoshita K. Microvascular decompres-

sion for trigeminal neuralgia with special reference to delayed recurrence. Neurol Med Chir (Tokyo) 1990; 30: 462–467.

* Graff-Radford SB, Simmons M, Fox L, White S, Solberg WK. Are bony cavities exclusively associated with atypical facial pain and trigeminal neuralgia? Proc. Western USA Pain Soc 1 1988.

* Grant FC. Alcohol injection in the treatment of major trigeminal neuralgia. JAMA 1936; 107: 771–774.

* Gregg JM, Small EW. Surgical management of trigeminal pain with radiofrequency lesions of peripheral nerves. J Oral Maxillofac Surg 1986; 44: 122–125.

* Hakanson S. Trigeminal neuralgia treated by the injection of glycerol into the trigeminal cistern. Neurosurgery 1981; 9: 638–646.

* Hamlyn PJ. Neurovascular Compression of the Cranial Nerves in Neurological and Systematic Disease. Elsevier, Amsterdam, 1999.

* Hamlyn PJ, King TT. Neurovascular compression in trigeminal neuralgia: a clinical and anatomical study. J Neurosurg 1992; 76: 948–954.

* Hanakita J, Kondo A. Serious complications of microvascular decompression operations for trigeminal neuralgia and hemifacial spasm. Neurosurgery 1988; 22: 348–352.

* Harris W. Neuritis and Neuralgia. Oxford University Press, Oxford, 1926, pp 150–222.

* Hasegawa T, Kondziolka D, Spiro R, Flickinger JC, Lunsford LD. Repeat radiosurgery for refractory trigeminal neuralgia. Neurosurgery 2002; 50: 494–502.

* Henderson WR. Trigeminal neuralgia: the pain and its treatment. Br Med J 1967; 1: 7–15.

** Ho M, Pazin GJ, Armstrong JA, Haverkos HS, Dummer JS, Jannetta PJ. Paradoxical effects of interferon on reactivation of oral infection with herpes simplex virus after microvascular decompression for trigeminal neuralgia. J Infect Dis 1984; 150: 867–872.

* Hochman MS. Jaw clenching following Gamma Knife treatment for trigeminal neuralgia. Neurology 1998; 50(4): 1193–1194.

* Hooge JP, Redekop WK. Trigeminal neuralgia in multiple sclerosis. Neurology 1995; 45: 1294–1296.

* Horrax G, Poppen JL. Trigeminal neuralgia. Experiences with and treatment employed in 468 patients during the past 10 years. Surg Gynecol Obst 1935; 61: 394–402.

* Iannone A, Baker AB, Morrell F. Dilantin in the treatment of trigeminal neuralgia. Neurology 1958; 8: 126–128.

* Ischia S, Luzzani A, Polati E, Ischia A. Percutaneous controlled thermocoagulation in the treatment of trigeminal neuralgia. Clin J Pain 1990a; 6(2): 96–104.

* Ischia S, Luzzani A, Polati E. Retrogasserian glycerol injection: a retrospective study of 112 patients. Clin J Pain 1990b; 6(4): 291–296.

* Jannetta PJ, Bissonette DJ. Management of the failed patient with trigeminal neuralgia. Clin Neurosurg 1985; 32: 334–347.

SR Jensen TS. Anticonvulsants in neuropathic pain: rationale and clinical evidence. Eur J Pain 2002; 6(Suppl A): 61–68.

* Jho HD, Lunsford LD. Percutaneous retrogasserian glycerol rhizotomy. Current technique and results. Neurosurg Clin N Am 1997; 8: 63–74.

* Kakizawa T, Shimizu T, Fukushima T. [Monitoring of auditory brainstem response (ABR) during microvascular decompression (MVD): results in 400 cases]. No To Shinkei 1990; 42: 991–998.

* Kanpolat Y, Savas A. Radiosurgery and trigeminal neuralgia. J Neurosurg 2001; 94: 1018–1019.

Katusic S, Beard CM, Bergstralh E, Kurland LT. Incidence and clinical features of trigeminal neuralgia, Rochester, Minnesota, 1945–1984. Ann Neurol 1990; 27: 89–95.

* Khan OA. Gabapentin relieves trigeminal neuralgia in multiple sclerosis patients. Neurology 1998; 51: 611–614.

*** Killian JM, Fromm GH. Carbamazepine in the treatment of neuralgia. Use of side effects. Arch Neurol 1968; 19: 129–136.

Kitt CA, Gruber K, Davis M, Woolf CJ, Levine JD. Trigeminal neuralgia: opportunities for research and treatment. Pain 2000; 85: 3–7.

* Klun B. Microvascular decompression and partial sensory rhizotomy in the treatment of trigeminal neuralgia: personal experience with 220 patients. Neurosurgery 1992; 30: 49–52.

* Kondo A. Follow-up results of microvascular decompression in trigeminal neuralgia and hemifacial spasm. Neurosurgery 1997; 40: 46–51; discussion 51–52.

*** Kondziolka D, Lemley T, Kestle JR, Lunsford LD, Fromm GH, Jannetta PJ. The effect of single-application topical ophthalmic anesthesia in patients with trigeminal neuralgia. A randomized double-blind placebo-controlled trial. J Neurosurg 1994a; 80: 993–997.

* Kondziolka D, Lunsford LD, Bissonette DJ. Long-term results after glycerol rhizotomy for multiple sclerosis-related trigeminal neuralgia. Can J Neurol Sci 1994b; 21: 137–140.

* Kondziolka D, Lunsford LD, Flickinger JC, Young RF, Vermeulen S, Duma CM, Jacques DB, Rand RW, Regis J, Peragut JC, Manera L, Epstein MH, Lindquist C. Stereotactic radiosurgery for trigeminal neuralgia: a multiinstitutional study using the gamma unit. J Neurosurg 1996; 84: 940–945.

* Kondziolka D, Lunsford LD, Habeck M, Flickinger JC. Gamma knife radiosurgery for trigeminal neuralgia. Neurosurg Clin N Am 1997; 8: 79–85.

Kondziolka D, Lacomis D, Niranjan A, Mori Y, Maesawa S, Fellows W, Lunsford LD. Histological effects of trigeminal nerve radiosurgery in a primate model: implications for trigeminal neuralgia radiosurgery. Neurosurgery 2000; 46: 971–976.

* Kuchta J, Moller AR, Wedekind C, Jannetta PJ. Delayed hearing loss after microvascular decompression of the trigeminal nerve. Acta Neurochir (Wien) 1998; 140: 94–97.

Kugelberg E, Lindblom U. The mechanism of the pain in trigeminal neuralgia. J Neurol Neurosurg Psychiatry 1959; 22: 36–43.

* Kureshi SA, Wilkins RH. Posterior fossa reexploration for persistent or recurrent trigeminal neuralgia or hemifacial

spasm: surgical findings and therapeutic implications. Neurosurgery 1998; 43: 1111–1117.

*Lahuerta J, Lipton S, Miles J. Percutaneous radio frequency gangliolysis in the treatment of trigeminal neuralgia. Eur Neurol 1985; 24: 272–275.

*Latchaw JP Jr, Hardy RW Jr, Forsythe SB, Cook AF. Trigeminal neuralgia treated by radiofrequency coagulation. J Neurosurg 1983; 59: 479–484.

***Lechin F, van der Dijs B, Lechin ME, Amat J, Lechin AE, Cabrera A, Gomez F, Acosta E, Arocha L, Villa S, Jienez V. Pimozide therapy for trigeminal neuralgia. Arch Neurol 1989; 46: 960–963.

Leksell I. The sterotaxis method and radiosurgery of the brain. Acta Chir Scand 1951; 102: 316–319.

*Liao JJ, Cheng WC, Chang CN, Yang JT, Wei KC, Hsu YH, Lin TK. Reoperation for recurrent trigeminal neuralgia after microvascular decompression. Surg Neurol 1997; 47: 562–568.

**Lichtor T, Mullan JF. A 10-year follow-up review of percutaneous microcompression of the trigeminal ganglion. J Neurosurg 1990; 72(1): 49–54.

Linderoth B, Hakanson S. Retrogasserian glycerol rhizolysis in trigeminal neuralgia. In: Schmidek HH, Sweet WH (eds) Operative Neurosurgical Techniques. W.B. Saunders, Philadelphia, PA, 1995.

**Lindstrom P, Lindblom V. The analgesic effect of tocainide in trigeminal neuralgia. Pain 1987; 28: 45–50.

*Linskey ME, Jho HD, Jannetta PJ. Microvascular decompression for trigeminal neuralgia caused by vertebrobasilar compression J Neurosurg 1994; 81: 1–9.

*Lobato RD, Rivas JJ, Sarabia R, Lamas E. Percutaneous microcompression of the gasserian ganglion for trigeminal neuralgia. J Neurosurg 1990; 72(4): 546–553.

Love S, Coakham HB. Trigeminal neuralgia: pathology and pathogenesis. Brain 2001; 124: 2347–2360.

*Lovely TJ, Jannetta PJ. Microvascular decompression for trigeminal neuralgia. Surgical technique and long-term results. Neurosurg Clin N Am 1997; 8: 11–29.

*Lunardi G, Leandri M, Albano C, Cultrera S, Fracassi M, Rubino V, Favale E. Clinical effectiveness of lamotrigine and plasma levels in essential and symptomatic trigeminal neuralgia. Neurology 1997; 48: 1714–1717.

Macdonald BK, Cockerell OC, Sander JW, Shorvon SD. The incidence and lifetime prevalence of neurological disorders in a prospective community-based study in the UK. Brain 2000; 123(Pt 4): 665–676.

*Maesawa S, Salame C, Flickinger JC, Pirris S, Kondziolka D, Lunsford LD. Clinical outcomes after stereotactic radiosurgery for idiopathic trigeminal neuralgia. J Neurosurg 2001; 94: 14–20.

*Maher CO, Pollock BE. Radiation induced vascular injury after stereotactic radiosurgery for trigeminal neuralgia: case report. Surg Neurol 2000; 54: 189–193.

**Majoie CB, Hulsmans FJ, Verbeeten BJ, Castelijns JA, van Beek EJ, Valk J, Bosch DA. Trigeminal neuralgia: comparison of two MR imaging techniques in the demonstration of neurovascular contact. Radiology 1997; 204: 455–460.

*Marbach JJ, Lund P. Depression, anhedonia and anxiety in temporomandibular joint and other facial pain syndromes. Pain 1981; 11: 73–84.

*Mason DA. Peripheral neurectomy in the treatment of trigeminal neuralgia of the second and third division. J Oral Surg 1972; 30: 113–120.

*Masur H, Papke K, Bongartz G, Vollbrecht K. The significance of three-dimensional MR-defined neurovascular compression for the pathogenesis of trigeminal neuralgia. J Neurol 1995; 242: 93–98.

Mathews ES, Scrivani SJ. Percutaneous stereotactic radiofrequency thermal rhizotomy for the treatment of trigeminal neuralgia. Mount Sinai J Med 2000; 67(4): 288–299.

*McCleane G. 200 mg daily of lamotrigine has no analgesic effect in neuropathic pain: a randomised, double-blind, placebo controlled trial. Pain 1999; 83: 105–107.

*McLaughlin MR, Jannetta PJ, Clyde BL, Subach BR, Comey CH, Resnick DK. Microvascular decompression of cranial nerves: lessons learned after 4400 operations. J Neurosurg 1999; 90: 1–8.

SR McQuay H. Neuropathic pain: evidence matters. Eur J Pain 2002; 6: 11–18.

SR McQuay H, Carroll D, Jadad AR, Wiffen P, Moore A. Anticonvulsant drugs for management of pain: a systematic review. BMJ 1995; 311: 1047–1052.

**Meaney JF, Eldridge PR, Dunn LT, Nixon TE, Whitehouse GH, Miles JB. Demonstration of neurovascular compression in trigeminal neuralgia with magnetic resonance imaging. Comparison with surgical findings in 52 consecutive operative cases. J Neurosurg 1995a; 83: 799–805.

*Meaney JF, Watt JW, Eldridge PR, Whitehouse GH, Wells JC, Miles JB. Association between trigeminal neuralgia and multiple sclerosis: role of magnetic resonance imaging. J Neurol Neurosurg Psychiatry 1995b; 59: 253–259.

*Melendez JC, McCrank E. Anxiety-related reactions associated with magnetic resonance imaging examinations. JAMA 1993; 270: 745–747.

**Melzack R, Terrence C, Fromm G, Amsel R. Trigeminal neuralgia and atypical facial pain: use of the McGill Pain Questionnaire for discrimination and diagnosis. Pain 1986; 27: 297–302.

*Mendoza N, Illingworth RD. Trigeminal neuralgia treated by microvascular decompression: a long-term follow-up study. Br J Neurosurg 1995; 9(1): 13–19.

*Miles JB, Eldridge PR, Haggett CE, Bowsher D. Sensory effects of microvascular decompression in trigeminal neuralgia. J Neurosurg 1997; 86: 193–196.

*Mittal B, Thomas DG. Controlled thermocoagulation in trigeminal neuralgia. J Neurol Neurosurg Psychiatry 1986; 49: 932–936.

*Moller AR, Moller MB. Does intraoperative monitoring of auditory evoked potentials reduce incidence of hearing loss as a complication of microvascular decompression of cranial nerves? Neurosurgery 1989; 24: 257–263.

Munoz M, Dumas M, Boutros-Toni F, Coquelle D, Vallat JM, Jauberteau MO, Ndzanga E, Boa F, Ndo D. A neuro-epidemiologic survey in a Limousin town. Rev Neurol (Paris) 1988; 144: 266–271.

* Murali R. Peripheral nerve injections and avulsions in the treatment of trigeminal neuralgia. In: Rovit RL, Murali R, Jannetta PJ (eds) Trigeminal Neuralgia. Williams and Wilkins, Baltimore, MD, 1990.

* Murali R, Rovit RL. Are peripheral neurectomies of value in the treatment of trigeminal neuralgia? An analysis of new cases and cases involving previous radiofrequency gasserian thermocoagulation. J Neurosurg 1996; 85: 435–437.

* Nicol B, Regine WF, Courtney C, Meigooni A, Sanders M, Young B. Gamma knife radiosurgery using 90 Gy for trigeminal neuralgia. J Neurosurg 2000; 93(Suppl 3): 152–154.

*** Nicol CF. A four year double-blind study of tegretol in facial pain. Headache 1969; 9: 54–57.

* Niemeyer FP. Neurovascular decompression in trigeminal neuralgia. Analysis of 70 cases. Arq Neuro-Psiquiatria 1983; 41(4): 321–331.

* North RB, Kidd DH, Piantadosi S, Carson BS. Percutaneous retrogasserian glycerol rhizotomy. Predictors of success and failure in treatment of trigeminal neuralgia. J Neurosurg 1990; 72: 851–856.

* Nugent GR. Radiofrequency treatment of trigeminal neuralgia using a cordotomy-type electrode. A method. Neurosurg Clin N Am 1997; 8: 41–52.

* Nugent GR, Berry B. Trigeminal neuralgia treated by differential percutaneous radiofrequency coagulation of the Gasserian ganglion. J Neurosurg 1974; 40: 517–523.

* Nurmikko TJ. Altered cutaneous sensation in trigeminal neuralgia. Arch Neurol 1991; 48: 523–527.

* Nurmikko TJ, Eldridge PR. Trigeminal neuralgia — pathophysiology, diagnosis and current treatment. Br J Anaesth 2001; 87: 117–132.

* Nurmikko TJ, Haggett CE, Miles J. Neurogenic vasodilation trigeminal neuralgia. In: Devor M, Rowbotham MC, Wiesnfeld-Hallin Z (eds) Proceedings of the 9th World Congress of Pain. IASP Press, Seattle, WA, 2000: 747–755.

* Ogungbo BI, Kelly P, Kane PJ, Nath FP. Microvascular decompression for trigeminal neuralgia: report of outcome in patients over 65 years of age. Br J Neurosurg 2000; 14: 23–27.

* Oturai AB, Jensen K, Eriksen J, Madsen F. Neurosurgery for trigeminal neuralgia: comparison of alcohol block, neurectomy, and radiofrequency coagulation. Clin J Pain 1996; 12: 311–315.

Patsolos PN. In: Zakrezewska JM (ed), Trigeminal Neuralgia. W.B. Saunders, London, 1995: pp. 80–107.

* Peiris JB, Perera GL, Devendra SV, Lionel ND. Sodium valproate in trigeminal neuralgia. Med J Aust 1980; 2: 278–279.

Penman J. In: Vinken PJ, Bruyn GN (eds), Handbook of Clinical Neurology. Elsevier Science, Amsterdam, 1968: pp. 269–322.

* Piatt JH Jr, Wilkins RH. Microvascular decompression for tic douloureux. Neurosurgery 1984; 15: 456.

* Politis C, Adriaensen H, Bossuyt M, Fossion E. The management of trigeminal neuralgia with cryotherapy. Acta Stomatol Belg 1988; 85: 197–205.

* Pollack IF, Jannetta PJ, Bissonette DJ. Bilateral trigeminal neuralgia: a 14-year experience with microvascular decompression. J Neurosurg 1988; 68: 559–565.

* Pollock BE, Phuong LK, Foote RL, Stafford SL, Gorman DA. High-dose trigeminal neuralgia radiosurgery associated with increased risk of trigeminal nerve dysfunction. Neurosurgery 2001; 49: 58–62.

* Puca A, Meglio M, Vari R, Tamburrini G, Tancredi A. Evaluation of fifth nerve dysfunction in 136 patients with middle and posterior cranial fossae tumors. Eur Neurol 35: 1995; 33–37.

* Rand RW. Leksell Gamma Knife treatment of tic douloureux. Neurosurg Clin N Am 1997; 8: 75–78.

* Rappaport ZH, Gomori JM. 1988; Recurrent trigeminal cistern glycerol injections for tic douloureux. Acta Neurochir (Wien) 90: 31–34.

* Rasmussen P. Facial Pain 1. A prospective survey of 1052 patients with a view of: definition, delimitation,classification, general data, genetic factors and previous diseases. Acta Neurochir (Wien) 1990a; 107: 112–120.

* Rasmussen P. Facial pain. II. A prospective survey of 1052 patients with a view of: character of the attacks, onset, course, and character of pain. Acta Neurochir (Wien) 1990b; 107: 121–128.

* Rasmussen P. Facial pain. III. A prospective study of the localization of facial pain in 1052 patients. Acta Neurochir (Wien) 1991a; 108: 53–63.

* Rasmussen P. Facial pain. IV. A prospective study of 1052 patients with a view of: precipitating factors, associated symptoms, objective psychiatric and neurological symptoms. Acta Neurochir (Wien) 1991b; 108: 100–109.

* Rath SA, Klein HJ, Richter HP. Findings and long-term results of subsequent operations after failed microvascular decompression for trigeminal neuralgia. Neurosurgery 1996; 39: 933–938; discussion 938–40.

* Ratner EJ, Person P, Kleinman DJ, Shklar G, Socransky SS. Jawbone cavities and trigeminal and atypical facial neuralgias. Oral Surg Oral Med Oral Pathol 1979; 48: 3–20.

* Regis J, Manera L, Dufour H, Porcheron D, Sedan R, Peragut JC. Effect of the Gamma Knife on trigeminal neuralgia. Stereotact Funct Neurosurg 1995; 64(Suppl 1): 182–192.

* Remillard G. Oxcarbazepine and intractable trigeminal neuralgia. Epilepsia 1994; 35: s28–s29.

* Resnick DK, Jannetta PJ, Lunsford LD, Bissonette DJ. Microvascular decompression for trigeminal neuralgia in patients with multiple sclerosis. Surg Neurol 1996; 46: 358–361.

* Rogers CL, Shetter AG, Fiedler JA, Smith KA, Han PP, Speiser BL. 2000; Gamma knife radiosurgery for trigeminal neuralgia: the initial experience of The Barrow Neurological Institute. Int J Radiat Oncol Biol Phys 47: 1013–1019.

Rothman KJ, Monson RR. Epidemiology of trigeminal neuralgia. J Chron Dis 1973a; 26: 3–12.

Rothman KJ, Monson RR. Survival in trigeminal neuralgia. J Chron Dis 1973b; 26: 303–309.

Rothman KJ, Beckman TM. Epidemiological evidence for two types of trigeminal neuralgia. Lancet 1974; 1: 7–9.

Rothman KJ, Wepsic JG. Side of facial pain in trigeminal neuralgia. J Neurosurg 1974; 40: 514–523.

Rovit RL. Trigeminal neuralgia. [Review]. Compr Ther 1992; 18: 17–21.

* Royal M, Wienecke G, Movva V, Ward S, Bhakta B, Jensen, M, Gunyea I. Open label trial of oxcarbazepine in neuropathic pain. Pain Med 2001; 2: 250–251.

* Rushton JG, Macdonald HNA Trigeminal neuralgia. Special considerations of nonsurgical treatment. JAMA 1957; 165: 437–440.

Sahni KS, Pieper DR, Anderson R, Baldwin NG. Relation of hypesthesia to the outcome of glycerol rhizolysis for trigeminal neuralgia. J Neurosurg 1990; 72: 55–58.

* Saini SS. Retrogasserian anhydrous glycerol injection therapy in trigeminal neuralgia: observations in 552 patients. J Neurol Neurosurg Psychiatry 1987; 50: 1536–1538.

* Schvarcz JR. Percutaneous thermocontrolled differential retrogasserian rhizotomy for idiopathic trigeminal neuralgia, Acta Neurochir (Wien) 1982; 64(1–2): 51–58.

* Shuhan G, Benren X, Yuhuan Z. Treatment of primary trigeminal neuralgia with acupuncture in 1500 cases. J Tradit Chin Med 1991; 11: 3–6.

* Sindou M, Mertens P. Microsurgical vascular decompression (MVD) in trigeminal and glosso-vago-pharyngeal neuralgias. A twenty year experience. Acta Neurochir Suppl (Wien) 1993; 58: 168–170.

* Sindou M, Amrani F, Mertens P. [Microsurgical vascular decompression in trigeminal neuralgia. Comparison of 2 technical modalities and physiopathologic deductions. A study of 120 cases]. Neurochirurgie 1990; 36: 16–25.

* Sindou M, Amrani F, Mertens P. Does microsurgical vascular decompression for trigeminal neuralgia work through a neocompressive mechanism? Anatomical–surgical evidence for a decompressive effect. Acta Neurochir Suppl (Wien) 1991; 52: 127–129.

SR Sindrup SH, Jensen TS. Efficacy of pharmacological treatments of neuropathic pain: an update and effect related to mechanism of drug action. Pain 1999; 83: 389–400.

* Sist T, Filadora V, Miner M, Lema M. Gabapentin for idiopathic trigeminal neuralgia: report of two cases. Neurology 1997; 48: 1467.

* Skirving DJ, Dan NG. A 20-year review of percutaneous balloon compression of the trigeminal ganglion. J Neurosurg 2001; 94: 913–917.

* Slettebo H, Eide PK. A prospective study of microvascular decompression for trigeminal neuralgia, Acta Neurochir (Wien) 1997; 139(5): 421–425.

* Slettebo H, Hirschberg H, Lindegaard KF. Long-term results after percutaneous retrogasserian glycerol rhizotomy in patients with trigeminal neuralgia. Acta Neurochir (Wien) 1993; 122: 231–235.

* Smirne S, Scarlato G. Clonazepam in cranial neuralgias. Med J Aust 1977; 1: 93–94.

* Solaro C, Messmer UM, Uccelli A, Leandri M, Mancardi GL. Low-dose gabapentin combined with either lamotrigine or carbamazepine can be useful therapies for trigeminal neuralgia in multiple sclerosis. Eur Neurol 2000; 44: 45–48.

* Solaro C, Uccelli MM, Brichetto G, Gaspperini C, Mancardi G. Topiramate relieves idiopathic and symptomatic trigeminal neuralgia. J Pain Symptom Manage 2001; 21: 367–368.

* Spaziante R, Cappabianca P, Peca C, de Divitiis E. Subarachnoid hemorrhage and 'normal pressure hydrocephalus': fatal complication of percutaneous microcompression of the gasserian ganglion. Case report. Neurosurgery 1988; 22(1 Pt 1): 148–151.

* Spaziante R, Cappabianca P, Saini M, Peca C, Mariniello G, de Divitiis E. Treatment of trigeminal neuralgia by ophthalmic anesthetic [letter]. J Neurosurg 1992; 77: 159–160.

*** Stajcic Z, Juniper RP, Todorovic L. Peripheral streptomycin/lidocaine injections versus lidocaine alone in the treatment of idiopathic trigeminal neuralgia. A double blind controlled trial. J Craniomaxillofac Surg 1990; 18: 243–246.

* Steardo L, Leo A, Marano E. Efficacy of baclofen in trigeminal neuralgia and some other painful conditions. A clinical trial. Eur Neurol 1984; 23: 51–55.

* Steiger HJ. Prognostic factors in the treatment of trigeminal neuralgia. Analysis of a differential therapeutic approach. Acta Neurochir (Wien) 1991; 113: 11–17.

* Sun SY, Yin JZ, Qiu LL. Microvascular decompression for trigeminal neuralgia. Chin Med J (Engl) 1994; 107: 286–288.

Sweet WH. Complications of treating trigeminal neuralgia: an analysis of the literature and response to questionnaire. In: Rovit RL, Murali R, Jannetta PJ (eds) Trigeminal Neuralgia. Williams and Wilkins, Baltimore, MD, 1990.

* Sweet WH, Poletti CE. Problems with retrogasserian glycerol in the treatment of trigeminal neuralgia. Appl Neurophysiol 1985; 48: 252–257.

* Sweet RL, Poletti CE. Complications of percutaneous rhizotomy and microvascular decompression operations for facial pain. In: Schmidek HH, Sweet WH (eds) Operative Neurosurgical Techniques. W.B. Saunders, Philadelphia, PA, 1995: 1543–1546.

Sweet WH, Wepsic JG. Controlled thermoregulation of trigeminal ganglion and rootlets for differential destruction of pain fibres, part 1. Trigeminal neuralgia. J Neur Surg 1974; 143–158.

* Sweet WH, Poletti CE, Roberts JT. Dangerous rises in blood pressure upon heating of trigeminal rootlets; increased bleeding times in patients with trigeminal neuralgia. Neurosurgery 1985; 17: 843–844.

* Szapiro J Jr, Sindou M, Szapiro J. Prognostic factors in microvascular decompression for trigeminal neuralgia. Neurosurgery 1985; 17: 920–929.

* Tacconi L, Miles JB. Bilateral trigeminal neuralgia: a therapeutic dilemma. Br J Neurosurg 2000; 14: 33–39.

* Taha JM, Tew JM Jr. Comparison of surgical treatments for trigeminal neuralgia: reevaluation of radiofrequency rhizotomy. Neurosurgery 1996; 38: 865–871.

* Taha JM, Tew JM. Radiofrequency trigeminal rhizolysis. Tech Neurosurg 1999; 5: 218–224.

* Taha JM, Tew JM Jr, Buncher CR. A prospective 15-year follow up of 154 consecutive patients with trigeminal neuralgia treated by percutaneous stereotactic radiofrequency thermal rhizotomy. J Neurosurg 1995; 83: 989–993.

* Taylor JC, Brauer S, Espir MLE Long-term treatment of trigeminal neuralgia. Postgr Med J 1981; 57: 16–18.

* Tew JM, Taha JM. Percutaneous rhizotomy in the treatment of intractable facial pain (trigeminal, glossopharyngeal and vagal nerves). In: Schmidek HH, Sweet WH (eds) Operative Neurosurgical Techniques. W.B. Saunders, Philadelphia, PA, 1995: 1469–1484.

* Tronnier VM, Rasche D, Hamer J, Kienle AL, Kunze S. Treatment of idiopathic trigeminal neuralgia: comparison of long-term outcome after radiofrequency rhizotomy and microvascular decompression. Neurosurgery 2001; 48: 1261–1267.

* Tyler-Kabara EC, Kassam AB, Horowitz MH, Urgo L, Hadjipanayis C, Levy EI, Chang YF. Predictors of outcome in surgically managed patients with typical and atypical trigeminal neuralgia: comparison of results following microvascular decompression. J Neurosurg 2002; 96: 527–531.

* Urgosik D, Vymazal J, Vladyka V, Liscak R. Gamma knife treatment of trigeminal neuralgia: clinical and electrophysiological study. Stereotact Funct Neurosurg 1998; 70(Suppl 1): 200–209.

* Valzania F, Strafella AP, Nassetti SA, Tropeani A, Tassinari CA. Gabapentin in idiopathic trigeminal neuralgia. Neurology 1998; 50(4): A379.

* Vassilouthis J. Relief of trigeminal neuralgia by proparacine. J Neurol Neurosurg Psychiatry 1994; 57: 121.

*** Vilming ST, Lyberg T, Latase X. Tizanidine in the management of trigeminal neuralgia. Cephalalgia 1986; 6: 181–182.

* Vladyka V, Subrt O. The possibility of retrogasserian thermocoagulation, glycerol radiculolysis and balloon compression in Meckel's cavity with a single surgical instrumentarium. Zentralbl Neurochir 1989; 50: 149–152.

* Walchenbach R, Voormolen JH, Hermans J. Microvascular decompression for trigeminal neuralgia: a critical reappraisal. Clin Neurol Neurosurg 1994; 96(4): 290–295.

* Walker J. Relief from chronic pain by low power laser irradiation. Neurosci Lett 1983; 43: 339–344.

* Walker JB, Akhanjee LK, Cooney MM, Goldstein J, Tamayoshi S, Segal-Gidan F. Laser therapy for pain of trigeminal neuralgia. Clin J Pain 1988; 3: 183–187.

* Weddington WW Jr, Blazer D. Atypical facial pain and trigeminal neuralgia: a comparison study. Psychosomatics 1936; 20: 348–349.

Wiffen P, McQuay H, Carroll D, Jadad A, Moore A. Anticonvulsant drugs for acute and chronic pain. Cochrane Database Syst Rev 2000; 2, CD001133.

* Wilkins RH. Historical overview of surgical techniques for trigeminal neuralgia. Tech Neurosurg 1999; 5: 202–217.

* Wilkinson HA. Trigeminal nerve peripheral branch phenol/glycerol injections for tic douloureux. J Neurosurg 1999; 90: 828–832.

* Yamaki T, Hashi K, Niwa J, Tanabe S, Nakagawa T, Nakamura T, Uede T, Tsuruno T. Results of reoperation for failed microvascular decompression. Acta Neurochir (Wien) 1992; 115: 1–7.

* Yoon KB, Wiles JR, Miles JB, Nurmikko TJ. Long-term outcome of percutaneous thermocoagulation for trigeminal neuralgia. Anaesthesia 1999; 54: 803–808.

* Young RF, Vermeulen SS, Grimm P, Blasko J, Posewitz A. Gamma Knife radiosurgery for treatment of trigeminal neuralgia: idiopathic and tumor related. Neurology 1997; 48: 608–614.

* Young RF, Vermulen S, Posewitz A. Gamma knife radiosurgery for the treatment of trigeminal neuralgia. Stereotact Funct Neurosurg 1998; 70(Suppl 1): 192–199.

Zakrzewska JM. Trigeminal Neuralgia. W.S. Saunders, London, 1995.

* Zakrzewska JM. Consumer views on management of trigeminal neuralgia. Headache 2001; 41: 369–376.

SR Zakrzewska JM. Diagnosis and differential diagnosis of trigeminal neuralgia. Clin J Pain 2002a; 18: 14–21.

SR Zakrzewska JM. Trigeminal neuralgia. Clin Evidence 2002b; 7: 1221–1231.

SR Zakrzewska JM, Hamlyn PJ. Facial pain. In: Crombie IKCPR, Linton SJ, LeResche L, Von Korff M (eds) Epidemiology of Pain. IASP, Seattle, WA, 1999: 171–202.

* Zakrzewska JM, Nally FF. The role of cryotherapy (cryoanalgesia) in the management of paroxysmal trigeminal neuralgia: a six year experience. Br J Oral Maxillofac Surg 1988; 26: 18–25.

* Zakrzewska JM, Patsalos PN. Long-term cohort study comparing medical (oxcarbazepine) and surgical management of intractable trigeminal neuralgia. Pain 2002; 95: 259–266.

* Zakrzewska JM, Thomas DG. Patient's assessment of outcome after three surgical procedures for the management of trigeminal neuralgia. Acta Neurochir (Wien) 1993; 122: 225–230.

*** Zakrzewska JM, Chaudhry Z, Nurmikko TJ, Patton DW, Mullens EL. Lamotrigine (lamictal) in refractory trigeminal neuralgia: results from a double-blind placebo controlled crossover trial. Pain 1997; 73: 223–230.

* Zakrzewska JM, Jassim S, Bulman JS. A prospective, longitudinal study on patients with trigeminal neuralgia who underwent radiofrequency thermocoagulation of the Gasserian ganglion. Pain 1999; 79: 51–58.

* Zvartau-Hind M, Din MU, Gilani A, Lisak RP, Khan OA. Topiramate relieves refractory trigeminal neuralgia in MS patients. Neurology 2000; 55: 1587–1588.

Assessment and Management of Orofacial Pain
Pain Research and Clinical Management, Vol. 14
Edited by J.M. Zakrzewska and S.D. Harrison
© *2002 Elsevier Science B.V. All rights reserved*

CHAPTER 16

Burning mouth

Joanna M. Zakrzewska[*]

Department of Clinical and Diagnostic Oral Sciences, Oral Medicine Unit, Dental Institute, Barts and the London Queen Mary's School of Medicine and Dentistry, Turner Street, London E1 2AD, UK

Objectives for this chapter:

This chapter will enable you to:
- distinguish between burning mouth syndrome (BMS) and burning mouth as a symptom of disease
- list common causes of burning mouth which should be looked for and eliminated before making the final diagnosis of burning mouth syndrome
- recognise the clinical features of burning mouth syndrome patients and know how to investigate them
- suggest treatments for burning mouth syndrome which are based on a systematic review
- appreciate the need for more research if treatment is to be based on good quality evidence

1. Definition

The IASP classification defines glossodynia and sore mouth as "a burning pain in the tongue or other mucous membranes". This is a very broad definition which needs to be more carefully defined. The range of words that are used when searching the literature for articles on this topic is ample evidence that widely differing terminology is used and interpreted differently which has led to confusion both for those trying to find some literature on the topic and those doing systematic reviews. Two review articles have commented on this lack of agreed terminology and suggest clearer criteria which would enable consistencies between studies to be achieved (Tourne and Fricton, 1992; Bergdahl and Anneroth, 1993). The

TABLE 1

KEY FACTS: definition of burning mouth and alternative terminology

- Burning mouth is said to be a symptom of another disease when local or systemic factors are found to be implicated and their treatment results in resolution of burning mouth.

- Burning mouth syndrome is an intraoral burning sensation for which no medical or odontological causes can be found and in which the oral mucosa is of grossly normal appearance. Many will also have subjective dryness, parasthesia and altered taste.

Other words used: burning mouth or tongue, sore tongue, glossodynia, oral dysesthesia, stomatodynia, glossopyrosis and burning mouth syndrome

definition of the burning mouth syndrome and alternative terminology is given in Table 1.

[*] Tel. +44-20-7377-7053; Fax: +44-20-7377-7627;
E-mail: j.m.zakrzewska@qmul.ac.uk

The complaint of a burning sensation in the mouth which can be localised to the lips or tongue or be more widespread within the mouth can be a symptom of another disease or a syndrome in its own right of unknown aetiology. In other patients, however, no underlying dental or medical causes are identified and no gross oral signs are found and it is in these instances that the term burning mouth syndrome (BMS) should be used. The word syndrome is justified in that many patients will also have subjective xerostomia (dryness), oral paraesthesia and altered taste or smell. Bogetto et al. (1998) further divide these patients into those who have or have not got comorbid diagnosis especially of a psychiatric type.

2. Epidemiology

The epidemiological data on BMS are generally poor due, in part, to lack of strict adherence to diagnostic criteria. We did a systematic review on the epidemiology of BMS in 1997 and the data given below are from that review (Zakrzewska and Hamlyn, 1999). We found that prevalence rates in general populations varied from 0.7% to 15%. The reason for the wide variation was due to the fact that most surveys carried out in the community relate to burning mouth as a symptom rather than the syndrome. Tammiala-Salonen et al. (1993) carried out their survey in the Finish community using a sample of 600. Those reporting burning mouth as a symptom were then contacted and a fuller history and examination were performed. After completion of all investigations and treatments the number of patients still with a complaint of burning mouth was down from 15% to 1%. This latter group probably represents those patients with burning mouth syndrome (BMS). What data is available seems to indicate that BMS affects predominantly females with an increased prevalence with age and following menopause (Zakrzewska and Hamlyn, 1999). The natural history of BMS has not clearly been defined and there are no reports of longitudinal cohort studies. Risk factors and high risk patients have not been identified although it would appear that post-menopausal women are at highest

risk. There are anecdotal reports of at least partial spontaneous remission in approximately half of these patients within 6 to 7 years (Grushka et al., 1986a).

3. Aetiology

The cause of burning mouth syndrome is essentially unknown, although a wide range of factors has been suggested as a possible cause of burning but none have been the subject of high quality research and the level of evidence is at best at level 4 (Chapter 1). Proposed causes of burning as suggested in reviews (not systematic) are shown in Table 2 (Tourne and Fricton, 1992; Bergdahl and Anneroth, 1993).

These small case series, some only single case reports, uncontrolled in most instances, lacking replication and standardised outcome measures to determine

TABLE 2

KEY FACTS: proposed causes of the symptom burning mouth

Site	Cause
Local	fungal — candidiasis
	xerostomia — mucositis, immunological diseases
	geographic tongue
	oral parafunctional habits especially tongue thrusting
	oesophageal reflux
	poor denture design
	allergy to denture material, foodstuffs, fillings
	nerve damage — chordi tympani during extractions
Systemic	climacteric
	vitamin B_{12} deficiency
	folate deficiency
	iron deficiency
	immunologically mediated diseases, e.g. Sjogren's
	psychogenic — anxiety, depression, personality
	diabetes indirectly due to candidiasis
	cancerphobia
	psychosocial stressors — life events
	drugs, e.g. ACE inhibitors

whether corrections result in resolution of symptoms, add little to our knowledge and confuse the unwary reader. You can find a recent review on this in a book reporting the proceedings of the third World Workshop on Oral Medicine (Truelove et al., 2000). Although standard examination in patients with BMS reveals no abnormalities, more sophisticated testing indicates that neuronal mechanisms may be involved. Grushka et al. (1987a) and Svensson et al. (1993) have suggested that these patients may have altered sensory and pain threshold and Jääskeläinen et al. (1997) have found abnormal blink reflexes in chronic burning mouth patients. Cekic-Arambasin et al. (1990) have shown temperature changes on the tongue in BMS patients as compared to controls.

Patients with BMS often complain of phantom tastes and this has led to the theory that patients with BMS are so called supertasters and have sustained damage to the VII nerve (Grushka and Bartoshuk, 2000). Bartoshuk (2000) has identified groups of people, more frequently females, as being 'supertasters'. These people taste PROP (6-*n*-propylthiouracil) as intensely bitter and have the highest density of fungiform papillae on the dorsum of the tongue which are responsible for taste. Supertasters not only have a heightened sensation of taste but they are also more likely to react to noxious stimuli. They have also suggested that VII (taste of the anterior part of the tongue) normally inhibits IX (taste of the posterior part of the tongue) but if the VII is damaged or anaesthetised the inhibitions are released and so give rise to phantom tastes. They suggest that a similar mechanism is present between the VII and V. Bartoshuk et al. (1999) hypothesise that BMS patients have sustained damage to VII and are supertasters. In their study of BMS patients (postmenopausal 17, premenopausal 5, male 9), the peak intensity of burning correlated with the number of fungiform papillae ($r = 0.8$, $p < 0.0001$). That is, the most intense burn was experienced by supertasters. BMS patients showed severe damage to VII, particularly for bitter, as compared to 72 young adult controls.

A study on 53 patients who sustained damage to their lingual nerve during wisdom tooth surgery reported that 64% of them complain of taste distur-

bance and that post-repair more fungiform papillae are detected on the affected side than pre-operatively (pre-operatively 74% have fewer fungiform papillae than on the opposite side and this changed to 45% post-operatively). In the long term it is not known whether these patients develop BMS later in life although 47% report oral dysaesthesiae (Robinson et al., 2000).

Many of these patients show evidence of anxiety, depression, somatisation and personality disorders as discussed under clinical features. Some of these may be as a result of the frustration of coping with the condition rather than predisposing factors. Patients with BMS are more likely to have other health problems (Svensson and Kaaber, 1995; Bogetto et al., 1998; Bergdahl and Bergdahl, 1999).

4. Clinical features

Before reading the text on clinical features look through the case studies in Table 3 and see if you can come to a diagnosis.

4.1. History

The diagnosis is made mainly on history and only those studies based on prospective studies with adequate control data or epidemiological surveys with clear diagnostic criteria are quoted (Grushka, 1987; Grushka et al., 1987a,b; Tammiala-Salonen et al., 1993; Eli et al., 1994a,b; Svensson and Kaaber, 1995; Bogetto et al., 1998; Bergdahl and Bergdahl, 1999). The level of evidence ranges from 3b to 4 (see Chapter 1). There are several other reports on the clinical features but the findings may be biased due to lack of control data. The key features are summarised in Table 4, whereas Table 5 describes the studies that have been used to contribute to the characterisation of the syndrome.

Many patients present with a chronic history. Around two third of patients cannot relate the onset of their symptoms to any factors but others will relate it to either dental treatment or some other illness such as upper respiratory tract infection (Grushka, 1987;

TABLE 3

Case studies 1 and 2

List what you would consider some key features of BMS to be. Now read the two case reports and based on your list decide if they should be considered to be BMS. A fuller explanation of the measures used and their significance can be found in Chapter 6.

CASE 1

Name	EW
Age	89
Gender	female
Development of pain	slowly developed over the last year and not associated with any illness
Character	sore, hot, tender, annoying, numb, nauseating, not a pain
Site/radiation	tongue only in all areas
Severity 0–10	from Brief Pain Inventory (BPI) current 7, worse 8, least 6
Duration and periodicity	continuous and tends to be worse towards the end of the day, varies in severity daily, may wake at night, no pain-free periods
Provoking factors	eating sharp foods such as toast
Relieving factors	nothing
Associated factors	altered taste, dry mouth, clenches teeth, cheeks feel rough, headaches, neck and back pains
Medical history	angina, high blood pressure, diverticulitis, recent carpal tunnel operations
Current drugs	isosorbide, calcium channel blocker, diuretic, iron, folic acid
McGill Pain Questionnaire (MPQ)	pain rating index (PRI) total 9, sensory 4, affective 0, evaluative 1, misc. 4, number of words chose (NWC) 6, present pain intensity 3
Hospital anxiety and depression (HAD) scores 0–21	anxiety 12, depression 13 — indicates possible presence of anxiety and depression
Brief Pain Inventory (BPI) scores 0–10 on quality of life	mood, sleep, enjoyment all scored 3, rest of interference 0
Social factors	widowed 22 years, lives with daughter, last three years marked deterioration of health which has restricted her social life; all 8 of her siblings have died, sister 10 years her junior died 2 years ago from cancer of the ear
Health beliefs	may have oral cancer
Examination	full denture wearer, geographic tongue

CASE 2

Name	SD
Age	58
Gender	female
Development of pain	most of her symptoms began 3 years ago after dental treatment; her taste problem has been present for 30 years; the problem is getting worse
Character	tingling, burning
Site and radiation	all parts of the mouth including tongue and lips and spreads to her throat
Severity 1–10	from BPI current 8, worse 8, least 6, average 7
Duration/periodicity	intermittent, weeks when pain-free
Provoking factors	none
Relieving factors	courses of antibiotics
Associated factors	altered taste, especially fruit taste bad or no taste present for 30 years, dry mouth, dry eyes, dry skin
Medical history	severe arthritis
Current drugs	analgesics
HAD scores 0–21	anxiety 10, depression 12
BPI scores 1–10	activity 8, mood 10, walking 2, work 7, relationships 9, sleep 10, enjoyment 10
Social factors	widowed 18 years ago, death of 16-year-old daughter 16 years ago, 2 other children, retired on medical grounds 2 years ago

Please see Table 13 at the end of the chapter for the answers.

TABLE 4

KEY FACTS: clinical features of burning mouth syndrome

Duration	mean time to development 3 years, builds up gradually
Periodicity	some patients have continuous symptoms, in others the sensation builds up over the day being worse in the evening
Character	may be described as a pain or discomfort, burning, smarting, tender and annoying
Site	often more than one site, tongue most common, cheeks, gingiva, palate
Radiation	remains in the mouth
Severity	ranges from mild to moderate
Provoking factors	tension, fatigue
Relieving factors	sleep, cold foods, distraction
Associated factors	taste changes, mood changes, tongue thrusting, dryness
Examination	in BMS no gross changes found, although may be some dryness

TABLE 5

Clinical features of burning mouth syndrome (BMS) as described in published studies

Duration	mean time 3 years or over (3 months to 18 years) [1,5,7]; mean time 2.3 years (2 months to 10 years) [6]; less than 1 year 47% [2]
Periodicity	builds up over the day, worse in the evening 75% [1], 33% [5]; continuous once started 100% [1], 85% [6], 65% [5]; intermittent 85% [2,3], 30% [5], 14% [7]
Character	McGill descriptions: burning 85% [4], 62% [7], smarting 55% [7], tender 51% [4,7], annoying 51% [4,7], tiring 37% [4], 34% [7], nagging 37% [4], pricking 34% [7]; others: burning 76% [5], 64% [6]; itchy 27%, dull 25%, stinging 25% [5]
Site	often more than one site 92% [1], 57% [5], 38% [2], 34% [3]; tongue (especially tip) 78% [1,5], 70% [7], 67% [3]; gingiva 25% [1], 11% [3], 60% [5]; whole mouth 8% [3]; anterior hard palate 65% [7], 49% [1,5], 6% [3]; lips 49% [1], 45% [5], 38% [7], 6% [3]
Radiation	none
Severity	mild to moderate 73% [2]; mean 6.3, range 2.1–10.5 on VAS 1–150 cm [1]; mean 4.6 [3], 5.2 [7], 7.2 [6], range 2–9 on VAS of 1–10 cm
Provoking factors	tension 78%, fatigue 54%, speaking 44%, hot foods 38% [1]
Relieving factors	sleep 69%, cold foods 52%, eating 58%, working 52%, distraction 48%, alcohol 27% [1]
Associated factors	taste changes 69% [1], 40% [2,7], 25% [5], 11% [3]; dryness 63% [1], 66% [3], 55% [5], 53% [7]; difficulty falling asleep 75%, mood changes 71%, nausea 17%, headaches 21%, dizziness 19% [1]; tongue thrusting 60%, clenching 9% [5]; neurotic trait with depression on MMPI [4,5]; high scores on SCL90 [6], see Chapter 6 for explanation; female over 50 years [1,2,3,5,7]; menopausal symptoms rated more severe than controls [1]; more than one other pain complaint 81% [1,7]; lifetime history of psychiatric disorder 70% [5]

[1] Grushka (1987): case control 72 BMS, 43 age, gender matched.
[2] Tammiala-Salonen et al. (1993): 600 patients in epidemiological survey, 34 BMS.
[3] Bergdahl and Bergdahl (1999): 1000 patients of which 53 BMS.
[4] Grushka et al. (1987b): case control, 72 BMS, 43 gender, age same group as foot note 1.
[5] Bogetto et al. (1998): case control 102 BMS, divides into groups with or without co-morbid conditions and use mean, 102 age, gender, marital status, education, social class matched.
[6] Eli et al. (1994a): case control 45 BMS, 45 age, gender, race, education matched.
[7] Svensson and Kaaber (1995): case control 30 BMS with dentures, 26 gender, age, denture matched.
MMPI Minnesota Multiphasic Personality Inventory (see Chapter 6 for details). SCL-90 (see Chapter 6 for details).

Tammiala-Salonen et al., 1993). Eli et al. (1994b) found that significant life events did not appear to correlate with the onset of symptoms, whereas Svensson and Kaaber (1995) did. However, Bogetto et al. (1998) using controls suggest that severity rather than number of life events was significantly associated with BMS. 17% of BMS had at least one severe life event compared with 9% in controls and so life events may play a role in the precipitation of BMS. The onset may be sudden or come on gradually over a period of months (Grushka, 1987).

The burning may be described as a discomfort rather than a pain which is present in all parts or selected areas of the mouth but most consistently in the lips, tongue. In two case control studies numbering 72 and 29 BMS the McGill Pain Questionnaire (see Chapter 6 for further details) was used to assess the pain (Grushka et al., 1987a,b; Svensson and Kaaber, 1995) and the results are shown in Table 6.

The words chosen differed significantly from patients with toothache (tender, sharp, annoying) but their overall intensity was comparable to toothaches, menstrual disorders and arthritis but lower than headache, cancer pain, post-herpetic neuralgia and back pain (Grushka et al., 1987a,b). The affective

scores are similar to toothaches or other organic pains suggesting a lack of psychological component when reporting pain. This may suggest that the reported psychological factors found in BMS patients are a result of the pain rather than its cause (Grushka et al., 1987a,b). The burning may be continuous or intermittent and occur at different times of the day and attempts have been made at categorising patients on this characteristic but the studies are anecdotal and not controlled.

In most studies over 50% of patients experience oral dryness (Grushka, 1987; Bergdahl et al., 1994; Svensson and Kaaber, 1995; Bogetto et al., 1998), which is often subjective and could also be related to medication, systemic diseases and psychological factors. Increased thirst is also reported (Grushka, 1987).

Associated with burning, patients will often also complain of alteration in their perception of taste or a persistent altered taste (dysgeusia) or even a combination of both (Grushka et al., 1998; Bartoshuk et al., 1999). The persistent taste most frequently reported is bitter (33%) and metallic (27%) and eating reduces the symptoms in many patients (Grushka, 1987). Alterations in taste perception are most frequently reported in relation to salt (70%), sweet and sour (40% each). The salt perception may be either stronger or weaker (Grushka, 1987). Patients report mood changes, alterations in eating and sleep habits and reduced socialising (Grushka, 1987). Svensson and Kaaber (1995) especially looked at BMS in patients with dentures and they found that compared with controls BMS patients were less likely to wear dentures, had decreased tongue space, incorrect occlusal plane and reduced vertical dimension (see Chapter 4 on history taking for more details of questions to ask).

4.2. Psychiatric findings

There is a considerable amount of literature on the presence of psychiatric morbidity in BMS patients. Eli et al. (1994a,b) have shown that BMS patients score significantly higher on scales of somatisation, obsession–compulsion, personal sensitivity, depres-

TABLE 6

Patients with BMS description of their symptoms on the McGill Pain Questionnaire

Measure	Grushka et al., 1987a	Svensson and Kaaber, 1995
Pain Rating Index (PRI) total	17.6	15
PRI sensory	10	9
PRI affective	2.3	2
PRI evaluative	2	1
PRI miscellaneous	3.4	3.1
Number of words chosen	8.5	7
Present pain intensity	2.3	2.5
Words chosen:		
burning	85%	65%
tender	51%	51%
annoying	51%	51%
tiring	37%	34%

sion, anxiety, hostility, phobic anxiety and psychoticism when compared to controls. They also found that BMS patients had a greater tendency to have had psychological treatment as compared to controls. Hampf et al. (1987) attempted to assess psychiatric disorders in a variety of facial pain patients as compared with controls and in the burning mouth group found that 8 out of 18 patients refused to attend for psychiatric interview, of those who attended dependent personalities were found in 5. Bergdahl et al. (1995b) showed in a group of 32 patients who were matched for age and gender that there were significant differences in relation to personality and psychological functioning including socialization, anxiety, tension, fatigue and concern with health. Browning et al. (1987), Zilli et al. (1989), Paterson et al. (1995) and Bogetto et al. (1998) all reported a higher percentage of patients with depression, anxiety or mood changes than controls. It could be argued that many of the reported associated factors are common to other pain patients and are not specific to BMS patients (Grushka, 1987). Quality of life as measured on 14 questions using a Likert type format showed no difference between BMS and controls (Eli et al., 1994b).

4.3. Examination

In the burning mouth syndrome no oral mucosal changes will be detected. However, a careful examination is essential to look for other causes of burning mouth; a summary of these appearances are described in Table 7. How many of these clinical changes consistently cause burning is not known and the level of evidence is low (4, Chapter 1).

The most common oral finding would be candidiasis of which four major forms are recognised: denture stomatitis, pseudomembranous, hyperplas-

TABLE 7

KEY FACTS: possible oral findings in patients with a complaint of burning but not BMS

Appearance	Likely diagnosis	Possible causes
Redness under a denture	Denture stomatitis	Denture wear, uncontrolled diabetes
Generalised redness in the palate	Atrophic candidiasis	Inhaler use, antibiotics, post radiotherapy, immunocompromised patients, allergy to denture material
	Allergy	
Creamy white plaques that rub off leaving red patches multiple sites	Pseudomembranous candidiasis	Immunocompromised patients, uncontrolled diabetics
White patches that do not rub off	Hyperplastic candidiasis	Immunocompromised patients, smokers, precancerous lesions
	Leukoplakia	
White patches bilaterally in line of occlusion	Frictional keratosis	Bruxism
Scalloped tongue edges	Variation of normal appearance	Bruxism, parafunctional habits
Changing red patches surrounded by white elevated margins on the dorsum of the tongue	Geographic tongue	May be associated with candidiasis and so cause burning
Fissured tongue	Variation of normal, seen often in patients with dry mouths	Normal but may indicate Sjogren's syndrome
Red smooth tongue due to loss of papilla	Post inflammatory, haematological deficiency	Post-erosive lichen planus, vitamin B_{12} or folate deficiency
Dry mouth, lack of pooling in the floor	Sjogrens's syndrome, anxiety, drugs	Sjogren's syndrome, drugs

tic and atrophic forms which can present either as red areas or milky yellow curd-like spots that will partially rub off. Denture stomatitis which is found under dentures, especially in those not taking them out at night, is by far the commonest and is least likely to result in a burning sensation. On the other hand pseudomembranous candidiasis is often acute and causes intense burning. It is especially seen in patients who are immunocompromised or taking large doses of systemic steroids. The atrophic form in the absence of dentures presents as a redness and is often associated with use of inhalers or broad spectrum antibiotics for long periods. Allergy to denture material is very rare but will cause a redness under the denture and may cause a burning sensation which improves when the dentures are left out.

Parafunctional habits, especially tongue thrusting and clenching, can be detected by the scalloped edges of the tongue which reflect the arrangement of the teeth and also often result in white patches on the lateral border of the tongue and side of the cheeks in the line of occlusion. Excessive tooth wear and faceting on teeth can also be seen in these patients (Paterson et al., 1995). If patients wear dentures it is worth checking their overall appearance, the vertical dimension, tongue space and occlusal balance as these could play a role in the development of burning (Svensson and Kaaber, 1995). You may consider a referral to a prosthodontist useful as it is important that dentures are changed regularly to reflect ageing changes in the mouth.

Although haematological deficiencies are said to cause a variety of changes in the mouth including a beefy red tongue, smooth tongue or even ulceration there is no good evidence from case control studies to substantiate these observations. A smooth tongue is seen much more frequently in patients who have had severe lichen planus of the tongue which has healed. Personally, I have not had any patients with post-inflammatory tongue changes complain of burning. It is worth noting the oral hygiene status and the dentition in terms of its completeness and restoration as detailed in Chapter 5. The mouth may be dry with very severe dryness being manifest by the inability to slide dental instruments smoothly over the mucosa and a lack of pooling of saliva in the floor of the mouth. The salivary glands need to be palpated and their function tested. All glands should secrete clear saliva which should not be too viscous and any colour changes indicate infection. Taste can be tested using four basic solutions but this may not be sufficient to discriminate between patients. More sophisticated testing as suggested by Bartoshuk et al. (1999) is not feasible in the busy clinic. Svensson and Kaaber (1995) showed that BMS patients reported more tenderness and pain in their facial and neck muscles when compared to controls.

5. Investigations

Work through case study 3 in Table 8 on investigations of a burning mouth.

Investigations are aimed at eliminating possible causal factors and could include those listed in Table 9, but should only be done if indicated by history and examination. Many of the tests have low sensitivity and specificity and will not help to rule a condition in or out. See Chapter 7 for more details on tests.

Grushka (1987) showed that 58% of patients with BMS had some abnormal immunological test as compared with controls and these included positive ANF, RF, low C4. Follow-up studies on 27 patients with BMS and abnormal immunological tests showed that 12 had evidence of connective tissue disorders such as Sjogren's syndrome (Grushka et al., 1986b).

TABLE 8

Case study 3

You have taken a history and examined a 60-year-old lady who you think has got burning mouth syndrome. What investigations are you going to perform which may have a bearing on the way she is managed?

See Table 14 the end of the chapter for the answer or continue reading below.

TABLE 9

KEY FACTS: investigations to be considered in patients with burning mouth symptoms

- Full blood count and differential
- Iron status — serum ferritin
- Vitamin B_{12} and red cell folate levels
- Random blood glucose or glycosylated haemoglobin
- Salivary flow
- Oral swabs
- Oral biopsy
- Allergy testing
- Denture functioning
- Immunological–rheumatoid factor, complement, antinuclear factor
- Psychological — anxiety, depression
- Quality of life, coping strategies

Salivary flow rates can be measured and have on the whole been reported as being unaltered but the studies are not controlled. Svensson and Kaaber (1995) showed a reduction in salivary flow in BMS patients in comparison to controls but they did not indicate how the saliva was measured and how it correlated with clinical findings. Research-orientated investigations, not currently clinically relevant, have shown some chemical composition changes in saliva (Glick et al., 1976) but others have not found any difference in protein composition which could affect protection and lubrication of the oral mucosa (Tammiala-Salonen and Soderling, 1993).

Serum zinc levels have been found to be lowered in a small study with controls (Maragou and Ivanyi, 1991). Taste testing and its evaluation is complex and probably not feasible on busy clinics at present (Bartoshuk, 2000).

All patients whom you are going to treat should have some repeatable baseline assessments done such as character and severity of the symptoms as well as psychosocial assessments as described in Chapter 6.

6. Management

This is initially based on reassurance and correction of all contributing factors. Treatment and prevention of oropharyngeal candidiasis is covered in *Clinical Evidence* which is regularly updated (Pankhurst, 2001). Remember to assess patients' drug therapy as many drugs cause xerostomia which can then lead to candidiasis and burning. Patients with mucositis-related burning need to be treated according to local guidelines (see end of chapter). If treatment of all local causes does not result in resolution and there are no signs of oral mucosa disease then you can assume that the patient has burning mouth syndrome. To date there have been no high quality randomised controlled trials reported in this field, so making management difficult. A summary is shown in Table 10 which is based on a Cochrane systematic review.

The Cochrane systematic review (Zakrzewska et al., 2001) and a paper in *Clinical Evidence* (Buchanan and Zakrzewska, 2002) on interventions in BMS are regularly updated. The only treatment that has shown some benefit is cognitive behaviour therapy (Bergdahl et al., 1995a). Others have attempted to give female patients hormone replacements or massaged oestrogen locally but none are conclusive. Vitamin replacements have been tried but the trials are inconclusive. Antidepressants are used but often BMS patients have not been analysed separately from other facial pain patients so their individual outcomes are not known.

A novel approach which tries to manage BMS along the lines of other neuropathic pains is the use of low dose clonazepam (mean 1 mg daily) used either topically (Woda et al., 1998) or systemically (Grushka et al., 1998). Both case series reports of 30 and 25 patients suggest that up to a third of the patients may be helped without undue side effects and the improvement is seen especially in taste. Randomised controlled trials are awaited. It is suggested that clonazepam is a GABA (gamma-amino butyric acid) receptor agonist and so may facilitate the inhibitory action of GABA and hence lead to improved taste.

TABLE 10

KEY FACTS: management of BMS based on systematic review. Levels of evidence as discussed in Chapter 1, Table 10.

Drug/treat	Level of evidence	Therapy, number	Efficacy	Side effects/adverse	References	Comments
Cognitive behaviour therapy	2b	Placebo controlled, 12–15 sessions of CBT, 30	At six months 27% in active group pain-free	None	Bergdahl et al., 1995a	VAS was not validated, no details whether groups were comparable
Antidepressant	1b	Trazodone 200 mg, placebo, 37	No improvement	Dizziness 11, drowsiness in 9	Tammiala-Salonen and Forssell, 1999	RCT, good outcome measures
	4	Clomipramine 75–100 mg, mianserin 30–60 mg, placebo 77 patients	No improvement	Drop outs due to side effects	Loldrup et al., 1989	No blinding, lack of follow-up, other types of pain included
	4	Paroxitine 20 mg, amitriptyline 25 mg, clordemetildiazepam 1 mg, amisulpride 50 mg, 121	No significant differences	Side effects resulted in 24 drop-outs	Bogetto et al., 1999	Open trial
Analgesic topical	1b	Benzydamine mouth rinse, placebo and no treatment, 30	No improvement	Nil	Sardella et al., 1999	RCT, small, good outcome measures, last group not blinded
Vitamin B replacement	2b	Alpha-lipoic acid 600 mg, placebo, 42	Slight improvement, 16/21 active vs 3/21 placebo	None	Femiano et al., 2000	Assessment not blinded
Hormone replacement	3b	Estrone ointment, estrone and progesterone ointment, placebo, 22	No significant improvement	None	Pisanty et al., 1975	No randomisation, poor criteria, lack of follow-up
	4	Mestranol 40 μg, placebo, 145	No significant oral improvements	None reported	Ferguson et al., 1981	No randomisation, no criteria, poor follow-up
	4	Hormone replacement, placebo, 27	No valid results	None reported	Forabosco et al., 1992	Not randomised, not blinded, unclear criteria, lack of follow-up

Patients who complain of a dry mouth may be offered a variety of saliva substitutes which have not been evaluated in randomised controlled trials.

7. Prognosis

All patients can be reassured and told that improvement can be expected in about one third of cases but that this may not resolve for 6 to 7 years (Grushka et al., 1986a). They showed that patients with intermittent symptoms were more likely to improve and that partial improvement is often due to pain becoming cyclical rather than constant. A survey done in the Netherlands where there is a support group for patients with burning mouths indicates that 88% wanted more information from their health-care workers and up to 57% said they were poorly informed by either dentist or physician (Van der Ploeg et al., 1987). This is something that all of you should now be able to do! Now try your skills at solving the cases in Table 11 and look for the answers at the end of the chapter.

8. Algorithm for management

As you have seen there is very little good quality evidence and most is based on case reports and expert opinions. It is therefore difficult to call the schemata presented in Fig. 1 as anything more than a suggestion based on the author's reading of the current literature and her own clinical practise.

TABLE 11

Case studies

Given the cases studies 1 and 2 in Table 3, how would you manage the two patients based on the evidence available to date?

Please see Table 16 at the end of chapter for answers.

9. Summary

A summary of the chapter is shown in Table 12. Tables 13–15 give the answers to the case studies.

TABLE 12

Summary of the chapter

1. Burning mouth as a symptom is common but burning mouth syndrome (BMS) is relatively rare, commonest in females over 50 years, unproven aetiology

2. Key features of BMS
   - gradual onset over 1 to 3 years
   - present throughout day, worse p.m.
   - pain/discomfort may be continuous or intermittent
   - burning 64–85%, tender and annoying
   - moderate severity
   - more than one site involved but tongue is the commonest
   - can be provoked or relieved by eating
   - taste changes 69–11%
   - dryness in over 60%
   - psychosocial morbidity
   - no oral signs

3. Investigations for exclusion, dictated by findings in the history and examination

4. Measure character, intensity, anxiety, depression and effect on quality of life

5. Management
   - eliminate possible causes of burning mouth
   - reassure, written information
   - counsel
   - cognitive behaviour therapy
   - antidepressants

6. Future research
   - assessment of the role of taste and nerve trauma in BMS
   - consensus view on diagnostic criteria and outcome measures
   - large multicentred randomised controlled trials for range of agents used in neuropathic pains including clonazepam

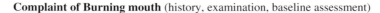

Complaint of Burning mouth (history, examination, baseline assessment)

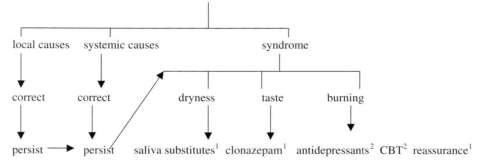

1 level of evidence C (see Chapter 9, Table 9)
2 level of evidence B (see Chapter 9, Table 9)
CBT cognitive behaviour therapy

Fig. 1. Algorithm for management.

TABLE 13

Answer to case studies 1 and 2 in Table 3

Mrs W has many of the classical features of BMS but interestingly does not use the word burning when describing her symptoms. She describes life events and recent deterioration in health which could be factors leading to the development of burning. It is probably the lack of good health rather than her burning mouth that is causing her depression. However, she has a number of possible causes for her burning mouth (see Table 15) which may need excluding. We investigated her and all findings were negative and so she was diagnosed as having BMS.

Mrs SD again has a number of possible causes for her burning mouth and the one that should be at the top of the list is Sjogren's syndrome given the dry eyes, mouth and arthritis. There does not appear to be any evidence for oral infections. All Mrs SD's investigations proved negative for Sjogren's syndrome and no deficiency states were identified. She was therefore diagnosed as having BMS.

TABLE 14

Answer to case study 3, Table 8

Although you will find a whole list of investigations in Table 9, there is no evidence to substantiate their performance if the history or examination does not suggest them. In patients who are at high risk for certain systemic conditions it may be validated, e.g. older Bengali women are at risk of developing maturity onset diabetes. Immunological tests may be worth pursuing as these have been found to be abnormal in up to 58% of patients with BMS especially if there is a history of dryness and connective tissue disease (Grushka et al., 1986a). Psychological and quality of life tests are important as they will indicate the effect the symptoms are having on the life of the patient and should be used as outcome measures in any treatment given.

TABLE 15

Answer to case studies in Table 11

Mrs EW (case 1) was reassured that she had no cancer, the symptoms were explained to her. She was started on antidepressants and given some counselling on how to cope. She showed marked improvement at her next appointment in 3 months.

Mrs SD (case 2) was given saliva substitutes for her dry mouth and antidepressants. Six weeks later she returned saying she had not noticed any improvement and her pain scores were the same as on the first visit; there was some improvement in mood but her anxiety and depression had worsened. She was told that all her results were within the normal range and that she was suffering from BMS. We counselled her and explained the importance of developing coping strategies and seeing whether stress played a role in her symptoms. In view of her depression we suggested to her to continue her antidepressant and we considered referring her for cognitive behaviour therapy (CBT). Three months later she failed her follow-up appointment. Mrs SD illustrates many of the problems we encounter when treating these patients. We do not have easy access to CBT and were concerned that she would not be motivated to attend a full course. New lines of treatment are needed as this patient has considerable disability from this condition.

10. Further reading

(1) Anonymous. Classification and diagnostic criteria for headache disorders, cranial neuralgias and facial pain. Headache Classification Committee of the International Headache Society. Cephalalgia 1988; 8(Suppl 7): 1–96.

(2) Merskey H, Bogduk N (eds). Classification of Chronic Pain. Descriptors of Chronic Pain Syndromes and Definitions of Pain Terms, 2nd ed. IASP Press, Seattle, WA, 1994.

(3) Clinical Guidelines on management of mucositis are available on the web site of the Royal College of Surgeons Engl (Faculty of Dental Surgery) but no information is available as to the authors or when it was last updated or due for update.

References

Marked as regards quality according to criteria set by author.
* Poorer quality studies but only ones in the field.
** Cohort studies, high quality case series with controls.
*** Randomised controlled trials, high quality original studies.

* Bartoshuk LM. Comparing sensory experiences across individuals: recent psychophysical advances illuminate genetic variation in taste perception. Chem Senses 2000; 25: 447–460.
* Bartoshuk LM, Grushka M, Duffy VB, Fast K, Lucchina L, Prutkin JSD. Burning mouth syndrome: damage to CN VII and pain phantoms in CN V. Chem Senses 1999; 24: 609.
* Bergdahl J, Anneroth G. Burning mouth syndrome: literature review and model for research and management. J Oral Pathol Med 1993; 22: 433–438.
*** Bergdahl M, Bergdahl J. Burning mouth syndrome: prevalence and associated factors. J Oral Pathol Med 1999; 28: 350–354.
** Bergdahl BJ, Anneroth G, Anneroth I. Clinical study of patients with burning mouth. Scand J Dent Res 1994; 102: 299–305.
*** Bergdahl J, Anneroth G, Perris H. Cognitive therapy in the treatment of patients with resistant burning mouth syndrome: a controlled study. J Oral Pathol Med 1995a; 24: 213–215.
** Bergdahl J, Anneroth G, Perris H. Personality characteristics of patients with resistant burning mouth syndrome. Acta Odontol Scand 1995b; 53: 7–11.
*** Bogetto F, Maina G, Ferro G, Carbone M, Gandolfo S. Psychiatric comorbidity in patients with burning mouth syndrome. Psychosom Med 1998; 60: 378–385.
* Bogetto F, Revello RB, Ferro G, Maina G, Ravizza L. Psychopharmacological treatments of burning mouth (BMS). A study sample of 121 patients (in Italian). Minerva Psichiatr 1999; 40: 1–10.
** Browning S, Hislop S, Scully C, Shirlaw P. The association between burning mouth syndrome and psychosocial disorders. Oral Surg Oral Med Oral Pathol 1987; 64: 171–174.
*** Buchanan J, Zakrzewska J. Burning mouth syndrome. Clin Evidence 2002; 7: 1239–1243.
** Cekic-Arambasin A, Vidas I, Stipetic-Mravak M. Clinical oral test for the assessment of oral symptoms of glossodynia and glossopyrosis. J Oral Rehabil 1990; 17: 495–502.
** Eli I, Baht R, Littner MM, Kleinhauz M. Detection of psychopathologic trends in glossodynia patients. Psychosom Med 1994a; 56: 389–394.
*** Eli I, Kleinhauz M, Baht R, Littner M. Antecedents of burning mouth syndrome (glossodynia) — recent life events

vs. psychopathologic aspects. J Dent Res 1994b; 73: 567–572.

**Femiano F, Gombos F, Scully C, Busciolano M, Luca PD. Burning mouth syndrome (BMS): controlled open trial of the efficacy of alpha-lipoic acid (thioctic acid) on symptomatology. Oral Dis 2000; 6: 274–277.

**Ferguson MM, Carter J, Boyle P, Hart DM, Lindsay R. Oral complaints related to climacteric symptoms in oophorectomized women. J R Soc Med 1981; 74: 492–498.

**Forabosco A, Criscuolo M, Coukos G, Uccelli E, Weinstein R, Spinato, S, Botticelli A, Volpe A. Efficacy of hormone replacement therapy in postmenopausal women with oral discomfort. Oral Surg Oral Med Oral Pathol 1992; 73: 570–574.

**Glick D, Ben-Aryeh H, Gutman D, Szargel R. Relation between idiopathic glossodynia and salivary flow rate and content. Int J Oral Surg 1976; 5: 161–165.

***Grushka M. Clinical features of burning mouth syndrome. Oral Surg Oral Med Oral Pathol 1987; 63: 30–36.

Grushka M, Bartoshuk LM. Oral dysesthesia and burning mouth syndrome: taste is a piece of the puzzle. Can J Diagnosis, 2000; 99–109.

***Grushka M, Sessle BJ. Applicability of the McGill Pain Questionnaire to the differentiation of 'toothache' pain. Pain 1984; 19: 49–57.

**Grushka M, Sessle B. Taste dysfunction in burning mouth syndrome. Gerodontics 1988; 4: 256–258.

**Grushka M, Katz RL, Sessle BJ. Sontaneous remission in burning mouth syndrome. J Dent Res 1986a; 274 (abstract 1341).

**Grushka M, Shupak R, Sessle BJ. A rheumatological examination of 27 patients with burning mouth syndrome (BMS). J Dent Res 1986b; 26: 533.

***Grushka M, Sessle BJ, Howley TP. Psychophysical assessment of tactile, pain and thermal sensory functions in burning mouth syndrome. Pain 1987a; 28: 169–184.

***Grushka M, Sessle BJ, Miller R. Pain and personality profiles in burning mouth syndrome. Pain 28: 1987b; 155–167.

**Grushka M, Epstein J, Mott A. An open-label, dose escalation pilot study of the effect of clonazepam in burning mouth syndrome. Oral Surg Oral Med Oral Pathol Oral Radiol Endod 1998; 86: 557–561.

**Hampf G, Vikkula J, Ylipaavalniemi P, Aalberg V. Psychiatric disorders in orofacial dysaesthesia. Int J Oral Maxillofac Surg 1987; 16: 402–407.

**Jääskeläinen SK, Forssell H, Tenovuo O. Abnormalities of the blink reflex in burning mouth syndrome. Pain 1997; 73: 455–460.

**Loldrup D, Langemark M, Hansen HJ, Olesen J, Bech P. Clomipramine and mianserin in chronic idiopathic pain syndrome. A placebo controlled study. Psychopharmacology 1989; 99: 1–7.

**Maragou P, Ivanyi L. Serum zinc levels in patients with burning mouth syndrome. Oral Surg Oral Med Oral Pathol 1991; 71: 447–450.

***Pankhurst C. Oropharyngeal candidiasis. Clin Evidence 2001; 6: 1053–1066.

*Paterson AJ, Lamb AB, Clifford TJ, Lamey PJ. Burning mouth syndrome: the relationship between the HAD scale and parafunctional habits. J Oral Pathol Med 1995; 24: 289–292.

**Pisanty S, Rafaely B, Polishuk, A. The effect of steroid hormones on buccal mucosa of menopausal women. Oral Surg Oral Med Oral Pathol 1975; 40: 346–353.

**Robinson PP, Loescher AR, Smith KG. A prospective, quantitative study on the clinical outcome of lingual nerve repair. Br J Oral Maxillofac Surg 2000; 38: 255–263.

***Sardella A, Uglietti D, Demarosi F, Lodi G, Bez C, Carrassi A. Benzydamine hydrochloride oral rinses in management of burning mouth syndrome. A clinical trial. Oral Surg Oral Med Oral Pathol Oral Radiol Endod 1999; 88: 683–686.

**Svensson P, Kaaber S. General health factors and denture function in patients with burning mouth syndrome and matched control subjects. J Oral Rehabil 1995; 22: 887–895.

**Svensson P, Bjerring P, Arendt-Nielsen L, Kaaber S. Sensory and pain thresholds to orofacial argon laser stimulation in patients with chronic burning mouth syndrome. Clin J Pain 1993; 9: 207–215.

***Tammiala-Salonen T, Forssell H. Trazodone in burning mouth pain: a placebo-controlled, double-blind study. J Orofac Pain 1999; 13: 83–88.

***Tammiala-Salonen T, Soderling E. Protein composition, adhesion, and agglutination properties of saliva in burning mouth syndrome. Scand J Dent Res 1993; 101: 215–218.

***Tammiala-Salonen T, Hiidenkari T, Parvinen T. Burning mouth in a Finnish adult population. Community Dent Oral Epidemiol 1993; 21: 67–71.

*Tourne LP, Fricton JR. Burning mouth syndrome. Critical review and proposed clinical management. Oral Surg Oral Med Oral Pathol 1992; 74: 158–167.

Truelove EL, Blasberg B, de Pont L, Dionne RA, Dworkin SF, Epstein J, Grushka M, Lamey PJ, Sessle B, Zakrzewska JM. In: Millard HD, Mason DK (eds) Perspectives on World Workshop on Oral Medicine III 1998. University of Michigan, Ann Arbor, 2000; pp. 137–273.

*Van der Ploeg HM, Van der Wal N, Eijkman MA, Van der Waal I. Psychological aspects of patients with burning mouth syndrome. Oral Surg Oral Med Oral Pathol 1987; 63: 664–668.

Woda A, Navez ML, Picard P, Gremeau C, Pichard-Leandri E. A possible therapeutic solution for stomatodynia (burning mouth syndrome). J Orofac Pain 1998; 12: 272–278.

***Zakrzewska JM, Hamlyn PJ. In: Crombie IKCPR, Linton SJ, LeResche L, Von Korff M (eds) Epidemiology of Pain. IASP, Seattle, WA, 1999; pp. 171–202.

***Zakrzewska JM, Glenny AM, Forssell H. Interventions for the treatment of burning mouth syndrome (Cochrane Review). The Cochrane Library (3), Oxford Update Software, 2001.

**Zilli C, Brooke RI, Lau CL, Merskey H. Screening for psychiatric illness in patients with oral dysesthesia by means of the General Health Questionnaire twenty-eight item version (GHQ-28) and the Irritability, Depression and Anxiety Scale (IDA). Oral Surg Oral Med Oral Pathol 1989; 67: 384–389.

Assessment and Management of Orofacial Pain
Pain Research and Clinical Management, Vol. 14
Edited by J.M. Zakrzewska and S.D. Harrison
© *2002 Elsevier Science B.V. All rights reserved*

CHAPTER 17

Other neurological causes of head and face pain

M.S. Chong [*]

The Medway Hospital NHS Trust, Gillingham, Kent, and King's College Hospital NHS Trust London, Mapother House, London SE5 9AZ, UK

Objectives for this chapter:

At the end of this chapter you will be able to:
- make a diagnosis and investigate and manage a patient with suspected Giant Cell Arteritis (GCA)
- recognise the similarities and differences between glossopharyngeal neuralgia and trigeminal neuralgia and may present with referred
- recognise rare syndromes such as Raeder's, Tolosa–Hunt and pre-trigeminal neuralgia
- appreciate that connective tissue disorders may present with painful trigeminal neuropathy

1. Giant cell arteritis (GCA)

Giant cell arteritis is a condition that should be considered in any elderly person with recent on-set headache or facial pain. There is considerable overlap between GCA and polymyalgia rheumatica (PMR) and this condition is often treated as opposite spectrums of a single entity. GCA is also known by different names including Horton's arteritis and temporal arteritis. Although the temporal arteries are the commonest vessels involved, this condition is not confined to this anatomical location (see below). In addition, there is a pathognomonic histological appearance of mononucleated giant cells in the blood vessel involved, and GCA is the preferred term for this condition.

1.1. Definition

The IASP classification of pain (Merskey and Bogduk, 1994) has defined GCA as a "unilateral or bilateral headache, mainly continuous with aching or throbbing pain, sometimes very intense, usually in the elderly, with signs of temporal artery involvement. . . ". This is an imprecise diagnosis that takes little account of the pathology of this condition. The American College of Rheumatology has proposed a more restrictive set of findings for making this diagnosis (see Table 1). It is estimated that the presence of three or more out of these five features gives a predictive sensitivity and specificity of over 90% (Hunder et al., 1990; Table 1). A second method of coming to a diagnosis of GCA is by using the 'tree format' which starts with the clinical findings and uses other criteria to formulate the final decision (for a discussion of these two methods see Hunder, 2000). Both these methods are equally valid as clinical aids.

* E-mail: mschong@doctors.org.uk

TABLE 1

American College of Rheumatology criteria for the classification of giant cell arteritis (Hunder et al., 1990)

- Age 50 years or greater at onset of symptoms
- New onset of localized headache
- Tenderness or decreased pulse of temporal artery
- Elevated erythrocyte sedimentation rate 50 mm/h or greater
- Temporal artery biopsy showing necrotising arteritis with predominance of mononuclear cell infiltrate or granulomatous process with multinucleated giant cells

1.2. Epidemiology

The incidence of biopsy-proven GCA ranged from around 10.24 per 100,000 population over the age of 50 in northwest Spain (González-Gay et al., 2001) to 29.1 per 100,000 persons of the same age group in southern Norway (Haugeberg et al., 2000). There appears to be a geographical variation in the incidence of GCA/PMR and southern Norway has the highest reported prevalence of this condition in the world. This disparity of incidence points towards a possible racial predisposition to the development of GCA. In a retrospective study over 12 years of 121 patients who underwent temporal artery biopsy, Liu et al. (2001) found no cases amongst Afro-American and Hispanic patients. The incidence was 11% amongst Asian patients and 29% in those from white racial origin. This epidemiological link has been confirmed by studies where GCA has been found to be more common in persons with HLA-DRB1 [*]04 alleles. It has also been proposed that other factors like genetic polymorphism for ICAM-1 (InterCellular Adhesion Molecule), RANTES (Regulated upon Activation Normal T-cell Expressed Secreted) and Interleukin-1 receptors may also alter susceptibility to developing GCA (González-Gay et al., 2001).

In an epidemiology study over 18 years reported by González-Gay et al. (2001) there is also a steady increase in the incidence of GCA throughout that period. This appears to reflect a true increase in the incidence of this condition of nearly 10% a year rather than better access to health care and improved diagnostic acumen of doctors.

1.3. Aetiology and pathophysiology

The pathogenesis of GCA primarily involves cell mediated immune damage. This is caused by activated CD4 helper T-cells responding to an antigen challenge. The most intense inflammatory response centres are around the arterial internal elastic lamina where multinucleated giant cells are formed. Elastic fibre fragments are reported to be isolated from these giant cells (Banks et al., 1983), adding support to the speculation that elastin is the primary antigen that triggers this inflammatory process. The assertion that GCA primarily affects the internal elastic lamina also explains why intracranial arteries that do not possess an internal elastic lamina are spared in this condition. In spite of extensive investigations, however, no specific antigen has been identified as the primary culprit. Recent investigations have focused on antigens from infective agents as possible triggers. Polymerase chain reaction amplification techniques on DNA extracted from temporal artery biopsy specimens, however, have failed to find a link between GCA and Chlamydia, parvovirus and eight human herpes viruses (Helweg-Larsen et al., 2002). The pathogenesis of CGA remains unknown except that it is more common amongst people of Nordic origin (for a review of pathogenesis of GCA see Weyand and Goronzy, 2002).

1.4. Clinical features

1.4.1. Pain characteristics
GCA commonly affects the temporal arteries, so pain in both temples, moderate to severe in intensity, dull and aching in character that is persistent, is thought to be the most common manifestation of this condition (Merskey and Bogduk, 1994). In a large series of 166 patients with biopsy-proven GCA, Caselli and co-workers reported that headache was the initial symptom in one third of patients and over 70% of patients reported this symptom (Caselli

and Hunder, 1997). The headache was described as throbbing, generalised and continuous, affecting the temples and occipital regions. Unfortunately, this is not always the case and the pain of GCA appears to be able to take on many forms. There are few studies that specifically investigated the pain characteristics of GCA. One such study was reported by Solomon and Cappa (1987), who performed a retrospective analysis of the headache characteristics of 24 patients with biopsy-proven GCA. The temple was the sole site of pain in 6/24 patients. The majority of patients either had a generalised headache or pain affecting another part of their heads. Seven patients had no pain in the temples at all and two patients did not even experience headaches.

A new onset headache in patients over the age of 50, however, can be useful for diagnosing GCA. In the original American College of Rheumatology criteria (1990) these two features were included into the diagnostic features with high sensitivity and specificity. Therefore, a high index of suspicion in these patients together with a careful search for the associated features remains the most accurate method of diagnosing GCA. Kantor (1999) has attempted to give some estimates of the sensitivity of the different clinical manifestations and these are summarised in Tables 2 and 3.

1.4.2. Associated features

The list of clinical symptoms associated with GCA is extensive and often seems to be non-specific. There are some features that are not reported by all patients but when present, are highly specific for this disorder. It is estimated that jaw and tongue claudication is only present in 40% of patients with GCA. If present, however, it can provide confirmatory evidence of up to 98% specificity (Hunder et al., 1990). Where the lingual artery is affected, infarction of the tongue has been described. Similarly, polymyalgia rheumatica as mentioned above is only found in half of patients with GCA. However, if a patient with polymyalgia also complains of new onset headache, there is a chance of up to 80% that this is caused by GCA (Hunder et al., 1990; Rodríguez-Valverde et al., 1997). It is estimated that constitutional symp-

---

TABLE 2

KEY FACTS: clinical symptoms and signs in patients with GCA

Site and radiation: temples, but may be other sites, bilateral
Severity: moderate to severe
Character: dull, aching, throbbing, tender
Periodicity: continuous, sudden onset
Provoking factors: chewing
Tender temporal artery with reduced or absent pulsation in 20–40%
Scalp tenderness with nodules, ischaemic ulcers
Ophthalmic: visual field constriction, visual loss, optic atrophy, scleritis, episcleritis, proptosis, ptosis, diplopia
Neurological: signs of posterior circulation stroke or transverse myelitis
Limb ischaemia with possible tender limb arteries, bruits, pulse asymmetry
Congestive cardiac failure

TABLE 3

Associate symptoms of GCA and the % occurrence (Kantor, 1999)

Jaw and tongue claudication especially when chewing, 11–38%
Polymyalgia, 20–52%
Constitutional upset: pyrexia (45–67%), fatigue, weight loss and anorexia (20–79%)
Ophthalmic: 22–41% visual blurring, diplopia, visual obscuration, amaurosis fugax
Neurological: vertigo, unsteadiness, numbness, paraesthesia, depression (12–25%)
Ischaemic limb pain
Angina, dyspnoea

---

toms like fever, fatigue, anorexia and weight loss (Calamia and Hunder, 1981) may be present in a third of patients with polymyalgia. Other less common neurological symptoms include vertigo, tinnitus, unsteadiness, numbness and paraesthesia (Reich et al., 1990). The anterior spinal artery may also be involved in GCA, causing spinal cord infarction and myelopathy (Caselli and Hunder, 1993).

The arteritis can also affect numerous vessels in GCA. Where the aorta is involved, this may cause aortic aneurysms and dissection, which are known complications of GCA (Perruquet et al., 1986; Evans et al., 1995; Evans and Hunder, 1997). Patients with involvement of the limb vessels will complain of ischaemic rest pain and claudication (Klein et al., 1975; Le Hello et al., 2001). Very rarely, GCA can affect the coronary arteries and may cause angina, myocardial infarction and congestive cardiac failure (Morris and Scheib, 1994).

1.4.3. Examination

Abnormalities in the temporal artery are the most common physical finding in GCA. In near 60% of patients, temporal artery tenderness, reduced pulsation and even a hard rigid cord of a partly thrombosed vessel may be found. The specificity of this finding has been estimated to be over 90% for GCA (Hunder et al., 1990). Tenderness of the scalp including painful nodules from ischaemia and even ischaemic scalp ulceration may be seen in nearly half of patients with GCA.

The other abnormalities which may be found on examination are a result of complications of GCA. Ophthalmological signs in patients with GCA include constriction of the peripheral visual fields, optic pallor and atrophy, diplopia and, less commonly, scleritis, episcleritis, proptosis and ptosis. Patients may have neurological signs from strokes affecting the posterior circulation as the vertebral arteries are commonly affected by GCA. Cranial nerve palsies, nystagmus and ataxia may result from these strokes. Limb ischaemia, tenderness and abnormalities of the large and medium size limb vessels are also seen where GCA affects other blood vessels. Where coronary arteries are affected, the patients may suffer heart failure.

Unless several specific findings are present the pre-test probability based on history and examination is typically less than 50%, but if you have a cluster of symptoms such as new headache, jaw claudication and abnormal arteries the sensitivity becomes 34% and specificity over 99% with a positive likelihood ratio of 47 (Rodríguez-Valverde et al., 1997). Jaw claudication correlates strongly with a positive biopsy and increases the likelihood ninefold (Hayreh et al., 1997).

1.5. Complications

The complications of GCA are those related to the associated signs and symptoms. Visual loss is the most common and worrying complication. This can occur very rapidly and is usually from an anterior ischaemic optic neuropathy (AION). In a prospective study of 174 patients, the risk factor for visual loss was a history of transient visual ischaemic symptoms and a higher platelet count (Liozon et al., 2001). This has led to a call for more aggressive antiplatelet therapy or anticoagulation in patients with AION who are at risk of becoming blind. Constitutional symptoms, polymyalgia, are associated with a reduced risk, presumably because these symptoms may alert clinicians to an earlier diagnosis. There is no doubt that early treatment with corticosteroids prevents blindness, and intravenous methylprednisolone is the treatment of choice because it appears to be more effective at saving sight (Chan et al., 2001).

1.6. Investigations

The investigation of choice is an assay of the erythrocyte sedimentation rate (ESR). In the criteria of the American College of Rheumatology a level of 50 mm/h was used and this had a sensitivity of nearly 90% but a specificity of less than 50% for making a diagnosis of GCA (Hunder et al., 1990). Clinicians are always worried about missing the diagnosis of GCA especially in patients with an apparent normal ESR (González-Gay et al., 1997). In the report of 238 patients by Martinez-Toboada et al. (2000), 10 patients or 4.2% of this sample had an ESR of less than 50. In another 167 patients reported by Salvarani and Hunder (1999), 9 of their patients or 5.4% had an ESR of less than 40 mm/h. It has been suggested that in patients with typical clinical symptoms, a cut-off ESR of 30 mm/h is used as the diagnostic criteria for GCA-PMR (Martinez-Toboada et al., 2000). Unfortunately, this level would still miss the 9 patients from the case series reported by

TABLE 4

Laboratory tests for GCA and their specificity and sensitivity

Test	Sensitivity	Specificity	Likelihood ratio	
			positive	negative
Erythrocyte sedimentation rate over 50 mm/h	99	50–70	2.5	0.02
C-reactive protein over 0.5 mg/dl	93–100	74–88		
Doppler flow studies	80–93			
Temporal artery biopsy	80	95	16	0.21

Salvarani and Hunder (1999) where the mean ESR was 19 mm/h and after 1 week of steroid therapy, dropped to 3 mm/h. The near normal level of ESR in these patients appears to be peculiar to the patients rather than that they may have a different variety of GCA. These patients appear to have a different inflammatory response and would still have a normal ESR even if they are challenged by another inflammatory event (Salvarani and Hunder, 1999). You need to remember that ESR can be elevated by many infectious, inflammatory or rheumatic disorders and increases with age. A normal ESR rules out GCA but a high one does not rule it in. The specificity and sensitivity of these tests is shown in Table 4.

Other laboratory parameters associated with GCA-PMR include mild anaemia, thrombocytopaenia, elevated serum enzymes like aspartate transaminase and alkaline phosphatase. A raised level of C-reactive protein is also common (Cantini et al., 2000) and sometimes may be more accurate than just an assay of the ESR.

The most important test for making a diagnosis of GCA remains the temporal artery biopsy (Hayreh et al., 1997). This is vital for making an accurate diagnosis before subjecting the patient to a prolonged period of immunosuppression. Histological evidence of GCA is present for up to 6 weeks after initiation of treatment with corticosteroids (Achkar et al., 1994). The length of biopsy is critical. Skip lesions (Hall et al., 1983) have been reported and a 4–6 cm segment of temporal artery should be removed. This was estimated to give a positive diagnosis in 86% of patients with GCA (Hall et al., 1983). Where the

initial biopsy was negative and clinical suspicion was high, biopsy of the contralateral temporal artery has been advocated. In a study by Danesh-Meyer et al. (2000) this was not found to be useful. They found that a second biopsy has very low yield and that the concordance rate between temporal artery biopsy specimens from the two sides was as high as 98.9%.

Doppler studies of the temporal artery can also be useful in skilled hands. The main use of this was to select the appropriate segment of temporal artery for a biopsy to be carried out (Barrier et al., 1982). With more sophisticated technology, the different patterns of Doppler abnormality is starting to be recognised and it is estimated that this method of investigation has a specificity of 80% for coming to a diagnosis of GCA (Ho et al., 1994). However, it is unlikely that this will substitute the use of temporal artery biopsy and the main use will still be as an aid for the surgeon to localise the segment to be biopsied.

1.7. Treatment and prognosis

Oral corticosteroids remain the treatment of choice in patients with GCA. A starting dose of 0.5–1 mg/kg body weight is advocated. In patients with an acute neurological or ophthalmological syndrome or who are at a risk of serious complications of GCA, intravenous methylprednisolone of 1 g/day for 3–5 days is the treatment of choice (Chevalet et al., 2000). There is evidence that this can reduce the risk of blindness (Chan et al., 2001), but whether this is better than a higher dose of prednisolone (2 mg/kg body weight) has not been systematically investigated. The dose of steroids is then slowly reduced to around 40 mg/day within 4–6 weeks of initiating therapy. Rapid resolution of headache and constitutional symptoms within days is a good indicator that the diagnosis is correct. Jaw claudication and neurological complications, however, may persist for a few weeks after initiation of therapy (Caselli et al., 1988). The resolution of these symptoms can be useful to help guide the tapering of steroid treatment. Reductions in steroid dosage can be made by 2.5–5 mg a day every 2–4 weeks and guided by the patient's symptoms and regular checking of the ESR.

Long-term treatment with steroids can cause considerable side effects. Weight gain, hyperglycaemia and even diabetes mellitus can result from steroid therapy. Patients should be advised about this and asked to modify their diet to reduce the risk of this complication. To reduce the risk of osteoporosis, patients should undergo a DEXA (Dual Energy X-ray Absorptiometry) scan to assess bone density. Preventative drug therapy and diet modification are once again advocated. It is useful for patients to be counselled about the other risk of long-term steroid therapy as well, which includes susceptibility to infection, adrenal insufficiency and gastric irritation. Other immunosuppressants may also be used in place of steroids. Azathioprine is well known as a steroid sparing drug and is extensively used by neurologists for the treatment of myasthenia gravis. It is a useful alternative and has been assessed by double-blind studies (De Silva et al., 1986).

The drug of choice, however, is methotrexate at a dose of 7.5–12.5 mg weekly. In a placebo-controlled study of 42 patients, the addition of methotrexate to prednisolone nearly halved the relapse rate and allowed the cumulative dose of steroids to be reduced (Jover et al., 2001). Therefore, methotrexate appears to be the drug of choice with the best evidence, but it must not be forgotten that methotrexate should be co-prescribed with 10 mg folic acid to reduce the risk of side-effects which include oral ulcers.

The long-term outcome for patients with GCA is good with prompt treatment and careful follow-up. Relapses when patients are on a lower dose of steroid treatment do occur. In a retrospective long-

term follow-up study of 133 patients, Hachulla et al. (2001) found that relapse during tapering of steroid therapy occurred in 62% of the patients with a mean relapse rate of 1.5. The ESR at presentation was the only factor that could be correlated with the risk of relapse. Of the 56 patients in their cohort that managed to come off all treatment, 48% relapsed and this may occur at any time between 1 and 35 months after discontinuation of therapy. Analysis of survival using the Kaplan–Meier curve showed that 30.7% of their patients died and this was more likely to happen for those who became permanently blind or who needed larger doses of steroids to control their symptoms. Fig. 1 summarises the management of giant cell arteritis (GCA).

In summary, GCA is a treatable condition that may present with facial pain as well as numerous non-specific symptoms. Making a diagnosis is important because prompt treatment can reduce the risk of complications. There are well described criteria that help to make a diagnosis of GCA but a high level of clinical suspicion remains the most important practical factor.

This is such an important diagnosis to be correctly made that I do not hesitate to repeat findings from the literature. Smentana and Shmerling (2002) reported that:

- Jaw claudication was an important clue to the diagnosis of GCA.
- The positive predictive findings on physical examination were temporal artery beading, prominence and tenderness.
- A normal ESR was the best negative predictor of GCA.
- Where the clinical suspicion is high, the patients should be treated with steroids immediately after blood samples are taken for investigations.
- A temporal artery biopsy should then be arranged and carried out within 2 weeks.
- Patients with a diagnosis of GCA need long-term careful follow-up.
- Even when there is an apparent resolution of the condition with discontinuation of therapy, relapses may occur years later.

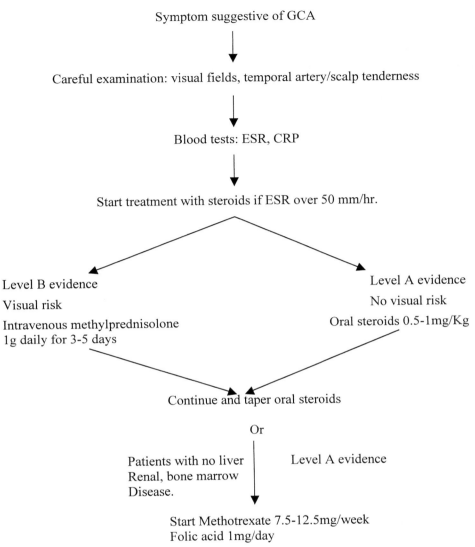

Symptom suggestive of GCA

Careful examination: visual fields, temporal artery/scalp tenderness

Blood tests: ESR, CRP

Start treatment with steroids if ESR over 50 mm/hr.

Level B evidence

Visual risk

Intravenous methylprednisolone
1g daily for 3-5 days

Level A evidence

No visual risk

Oral steroids 0.5-1mg/Kg

Continue and taper oral steroids

Or

Patients with no liver
Renal, bone marrow
Disease.

Level A evidence

Start Methotrexate 7.5-12.5mg/week
Folic acid 1mg/day

Fig. 1. Management of giant cell arteritis (GCA). Levels of evidence as shown in Chapter 9, Table 9.

2. Glossopharyngeal neuralgia

This is an uncommon condition with pain mainly in the throat and neck. It is included as a differential diagnosis of head and facial pain because the pain may radiate to the ipsilateral ear and there are cases where glossopharyngeal neuralgia co-exists with trigeminal neuralgia. Weisenberg (1910) first described a form of secondary glossopharyngeal neuralgia in a patient with pain symptoms similar to trigeminal neural-

gia but caused by a pontine tumour affecting the glosopharyngeal nerve.

2.1. Definition

In the IASP classification of chronic pain, glossopharyngeal neuralgia is defined as sudden, severe, brief, recurrent pains in the distribution of the glossopharyngeal nerve. This was given the code of 006.X8b (IASP Task Force on Taxonomy, 1994).

2.2. Epidemiology

This is such an uncommon condition that it is difficult to know the true incidence and prevalence. The Rochester, Minnesota study remains one of the few reports where the incidence of glossopharyngeal neuralgia was estimated. In this study, between 1945 and 1984, the incidence of glossopharyngeal neuralgia was compared to that of trigeminal neuralgia. The incidence rate for glossopharyngeal neuralgia was 0.8 per 100,000 of the population per year. In the study of this population, it is estimated that trigeminal neuralgia is six times more common that glossopharyngeal neuralgia. The greater incidence rate for glossopharyngeal neuralgia compared to trigeminal neuralgia was seen regardless of age and gender. In their study of 217 patients diagnosed with glossopharyngeal neuralgia seen at the Mayo Clinic over a 55-year period, Rushton et al. (1981) reported that this condition is only slightly more common in patients over the age of 50. They also noted the co-existence of trigeminal neuralgia and glossopharyngeal neuralgia in over 10% of their patients. Patel et al. (2002), in their series of over 200 patients with glossopharyngeal neuralgia treated by microvascular decompression (see below), reported that like trigeminal neuralgia, glossopharyngeal neuralgia is more common in women with a ratio of around 2 : 1. The mean age of these patients was 50.2 and symptoms of glossopharyngeal neuralgia were more commonly found on the left (55%) than on the right side (45%). Glossopharyngeal neuralgia has also been reported in children (Childs et al., 2000).

2.3. Aetiology and pathophysiology

The exact cause of primary glossopharyngeal neuralgias is unknown. There are undoubted similarities between glossopharyngeal neuralgia and trigeminal neuralgia. Vascular compression of these nerves has been postulated in the pathogenesis of both conditions (see Chapter 2). For glossopharyngeal neuralgia, this is supported by visualisation of nerve–blood vessel contact on magnetic resonance imaging (Boch et al., 1998) and numerous studies reporting the efficacy of microvascular decompression (Kondo, 1998; McLaughlin et al., 1999; Patel et al., 2002). There is also some histological evidence that trigeminal and glossopharyngeal neuralgias are caused by the same pathological process. Devor and colleagues examined biopsy samples of the nerve in a patient with glossopharyngeal neuralgia (Devor et al., 2002). They found areas of demyelinated and dysmyelinated axons similar to that seen in patients with trigeminal neuralgia (see Chapter 2).

There are also many case reports of secondary causes of glossopharyngeal neuralgia. Other secondary causes of glossopharyngeal neuralgia include congenital abnormalities, like an Arnold-Chiari malformation (Aguiar et al., 2002), multiple sclerosis (Minagar and Sheremata, 2000), malignancies of the neck (Metheetrairut and Brown, 1993) and neck trauma with foreign body impaction (Webb et al., 2000).

2.4. Clinical characteristics

There are no published case control series which would help to validate the clinical features.

2.4.1. Characteristics and timing

Glossopharyngeal neuralgia is usually described as sharp, stabbing, lancinating pain. The pain comes on very suddenly like trigeminal neuralgia and may persist for seconds or a maximum of 1–2 min (Rushton et al., 1981; Katusic et al., 1991; Minagar and Sheremata, 2000).

2.4.2. Site and radiation

The site of pain is usually in the back of the throat, involving the tonsillar fossa and radiating to the auditory channel and sometimes to the neck. As previously mentioned, glossopharyngeal neuralgia is more commonly reported on the right compared to trigeminal neuralgia (see Chapter 9). Glossopharyngeal neuralgia is also more likely to be bilateral (Rushton et al., 1981; Katusic et al., 1991). In the series of patients reported by Rushton and colleagues (1981), 12% of their patients had bilateral glossopharyngeal neuralgia, primarily in the throat and areas innervated by the glossopharyngeal nerve. The pain may radiate to the inner ear (otic variety) or the neck (cervical variety).

2.4.3. Severity of pain

There is no published case series of patients where this was specifically investigated. However, in patients with coexistence of glossopharyngeal and trigeminal neuralgias, the severity of pain is described in comparable terms for both conditions.

2.4.4. Trigger factors

Similar to that for trigeminal neuralgia, i.e. light touch provoked. These include swallowing and on occasions sneezing or yawning; other mechanical contact, particularly by cold or acidic fluids such as orange juice, can also trigger a severe attack (Minagar and Sheremata, 2000).

2.4.5. Associated features

Cardiac dysrhythmias and syncope associated with glossopharyngeal neuralgia are well described (Johnston and Redding, 1990; Marks and Purchas, 1992; Metheetrairut and Brown, 1993; Ferrante et al., 1995; Ceylan et al., 1997). However, the exact incidence of this potentially life threatening association is unknown. Rushton and colleagues reporting the symptomatology of 217 patients with glossopharyngeal neuralgia found that syncope was not a common association (Rushton et al., 1981). Cardiac syncope was thought to be caused by discharges from parasympathetic axons within the glossopharyngeal nerve, provoking bradycardia leading to hypotension and syncope (Marks and Purchas, 1992; Ferrante et al., 1995). As mentioned above, there is also a known combination of glossopharyngeal and trigeminal neuralgia

2.4.6. Physical examination

In primary cases, the physical examination is essentially normal apart from a trigger area in the back of throat when the patient is undergoing a period of exacerbation of pain. In patients with secondary causes of glossopharyngeal neuralgia there may be coexistence of other cranial nerve palsies (Table 5).

2.5. Natural history

Usually episodes will last for weeks to months, but may subside spontaneously. The epidemiological studies seem to suggest that glossopharyngeal neuralgia is a milder disease than trigeminal neuralgia, with less episodes or recurrence (Katusic et al., 1991). Rushton and colleagues in their series of 200 cases of glossopharyngeal neuralgia reported spontaneous remission in nearly 75% of the cases.

2.6. Investigation

An ECG would be useful to exclude cardiac dysrhythmias associated with this condition. Am MRI scan is the investigation of choice to look at the posterior fossa and also the upper cervical spine. As mentioned above, glossopharyngeal neuralgia may be the presenting symptom of head and neck tumours. More specialised imaging techniques involving magnetic resonance angiography may also reveal any neurovascular contact (Schmitz et al., 1999). None of these are based on any good quality evidence.

2.7. Management

2.7.1. Medical

There are no large placebo-controlled studies to guide the choice of therapy. Pharmacotherapy for glossopharyngeal neuralgia is the same as that for trigeminal neuralgia with the predominant use of anticonvulsants. Although phenytoin has been reported to be successful in treating glossopharyngeal neuralgia (Metheetrairut and Brown, 1993), carbamazepine remains the treatment of choice. The preference for carbamazepine comes from the reports of large series of patients like the Mayo Clinic study, where carbamazepine was the treatment of choice (Rushton et al., 1981) and case studies (Johnston and Redding, 1990; Minagar and Sheremata, 2000). Another medication reported to be effective for treating glossopharyngeal neuralgia is ketamine administered orally (Eide and Stubhaug, 1997). This is however only in one patient in an $n = 1$ placebo-controlled

TABLE 5

KEY FACTS: clinical features of glossopharyngeal neuralgia

Character	sharp, searing
Site and radiation	tonsillar bed radiating to inner ear and neck
Periodicity/onset/duration	brief, multiple recurrent episodes of pain during an exacerbation
Severity	comparable to the pain of trigeminal neuralgia
Provoking factors	swallowing, coughing, touching back of throat
Relieving factors	prophylaxis: phenytoin, carbamezepine
Associated factors	syncope and cardiac dysrhythmias described but uncommon
Clinical examination	normal in between attacks; trigger area in throat during exacerbation
Prognosis	episodes for weeks to months with long-term spontaneous remission in up to 75% of cases

study. The side-effects of ketamine remain the main limiting factor for choosing this treatment. In patients where cardiac syncope is a profound symptom, transvenous cardiac pacing may be necessary (Johnston and Redding, 1990; Marks and Purchas, 1992; Ferrante et al., 1995; Ceylan et al., 1997; Minagar and Sheremata, 2000).

2.7.2. Surgical therapy
Early surgical treatment was by avulsion of the glossopharyngeal nerve or section of the nerve at the jugular foramen (Rushton et al., 1981). In their review of over 200 cases, Rushton and colleagues reported pain relief in only half of their patients after such a procedure. This treatment method has now been superseded by other surgical techniques. For some patients with poor long-term prognosis, percutaneous rhizotomy may also be effective in alleviating pain. Arbit and Krol (1991) described computed tomography-guided percutaneous radiofrequency rhizotomy with neoplasm. Like trigeminal neuralgia, the outcome after microvascular decompression (MVD) appears to be the best for glossopharyngeal neuralgia. However, this evidence only comes from uncontrolled reported case series with relatively short follow-up periods. Patel et al. (2002) have reported over 200 cases where this was performed. In their retrospective analysis, their immediate success rate was over 90%, but the follow-up period was limited. They reported that MVD was effective for pain relief in patients with typical glos-

sopharyngeal neuralgia with pain restricted to the throat and palate. A longer follow-up period was reported by Kondo (1998) but in only 16 patients. Five years after MVD, all patients were pain-free but two patients complained of a hoarse voice and two had episodes of persistent unprovoked coughing.

2.7.3. Summary
With an estimated spontaneous resolution rate of over 75% (Katusic et al., 1991), it would be difficult to judge the efficacy of any medical or surgical intervention for the treatment of glossopharyngeal neuralgia. First of all, refining the diagnosis would be very helpful. To improve this, Matsushima and colleagues have reported an endovascular method of confirming the syndrome (Matsushima et al., 1999). In their single reported patient with glossopharyngeal neuralgia, insertion of a microcatheter into the correct artery provoked a typical attack. Whether this can be employed in all patients with glossopharyngeal neuralgia (or even trigeminal neuralgia) would need further studies. Next, large placebo-controlled trials with careful pre- and post-treatment follow-up assessment as that called for in treating trigeminal neuralgia would be required (see Chapter 15). Until then, unbiased counselling of the patients would be best to help them choose the treatment of choice for their glossopharyngeal neuralgia. Obviously, careful cardiac monitoring would be necessary in those symptomatic with unexplained syncope. For the subgroup of patients with 'cardiac' glossopharyngeal

neuralgia it is also uncertain whether pharmacotherapy can be combined with a pacemaker or a surgical procedure; either MVD or partial rhizotomy is the treatment of choice.

3. Other causes of facial pain

The causes of facial pain are extensive and include a long list of conditions giving rise to both somatic and visceral pain. It is important to realise that retro-orbital pain, which makes up a large portion of causes of facial pain, may be referred to pain arising from meningeal irritation in the middle cranial fossa. The list provided in Table 6 is not meant to be comprehensive but to illustrate the multitude of causes of direct and referred facial pain. Please also see Chapter 8 on classification. Post-herpetic neuralgia has not been included as it is a subject of a separate book in the series. Trigeminal post-herpetic neuralgia has the same characteristics as other sites. Amongst the many causes of facial pain I have chosen the four mentioned below for discussion in a little more detail because they are much quoted and often misunderstood.

4. Tolosa–Hunt syndrome

The reported case of a patient with unilateral ophthalmoplegia and retro-orbital pain caused by non-specific granulomatous inflammatory infiltration into the ipsilateral cavernous sinus was described by the Spanish neurosurgeon Tolosa (1954). The American neurosurgeon Hunt then described six cases of recurrent painful ophthalmoplegia responsive to treatment with corticosteroids (Hunt et al., 1961). It was the amalgamation and recognition of these two reports that gave rise to the eponymous name of Tolosa–Hunt syndrome.

4.1. Definition

The 1988 International Headache Society defined the Tolosa–Hunt syndrome as a syndrome of episodic

TABLE 6
Secondary causes of facial pain (many are rare)

- Acute angle glaucoma
- Tolosa-Hunt syndrome
- Giant cell arteritis
- Raeder's syndrome
- Pre-trigeminal neuralgia
- Local and metastatic neoplasms including:
- Lymphomas
- Nasopharyngeal carcinoma
- Trigeminal nerve neurofibromas/schwanomas
- Referred pain from meningiomas, chordomas, pituitary adenomas
- Painful trigeminal neuropathy
- Sinus mucocoeles
- Sinusitis
- Petrous apex infection/inflammation: Gradenigo's syndrome
- Post-herpetic neuralgia
- Mucormycosis
- Cavernous sinus thrombosis
- Carotid-cavernous fistula
- Carotid artery dissection
- Intracranial aneurysms

unilateral orbital pain for an average of 8 weeks if untreated, associated with paralysis of one or more of the third, fourth and sixth cranial nerves (Table 7). There should also be a prompt response to treatment with steroids and adequate imaging must be carried out to exclude other pathological conditions affecting the cavernous sinus (IHS, 1988).

4.2. Aetiology and pathophysiology

The precise pathology of this condition is unclear. In the original reports by Tolosa and Hunt it was that of an inflammatory granulomatous mass with

TABLE 7

KEY FACTS: IHS definition of the Tolosa–Hunt syndrome

1.	One or more episodes of a unilateral orbital pain for about 8 weeks if untreated
2.	Simultaneous or within the first 2 weeks, paresis of one or more of the cranial nerves III, IV, and VI may occur.
3.	Pain disappears within 72 h after the beginning of steroid therapy
4.	Other diseases excluded by CT or MRI

TABLE 8

KEY FACTS: key features Tolosa–Hunt syndrome

- This syndrome describes the symptoms of unilateral orbital pain with ocular motor nerve palsies of cranial nerves III, IV and VI
- The anatomical site of this syndrome is in the posterior supraorbital fissure and/or anterior cavernous sinus
- The original pathological entity of this syndrome is that of a non-specific inflammatory infiltrate
- Other pathological processes in this anatomical site can cause identical symptoms
- Treatment of this condition is with high dose steroids
- Extensive investigations with repeated MRI scans are recommended for any patients presenting with these symptoms

no obvious specific pathological trigger. Goadsby and Lance (1989) have reported such a case of Tolosa–Hunt syndrome with proptosis, recurrent pain, sixth and third nerve palsies and initial response to treatment with steroids. The patient underwent multiple surgical procedures until the removal of a non-caseating granuloma from the cavernous sinus lead to resolution of these symptoms. Many case series have since been reported describing the clinical syndrome without adding to our knowledge of the precise histopathology of this condition (146 patients summarised by Kline, 1982).

It must be emphasised that many other pathological processes can cause a lesion in this anatomical site leading to the same symptoms as the Tolosa–Hunt syndrome. Sarcoidosis, systemic lupus erythematosus, Wegener's granulomatosis, rheumatoid arthritis as well as primary and secondary neoplasms (Harnett et al., 1999; Esmaeli et al., 2000) have been reported to cause a painful opthalmoplegia with cranial nerve palsies.

There has been a recent call for the Tolosa–Hunt syndrome to be redefined using much stricter criteria. In particular, it has been emphasised that more extensive investigations must be undertaken. These should include extensive serological tests and CSF examination to exclude another pathological process in the cavernous sinus. Where initial investigations appear to be negative it is recommended that radi-

ological follow-up with repeated scans at different time intervals for at least 2 years be carried out. This is to make sure that an underlying lesion, especially a neoplasm, has not been missed (Forderreuther and Straube, 1999; Table 8).

4.3. Clinical features

There has not been any large reported systematic study of the pain characteristics in patients with the Tolosa–Hunt syndrome. The site of pain is accepted and generally recognised as being experienced in the orbit or retro-orbital area. However, pain descriptors used by patients in different case series vary from pressure, boring, steady to pulsating, or even sharp and stabbing (Hannerz, 1985; Gonzales, 1998). Many case series emphasised the recurrent nature of pain and the rapid alleviation with steroid treatment (Kline, 1982; Hannerz, 1999) Once again, this can cause diagnostic pitfalls as other pathological entities like lymphomas, sarcoidosis, myelomas and various solid tumours may also respond to treatment with steroids.

The natural history of this condition is unknown. As defined within the IHS diagnostic criteria, the symptoms may recover spontaneously within 8 weeks but may then recur months or even years later (Hannerz, 1999).

4.4. Management

As mentioned above, extensive investigations should be undertaken in any patient with painful opthalmoplegia and cranial nerve palsies. Magnetic resonance imaging with contrast enhancement is the neuroimaging of choice. If no lesion is found, repeated scans should be performed with a follow-up period of at least 2 years. Serological markers for other inflammatory conditions with cerebrospinal fluid examination should also be carried out. Angiography should be carried out if the MRI scan provides an indicator that there may be an underlying vascular lesion.

   Treatment for this condition is with high-dose corticosteroids equivalent to 80–100 mg prednisolone a day. Response to treatment is usually very rapid although non-specific. As mentioned above, other pathological entities that mimic this syndrome may also respond in the same way. A high dose of steroids is usually continued for 1–2 weeks with gradual tapering of the dose. In patients with recurrent symptoms, steroid therapy may be prolonged. Exactly how long treatment should continue is unknown and the use of steroid sparing immunosuppression like azathioprine, methotrexate or cyclophosphamide has not been subjected to any systematic investigation. Where repeated neuroimaging was performed, the abnormal inflammatory lesion may persist for 3–6 months (De Arcaya et al., 1999) and this invariably leads to doubts regarding the accuracy of diagnosis and a call for biopsies to be undertaken to verify the pathological diagnosis.

5. Raeder's syndrome

Raeder first described five patients with trigeminal nerve dysfunction associated with sympathetic dysfunction in the eye, with miosis in all five and ptosis in four patients (Raeder, 1924; Table 9). Since then,

---

TABLE 9

KEY FACTS: Raeder's syndrome

- This syndrome describes ptosis, miosis or both together with first division trigeminal neuropathic pain or sensory loss.
- The constellation of these symptoms point to an anatomical localisation in the middle cranial fossa.
- This syndrome is not specific to any pathological entity.
- Neuroimaging is important and repeated if necessary to determine the underlying abnormality.
- The eponymous name to this syndrome may be replaced by paratrigeminal oculosympathetic syndrome (POSS).

---

this eponymous name has been used very loosely to describe numerous patients with lesions affecting both the trigeminal and sympathetic nerves. Because of the imprecise use of this eponymous name for this syndrome, there is a suggestion for this name to be abandoned (Solomon and Lustig, 2001).

   Goadsby in a recent paper has attempted to clarify this and suggests that the eponymous name of Raeder could perhaps be dropped but the important lesson regarding the applied anatomy of this condition ought to be remembered (Goadsby, 2002). In patients where the ocular sympathetic system is affected as evidenced by miosis, ptosis or both (but with normal forehead sweating) and symptoms of trigeminal nerve involvement that manifest as either sensory loss or neuropathic pain, it should still be known as the paratrigeminal oculo-sympathetic syndrome (POSS). The anatomical localisation for a lesion causing POSS would be in the middle cranial fossa medial to the trigeminal ganglion and lateral to the anterior clinoid process. Thus, the important clinical point about this constellation of signs and symptoms is that a careful search ought to be made to look for a lesion in this site. If initial investigations are normal, then repeated neuroimaging, probably MRI scan, ought to be performed over a period of time to make sure that no lesions have been missed. Many pathological conditions, including both primary and secondary tumours, can affect this area and neither Raeder's syndrome or the para-trigeminal ocular sympathetic syndrome is confined to any pathological entity.

6. Pre-trigeminal neuralgia

This condition was first described by Symonds (1949). Later, Mitchell (1980) called it pre-trigeminal neuralgia, being a prodromal dull aching pain in the mouth which precedes trigeminal neuralgia. Fromm et al. (1990) also described some cases so the total number of patients reported is 62. There are no case-controlled studies and the diagnosis is often made in retrospect and so is of doubtful usefulness.

6.1. Clinical features

The mean age and gender are the same as for trigeminal neuralgia: middle age, female. The key features are summarised in Table 10. The patients compare the pain to toothache or sinusitis as it is a well localised pain. It has a dull aching quality and is also light touch provoked. The pain is episodic and trigeminal neuralgia may develop 1–11 months later, although Fromm et al. (1990) report one occurring 12 years later.

TABLE 10

KEY FACTS: pre-trigeminal neuralgia

- Pre-dromal condition preceding classical trigeminal neuralgia
- Moderately severe, dull toothache-like pain
- Unilateral, often one division of trigeminal nerve
- Paroxysmal, short lasting
- Provoked by light touch
- Relieved by anticonvulsants
- Nil found on examination

6.2. Management

The condition is often not recognised and patients may either undergo unnecessary dental treatment or be treated for atypical odontalgia. As with trigeminal neuralgia the pain responds to carbamazepine.

7. Trigeminal neuropathy associated with connective tissue disease

Trigeminal sensory neuropathy with and without pain is known to be associated with numerous connective tissue disorders (Table 11). Case reports of patients with scleroderma, Sjogren's syndrome, mixed connective tissue diseases, systemic lupus erythematosus, rheumatoid arthritis and dermatomyositis have been reported in the literature to be associated with trigeminal nerve dysfunction.

The largest published series of patients with this condition is from Hagen et al. (1990). They carried out a search of the case notes from the Mayo Clinic from 1970 to 1986 and found 81 patients with trigeminal nerve dysfunction associated with connective tis-

---

TABLE 11

KEY FACTS: trigeminal neuropathy with connective tissue disorders

- Atypical facial pain may be caused by trigeminal neuropathy associated with a connective tissue disorder.
- Symptoms of the neuropathy may precede the underlying connective tissue disorder.
- Serological tests for an underlying connective tissue disorder include ESR (erythrocyte sedimentation rate), ANA (antinuclear antibodies) and ENA's (extractable nuclear antigen antibodies).
- Symptoms of neuropathy may also precede some of the positive serological tests.
- Treating the underlying connective tissue disorder does not always alleviate the symptoms of trigeminal neuropathy.

sue diseases. It was interesting to note that the trigeminal neuropathy may precede symptoms of connective tissue disease and this was certainly the case in sixteen of their patients. In this series of patients, the most common manifestation of trigeminal nerve dysfunction was numbness in the face and was present in 64 patients. Most of their patients experienced initial unilateral symptoms that progressed to eventual bilateral involvement. The maxillary division of the trigeminal nerve was the most commonly affected site. The next most common symptom was pain, which was reported by 49 patients. Their patients described their pain as burning, lancinating in quality, and it was emphasised by the authors that no patients had symptoms consistent with typical trigeminal neuralgia. The severity of pain was described as severe in 13 patients and moderate in 33 patients.

The connective tissue disorder underlying trigeminal neuropathy was varied. Nearly half of the patients were diagnosed as undifferentiated connective tissue disease. The next most common diagnosis was mixed connective tissue disease (MCTD) (21 patients), scleroderma (15 patients) Sjogren's (2 patients), rheumatoid arthritis (2 patients) and systemic lupus erythomatosis (SLE, 2 patients). In this series of patients, the prognosis was poor with the majority of these patients having experienced pain for years and having responded poorly to various neuropathic medications.

The underlying pathology for trigeminal nerve dysfunction in patients with connective tissue disease is unknown. Nerve biopsy in one patient yielded evidence of severe loss of myelinated fibres with evidence of inflammatory changes (Lacky et al., 1987). It is possible that the numbness and/or pain is caused by a form of isolated vasculitis affecting the trigeminal nerve and ganglia.

In summary (see Table 11), trigeminal neuropathy associated with mixed connective tissue disease remains a differential diagnosis in patients with atypical facial pain. This is the case even when there is no clinical evidence of an underlying connective tissue disorder. As mentioned above, the trigeminal neuropathy may precede the appearance of signs and symptoms of a connective tissue disorder. Testing for serological markers for connective tissue disorders is

TABLE 12

Serological markers for connective tissue disorder adapted from the series of 81 patients reported by Hagen et al., 1990

Serological test	No. positive
Erythrocyte sedimentation rate over 20 mm/h	63/80
Positive antinuclear antibodies	68/74
Extractable nuclear antigen antibodies (ENA's)	
Anti-RNP antibody	28/42
Anti-SSA antibody	3/8
Anti SSB antibody	1/30
Anti-DNA antibody	11/44
Anti-SM antibody	3/41

important to narrow down the precise diagnosis (see Table 12). It is important to realise that these serological markers may be absent in the initial phase of the illness. For example, Alfaro-Giner et al. (1992) reported the case of a patient with mixed connective tissue disorder (MCTD) and facial pain, where antinuclear antibodies appeared 2 months after treatment with steroids. It is therefore useful to retest the serological markers for patients with atypical facial pain, particularly when the erythrocyte sedimentation rate is raised. It is unclear whether immunosuppressive treatment of the underlying connective tissue disorder will make any significant difference to the neuropathic pain. There are case studies where this was reported (Bennet et al., 1978; Searles et al., 1978; Alfaro-Giner et al., 1992,) but this was not seen in the patients reported by Hagen et al. (1990) and no systematic studies have been carried out to test this hypothesis.

Now it is time to test your skills. Please read through the case study in Table 13.

8. Summary

The chapter is summarised in Table 14. Table 15 gives the answer to the case study in Table 13.

TABLE 13

Case study

Mrs NB is a 56-year-old retired secretary who has experienced headaches for over 20 years. 4 months ago, she noticed a new type of pain in her face. This is episodic, centred around the forehead and both eyes. The pain is described as dull aching and normally lasts 30 min. The pain wakes her in the middle of the night and within 2 months has changed from being intermittent to a continuous throb. This pain was associated with intermittent blurring of vision. On direct questioning, there was no temporal tenderness or jaw claudication. She does complain of sensitivity of her scalp with discomfort brushing her hair. On examination, Mrs. NB is an overweight Guyanese woman of Oriental extraction. Her visual field and blind spot were normal and her acuity was correctable with a pinhole. There is no papilloedema, the retina looks normal. The temporal arteries were pulsatile but tender.

What investigations should be performed and how should she be treated? Please see Table 15 for the answer.

TABLE 14

Summary of the chapter

- Giant cell arteritis (GCA) is an important differential diagnosis of facial pain that may present insidiously and should be suspected in patients over 50 years, new onset of headache, visual disturbance, jaw claudication, generalised malaise, high ESR.

- GCA is confirmed by temporal artery biopsy.

- There is class A evidence that steroid therapy and methotrexate reduce the relapse and complications of GCA.

- Glossopharyngeal neuralgia has many common features to trigeminal neuralgia and may present with referred ear and face pain.

- Connective tissue disorders may present with painful trigeminal neuropathy.

TABLE 15

Answer to case study

This woman's GP arranged for an urgent ESR test which was raised at 42 mm/h. After discussion with the local neurologist, she was treated with prednisolone 60 mg daily and a temporal artery biopsy was performed. This confirmed the diagnosis of temporal arteritis. Methotrexate was initiated at the same time to reduce steroids as much as possible.

Learning points from this case:
- Temporal arteritis can cause intermittent pain

- Not all symptoms are present and a high index of suspicion must be raised in any patient with new onset facial pain or headache over the age of 50.

- Visual blurring in this woman is probably not related to the arteritis. She appears to have a refractive error which corrects completely with a pin hole. Where visual symptoms attributable to arteritis are present like visual obscuration, greying out, constriction of visual fields are present, there is an argument for treating with intravenous steroids.

- The ESR may not be very high and it is recommended that where suspicious symptoms are present, biopsies should be performed to confirm the diagnosis.

- Treatment should not be delayed while a biopsy is being organised. The biopsies should however be performed within 7 days of starting steroid therapy.

- Steroids remain the mainstay of therapy although azathioprine or methotrexate has been reported to be useful too.

- Biopsies are important to confirm the diagnosis because patients are committed to years of treatment with immunosuppressive agents with serious side effects.

9. Further reading

(1) Matharu MS, Goadsby PJ. Trigeminal autonomic cephalgias. J. Neurol Neurosurg Psychiatry 2002; 72(Suppl 1): ii19–ii26 (a useful overview of these types of pain; the rest of this supplement contains other articles on headaches which are aimed at trainees).

References

Achkar AA, Lie JT, Hunder GG, O'Fallon WM, Gabriel SE. How does previous corticosteroid treatment affect the biopsy findings in giant cell (temporal) arteritis? Ann Intern Med 1994; 120: 987–992.

Aguiar PH, Tella OI Jr, Perera CU, Godinho F, Simm R. Chiari Type I, presenting as left glossopharyngeal neuralgia with cardiac syncope. Neurosurg Rev 2002; 25, 99–102.

Alfaro-Giner A, Penarrocha-Diago M, Bagan-Sebastian JV. Orofacial manifestation of mixed connective tissue disease with an uncommon serological evolution. Oral Surg Oral Med Oral Pathol 1992; 73: 441–444.

Arbit E, Krol G. Percutaneous radiofrequency neurolysis guided by computed tomography for the treatment of glossopharyngeal neuralgia. Neurosurgery 1991; 29: 580–582.

Banks PM, Cohen MD, Ginsburg WW, Hunder GG. Immunohistologic and cytochemical studies of temporal arteritis. Arthritis and Rheum 1983; 26: 1201.

Barrier J, Potel G, Renaut-Hovasse H, Hanh TH, Peltier P, Chamary V. et al. The use of Doppler flow studies in the diagnosis of giant cell arteritis. Selection of temporal artery biopsy site is facilitated. JAMA 1982; 248: 2158–2159.

Bennet RM, Bong DM, Spergo BH. Neuropsychiatric problems with mixed connective tissue disease. Am J Med 1978; 65: 955–962.

Boch AL, Oppenheim C, Biodi A, Marsault C, Phillipon J. Glossopharyngeal neuralgia associated with a vascular loop demonstrated by magnetic resonance imaging. Acta Neurochir 1998; 140: 813–818.

Calamia KT, Hunder GG. Giant cell arteritis (temporal arteritis) presenting as fever of undetermined origin. Arthritis Rheum 1981; 24: 1414–1418.

Cantini F, Salvarani C, Olivieri I, Macchioni L, Ranzi A, Niccoli L et al. Erythrocyte sedimentation rate and C-reactive protein in the evaluation of disease activity and severity in polymyalgia rheumatica: a prospective follow-up study. Semin Arthritis Rheum 2000; 30: 17–24.

Caselli RJ, Hunder GG. Neurologic aspects of giant cell (temporal) arteritis. Rheum Dis Clin North Am 1993; 19: 941–953.

Caselli RJ, Hunder GG. Giant cell (temporal) arteritis. Neurol Clin 1997; 15: 893–902.

Caselli RJ, Hunder GG, Whisnant JP. Neurologic disease in giant cell (temporal) arteritis. Neurology 1988; 38: 352.

Ceylan S, Karakus A, Duru S, Baykal S, Koca O. Glossopharyngeal neuralgia: a study of 6 cases. Neurosurg Rev 1997; 20: 196–200.

Chan CC, Paine M, O'Day J. Steroid management in giant cell arteritis. Br J Ophthalmol 2001; 85: 1061–1064.

Chevalet P, Barrier JH, Pottier P, Magadur-Joly G, Pottier MA, Hamidou M et al. A randomized, multicenter, controlled trial using intravenous pulses of methylprednisolone in the initial treatment of simple forms of giant cell arteritis: a one year follow-up study of 164 patients. J Rheumatol 2000; 27: 1484–1491.

Childs AMN, Meaney JF, Ferrie CD, Holland PC. Neurovascular compression of the trigeminal and glossopharyngeal nerve: three case reports. Arch. Dis Child 2000; 82: 311–315.

Danesh-Meyer HV, Savino PJ, Eagle RC Jr, Kubis KC, Sergott RC. Low diagnostic yield with second biopsies in suspected giant cell arteritis. J Neuroophthalmol 2000; 20: 213–215.

De Arcaya AA, Cerezal L, Canga A, Polo JM, Berciano J, Pascual J. Neuroimaging diagnosis of Tolosa–Hunt syndrome: MRI contribution. Headache 1999; 39: 321–325.

De Silva M, Hazleman BL. Azathioprine in giant cell arteritis/polymyalgia rheumatica: a double-blind study. Ann Rheum Dis 1986; 45(2): 136–138

Devor A, Govrin-Lippmann R, Rappaport ZH, Tasker RR, Dovstrovsky JO. Cranial root injury in glossopharyngeal neuralgia: electron microscopic observations. Case report. J Neurosurg 2002; 96: 603–606.

Eide PK, Stubhaug A. Relief of glossopharyngeal neuralgia by ketamine-induced *N*-methyl-aspartate receptor blockade. Neurosurgery 1997; 42: 505–508.

Esmaeli B, Ginsberg L, Goepfert H, Deavers M. Squamous cell carcinoma with perineural invasion presenting as a Tolosa–Hunt-like syndrome: a potential pitfall in diagnosis. Ophthalmic Plast Reconstr Surg 2000; 16: 450–452.

Evans J, Hunder GG. The implications of recognizing large-vessel involvement in elderly patients with giant cell arteritis. Curr Opin Rheumatol 1997; 9: 37–40.

Evans JM, O'Fallon WM, Hunder GG. Increased incidence of aortic aneurysm and dissection in giant cell (temporal) arteritis. A population-based study. Ann Intern Med 1995; 122: 502–507.

Ferrante L, Artico M, Nardacci B, Fraioli B, Consentino F, Fortuna A. Glossopharyngeal neuralgia with cardiac syncope. Neurosurgery 1995; 36: 58–63.

Forderreuther S, Straube A. The criteria of the International Headache Society for Tolosa–Hunt syndrome need to be revised. J Neurol 1999; 246: 371–377.

Fromm GH, Graff-Radford SB, Terrence CF, Sweet WH. Pretrigeminal neuralgia. Neurology 1990; 40: 1493–1495.

Goadsby PJ. Paratrigeminal paralysis of the oculopupillary sympathetic system. J Neurol Neurosurg Psychiatry 2002; 72: 297–299.

Goadsby PJ, Lance JW. Clinical correlation in a case of Painful

Ophthalmoplegia Tolosa–HUNT Syndrome. J Neurol Neurosurg Psychiatry 1989; 52: 1290–1293.

Gonzales GR. Pain in Tolosa–Hunt syndrome. J Pain Symptom Manage 1998; 16: 199–204.

González-Gay MA, Rodríguez-Valverde V, Blanco R, Fernández-Sueiro JL, Armona J, Figueroa M et al. Polymyalgia rheumatica without significantly increased erythrocyte sedimentation rate. A more benign syndrome. Arch Intern Med 1997; 157: 317–320.

González-Gay MA, Blanco R, Rodríguez-Valverde V, Martínez-Taboada VM, Delgado-Rodriguez M, Figueroa M et al. Permanent visual loss and cerebrovascular accidents in giant cell arteritis: predictors and response to treatment. Arthritis Rheum 1998; 41: 1497–1504.

González-Gay MA, Garcia-Porrua C, Rivas MJ, Rodríguez-Ledo P, Llorca J. Epidemiology of biopsy proven giant cell arteritis in northwestern Spain: trend over an 18 year period. Ann Rheum Dis 2001; 60: 367–371.

Hachulla E, Boivin V, Pasturel-Michon U, Fauchais AL, Bouroz-Joly J, Perez-Cousin M, Hatron PY, Devulder B. Prognostic factors and long-term evolution in a cohort of 133 patients with giant cell arteritis. Clin Exp Rheumatol 2001: 171–176.

Hagen NA, Stevens JC, Michet CJ. Trigeminal sensory neuropathy associated with connective tissue diseases. Neurology 1990; 40: 891–896.

Hall S, Persellin S, Lie JT, O'Brien PC, Kurland LT, Hunder GG. The therapeutic impact of temporal artery biopsy. Lancet 1983; 2: 1217–1220.

Hannerz J. Pain characteristics of painful opthalmoplegia (the Tolosa–Hunt syndrome). Cephalalgia 1985; 9: 103–106.

Hannerz J. Recurrent Tolosa–HUNT Syndrome. Report of Ten New Cases. Cephalalgia 1999; 19(Suppl 25): 33–35.

Harnett AN, Kemp EG, Fraser G. Metastatic breast cancer presenting as Tolosa–Hunt syndrome. Clin Oncol 1999; 11: 407–408.

Haugeberg G, Paulsen PQ, Bie RB. Temporal arteritis in Vest Agder County in Southern Norway: incidence and clinical findings. J Rheumatol 2000; 27: 2624–2627.

Hayreh SS, Podhajsky PA, Raman R, Zimmerman B. Giant cell arteritis: validity and reliability of various diagnostic criteria. Am J Ophthalmol 1997; 123: 285–296.

Helweg-Larsen J, Tarp B, Obel N, Baslund B. No evidence of parvovirus B19, Chlamydia pneumoniae or human herpes virus infection in temporal artery biopsies in patients with giant cell arteritis. Rheumatology 2002; 41: 445–449.

Hernández-García C, Soriano C, Morado C, Ramos P, Fernández-Gutiérrez B, Herrero M et al. Methotrexate treatment in the management of giant cell arteritis. Scand J Rheumatol 1994; 23: 295–298.

Ho AC, Sergott RC, Regillo CD, Savino PJ, Lieb WE, Flaharty PM et al. Color Doppler hemodynamics of giant cell arteritis. Arch Ophthalmol 1994; 112: 938–945.

Hunder GG. Classification/diagnostic criteria for GCA/PMR. Clin Exp Rheumatol 2000; 18(Suppl. 20); S4–S5.

Hunder GG, Bloch DA, Michel BA, Stevens MB, Arend WP, Calabrese LH, Edworthy SM, Fauci AS, Leavitt RY, Lie JT. The American College of Rheumatology 1990 criteria for the classification of giant cell arteritis. Arthritis Rheum 1990; 33: 1122–1128.

Hunt WE, Meagher JN, LeFever HE, Zeman W. Painful ophthalmoplegia: its relation to indolent inflammation of the cavernous sinus. Neurology 1961; 11: 56.

Johnston RT, Redding VJ. Glossopharyngeal neuralgia associated with cardiac syncope: long term treatment with permanent pacing and carbamazepine. Br Heart J 1990; 64: 403–405.

Jover JA, Hernández-García C, Morado IC, Vargas E, Bañares A, Fernández-Gutiérrez B. Combined treatment of giant-cell arteritis with methotrexate and prednisone. A randomized, double-blind, placebo-controlled trial. Ann Intern Med 2001: 134: 106–114.

Kantor SM. Diagnostic strategies — temporal arteritis. In: ER Black, DR Bordley, TG Tape, RJ Panzer (Eds.), Diagnostic Strategies for Common Medical Problems (2nd ed.). American College of Physicians/American Society of Internal Medicine, Philadelphia, PA, 1999, pp. 429–437.

Katusic S, Williams DB, Beard CM, Bergstralh EJ, Kurland LT. Epidemiology and clinical features of idiopathic trigeminal neuralgia and glossopharyngeal neuralgia: similarities and differences, Rochester, Minnesota, 1945–1984. Neuroepidemiology 1991; 10: 276–281.

Klein RG, Hunder GG, Stanson AW, Sheps SG. Large artery involvement in giant cell (temporal) arteritis. Ann Intern Med 1975; 83: 806–812.

Kline LB. The Tolosa–Hunt syndrome. Surv Ophthalmol 1982; 27: 79–95.

Kondo A. Follow-up results of using microvascular decompression for treatment of glossopharyngeal neuralgia. J Neurosurg 1998; 88: 221–225.

Krall PL, Mazanec DJ, Wilke WS. Methotrexate for corticosteroid-resistant polymyalgia rheumatica and giant cell arteritis. Cleve Clin J Med 1989; 56: 253–257.

Lacky BR, Hughes R, Murray NM. Trigeminal sensory neuropathy — a study of 22 cases. Brain 1987; 110: 1463–1485.

Le Hello C, Lévesque H, Jeanton M, Cailleux N, Galateau F, Peillon C et al. Lower limb giant cell arteritis and temporal arteritis: follow-up of 8 cases. J Rheumatol 2001; 28: 1407–1412.

Liozon E, Loustaud V, Ly K, Vidal E. Association between infection and onset of giant cell arteritis: can seasonal patterns provide the answer? J Rheumatol 2001; 28: 1197–1198.

Liu NH, LaBree LD, Feldon SE, Rao NA. The epidemiology of giant cell arteritis: a 12-year retrospective study. Ophthalmology 2001; 108: 1145–1149.

Marks PV, Purchas H. Life threatening glossapharyngeal neuralgia. Aust N Z J Surg 1992; 62: 660–661.

Martinez-Toboada VM, Blanco R, Armona J, Uriarte E, Figueroa M, González-Gay MA, Rodríguez-Valverde V. Giant cell arteritis with an erythrocyte sedimentation rate lower than 50. Clin Rheumatol 2000; 19: 73–75.

Matsushima T, Goto Y, Ishioka H, Mihara F, Fukui M. Possible role of an endovascular test in the diagnosis of glossopharyngeal neuralgia as a vascular compression syndrome. Acta Neurochir 1999; 141: 1229–1232.

McLaughlin MR, Jannetta PJ, Clyde BL, Subach BR, Comey CH, Resnick DK. Microvascular decompression of cranial nerves: lessons learned after 4400 operations. J Neurosurg 1999; 90: 1–8.

Merskey H, Bogduk N. Classification of Chronic Pain. Descriptors of Chronic Pain Syndromes and Definitions of Pain Terms. IASP Press, Seattle, WA, 1994.

Metheetrairut C, Brown DH. Glossapharyngeal neuralgia and syncope secondary to neck malignancy. J Otolaryngol 1993; 22: 18–20.

Minagar A, Sheremata WA. Glossopharyngeal neuralgia in MS. Neurology 2000; 54: 1368–1370.

Mitchell RG. Pre-trigeminal neuralgia. Br Dent J 1980; 149: 167–170.

Morris CR, Scheib JS. Fatal myocardial infarction resulting from coronary arteritis in a patient with polymyalgia rheumatica and biopsy-proved temporal arteritis. A case report and review of the literature. Arch Intern Med 1994; 154: 1158–1160.

Patel A, Kasam A, Horowitz M, Chang YF. Microvascular decompression in the management of glossopharyngeal neuralgia: analysis of 217 cases. Neurosurgery 2002; 50: 705–710.

Perruquet JL, Davis DE, Harrington TM. Aortic arch arteritis in the elderly. An important manifestation of giant cell arteritis. Arch Intern Med 1986; 146: 289–291.

Raeder JG. Paratrigeminal paralysis of oculo-pupillary sympathetic. Brain 1924; 47: 149–158.

Reich KA, Giansiracusa DF, Strongwater SL. Neurologic manifestations of giant cell arteritis. Am J Med 1990; 89: 67–72.

Rodríguez-Valverde V, Sarabia JM, González-Gay MA, Figueroa M, Armona J, Blanco R et al. Risk factors and predictive models of giant cell arteritis in polymyalgia rheumatica. Am J Med 1997; 102: 331–336.

Rushton JG, Stevens JC, Miller RH. Glossopharyngeal (vagoglossopharyngeal) neuralgia: a study of 217 cases. Arch Neurol 1981; 38: 201–205.

Salvarani C, Hunder GG. Musculoskeletal manifestations in a population-based cohort of patients with giant cell arteritis.

Arthritis Rheum 1999; 42: 1259–1266.

Schmitz SA, Hohenbleicher H, Koennecke HC, Offermann R, Offermann J, Branding G, Wolf KJ, Distler A, Sharma AM. Neurogenic hypertension. A new MRI protocol for the evaluation of neurovascular compression of the cranial nerves IX and X root-entry zone. Invest Radiol 1999; 34: 774–780.

Searles RP, Mlandinich EK, Messner RP. Isolated trigeminal sensory neuropathy: early manifestation of mixed connective tissue disease. Neurology 1978; 28: 1286–1289.

Smentana GW, Shmerling RH. Does this patient have temporal arteritis? JAMA 2002; 287: 92–101.

Soh KB. The glossopharyngeal nerve, glossopharyngeal neuralgia and Eagles syndrome — current concepts in management. Singapore Med J 1999; 40: 659–665.

Soles RP, Malandinich EK, Messner RP. Isolated trigeminal neuropathy — early manifestation of mixed connective tissue disease. Neurology 1978; 28: 1286–1289.

Solomon S, Cappa KG. The headache of temporal arteritis. J Am Geriatr Soc 1987; 35: 163–165.

Solomon S, Lustig JP. Benign Raeder's syndrome is probably a manifestation of carotid artery disease. Cephalalgia 2001; 21(1): 1–11.

Symonds C. Facial pain. Ann R Coll Surg Engl 1949; 4: 206–212.

Tolosa E. Periarteritic lesions of the carotid siphon with the clinical features of a carotid infraclinoid aneurysm. J Neurol Neurosurg Psychiatry 1954; 17: 300.

Van der Veen MJ, Dinant HJ, Van Booma-Frankfort C, Van Albada-Kuipers GA, Bijlsma JW. Can methotrexate be used as a steroid sparing agent in the treatment of polymyalgia rheumatica and giant cell arteritis? Ann Rheum Dis 1996; 55: 218–223.

Webb CJ, Makura ZG, McCormick MS. Glossopharyngeal neuralgia following foreign body impaction in the neck. J Laryngol Otol 2000; 114: 70–72.

Weisenburg TH. Cerebello-pontine tumour diagnosed for six years as tic douloureaux. The symptoms and irritation of the 9th and 12th cranial nerves. JAMA 1910; 54: 1600–1604.

Weyand CM, Goronzy JJ. Pathogenic mechanisms in giant cell arteritis. Cleve Clin J Med 2002; 69(Suppl 2): SII28–SII32.

Wilke WS, Hoffman GS. Treatment of corticosteroid-resistant giant cell arteritis. Rheum Dis Clin North Am 1995; 21: 59–71.

Assessment and Management of Orofacial Pain
Pain Research and Clinical Management, Vol. 14
Edited by J.M. Zakrzewska and S.D. Harrison
© 2002 Elsevier Science B.V. All rights reserved

Subject Index [1]

---

[1] Subjects listed are discussed in the chapters that start on pages referenced here.